# Emerging Topics in Statistics and Biostatistics

More information about this series at http://www.springer.com/series/16213

Yichuan Zhao • Ding-Geng (Din) Chen
Editors

# Statistical Modeling in Biomedical Research

Contemporary Topics and Voices in the Field

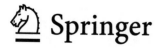 Springer

*Editors*
Yichuan Zhao
Math and Statistics, 1342
Georgia State University
Atlanta, GA, USA

Ding-Geng (Din) Chen
School of Social Work
University of North Carolina
Chapel Hill, NC, USA

ISSN 2524-7735 ISSN 2524-7743 (electronic)
Emerging Topics in Statistics and Biostatistics
ISBN 978-3-030-33418-5 ISBN 978-3-030-33416-1 (eBook)
https://doi.org/10.1007/978-3-030-33416-1

This Springer imprint is published by the registered company Springer Nature Switzerland AG.
The registered company address is: Gewerbestrasse 11, 6330 Cham, Switzerland

# Preface

The purpose of this book is to reflect the frontiers of statistical modeling in biomedical research, stimulate new research, and provide great opportunities for further collaborations. We received high-quality papers from distinguished researchers in biostatistics and biomedical research and have invited them to prepare book chapters. Finally, we selected 19 excellent papers for this book. All of the book chapters have been thoroughly peer-reviewed and revised several times before the final publication. This timely volume presents new developments in biomedical research, introduces innovative procedures, presents interesting applications in statistics and biomedical investigations, and contains the potential to impact statistics and biomedical research. This book makes contributions to biomedical studies in the data science era and provides new insights for biomedical researchers, postdocs, graduate students, applied investigators, and industry practitioners.

The 19 chapters are organized into five parts: Part I includes four chapters, which present next-generation sequence data analysis. Part II consists of three chapters on deep learning, precision medicine, and applications. Part III is composed of four chapters that present large-scale data analysis and its applications. Part IV outlines the biomedical research and the modeling. Part V consists of three chapters on survival analysis with complex data structures and its applications. The chapters are organized as self-contained units. In addition, we have included references at the end of each chapter. Furthermore, readers can easily request from us or the chapter authors computer programs or data sets used to facilitate the application of these statistical approaches in practice.

## Part I: Next-Generation Sequence Data Analysis (Chapters 1–4)

The chapter, "Modeling Species-Specific Gene Expression Across Multiple Regions in the Brain," presents a new statistical approach for identifying genes with species-specific expression. This new approach avoids multiple pairwise comparisons and can be susceptible to small changes in expression as well as intransitivity. In this chapter, Diao, Zhu, Sestan, and Zhao show that the proposed model can better identify human-specific genes than the naive approach. The authors also show that the new approach produces more robust gene classifications across regions and greatly reduces the number of human-specific genes.

In the chapter, "Classification of EEG Motion Artifact Signals Using Spatial ICA," Huang, Condor, and Huang proposed a new procedure, which reduces dimension by applying spatial independent component analysis (SICA) and classifies the gait speed for a given subject by the projected EEG motion artifact signals. The authors use SICA and principal component analysis for the dimensionality reduction before applying classifiers such as support vector machines, naïve Bayes, and multinomial logistic regression.

In the chapter, "Weighted K-means Clustering with Observation Weight for Single-Cell Epigenomic Data," Zhang, Wangwu, and Lin develop a weighted K-means algorithm. By down-weighting cells, the authors show that the new algorithm can lead to the improved detection of rare cell types. The authors finally investigated the proposed methods using extensive simulation studies.

In the chapter, "Discrete Multiple Testing in Detecting Differential Methylation Using Sequencing Data," Hao and Lin present the multiple testing issue in detecting differential methylation in next-generation sequencing studies. The existing FDR control procedures are often underpowered in methylation sequencing data analysis due to the discreteness. In this chapter, the authors also discussed several FDR control methods that can accommodate such discreteness.

## Part II: Deep Learning, Precision Medicine, and Applications (Chapters 5–7)

The chapter, "Prediction of Functional Markers of Mass Cytometry Data via Deep Learning," presents a novel deep learning architecture for predicting functional markers in the cells given data on surface markers. The proposed approach can automate measurements of functional markers across cell samples, and the proposed procedure demonstrates the improved prediction performance of the deep learning architecture.

In the chapter, "Building Health Application Recommender System Using Partially Penalized Regression," the authors proposed to estimate the optimal policy, which maximizes the expected utility by partial regularization via orthogonality using the adaptive Lasso (PRO-aLasso). The chapter also shows that PRO-aLasso estimators share the same oracle properties as the adaptive Lasso.

In the chapter, "Hierarchical Continuous-Time Hidden Markov Model, with Application in Zero-Inflated Accelerometer Data," Xu, Laber, and Staicu propose a flexible continuous-time hidden Markov model to extract meaningful activity patterns from human accelerometer data and derive an efficient learning algorithm for the proposed model. In this chapter, the authors also develop a bootstrap procedure for interval estimation.

# Part III: Large-Scale Data Analysis and Its Applications (Chapters 8–11)

In the chapter, "Privacy-Preserving Feature Selection via Voted Wrapper Method for Horizontally Distributed Medical Data," Lu and Zhang propose a privacy-preserving feature selection method, "privacy-preserving feature selection algorithm via voted wrapper methods (PPFSVW)." The experimental results show that the new algorithm workflow can work effectively to improve classification performance by selecting informative features and genes and can also make the classifier achieve the higher classification accuracy.

The chapter, "Improving Maize Trait Through Modifying Combination of Genes," proposes a computational method for detecting complex traits associated with gene interactions using a combination of gene expression and trait data across a set of maize hybrids. This new method represents changes of expression patterns in a gene pair and employs network topology to describe the inherent genotype–phenotype associations. In this chapter, the authors also investigate the proposed method on several phenotypic traits and achieved consistent results.

In the chapter, "Molecular Basis of Food Classification in Traditional Chinese Medicine," the authors used machine learning methods by using food molecular composition to predict the hot, neutral, or cold label of food, and achieved more than 80% accuracy, which indicated that TCM labels have a significant molecular basis. This research is the first study to quantitatively investigate the relationship between TCM labels and the molecular composition of food.

The chapter, "Discovery Among Binary Biomarkers in Heterogeneous Populations," presents jointly modeled binary and continuous disease outcomes when the association between predictors and these outcomes exhibits heterogeneity. In this chapter, Geng and Slate use ideas from logic regression to find Boolean combinations of these biomarkers and adopt a mixture-of-finite-mixtures fully Bayesian approach to simultaneously estimate the number of subgroups, the subgroup membership structure, and the subgroup-specific relationships between outcomes and predictors.

# Part IV: Biomedical Research and the Modeling (Chapters 12–16)

In the chapter, "Heat Kernel Smoothing on Manifolds and Its Application to Hyoid Bone Growth Modeling," Chung, Adluru, and Vorperian propose a unified heat kernel smoothing framework for modeling 3D anatomical surface data extracted from medical images. In this chapter, the authors apply the proposed method in characterizing the 3D growth pattern of human hyoid bone between ages 0 and 20 obtained from CT images. A significant age effect is detected on localized parts of the hyoid bone.

In the chapter, "Optimal Projections in the Distance-Based Statistical Methods," Yu and Huo propose a new way to calculate distance-based statistics, particularly when the data are multivariate. The main idea is to pre-calculate the optimal projection directions given the variable dimension and to project multidimensional variables onto these pre-specified projection directions. In this chapter, the authors also show that the exact solution of the nonconvex optimization problem can be derived in two special cases and propose an algorithm to find some approximate solutions.

The chapter "Kernel Tests for One, Two, and K-Sample Goodness-of-Fit: State of the Art and Implementation Considerations," discusses statistical distances in the goodness-of-fit and reviewed multivariate two-sample goodness-of-fit tests from machine learning point of view. In this chapter, Chen and Markatou introduce a class of one- and two-sample tests constructed using the kernel-based quadratic distance. The implementation of these tests, with emphasis on the kernel-based two-sample test, is provided.

The chapter, "Hierarchical Modeling of the Effect of Pre-exposure Prophylaxis on HIV in the US," centers on the effectiveness of chemical prophylaxis on the populations involved in the HIV epidemic in the US. In this chapter, the authors use a system of nonlinear differential equations to represent the system of populations involved in the HIV epidemic and define model parameters for both the national and the urban case, representing low and high sexual network densities. These results indicate that the undiagnosed high-risk infected group is the largest contributor to the epidemic under both national and urban conditions.

The chapter, "Mathematical Model of Mouse Ventricular Myocytes Overexpressing Adenylyl Cyclase Type 5," studies a new model of transgenic (TG) mouse ventricular myocytes overexpressing adenylyl cyclase type 5. The proposed model describes $\beta_1$- and $\beta_2$-adrenergic signaling systems very well. In this chapter, Bondarenko finds that the overexpression of AC5 results in an increased basal cAMP production.

## Part V: Survival Analysis with Complex Data Structure and Its Applications (Chapters 17–19)

The chapter, "Non-parametric Maximum Likelihood Estimator for Case-Cohort and Nested Case–Control Designs with Competing Risks Data," assumed cause-specific hazards given by the Cox's regression model and provided non-parametric maximum likelihood estimators (NPMLEs) in the nested case–control or case-cohort design with competing risks data. In this chapter, the authors propose an iterative algorithm based on self-consistency equations to compute the NPMLE and established the consistency and asymptotic normality of the proposed estimators.

In the chapter, "Variable Selection in Partially Linear Proportional Hazards Model with Grouped Covariates and a Diverging Number of Parameters," Afzal and Lu proposed a hierarchical bi-level variable selection approach for censored survival data in the linear part of a partially linear proportional hazards model. The benefit of the proposed method is that it enables us to conduct a simultaneous group selection and individual variable selection within selected groups. The chapter also develops computational algorithms and establishes the selection consistency, and asymptotic normality of the proposed estimators.

The chapter, "Inference of Transition Probabilities in Multi-State Models using Adaptive Inverse Probability Censoring Weighting Technique," develops a model-specific, state-dependent adaptive IPCW (AIPCW) technique for estimating transition probabilities in multi-state models. In this chapter, Zhang and Zhang conduct intensive simulation studies and the results show that the proposed AIPCW procedure improves the accuracy of transition probability estimates compared to the existing SIPCW approach.

The two editors are so grateful to all of the people who have provided the great support for the publication of this book. We deeply thank all the chapter authors (in the "Contributors") for their excellent contributions to this book. We sincerely thank all the reviewers (in the "List of Chapter Reviewers") for their insightful and helpful reviews, which significantly improved the presentation of the book. Moreover, our deep appreciations go to the organizers of the 6th Workshop on Biostatistics and Bioinformatics since several book chapters are based on the presentations in this workshop. Last but not least, our sincere acknowledgments go to the wonderful support of Laura Aileen Briskman (Editor, Statistics, Springer Nature) from Springer New York and Gerlinde Schuster (Editorial Assistant, Statistics, Springer), who made this interesting book publish on time. We look forward to readers' comments on further improvements for the book. Please contact us: Dr. Yichuan Zhao (email: yichuan@gsu.edu) and Dr. Ding-Geng (Din) Chen (email: dinchen@email.unc.edu).

Atlanta, GA, USA
Chapel Hill, NC, USA

Yichuan Zhao
Ding-Geng (Din) Chen

# Contents

# Contributors

**Nagesh Adluru** Waisman Laboratory for Brain Imaging and Behavior, University of Wisconsin, Madison, WI, USA

**Arfan Raheen Afzal** Department of Mathematics and Statistics, University of Calgary, Calgary, AB, Canada
Tom Baker Cancer Centre, Alberta Health Services, Calgary, AB, Canada

**Vladimir E. Bondarenko** Department of Mathematics and Statistics, Georgia State University, Atlanta, GA, USA
Neuroscience Institute, Georgia State University, Atlanta, GA, USA

**I-Shou Chang** Institute of Cancer Research and Division of Biostatistics and Bioinformatics, Institute of Population Health Science, National Health Research Institutes, Zhunan Town, Miaoli County, Taiwan

**Yang Chen** Department of Biostatistics, University at Buffalo, Buffalo, NY, USA

**Yi-Hau Chen** Institute of Statistical Science, Academia Sinica, Nankang, Taipei, Taiwan

**Yingqing Chen** Biostatistics Program, Fred Hutchinson Cancer Research Center, Seattle, WA, USA

**Yu Chen** Bayer U.S. Crop Science, Monsanto Legal Entity, Chesterfield, MO, USA
Eli Lilly and Company, Lilly Corporate Center, Indianapolis, IN, USA

**Ken Cheung** Columbia University, New York, NY, USA

**Moo K. Chung** Department of Biostatistics and Medical Informatics, University of Wisconsin, Madison, WI, USA

**Aubrey Condor** Department of Statistics and Data Science, University of Central Florida, Orlando, FL, USA

**Renee Dale** Department of Biological Sciences, Louisiana State University, Baton Rouge, LA, USA

**Liyang Diao** Department of Biostatistics, Yale University, New Haven, CT, USA

**Junxian Geng** Boehringer Ingelheim Pharmaceuticals Inc., Ridgefield, CT, USA

**Xiaosong Han** Key Laboratory of Symbol Computation and Knowledge Engineering of Ministry of Education, College of Computer Science and Technology, Jilin University, Changchun, China

**Guanshengrui Hao** Washington University in St. Louis, St. Louis, MO, USA

**Hongyu He** Math Department, Louisiana State University, Baton Rouge, LA, USA
Fred Hutchinson Cancer Research Center, Seattle, WA, USA

**Maxwell Hostetter II** Georgia State University, Atlanta, GA, USA

**Helen J. Huang** Department of Mechanical and Aerospace Engineering, University of Central Florida, Orlando, FL, USA

**Hsin-Hsiung Huang** Department of Statistics and Data Science, University of Central Florida, Orlando, FL, USA

**Xiaoming Huo** School of Industrial and Systems Engineering, Georgia Institute of Technology, Atlanta, GA, USA

**Suprateek Kundu** Emory University, Atlanta, GA, USA

**Eric B. Laber** Department of Statistics, North Carolina State University, Raleigh, NC, USA

**Yanchun Liang** College of Computer Science and Technology, Jilin University, Changchun, China
Zhuhai Laboratory of Key Laboratory of Symbol Computation and Knowledge Engineering of Ministry of Education, Department of Computer Science and Technology, Zhuhai College of Jilin University, Zhuhai, China

**Nan Lin** Washington University in St. Louis, St. Louis, MO, USA

**Zhixiang Lin** Department of Statistics, The Chinese University of Hong Kong, Sha Tin, Hong Kong

**Jingdong Liu** Bayer U.S. Crop Science, Monsanto Legal Entity, Chesterfield, MO, USA

**Xuewen Lu** Department of Mathematics and Statistics, University of Calgary, Calgary, AB, Canada

**Yunmei Lu** Department of Computer Science, Georgia State University, Atlanta, GA, USA

**Marianthi Markatou** Department of Biostatistics, University at Buffalo, Buffalo, NY, USA

**Xin Ma** Emory University, Atlanta, GA, USA

**David C. Mohr** Northwestern University, Evanston, IL, USA

**Eun Jeong Oh** Columbia University, New York, NY, USA

**Chun-Hao Pan** Unimicron Technology Corporation, Guishan, Taoyuan, Taiwan

**Daniel Pimentel-Alarcón** Georgia State University, Atlanta, GA, USA

**Min Qian** Columbia University, New York, NY, USA

**Peng Qiu** Georgia Institute of Technology and Emory University, Atlanta, GA, USA

**Nenad Sestan** Department of Neuroscience, Yale University, New Haven, CT, USA

**Elizabeth H. Slate** Department of Statistics, Florida State University, Tallahassee, FL, USA

**Claudia Solís-Lemus** Emory University, Atlanta, GA, USA

**Ana-Maria Staicu** Department of Statistics, North Carolina State University, Raleigh, NC, USA

**Houri K. Vorperian** Vocal Tract Development Laboratory, Waisman Center, University of Wisconsin, Madison, WI, USA

**Duolin Wang** Department of Electric Engineering and Computer Science, and Christopher S. Bond Life Sciences Center, University of Missouri, Columbia, MO, USA

**Jie-Huei Wang** Department of Statistics, Feng Chia University, Taichung, Taiwan

**Juexin Wang** Department of Electric Engineering and Computer Science, and Christopher S. Bond Life Sciences Center, University of Missouri, Columbia, MO, USA

**Jiaxuan Wangwu** Department of Statistics, The Chinese University of Hong Kong, Sha Tin, Hong Kong

**Dong Xu** Department of Electrical Engineering and Computer Science, University of Missouri, Columbia, MO, USA
Christopher S. Bond Life Sciences Center, University of Missouri, Columbia, MO, USA

**Hao Xu** Key Laboratory of Symbol Computation and Knowledge Engineering of Ministry of Education, College of Computer Science and Technology, Jilin University, Changchun, China

**Zekun Xu** Department of Statistics, North Carolina State University, Raleigh, NC, USA

**Sean Yang** Bayer U.S. Crop Science, Monsanto Legal Entity, Chesterfield, MO, USA

**Yun Yang** Philocafe, San Jose, CA, USA

**Chuanping Yu** School of Industrial and Systems Engineering, Georgia Institute of Technology, Atlanta, GA, USA

**Qin Zeng** Bayer U.S. Crop Science, Monsanto Legal Entity, Chesterfield, MO, USA

**Mei-Jie Zhang** Medical College of Wisconsin, Milwaukee, WI, USA

**Wenyu Zhang** Department of Statistics, The Chinese University of Hong Kong, Sha Tin, Hong Kong

**Yanqing Zhang** Department of Computer Science, Georgia State University, Atlanta, GA, USA

**Ying Zhang** Merck & Co., Kenilworth, NJ, USA

**Haiyan Zhao** Centre for Artificial Intelligence, FEIT, University of Technology Sydney (UTS), Broadway, NSW, Australia

**Hongyu Zhao** Department of Biostatistics, Program in Computational Biology and Bioinformatics, Yale University, New Haven, CT, USA

**Ying Zhu** Department of Biostatistics, Yale University, New Haven, CT, USA Department of Neuroscience, Yale University, New Haven, CT, USA

# Part I
# Next Generation Sequence Data Analysis

# Modeling Species Specific Gene Expression Across Multiple Regions in the Brain

Liyang Diao, Ying Zhu, Nenad Sestan, and Hongyu Zhao

**Abstract** *Motivation*: The question of what makes the human brain functionally different from that of other closely related primates, such as the chimpanzee, has both philosophical as well as practical implications. One of the challenges faced with such studies, however, is the small sample size available. Furthermore, expression values for multiple brain regions have an inherent structure that is generally ignored in published studies.

*Results:* We present a new statistical approach to identify genes with species specific expression, that (1) avoids multiple pairwise comparisons, which can be susceptible to small changes in expression as well as intransitivity, and (2) pools information across related data sets when available to produce more robust results,

**Electronic Supplementary Material** The online version of this chapter (https://doi.org/10.1007/978-3-030-33416-1_1) contains supplementary material, which is available to authorized users.

**Availability and Implementation**: Code for estimating the Markov random field parameters and obtaining posterior probabilities for the MRF can be found in the data package attached. All code is written in R.

L. Diao
Department of Biostatistics, Yale University, New Haven, CT, USA

Y. Zhu
Department of Biostatistics, Yale University, New Haven, CT, USA

Department of Neuroscience, Yale University, New Haven, CT, USA
e-mail: ying.zhu@yale.edu

N. Sestan
Department of Neuroscience, Yale University, New Haven, CT, USA
e-mail: nenad.sestan@yale.edu

H. Zhao (⊠)
Department of Biostatistics, Program in Computational Biology and Bioinformatics, Yale University, New Haven, CT, USA
e-mail: hongyu.zhao@yale.edu

3

such as in the case of gene expression across multiple brain regions. We demonstrate through simulations that our model can much better identify human specific genes than the naive approach. Applications of the model to two previously published data sets, one microarray and one RNA-Seq, suggest a moderately large benefit from our model. We show that our approach produces more robust gene classifications across regions, and greatly reduces the number of human specific genes previously reported, which we show were primarily due to the noise in the underlying data.

**Keywords** Gene expression · R code · Posterior probabilities · Markov random field · RNA sequencing · Akaike · Bayes

## 1 Introduction

As the human genome was first being sequenced, a natural question began to emerge: Can we determine what parts of our genomes differentiate us from our closest primate relatives? The origins of characteristic human abilities, such as speech, social behaviors, and abstract thinking, might be uncovered by comparing the genomes of humans, chimpanzees, and outgroups such as gorillas and macaques. Beyond the questions of our innate "human-ness", comparisons of the genomic differences between humans and other great apes have potentially wide-ranging practical effects: see [27] for an extensive collection of possible phenotypic comparisons of interest, ranging from differences in female reproductive biology, to brain size, to control of fire, and to usage of toys and weapons. In addition to observational phenotypic differences, the authors also note widely different incidence rates for certain diseases in humans and chimpanzees which have long been known. Diseases such as the progression from HIV to AIDS, infection by *P. falciparum* malaria, and occurrence of myocardial infarction, for example, are common in humans yet very rare in the great apes. Alzheimer's disease is a neurodegenerative disease characterized by the presence of amyloid plaques and neurofibrillary tangles in the brain, resulting in memory loss, dementia, and eventually death. While the diagnosis of these symptoms in primates may be difficult, one comparison that can be made is in age-matched dissections of human and primate brains. In such studies, human brains show development of these signature plaques as well as the neurofibrillary tangles, whereas chimpanzee brains show neither [26].

There are many approaches to finding the differences between human and primate genomics, several of which are delineated in [27]. We could analyze various kinds of genomic differences, such as indels, chromosomal changes, gene duplications, and repetitive element insertions. In this manuscript we will focus on differences in gene expression as measured by microarray and RNA-Seq technologies, which have been used in several studies [4, 9, 13, 14]. In the first study [9], only a single region of the brain, the left prefrontal lobe (Brodmann area 9) was analyzed. However, all subsequent studies have sampled at least three regions of the brain. In these studies, the analysis was conducted by performing pairwise comparisons and setting a cutoff for whether a gene has human specific gene expression or not in each region.

There are some issues with this straightforward approach, one of which is due to issues arising with pairwise comparisons: When all three pairwise comparisons are performed among three species, for example, intransitive results can easily result. When pooled pairwise comparisons are performed, i.e. by pooling two species and comparing the pooled species against the remainder, results are highly subject to slight changes in expression, as demonstrated in the following. The second issue is related to the structure of the data. Namely, while there are sure to be genes with differential expression patterns across brain regions, we expect that most genes do not. Thus, instead of analyzing each region separately, we should be able to use the gene expression in other regions to inform the analysis of a given region. Particularly in the case of primate studies, samples are difficult to attain, so sample sizes tend to be very limited. By pooling information, we can obtain more robust estimates of differential gene expression.

In this manuscript, we propose a method which overcomes the two issues described above. The problem of intransitivity in pairwise comparisons is well known, and examples are detailed in [6, 7]. We follow the author's suggestion here and propose an information criterion based model selection approach, testing various information criteria for which performs best for small sample sizes. An additional benefit of using an information criterion is that it produces a relative class membership probability for each gene, for each class. This enables us to use a Markov random field (MRF) to "smooth" assigned class memberships across brain regions, so that in regions with less certainty, we can use information from neighboring regions to inform the decision.

We demonstrate through simulations that the Bayesian information criterion (BIC) performs best for small sample sizes, and that the addition of the MRF can significantly reduce the number of classification errors when the neighbor effect is moderate, particularly for those genes with high variance. We then apply our method to two recently published brain expression data sets, one microarray and one RNA-Seq [14]. In these data, three brain regions were sampled: the caudate nucleus (CN), frontal pole (FP), and hippocampus (HP). We find evidence of a moderate neighbor effect among the three regions, and demonstrate that the Markov random field is able to reduce the number of incorrect classifications compared to the naive approach. Among the top genes we identified as being human specific include those associated with various neurological disorders and neural function, which we did not find using the naive ANOVA approach described in the original paper.

## 2 Methods

### 2.1 Overview

### 2.2 Use of Information Criterion for Model Selection

For each gene, we determine the appropriate latent model based on its expression levels. The latent models are described in Table 1. For this model selection

**Table 1** Description of
latent classes for a three
species comparison

| Model | Description |
|-------|-------------|
| $M_1$ | $Hu = Ch = Ma$ |
| $M_2$ | $Ma \neq Hu = Ch$ |
| $M_3$ | $Hu \neq Ma = Ch$ |
| $M_4$ | $Ch \neq Hu = Ma$ |
| $M_5$ | $Hu \neq Ch \neq Ma$ |

step, we evaluate the performance of three types of information criteria: Akaike's information criterion (AIC), the small sample size corrected version of the AIC (AICc), and the Bayesian information criterion (BIC) [1, 11, 22]. These are given in Eqs. (1)–(3), where $L$ is the likelihood of the model, $k$ is the number of parameters in the model, and $n$ is the sample size.

$$AIC = -2 \cdot \ln(L) + 2 \cdot k \tag{1}$$

$$AICc = AIC + \frac{2k(k+1)}{n-k-1} \tag{2}$$

$$BIC = -2 \cdot \ln L + k \cdot \ln(n) \tag{3}$$

Let $\mathbf{I} = (I_1, \ldots, I_5)$ be the vector of information criteria calculated for each of the 5 models, for a particular gene $g$. Then the probability of $g$ belonging to model $i$ is given by

$$p_i = \frac{1}{W} \exp\left(0.5\left(min(\mathbf{I}) - I_i\right)\right) \tag{4}$$

where $W$ is the normalizing constant $W = \sum_i I_i$.

We choose to use information criteria as a natural approach to performing model selection. In particular, we choose to perform model selection in lieu of multiple pairwise comparisons because the latter can often result in intransitivity. For example, we may find that $B > A$, $A > C$, and yet $B = C$. With model selection, such a nonsensical result is not possible. Use of model selection was advocated in [6, 7], which also extensively pointed out the problem of intransitive decisions.

## 2.3 Estimating Prior Probabilties of Class Membership

For the information criteria described above, we must first determine which models to use for microarray and RNA-Seq data types. Differential expression testing for microarray data has often been carried out using the $t$-test, but this can be problematic particularly when sample sizes are small, as variance estimates become unstable. Several methods have attempted to pool information across multiple genes in order to better model the variance [8, 10, 24]. Jeanmougin et al. [12] found in a comparison of multiple methods that appropriate modeling of the variance can significantly reduce the number of false positives found.

Here we assume that the data follow a Gaussian distribution after appropriate normalization just as in the standard $t$-test, and do not perform any moderated estimates of variance. We therefore simply estimate standard deviations of the microarray data. In simulations we find that both the unmoderated $t$-test and the information criteria perform relatively well under reasonable variances.

RNA-Seq data are widely modeled according to the negative binomial model [18, 19]. We use DESeq2 [18] to estimate the mean and dispersion parameters of the negative binomial model for the RNA-Seq data.

Let $y_g$ be the vector of normalized microarray expression values for a given gene $g$, where we drop the subscript $g$ for clarity. In the remainder of this manuscript, we adopt the following shorthand when referencing the three species, human, chimp, and macaque: $Hu$, $Ch$, and $Ma$, respectively.

Then let $y_{Hu}$, $y_{Ch}$, and $y_{Ma}$ denote vectors of expression values for human, chimp, and macaque samples, respectively, for the given gene. We estimate the means $\mu$ and standard deviations $\sigma$ (likewise dispersions $\phi$) for each of seven species groupings separately. i.e., $\mu_{Ma}$ is the mean expression value for macaque samples, $\sigma_{Hu}$ the standard deviation of human samples, $\mu_{Hu,Ch}$ the mean of the pooled human and chimp samples, and so on. The seven species groupings are $Ma$, $Hu$, $Ch$, $\{Ma, Hu\}$, $\{Ma, Ch\}$, $\{Hu, Ch\}$, $\{Ma, Hu, Ch\}$.

Then the model likelihood can be computed as:

$$P(y|M_1) = P(y|\mu, \sigma)$$

$$P(y|M_2) = P(y_{Ma}|\mu_{Ma}, \sigma_{Ma}) \, P(y_{Hu,Ch}|\mu_{Hu,Ch}, \sigma_{Hu,Ch})$$

$$P(y|M_3) = P(y_{Hu}|\mu_{Hu}, \sigma_{Hu}) \, P(y_{Ch,Ma}|\mu_{Ch,Ma}, \sigma_{Ch,Ma})$$

$$P(y|M_4) = P(y_{Ch}|\mu_{Ch}, \sigma_{Ch}) \, P(y_{Hu,Ma}|\mu_{Hu,Ma}, \sigma_{Hu,Ma})$$

$$P(y|M_5) = P(y_{Ma}|\mu_{Ma}, \sigma_{Ma}) \, P(y_{Hu}|\mu_{Hu}, \sigma_{Hu}) \, P(y_{Ch}|\mu_{Ch}, \sigma_{Ch}) \qquad (5)$$

Here $P$ indicates Gaussian densities, e.g., the probability of observing microarray values $y_{Ma}$ for macaque samples, given mean and standard deviations $\mu_{Ma}$ and $\sigma_{Ma}$, respectively. We can obtain similar model likelihoods for the RNA-Seq data, with mean and dispersion parameters estimated using DESeq2, and based on negative binomial probability densities. The model is specified as:

$$y \sim NB(\text{mean} = \mu, \text{dispersion} = \alpha) \qquad (6)$$

$$\mu = sq \qquad (7)$$

$$\log(q) = \sum_r x_j \beta_j \qquad (8)$$

$s$ is a factor unique to each sample that accounts for differences in library size among samples, $x_j$ are covariates (species, batch effects, etc.), and $\beta_j$ are the corresponding coefficients. For the [14] RNA-Seq data, no batch effects were identified, so that $\log(q)$ simply equals $\beta$ for the species grouping.

## 2.4 Empirical Bayes Shrinkage Priors for Negative Binomial Model

For the negative binomial model, we find that using the DESeq2 estimate of $\mu$ can result in overfitting when the absolute count values are small, thus leading to genes with low expression and/or high variability being ranked as highly species specific. To avoid this, we propose a shrunken mean model, which is derived from the interpretation of the negative binomial distribution as a hierarchical gamma-Poisson mixture.

In particular, we assume that the counts for each gene $g$ arise from a Poisson distribution, whose mean itself is gamma distributed:

$$p(\mathbf{k_g}; \lambda_g) = \prod_{i=1}^{n} \frac{e^{-\lambda_g} \lambda_g^{k_{gi}}}{k_{gi}!} \tag{9}$$

$$\lambda_g \sim \Gamma(\alpha_g, \beta_g) \tag{10}$$

Here $n$ is the number of samples. We drop the subscript $g$ in the following for clarity, understanding that we are calculating the posterior mean for a particular gene $g$. Then the posterior mean of $\lambda = \lambda_g$ takes on the form

$$\hat{\lambda} = \frac{n}{n+\beta} \left( \frac{\sum k_i}{n} \right) + \frac{\beta}{n+\beta} \left( \frac{\alpha}{\beta} \right)$$

$$= \frac{n\mu}{n\mu + \alpha} \left( \frac{\sum k_i}{n} \right) + \frac{\alpha}{n\mu + \alpha} \mu \tag{11}$$

We get Eq. (11) by noting that the mean of $\Gamma(\alpha, \beta)$ is $\mu = \alpha/\beta$ and the dispersion parameter of the negative binomial is the same $\alpha$ in $\Gamma(\alpha, \beta)$. Thus, when the mean $\mu$ and/or sample size $n$ is large with respect to the dispersion $\alpha$, $\hat{\lambda}$ is shrunken towards the average count value, whereas if the dispersion parameter is large, it is shrunken towards the mean of the underlying $\Gamma$.

In practice, we must obtain $\hat{\lambda}$ while taking into consideration differences in library size among samples. To do this, we take the $k_i$ above to be $k_i^* = k_i/s_i$, where $s_i$ is the size factor for sample $i$.

## 2.5 Leveraging Gene Expression Profiles over Several Brain Regions Using a Markov Random Field

While different regions of the brain may have different expression patterns, in general we find that the correlation of gene expressions across different regions is very high (see Fig. S2). Further, when sample sizes are small, robust estimates of model parameters can be difficult to obtain, even when borrowing information across genes as both limma and DESeq2 do. We propose to address this issue by utilizing prior model probabilities in neighboring regions to obtain more stable posterior model probabilities.

To do so, assume that the underlying "true" states of the genes are an instantiation of a locally dependent Markov random field (MRF) [3]. Let $z_{g,r}$ denote the unknown true model membership of gene $g$ in region $r$, $z_{g,r} \in \{M_1, \cdots, M_5\}$. Intuitively, if $z_{g,r_1} = M_2$, then we are more likely to believe that $z_{g,r_2} = M_2$ as well, for regions $r_1, r_2 \in R$. Under this model, only the neighboring regions of $R$, $R \setminus \{r\}$, have an effect on $z_{g,r}$. We will assume that all brain regions are thus neighbors of each other.

Generally speaking, the issue of finding the most likely $Z$,

$$Pr(Z|Y) \propto l(Y|Z)Pr(Z) \tag{12}$$

is extremely difficult. We use the simulated field approximation proposed in [5], which produces a solution via the expectation-maximization (EM) algorithm, and which the authors showed performed favorably compared to other approaches.

Let the conditional probability $p(z_{gr} = M_i|R \setminus \{r\})$ be

$$p(z_{g,r} = M_i|V \setminus \{gr\}) \propto exp\left\{\alpha_i + \beta \sum_{r' \in R\setminus\{r\}} I_{M_i}(z_{g,r'})\right\} \tag{13}$$

where $I_{M_i}(z_i)$ is an indicator variable, such that $I_{M_i}(z_i) = 1$ if $z_i = M_i$ and 0 otherwise.

Thus we see that the probability of model membership is proportional to the number of neighbors belonging to the same model. The strength of this "neighbor effect" is given by $\beta$. In total we have five parameters that need to be estimated, denoted by $\Theta = \{\alpha_1^*, \alpha_2^*, \alpha_4^*, \alpha_5^*, \beta\}$ (here we have taken $\alpha_i^* = \alpha_i - \alpha_3$ to avoid identifiability issues).

The steps of the simulated field algorithm are as follows:

1. Initialization:

   (a) Set the initial parameters $\Theta$.
   (b) Obtain an initial estimate of the models $Z$. These are the states corresponding to maximum relative BIC prior probabilities.

2. For each gene $g$ and region $r$:

  (a) Calculate the model probability, for each model, of $z_{g,r}$.
  (b) Sample $z_{g,r}^*$ accordingly.
  (c) Move to the next region and/or gene and repeat.

3. Once we have obtained $Z^*$, an updated state matrix for all genes and regions, re-estimate the parameters $\Theta$.
4. Repeat 2–3 until convergence.

  We update the parameters $\Theta$ using the Newton Raphson method.

  After obtaining estimates of the MRF parameters, we can obtain the posterior model membership probabilities using Markov chain Monte Carlo (MCMC).

## *2.6 Simulations*

We perform three types of simulations to evaluate each of the following:

1. Best information criterion to use for model selection
2. Accuracy of estimation of Markov random field parameters using the simulated field algorithm
3. Reduction of classification errors due to implementation of Markov random field

In each set of simulations, we generate gene expression values based on the gene's classification into one of five latent models, listed in Table 1. We generate expression values for three simulated "species" according to a Gaussian distribution, with species means given in Table 2. We tested three values of $\sigma$: 0.15, 0.25, and 0.5. For each species, we simulate five samples, comparable to the number of samples present in the Konopka experimental data. Simulations by both the DESeq [2], DESeq2 [18], and a similar method edgeR [21] have shown that these negative binomial approaches model the variances well. Thus, we will assume that the parameter estimates produced by DESeq2 of the means and dispersions are reasonable, and so evaluation of the information criteria on Gaussian simulated data is sufficient.

**Table 2** Gaussian simulation parameters

| Model | $\mu_{Ch}$ | $\mu_{Hu}$ | $\mu_{Ma}$ |
|-------|------|------|------|
| $M_1$ | 2 | 2 | 2 |
| $M_2$ | 2 | 2 | 2.5 |
| $M_3$ | 2 | 2.5 | 2 |
| $M_4$ | 2.5 | 2 | 2 |
| $M_5$ | 1.5 | 2 | 2.5 |

We test $\sigma = 0.15$, 0.25, and 0.5

### 2.6.1 Selection of Information Criterion

We test three different information criteria to see how well they classify genes belonging to each of the five models $M_i$: the AIC, AICc, and BIC. Additionally, although they are not directly comparable, we use two types of $t$-tests as a benchmark against which to compare the information criteria: the pairwise $t$-test as well as the pooled $t$-test. In the pairwise $t$-test, a gene is determined to be human specific if the comparisons $Hu$ vs. $Ch$ and $Hu$ vs. $Ma$ are both significant, while $Ch$ vs. $Ma$ is not significant (at $p = 0.05$). Species specificity for the other two species is similarly defined. Note that in some cases a gene will not be classifiable by this method.

In the pooled $t$-test, a gene is determined to be human specific if the comparison $Hu$ vs. $Ch, Ma$ is significant. If more than one such comparison is significant, then the mean difference between $Hu$ and $Ch, Ma$ must be larger than the difference in means of the other comparison in order for the gene to be declared species specific. This is similar to the approach taken by [14].

Performance is assessed according to the percentage of misclassified genes, which we call the classification error. For the information criterion approaches, we choose $M_i$ with the highest probability. We perform 100 such simulations.

### 2.6.2 Estimation of Markov Random Field Parameters

To determine how well we are able to estimate the true parameters $\Theta$ of an MRF, we simulate the latent models according to an MRF model, then generate gene expression values as before, and see if we can recover $\Theta$.

The latent class matrix $Z$ of $G = 1000$ genes by $R = 3$ regions is generated as follows: first, we randomly assign to each $z_{gr}$ one of the five classes $M_1, \cdots, M_5$. Then, given MRF parameters $\Theta = \{\alpha_1^*, \alpha_2^*, \alpha_4^*, \alpha_5^*, \beta\}$, we update each element of the $Z$ matrix according to the probability given in Eq. (13). We perform five complete steps of updating to obtain the final $Z$ matrix. In practice, very few steps are required for the $Z$ matrix to converge.

We take $\alpha = (0.8, 0.3, 0.1, -0.1)$ and let $\beta$ vary as one of $(1, 1.5, 2)$.

From these simulations, we can determine how well $\Theta$ is estimated, given (a) the underlying Gaussians are known, and (b) the prior probabilities are determined using the BIC. The former gives us an indication of how well the simulated field algorithm is able to estimate the MRF parameters when the prior probabilities are "exact"; the latter introduces noise from "inexact" priors. We calculate "exact" priors by taking, for each $M_i$, the probability of observing the values $x$ given the known $\mu_i$ and $\sigma_i$ corresponding to $M_i$. i.e.,

$$p(M_i) = \frac{1}{W} \prod_x p(x|\mu_i, \sigma_i) \tag{14}$$

where $W$ is a normalizing constant. In theory it is possible that $I_i = I_j$ for $i \neq j$, though we did not observe this in practice. In such cases of tied values of information criteria, we can divide

We run 20 steps of the simulated field algorithm for parameter estimation, and 50 steps of burnin and 100 steps of sampling for posterior probability estimation. We perform 20 simulations for each value of $\beta$.

### 2.6.3 Improvement in Performance Due to Markov Random Field

In the previous section all expression values are generated from Gaussians with the same variance, and thus all are equally noisy. Conceivably, when data are very noisy to begin with, borrowing information from neighbors does not improve predicted classification. However, in the case where some genes are less noisy than others, we may expect to observe an improvement.

To evaluate this effect, we perform a similar set of simulations as in Sect. 2.6.2, but this time randomly selected genes to have different variances. Out of a total of $G \times R = 1000 \times 3 = 3000$ genes, we let 50% be generated from a Gaussian with means given in Table 2 and $\sigma = 0.15$, 30% be generated with $\sigma = 0.25$, and the remaining 20% be generated with $\sigma = 0.5$. All other simulation parameters follow those in Sect. 2.6.2.

## 2.7 Experimental Data

We analyze two data sets published in [14]. The authors collected samples from three regions in human, chimp, and macaque brains, and compared their expression patterns using two microarray platforms (Affymetrix and Illumina) as well as next-generation sequencing (NGS). Since the authors found in their original manuscript that the Affymetrix arrays were able to capture more genes than the Illumina arrays, here we focus our analysis on the Affymetrix microarray and Illumina NGS data.

We downloaded the log transformed and quantile normalized microarray data deposited at the NCBI Gene Expression Omnibus (GEO) under accession number GSE33010. For genes corresponding to more than one probe, we took the maximum value over all probes. We mapped probes to their appropriate gene symbols from the downloaded .soft file. The RNA-Seq expression counts table was downloaded from GEO under accession number GSE33587. Only genes that were uniquely aligned to the genome were retained.

Konopka et al. [14] filtered both microarray and RNA-Seq data to retain only those genes which they deemed "present". For the Affymetrix microarray data, they defined such genes to be those which had a detection score of 0.05 or less in all samples, for each region and species. For RNA-Seq data, a gene was considered "present" if for each individual of a species and in a brain region, at least 2 reads aligned to the gene. Additional details of the processing steps can be found in the Supplementary Experimental Procedures of the original manuscript.

Here we did not filter the RNA-Seq genes for "presence", or perform additional filtering of the microarray data. In total, we retained 18,458 genes in the microarray data and 16,036 in the RNA-Seq data. We used the same set of genes for analysis of each brain region.

# 3  Results

## 3.1  Simulation Results

### 3.1.1  BIC Produces Best Classifications Overall Under a Variety of Different Scenarios and Parameters

We evaluate five different criteria for model selection: the three information criteria (AIC, AICc, and BIC), as well as the pooled and pairwise $t$ tests. The $t$ tests we use here only as a benchmark with which to compare the information criteria, because such tests do not produce relative model likelihoods and thus are not useful for the Markov random field part of our model.

We noticed marked differences in classification error depending on the criterion used and $\sigma$ (see Figs. S3, S4, and S5). Additionally, some criteria are better at distinguishing particular classes of $M_i$ than others.

Unsurprisingly, all classifiers perform best for $\sigma = 0.15$, and poorly for $\sigma = 0.5$. In comparison, half of the estimated $\sigma$ over all genes and all models fitted in Table 1 were less than or equal to 0.2 for each of the three regions, with 95% of the estimated $\sigma$ being less than 0.61, suggesting that the classifiers should perform relatively well. In particular, we find that the pooled and pairwise $t$ test classifiers make virtually no errors for $\sigma = 0.15$ for any $M_i$. However, as $\sigma$ increases, we find that the pairwise $t$ test classifier performs substantially worse than the others at differentiating genes which are species specific to at least one species. The pooled $t$ test classifier has among the lowest classification error rates across all $\sigma$ tested and for all $M_i$ except $M_5$, which it is unable to distinguish.

Of the three information criteria, the AIC incurs the most errors at detecting nonspecific genes, and AICc is significantly worse at detecting genes of class $M_5$. Overall, the BIC model selection criterion maintains relatively low error across the five classes compared to the other methods under the various $\sigma$, with error rates similar to that of the pooled $t$ test classifier. Thus, we choose to use the BIC to determine prior probabilities for use in our downstream analyses. However, the best choice may change on a case to case basis, with considerations for sample size. In our particular case where the sample size is very small for each region and species, the BIC appears to perform the best.

### 3.1.2 Estimation of Markov Random Field Parameters is Precise for Exact Priors

We perform extensive simulations to study how well we are able to correctly estimate the parameters of the MRF using the simulated field algorithm, both for exact and BIC priors (see Sect. 2.6.2).

The value of $\beta$ and most values of $\alpha$ are well estimated for exact priors (Fig. S6). For larger values of $\beta$, we observe higher estimation error for $\alpha_i$. If we fix $\alpha = 0$, the estimate of $\beta$ does not suffer. In fact, we surprisingly observe a greater decrease in classification error of the MRF model compared to the naive prior model when we hold $\alpha$ fixed, compared to using the estimated $\alpha$. This is reasonable if we consider that, in the context of Eq. (13), the magnitude of $\alpha_i$ indicates the prior likelihood a gene is classified as class $M_i$ in the absence of any other information. Thus, incorrectly estimated values of $\alpha_i$ may skew the results. However, if we fix $\alpha = 0$, we are essentially only using the classifications of neighboring regions and not these prior beliefs to influence $p(z_{g,r} = M_i)$.

Overall the classification errors under the exact model are extremely low for $\sigma = 0.15$ and $\sigma = 0.25$, being less than 5%. However, when $\sigma$ is increased to 0.5, the classification error jumps to nearly 30%. In the latter case, the MRF model can significantly reduce the error, even for moderate values of $\beta$ (Fig. S9). For $\beta = 1$, 1.5, and 2, the reduction in classification error from nearly 30% is to 21%, 16%, and 11%, respectively.

The picture is less clear when using BIC priors. Notably, parameter estimates become significantly worse at $\sigma = 0.5$. This is unsurprising, as we saw in our previous simulations comparing the different information criteria and the pairwise classifier that all methods make many classification errors when $\sigma$ is large. Thus, when priors are very noisy, MRF parameter estimation is poor. In both cases of $\alpha$ free and fixed, we find a small reduction in classification errors for $\sigma = 0.25$ (Fig. S10). However, when $\sigma = 0.5$, we find no improvement for $\alpha$ fixed, and in fact find that the MRF model performs slightly worse for $\alpha$ free.

Parameter estimation and classification results for AICc priors are given in Figs. S8 and S11, respectively, to demonstrate that noisier priors produce poorer results: Here we find no improvement from the MRF model for $\sigma = 0.5$.

### 3.1.3 Markov Random Field Can Significantly Improve Classification Errors When Some Neighboring Genes Have Smaller Variance

In the previous section, we find that when the priors are noisy, the MRF model yields little improvement. However, that is under the assumption that all gene expression values arise from distributions with the same high variance. In reality this is not always the case, as a few randomly selected genes demonstrate (Fig. S12). It is thus reasonable to ask if the MRF can improve the classification of such genes, which have high variability in one region but lower variability in others.

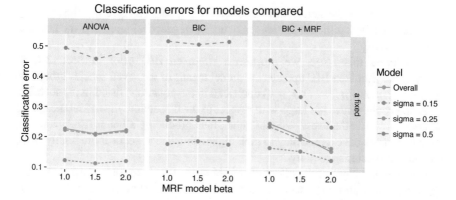

**Fig. 1** Classification error for the pooled $t$ test, the BIC, and the BIC + MRF models, when there is a mixture of genes of different $\sigma$. We simulate 50% of the genes from distributions with $\sigma = 0.15$, 30% from distributions with $\sigma = 0.25$, and the remaining 20% from distributions with $\sigma = 0.5$. We see that as the neighbor effect $\beta$ increases, the MRF model can dramatically reduce the classification error of high variability genes. Results shown are for $\alpha$ fixed, $\alpha = (0.8, 0.3, 0.1, -0.1)$. Results for $\alpha$ free, as well as $\alpha = (0.2, 0.8, -0.1, 0.2)$, are given in Fig. S13

We indeed find this to be the case, as seen in Fig. 1. For the pooled $t$ test and BIC, the classification error is high for genes simulated with $\sigma = 0.5$, as expected. However, the MRF is able to "rescue" these genes by borrowing information from neighbors which are less variable. Thus, when the neighbor effect is not negligible, we can achieve a dramatic decrease in classification error for these genes, and thus also a lower classification error overall.

The $\alpha$ tested in Fig. 1 may favor the pooled $t$ test because $\alpha_1^*$ is large, thereby increasing the number of genes classified as $M_1$. In Sect. 3.1.1 we find that the pooled $t$ test incurs fewer errors for genes of this class, and so we also tested a separate set of $\alpha$, $\alpha = (0.2, 0.8, -0.1, 0.2)$, and indeed find even greater improvements (Fig. S14). For both $\alpha$ we also tested the MRF model with AICc priors (Figs. S15 and S16). As expected, the AICc initially has lower classification error for genes generated from distributions with small $\sigma$, but the overall performance of the MRF model with AICc priors is not as good as with BIC priors, though there is still improvement over the naive pooled $t$ test model.

### 3.1.4 Shrunken Priors for RNA-Seq Data Produce More Consistent Results and Reduce the Number of Low-Abundance Genes Found to be Species Specific

Using BIC priors for the Konopka et al. [14] RNA-Seq data tended to give high species specific rankings for genes with low abundance. Thus, a gene may have low absolute counts, but fit a particular species specific model better than a gene with much higher absolute counts, though from a biological standpoint we are more interested in the latter. Similar to testing log fold changes in DESeq2 [18], even statistically significant findings may not be of practical interest if the absolute change is small.

To address this issue, we propose a shrunken BIC prior in Sect. 2.4. In essence, the shrunken BIC updates the model means of the seven species groupings $(\mu_R, \mu_H, \mu_P, \mu_{R,H}, \cdots, \mu_{R,H,P})$ described in the equations listed in (5) such that when the count values are large with respect to the dispersion, the model means are shrunken towards the average count value, thus producing a better fit. As a result, shrunken priors have a tendency to rank higher abundance genes more highly when it comes to species specificity.

One way to visualize the effect of the shrunken BIC is to look at the maximum expression over all three species of the genes classified as nonspecific, ordered by probability of being nonspecific. These genes are those which are the most highly species specific for at least one species. As we see in Fig. S17, by using the shrunken BICs the genes which are most nonspecific have higher maximum expression than if we used the naive BIC, as desired. Additionally, we find that the shrunken BIC leads to more consistent classifications across brain regions in the [14] data (Table S1).

### 3.1.5  Application to Experimental Data

We apply our BIC + MRF analysis method to the microarray and RNA-Seq data presented in [14]. For the microarrray data, we estimate mean and standard deviation of each of the seven species groupings as described in the equations of (5). For the sequencing data, we use DESeq2 to estimate the mean and dispersion parameters. Prior to doing this, we normalize the counts for library size using the relative log expression (RLE) method default for DESeq analyses using the full sequencing data set, including all regions and species. We then estimate the prior probabilities of each gene belonging to each model using the BIC and shrunken BIC, respectively for microarray and sequencing data. Finally, we estimate MRF parameters on these prior probabilities, and obtain posterior probabilities using MCMC. For these experimental data, we run 50 steps of the simulated field algorithm to estimate the MRF parameters, and also extend the burnin-in and sampling periods of the MCMC algorithm to 100 and 1000, respectively. The estimated parameters are given in Table 3.

**Table 3**  MRF parameters estimated from the microarray and RNA-Seq data sets

| Data | $\alpha$ | $\alpha_1^*$ | $\alpha_2^*$ | $\alpha_4^*$ | $\alpha_5^*$ | $\beta$ |
|---|---|---|---|---|---|---|
| Microarray | Free | 0.23 | 1.0 | 0.17 | 0.78 | 1.85 |
| | Fixed | – | – | – | – | 1.68 |
| RNA-Seq | Free | 0.86 | 0.40 | -0.26 | -0.99 | 1.93 |
| | Fixed | – | – | – | – | 1.59 |
| RNA-Seq (shrunken) | Free | 0.78 | 0.54 | -0.07 | -0.45 | 2.46 |
| | Fixed | – | – | – | – | 2.10 |

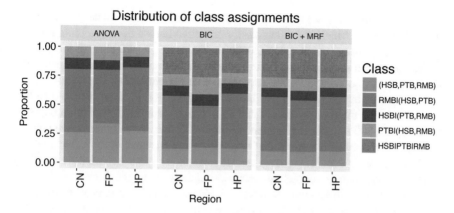

**Fig. 2** Classification breakdown of the 18,458 genes in the microarray data, for the ANOVA test as described in [14] and the BIC and BIC + MRF models described in this manuscript. As we see here, most genes are classified as macaque specific, regardless of the model used. Additionally, the BIC and BIC + MRF models identify a large number of genes with differential expression in all three species

First, we note that the value of $\beta$ estimated for both microarray and sequencing data fall between 1.6 and 2.1 for fixed $\alpha_i^*$, and is slightly higher for freely estimated $\alpha_i^*$. Based on our simulations, such values suggest that there is a moderate to large neighbor effect present in the data, which can benefit our MRF model. This is consistent with Fig. S2, which shows high expression correlation across regions within species. We also note that the values of the freely estimated $\alpha_i^*$ vary quite widely, particularly between the two data types. In particular, the values of the estimated $\alpha_5^*$ are 0.78 for the microarray data, $-0.99$ for RNA-Seq, and $-0.45$ for the shrunken BIC for RNA-Seq. This is consistent with what we observed in our simulations, which particularly showed that estimates of $\alpha_5^*$ could be problematic. Since it appears that the freely estimated $\alpha_i^*$ are highly variable and possibly unreliable, and our simulations show that in such cases fixing $\alpha = 0$ produce better results, we will discuss here only the results obtained from the fixed $\alpha_i^*$ analysis.

The proportion of genes classified into each of the five models for the microarray data is presented in Fig. 2. The figure also shows the discrepancy in these proportions among the ANOVA, BIC, and BIC + MRF models. Parallel results for the RNA-Seq data, for both the BIC and shrunken BIC, are given in Figs. S19 and S18. The two data types show distinctly different patterns. Firstly, there is a much smaller proportion of genes classified as $M_5$, and a much larger proportion of genes classified as $M_1$, in the RNA-Seq data than in the microarray data. There is also a much larger proportion of genes classified as macaque specific for the microarray data. Additionally, for the microarray data, the greatest difference we observe between the ANOVA and BIC classifications is that the BIC model classifies a large percentage ($\sim$25%) of the genes as $M_5$, or different for all species. Since the ANOVA model is unable to classify such genes, it is unsurprising that a discrepancy exists. However, the RNA-Seq data show very different model proportions.

For both data types, we find that the imposition of the MRF model decreases the number of genes which are differentially classified across the three brain regions, but does not destroy region specific patterns. For example, we observe more genes which are human specific in the frontal pole than in either the caudate nucleus or the hippocampus (see Table S2). We also observe an enrichment in $M_5$, i.e. all species specific, genes in the frontal pole. However, this is not the case for the ANOVA analysis for the microarray data (Table S3), where we in fact observe an opposite pattern, with 200 fewer genes human specific in FP than in the other two regions.

The microarray data suggest that most genes are macaque specific, whereas the RNA-Seq data suggest that most genes are not species specific. There are a variety of reasons why the microarray and RNA-Seq data types might show such different patterns. For one thing, both human and chimp microarray data were obtained using the Affymetrix U133 Plus 2.0 array, which is designed for humans, while the macaque data was obtained using a specially designed macaque array [14]. As [20] noted, using a chip designed for one species for another even closely related species, can cause biases in differential gene expression estimation. In this case of these data, two different microarray chips were used for three species. Namely, human and chimp data were both analyzed using a human chip, whereas macaque was analyzed using a macaque specific chip. The differences between these two chips likely inflated the observed differences among the species. Interestingly, in a PCA plot of the microarray data (Fig. S20), we observe a clear separation by brain region, which is much weaker in the RNA-Seq data.

On the other hand in cross-species comparisons using RNA-Seq data, transcripts which are mapped to more than a single position in the genome are often discarded. However, genomic differences between species encompass more than just base pair polymorphisms. For example, gene duplication events can affect whether or not a transcript is uniquely aligned. If in one species these transcripts are thrown out due to gene duplications, while in another species no such duplication exists, we may observe a systematic difference in what appears to be gene expression, but what is actually an artifact of data processing. See Supplementary text for a prominent example.

Comparing the ANOVA results with those genes found to be human specific by the MRF model yield a reasonable amount of overlap. For example, of the 1273 genes which are classified as $M_3$ (human specific) in the frontal pole by the BIC + MRF model and 1692 genes classified as such by the ANOVA method, 813 of the genes overlap. For the microarray data, the amount of overlap is comparable: Of 1534 and 1529 genes classified by the MRF + BIC and ANOVA models as $M_3$, respectively, 711 overlap. However, as we saw in our simulations, based on the $\sigma$ (average of 0.25) and $\beta$ (between 1.59 and 2.1) estimated from the data, we would expect that the BIC + MRF model to reduce the number of wrongly classified genes, and to make classifications more consistent across brain regions, the latter of which we directly observe.

It is reasonable that in addition to genes which are classified as $M_3$, we might also be interested in genes which are differentially expressed in all species, but for which the human gene has either highest or lowest expression compared to the other two species. This definition is more comparable to the ANOVA method described by the original authors. However, after including these genes as being human specific, we do not find a noticeably greater overlap. Rather, the greatest difference in results is in those genes which are human specific in only a single region (Table S4). We find noticeably fewer genes that are human specific in only a single brain region, while still finding an enrichment of human specific genes found in the frontal pole for both microarray and RNA-Seq data. The frontal pole is of particular interest to researchers because it is enlarged in humans compared to the other great apes, and has also been associated with human specific functions [14, 23, 25].

Among the top genes that we find to be human specific in the frontal pole using the RNA-Seq data are *TOMM20*, *LRRTM1*, *SPG7*, and *OPRL1*, which are associated with Perry syndrome (a neurodegenerative disorder associated with adult-onset parkinsonism and depression), schizophrenia, spastic paraplegia, drug dependence, and pain agnosia, respectively. Using the microarray data, top genes include *SHISA9*, *NEO1*, *BICD1*, *GBE1*, *SOX1*, and *DLGAP3*. *SHISA9*, *NEO1*, and *SOX1* are associated with neuronal synaptic plasticity, neural tube formation, and neural cell differentiation, while *BICD1*, *DLGAP3*, and *GBE1* are associated with various neurological disorders. The fact that we can find genes associated with neuron development and regulation, and psychiatric disorders, while we find very few such associations in the ANOVA analysis, suggests that our method is better at finding significant species-specific, cross-regional signals. A full list of results can be found Supplementary Table 2. Figure S21 gives us an indication of why that might be the case: in the ANOVA analysis, a gene may be found to be human specific in a single region due to slight variations in the expression of a single species, whereas our method is more robust to such variation.

# 4 Discussion

We have proposed a method for determining human specific genes using gene expression data sets from multiple brain regions and multiple species. The discovery of genes with human specific expression in the brain has biomedical implications: their involvement with neurological disorders and neural development could help us better understand the pathways involved, and point to important targets. While chimpanzees are most closely related to humans, an outgroup is needed in order to determine which differences formed between human and chimp divergence, and not before. This multi-species comparison poses some challenges for analysis, one of which is issues arising from multiple pairwise comparisons, and another of which is small sample size.

Our proposed analysis method of combining the Bayesian information criterion (BIC) for model selection and a Markov random field (MRF) produces classifications that are more robust to small sample sizes. The MRF has been used in a variety of biological contexts where multiple related data sets are available, for example for time series data [15–17, 28]. In the brain, we observe high expression correlation among the different regions of the brain sampled, suggesting that although there are almost certainly region-specific patterns in expression, it is reasonable to assume we can borrow information from neighboring regions to get more robust estimates of gene classifications.

We applied our method to a previous study with the same aim, published in [14]. The authors obtained both microarray and RNA-Seq expression data sets for three brain regions, and our analysis indicates that there is a moderate to strong neighbor effect among regions. According to our extensive simulations, this suggests that using a MRF can dramatically reduce the number of incorrect classifications. Noisy classifications in a single region will incur more genes incorrectly identified as being human specific in the frontal pole only. We find twice as many genes that are human specific in the frontal pole compared to the other two regions using the RNA-Seq data. We find the same pattern in the microarray data, though to a lesser degree, which is not found using the original ANOVA method. Thus, our analysis recapitulates some of the major patterns presented in the original study, but suggests that there are many fewer human specific genes.

While we have extensively demonstrated the performance of the BIC + MRF model here only on brain gene expression data, such a model can be applied to any group of datasets which one may believe are related in some way, whether by physical proximity, as is the case for the brain data, or some other measure. The model also demonstrates an approach to the analysis of multiple groups, in this case species, where we are interested in all pairwise comparisons of means. Instead of performing pairwise $t$ tests, for example, which frequently can lead to inconsistent results, using a model selection criteria such as the BIC can avoid such issues.

**Acknowledgements** We would like to thank Zhixiang Lin, for discussion of the Markov random field model and its applications.

**Funding** LD was supported by the National Library of Medicine Informatics training grant. HZ was supported in part by NIH R01 GM59507.

# References

1. Akaike, H. (1973). Information theory and an extension of the maximum likelihood principle. In B. N. Petrov & F. Csaki (Eds.). *Second International Symposium on Information Theory* (pp. 267–281). Budapest: Akadémiai Kiado.
2. Anders, S., & Huber, W. (2010). Differential expression analysis for sequence count data. *Genome Biology, 11*(10).
3. Besag, J. (1986). On the statistical analysis of dirty pictures. *Journal of the Royal Statistical Society, 48*(3), 259–302.
4. Cáceres, M., Lachuer, J., Zapala, M. A., Redmond, J. C., Kudo, L., Geschwind, D. H., et al. (2003). Elevated gene expression levels distinguish human from non-human primate brains. *Proceedings of the National Academy of Sciences of the United States of America, 100*(22), 13030–13035. ISSN 0027-8424. https://doi.org/10.1073/pnas.2135499100
5. Celeux, G., Forbes, F., & Peyrard, N. (2003). EM procedures using mean field-like approximations for Markov model-based image segmentation. *Pattern Recognition, 36*, 131–144.

6. Dayton, C. M. (1998). Information criteria for the paired-comparisons problem. *The American Statistician, 52*(2), 144–151.

7. Dayton, C. M. (2003). Information criteria for pairwise comparisons. *Psychological Methods, 8*(1), 61–71.

8. Delmar, P., Robin, S., Daudin, J., Delmar, P., Robin, S., & Daudin, J. (2005). *VarMixt: Efficient variance modelling for the differential analysis of replicated gene expression data.* ISSN 1367-4803. https://doi.org/10.1093/bioinformatics/bti023

9. Enard, W., Khaitovich, P., Klose, J., Zollner, S., Hessig, F., Giavalisco, P., et al. (2002). Intra- and interspecific variation in primate gene expression patterns. *Science, New York, NY, 296*(5566), 340–343. ISSN 0036-8075. https://doi.org/10.1126/science.1068996

10. Florence, J., Guillemette, M., Séverine, D., Isabelle, H., & Jean-Louis, F. (2007). A structural mixed model for variances in differential gene expression studies. p. 19. ISSN 0016-6723. https://doi.org/10.1017/S0016672307008646

11. Hurvich, C. M., & Tsai, C.-L. (1989). Regression and time series model selection in small samples. *Biometrika, 76*(2), 297–307.

12. Jeanmougin, M., de Reynies, A., Marisa, L., Paccard, C., Nuel, G., & Guedj, M. (2010). Should we abandon the t-test in the analysis of gene expression microarray data: A comparison of variance modeling strategies. *Plos One, 5*(9), e12336. https://doi.org/10.1371/journal.pone.0012336

13. Khaitovich, P., Muetzel, B., She, X., Lachmann, M., Hellmann, I., Dietzsch, J., et al. (2004). Regional patterns of gene expression in human and chimpanzee brains. *Genome Research, 14*(8), 1462–1473. ISSN 1088-9051. https://doi.org/10.1101/gr.2538704

14. Konopka, G., Friedrich, T., Davis-Turak, J., Winden, K., Oldham, M. C., Gao, F., et al. (2012). Human-specific transcriptional networks in the brain. *Neuron, 75*(4), 601–617. https://doi.org/10.1016/j.neuron.2012.05.034. http://www.ncbi.nlm.nih.gov/pubmed/22920253

15. Li, H., Wei, Z., & Maris, J. (2009). A hidden Markov random field model for genome-wide association studies. *Biostatistics, 11*(1), 139–150. https://doi.org/10.1093/biostatistics/kxp043

16. Lin, Z., Li, M., Sestan, N., & Zhao, H. (2016). A Markov random field-based approach for joint estimation of differentially expressed genes in mouse transcriptome data. *Statistical Applications in Genetics and Molecular Biology.* https://doi.org/10.1515/sagmb-2015-0070. http://www.ncbi.nlm.nih.gov/pubmed/26926866

17. Lin, Z., Sanders, S. J., Li, M., Sestan, N., State, M. W., & Zhao, H. (2015). A Markov random field-based approach to characterizing human brain development using spatial-temporal transcriptome data. *Annals of Applied Statistics, 9*(1), 429–451. https://doi.org/10.1214/14-AOAS802. http://www.ncbi.nlm.nih.gov/pubmed/26877824

18. Love, M. I., Huber, W., & Anders, S. (2014). Moderated estimation of fold change and dispersion for RNA-seq data with DESeq2. *Genome Biology, 15*(12), 550.

19. McCarthy, D. J., Chen, Y., & Smyth, G. K. (2012). Differential expression analysis of multifactor RNA-Seq experiments with respect to biological variation. *Nucleic Acids Research, 40*(10), 4288–4297.

20. Oshlack, A., Chabot, A. E., Smyth, G. K., & Gilad, Y. (2007). Using DNA microarrays to study gene expression in closely related species. *Methods of Biochemical Analysis, 23*(10), 1235–1242. ISSN 1367-4803. https://doi.org/10.1093/bioinformatics/btm111

21. Robinson, M. D., & Smyth, G. K. (2008). Small-sample estimation of negative binomial dispersion, with applications to sage data. *Biostatistics, 9*(2), 321–332.

22. Schwarz, G. (1978). Estimating the dimension of a model. *Annals of Statistics, 6*(2), 461–464, 03. https://doi.org/10.1214/aos/1176344136. http://dx.doi.org/10.1214/aos/1176344136

23. Semendeferi, K., Teffer, K.,Buxhoeveden, D. P., Park, M. S., Bludau, S., Amunts, K., et al. (2011). Spatial organization of neurons in the frontal pole sets humans apart from great apes. *Cerebral Cortex, 21*(7),1485–1497. https://doi.org/10.1093/cercor/bhq191

24. Smyth, G. K. (2004). Linear models and empirical Bayes methods for assessing differential expression in microarray experiments. *Statistical Applications in Genetics and Molecular Biology, 3*(1), 1–25. ISSN 1544-6115. https://doi.org/10.2202/1544-6115.1027

25. Tsujimoto, S., Genovesio, A., & Wise, S. P. (2010). Evaluating self-generated decisions in frontal pole cortex of monkeys. *Nature Neuroscience, 13*(1), 120–126. ISSN 1097-6256. https://doi.org/10.1038/nn.2453
26. Varki, A. (2000). A chimpanzee genome project is a biomedical imperative. *Genome Research, 10*(8), 1065-1070.
27. Varki, A., & Altheide, T. K. (2005). Comparing the human and chimpanzee genomes: Searching for needles in a haystack. *Genome Research, 15*(12), 1746–1758. ISSN 1088-9051. https://doi.org/10.1101/gr.3737405
28. Wei, Z., & Li, H. (2008). A hidden spatial-temporal Markov random field model for network-based analysis of time course gene expression data. *Annals of Applied Statistics, 2*(1), 408–429. https://doi.org/10.1214/07-AOAS145

# Classification of EEG Motion Artifact Signals Using Spatial ICA

Hsin-Hsiung Huang, Aubrey Condor, and Helen J. Huang

**Abstract** Using electroencephalography (EEG) data to extract information about cortical signals has become an increasingly explored task of interest in the field of computational neuroscience. In this paper, we proposed a novel procedure which reduce dimension by applying spatial Independent Component Analysis (SICA) on EEG motion artifact data and classify gait speed for a given subject by the projected EEG motion artifact signals. Whereas most applications of ICA in analyzing EEG data employ temporal ICA, we use SICA and Principal Component Analysis for dimension reduction before applying classifiers such as Support Vector Machines, Naive Bayes, and multinomial logistic regression to the extracted independent components. We evaluate and compare the classification models by using randomly selected channels from the multi-channel EEG motion artifact data as our test data. For practical application and interpretation, we treat the test channels as if they might come from a new trial for the given subject.

**Keywords** Classification · Brain signals · Time series · High-dimensional · Spatial dimension reduction

## 1 Introduction

Electroencephalography (EEG) has become more readily available as a method to analyze cortical activity due to its relatively low cost and high temporal resolution [10]. Although it can be convenient to collect EEG data, the dimensions of the

H.-H. Huang (✉) · A. Condor
Department of Statistics and Data Science, University of Central Florida, Orlando, FL, USA
e-mail: hsin.huang@ucf.edu; acondor99@Knights.ucf.edu

H. J. Huang
Department of Mechanical and Aerospace Engineering, University of Central Florida, Orlando, FL, USA
e-mail: hjhuang@ucf.edu

© Springer Nature Switzerland AG 2020
Y. Zhao, D.-G. (Din) Chen (eds.), *Statistical Modeling in Biomedical Research*, Emerging Topics in Statistics and Biostatistics,
https://doi.org/10.1007/978-3-030-33416-1_2

23

recorded electrical activity can become large very quickly, especially when using high-density EEG for trials recorded at lengthy time periods. Since EEG datasets are high-dimensional and noisy, thus it is difficult to use them for classifying subjects in terms of their movement characteristics. Therefore, it is important to develop methods for analyzing the EEG data with a reduced dimensional space where the variable information is still retained for classifying different gait movements for a given subject.

The purpose of this paper is to introduce a novel procedure which could classify movement characteristics with EEG motion artifact data projected by spatial Independent Component Analysis (SICA) for a given subject. The EEG motion artifact data did not actually contain electrophysiological signals from the body. Instead, the EEG motion artifact data consisted of signals that were recorded from an isolated conductive reference cap using an EEG system [17]. This EEG motion artifact recording method has enabled the development of new artifact rejection techniques to clean EEG signals [22] but these EEG motion artifact data could also potentially be used to classify movement characteristics.

ICA originates from a method to solve problems such as the "cocktail party" problem where one hopes to identify individual voices when many people are speaking simultaneously, recorded in multiple devices in different locations. In this case, the temporal ICA (TICA) algorithm assumes independence in time such that the original voices can be extracted from the mixtures [5]. Similar to the cocktail party problem, each electrode in EEG data is composed of the mixture of multiple electrophysiological signals that includes the true underlying cortical signals which are assumed to be temporally independent [6]. Therefore, TICA has been most commonly used to analyze EEG data [9]. Because TICA is most commonly used to analyze EEG data, the authors who recorded the first set of EEG motion artifact data in [17] applied TICA and source localization to the data and found that the independent components were mostly outside of the brain volume, which provided evidence that TICA could be used to partially distinguish motion artifact from electrophysiological signals [25]. However, the authors did not attempt to extract movement characteristics from the EEG motion artifact data, which inspired us to investigate that possibility in this paper.

In contrast to TICA, SICA assumes spatially independent components and has been used more commonly in literature which focuses on the analysis of functional magnetic resonance imaging (fMRI) data [7]. However, the temporal dimension of EEG data can be much larger than that of the spatial dimension in many cases [23]. Therefore, our aim is to reduce the temporal dimension and employ SICA on the reduced data instead of using TICA. Consequently, we propose a method which iteratively computes SICA on subsets of the partitioned data, and concatenates the independent components from each iteration.

The rest of this paper is organized as follows. We introduce the techniques of ICA, and then describe the examined data and the proposed data analysis procedure for dimension reduction. Furthermore, the classification methods: $k$-nearest neighbors, Support Vector Machines, Naive Bayes, and multinomial logistic regression are described. Finally, we discuss the results of our classification and further suggest the implications of our conclusions.

# 2 Classification Methods

We use the EEG motion artifact data projected by Spatial ICA with the following classifiers. (1) $k$-nearest neighbor ($k$-nn), (2) Support Vector Machines, (3) Naive Bayes, and (4) multinomial logistic regression. A brief description of each method is introduced as follows. Notice that $X$ is the matrix of predictors and $Y$ is the response vector of classification labels in this section.

## 2.1 k-Nearest Neighbor (k-nn)

We used the $k$-nearest neighbour classification method with $k = 3$, which determines the class by majority voting of each point's $k$ nearest neighbors. The $k$nn was fulfilled by knn3() function in package 'caret' in R were used in this study.

## 2.2 Support Vector Machines

In an approach to solve multi-class pattern recognition, we can consider the problem as many binary classification problems [8, 27]. If we consider the case of $K$ classes, $K$ classifiers are constructed. Each classifier builds a hyperplane between itself and the $K - 1$ other classes [27]. If our response, or the two classes, are represented by $Y \in \{-1, 1\}$, we can use a Support Vector Machine (SVM) to construct a hyperplane to separate the two groups such that the distance between the hyperplane and the nearest point, or the margin, is maximized [8].

The optimization problem seeks to minimize: $\phi(w, \xi) = \frac{1}{2}\|w\|^2 + C \sum_{i=1}^{n} \xi_i$ with constraints $y_i((w \cdot x_i) + b) \geq 1 - \xi_i, i = 1, \ldots, n$ and $\xi_i \geq 0, i = 1, \ldots, n$. We can solve the optimization problem by solving the dual problem, which consists of minimizing $W(\alpha) = \sum_{i=1}^{n} \alpha_i - \frac{1}{2} \sum_{i,j=1}^{n} y_i y_j \alpha_i \alpha_j K(x_i, x_j)$ under the constraints $0 \leq \alpha_i \leq C, i = 1, \ldots, n$ and $\sum_{i=1}^{n} \alpha_i y_i = 0$ The above gives the decision function: $f(x) = \text{sign} \left[ \sum_{i=1}^{n} (\alpha_i y_i K(x, x_i)) + b \right]$ [27].

There exist many different types of kernel functions to use in Support Vector Machine classification. Support vector machines (SVM) [8] with a linear kernel was used in this study. The cost parameters $C$ was tuned using cross validation [16] with package 'e1071' in R [21].

## 2.3 Naive Bayes

The Naive Bayes algorithm is a classification algorithm based on Bayes' rule and a set of conditional independence assumptions. Given the goal of learning $P(Y|X)$ where $X = X_1, \ldots, X_p$, the Naive Bayes algorithm makes the assumption that each feature $X_i$ is conditionally independent of each of the other $X_j$s given $Y = k$, and also independent of each subset of the other $X_j$s given $Y = k$ [15]. Bayes' rule states that the probability of some observed data, $x = (x_1, \ldots, x_p)$, belonging to class $k$ is $P(Y = k|x) = \frac{\pi_k f_k(x)}{\sum_{l=1}^{K} \pi_l f_l(x)}$, where $P(Y = k) = \pi_k$ and $f_k(x) = p(X = x|Y = k)$ is the probability density for $X$ in class $k$. For a given class $k$, Naive Bayes classification makes the assumption that all of the features, or $x_i$s are independent, or $f_k(x) = P(x_1, x_2, \ldots, x_p|Y = k) = \prod_{i=1}^{p} P(x_i|Y = k)$. Thus, the Naive Bayes classifier is as follows: $\arg\max_k \pi_k \prod_{i=1}^{p} f_k^i(x_i)$, where $f_k^i(x_i) = P(X_i = x_i|Y = k)$ [15]. We believe that, because we are reducing our data by Spatial ICA, Naive Bayes classification will provide the best results in terms of misclassification rate. We will use all other classification methods for a comparison to Naive Bayes.

## 2.4 Multinomial Logistic Regression

Logistic regression can be used as a method for modeling a categorical response variable by finding significant parameters. In the multinomial case, our $y$ response variable represents more than two categories. It does not require the assumption of statistical independence of predictors unlike the Naive Bayes classifier, but assumes collinearity between predictors. We used package 'glmnet' in R [11] to fulfill the multinomial logistic regression.

## 3 The EEG Motion Artifact Signals Data and Spatial ICA Methodology

We used the EEG motion artifact signals data that was collected in [17] and were analyzed using TICA in [25]. The method of recording isolated motion artifact in EEG is described in detail in [17]. Briefly, the isolated motion artifact data were collected using a 256 channel EEG system (ActiveTwo, Biosemi) from ten young and healthy participants. A non-conductive silicone swim cap was placed on each subject's head to block true electrophysiological signals. A simulated scalp consisting of a short wig soaked in conductive gel was placed over the silicone layer, and the EEG cap and electrodes were placed over the simulated scalp. Subjects sat (0 m/s) and walked at four different speeds (0.4 m/s, 0.8 m/s, 1.2 m/s, 1.6 m/s) on a treadmill. Each trial was 10 min in duration, and data were recorded at 512 Hz [25]. Ten subjects with complete data sets were used in analysis. In this study, we pre-processed data by vertically concatenating each of the subject's five speeds into one data file while creating a speed label for each signal. In terms of the temporal dimension, each recording consisted of 300, 000–310, 000 points for the 10 min of recorded signal. However, we used only points 1 through 300, 000 for consistency within and between the ten subjects. Therefore, for one of the ten subjects, we have total 1280 EEG motion artifact signals with dimension $p = 300,000$ in five speeds and the sample size $n = 256$ given a speed.

Independent Component Analysis (ICA) belongs to a class of methods often referred to as "Blind Source Separation" which aim to extract certain quantities from a mixture of other quantities [26]. ICA-unlike other statistical methods of dimension reduction that find mutually de-correlated signals such as Principle Component Analysis (PCA) or Factor Analysis (FA)- is based on the assumption of statistical independence [26]. ICA decomposes the data such that we are left with maximally independent signals by maximizing non-Gaussianity. One important distinction of ICA is that there is no order or ranking of the extracted components. It is also notable that the components do not recognize the difference of signs [18]. Since the EEG signals in our dataset have heavy-tailed and multimodal distributions, it is inadequate to apply PCA, which can not recover statistically independent source signals [13, 14].

Let us denote the observed data as an $n$ by $p$ matrix, $X$ where $n$ the number of spatial voxels and $p$ represents the number of time points. In Spatial ICA (SICA), we consider the $n$ vectors containing each of the $p$ instances to be our signals [3]. We can represent the SICA decomposition as follows. Assuming that $X$ is a mixture signals matrix from sources matrix $S$, and let $r = $ the number of components, $A$ is $n \times r$ and $S$ is $r \times p$, and then $X = AS + E$, where $E$ is defined using the smallest $(n - r)$ principal components (PCs). S = WKX is the estimated $n \times m$ matrix source matrix, $W$ is the estimated $m \times m$ un-mixing matrix, $K$ is the estimated $p \times m$ pre-whitening matrix projecting data onto the first $m$ principal components, where $n$ is the number of observations and $m$ is the number of independent components [3, 14]. In this study, the ordering of independent components is determined by Principal Component Analysis.

Before ICA is performed, it is necessary to first pre-process the data with reduction and whitening. For the purposes of data compression, SICA presumes that there are fewer independent sources than there are time points [7]. Reduction is first performed by PCA and the specified number of components are retained such that the maximum amount of variation is represented. ICA combined with PCA allows both whitening and achieving dimension reduction [23].

ICA supposes that the underlying sources are each not normally distributed. It follows that, sources can be extracted by making them as non-Gaussian as possible with the measure of negentropy. Given a covariance matrix, the distribution that has the highest entropy is the Gaussian distribution [4, 18]. Negentropy or differential entropy is a measure of deviation from normality expressed as

$$N(Z) = (EG(Z) - EG(Z_{Gaussian}))^2$$

where $Z$ is an arbitrary multivariate random variable and $Z_{Gaussian}$ is a multivariate Gaussian random variable of the same covariance matrix as $Z$, and the contrast function $G(u) = -\exp(-u^2/2)$ was used in our analysis [18]. There are several different algorithms that employ methods to estimate the independent components. The FastICA algorithm maximizes negentropy $N(X)$ [23]. We use the FastICA algorithm [13, 14] for SICA because it has been shown to outperform most other ICA algorithms in speed of convergence [23].

## 4  Data Analysis Procedure

The challenge of the examining EEG signals data is its high dimension. Since the dimension comes from the multiple time moments which records the EEG signals of the individuals walking on a treadmill at a given speed, we assume that the high dimensional ($p > n$) EEG motion artifact signals used in this study can be decomposed as $m < n$ independent components. Note that SICA cannot perform dimension reduction directly. Therefore, PCA is applied as a pre-process to determine the ordering of the importance of the components by the magnitude of the eigenvalues of the correlation matrix of $X$. To reduce the high dimensional signals, we transform the signals by using only the first four (which is $K - 1$, $K$ is the number of categories) independent components. We applied package FastICA in software R [20] for our data analysis. For each of the ten subjects, we split our data into training and testing subsets, such that we will use the training set to train our classification model, and the testing set to see how our model performs for new observations. We randomly select 256 channels out of the 1280 concatenated channels as our test set, and use the remaining 1024 channels as our training set. Although the channels for a given trial (or given speed) are receiving motion artifact signals simultaneously, we proceed in our analysis as if the selected test signals are recorded from another trial. The data analysis procedure is shown in the following algorithm. The proposed method is outlined, starting from the structure of the original data to the concatenated data, further into the training and testing split, and finishing with the SICA and PCA projected data.

For each of the ten subjects data, we first concatenate all records as a dataset with 1280 rows and 300,000 columns, and then partitioned the data as a training set (1024 records) and a test set (256 records) by random sampling. For each interval of 1000, we sampled a time point for both the training and test sets. The downsampling rate is equalled a duration of 1.95 s, since the original signals were collected by 512 Hz sampling rate (the unit of time is 1/512 or 0.00195 s). Then we applied SICA to the downsampled training set using the FastICA algorithm on the training data, since the five categories can be represented in a 4-dimensional space, each signal is compressed to the first four independent components. We then project the test data set onto the space of the first four independent components obtained from the training data. The plots in Figs. 1 and 2 show that most of the four independent components for the test set each subject have obvious clusters corresponding to the walking-speed categories.

We used the $k$-nearest neighbors with $k = 3$, SVM, Naive Bayes, and multinomial logistic regression for classification modeling. The accuracy rate is computed as the number of correctly categorized signals, over the total number of classified signals. We use the accuracy rates and the multi-class area under the curve

---

**Algorithm 1** Spatial ICA and classification of EEG motion artifacts signals

---

1: There are 10 subjects. Each subject has five EEG motion artifact signals datasets according to the five different walking speeds. Each dataset has 256 rows/space points (from 256 channels) and 300,000 columns/time points (recordings in sequential time points).
2: **procedure**
3:     Concatenate all records of the five speeds EEG motion artifact datasets corresponding to the subject walking speeds.
4:     Downsample the time points by keeping the first sample and then every 1000th sample after the first.
5:     Partition the data as training (1024 records) $X_{tr}$ and test sets (256 records) $X_{te}$ by random sampling.
6:     Apply SICA to the training set and extract 4 independent components by fastICA with type 'deflation' and the exponential contrast function. The components are extracted one at a time.
7:     The SICA outputs a source matrix $S_{tr}$, pre-whitening matrix $K$, and un-mixing matrix $W$.
8:     Obtain the source matrix of the test set by projection $S_{te} = X_{te}KW$
9:     Build classification models on $S_{tr}$ and evaluate by using $S_{te}$
10: **end procedure**
11: For comparisons, another analysis used randomly sampling 4 time points from $X_{tr}$ and $X_{te}$, and build classification models on the training and evaluation on the test set.

---

(AUC) to evaluate the proposed method with comparisons of randomly selecting four time points. Next we trained our Naive Bayes model for classification. For each subject, we use the projected SICA test data to compare the classified results with the true classifications and output the accuracy rate and AUC. Package 'naivebayes' in R was used for the Naive Bayes Classification [19]. Finally, we trained our last classification model with the training data using multinomial logistic regression [28]. We do not evaluate individual parameters for significance but instead simply use the fitted model for prediction of the test data to obtain the accuracy rates for each subject. We also provide a and 3. We provide the Area Under the Curve (AUC) values as well to show classification performance. These values give the total area under the Receiver Operating Curve (AUC) values were calculated with package HandTill2001 in R [12]. Classification results are presented in Tables 1 and 2. Table 3 is the comparison of the proposed SICA method versus random sampling four time points on the simulation data, which was generated by adding noises into the signals of Subject 1. The noises were sampled from uniformly distributed random variables with the range of $(-a, a)$, where $a$ is $\sqrt{3}$ signal-to-noise (SNR) ratio in order to make the simulated data have $SNR = 1$.

## 5 Classification Results

The aim of our study is to explore SICA as a method of dimension reduction for analyzing high dimensional EEG or EEG motion artifact datasets. We proposed an algorithm to downsample and perform SICA to the signals with a large number of time points such that sufficient information is still retained for classification. By using the first four independent components, the $k$-nn with $k = 3$, support vector

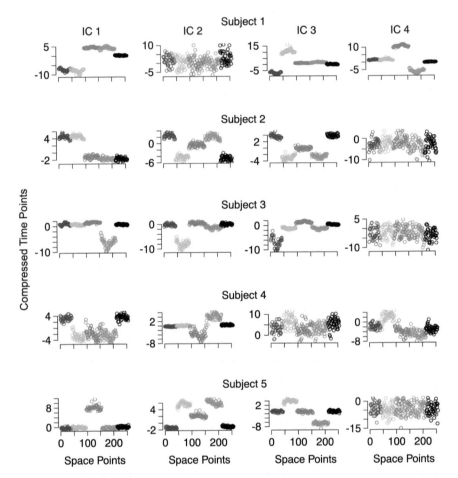

**Fig. 1** The first four projected independent components of the test set of each of subjects 1–5. In each plot, the $y$-axis is the component and the $x$-axis represents the space points (electrode channels) of the EEG motion artifacts signals. There are total 256 space points and five speeds (five categories). On average, each category contains about 51 space points. For each subject, most of the first four independent components clusters according to the subject's walking speed. The clusters are highlighted by different colored. The $x$-axis is the 256 space points in the test set, and the $y$-axis represents the values of the independent components, which are compressed time points

classifier with linear kernels, and multinomial logistic regression all successfully classify the EEG motion artifacts signals. The Naive Bayes method performed worse than the others. In contrast, the classification results are very poor when just using four randomly selected time points. The comparisons show that the proposed method effectively reduce the dimension of time with high classification accuracy. The scatter plots of the top four independent components (ICs) indicate that these ICs have different patterns with respect to their walking speeds (see Figs. 1 and 2).

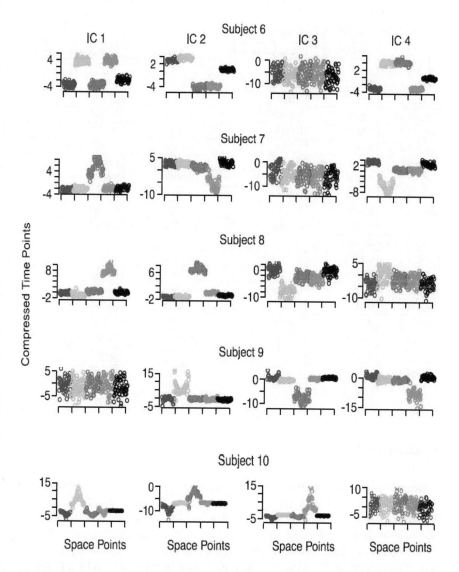

**Fig. 2** The first four projected independent components of the test set of each of subjects 6–10. In each plot, the $y$-axis is the component and the $x$-axis represents the space points of the EEG motion artifacts signals. There are total 256 space points and five speeds (five categories). On average, each category contains about 51 space points. For each subject, most of the first four independent components clusters according to the subject's walking speed. The clusters are highlighted by different colored. The $x$-axis is the 256 space points in the test set, and the $y$-axis represents the values of the independent components

**Table 1** Model comparisons in terms of accuracy rates

| Methods | knn ($k = 3$) | SVM (linear kernel) | Naive Bayes | Multinomial logistic |
|---|---|---|---|---|
| *SICA with four components* | | | | |
| Subject 1 | 0.9922 | 1.0000 | 0.8008 | 0.9961 |
| Subject 2 | 0.9219 | 0.9759 | 0.8242 | 0.9492 |
| Subject 3 | 0.8906 | 0.8789 | 0.7266 | 0.8945 |
| Subject 4 | 0.7891 | 0.9609 | 0.8056 | 0.9967 |
| Subject 5 | 0.8359 | 0.8906 | 0.8516 | 0.9180 |
| Subject 6 | 0.8320 | 0.8320 | 0.7578 | 0.8320 |
| Subject 7 | 0.9688 | 0.9141 | 0.9063 | 0.9531 |
| Subject 8 | 0.8125 | 0.8594 | 0.7539 | 0.9219 |
| Subject 9 | 0.7891 | 0.7852 | 0.8164 | 0.8359 |
| Subject 10 | 0.8984 | 0.8867 | 0.8320 | 0.8984 |
| *Random sampling four time points* | | | | |
| Subject 1 | 0.1211 | 0.1367 | 0.1406 | 0.1445 |
| Subject 2 | 0.1953 | 0.2148 | 0.2031 | 0.2188 |
| Subject 3 | 0.1133 | 0.1055 | 0.1563 | 0.0938 |
| Subject 4 | 0.2109 | 0.1445 | 0.1875 | 0.1758 |
| Subject 5 | 0.3047 | 0.3594 | 0.3281 | 0.3359 |
| Subject 6 | 0.2148 | 0.2305 | 0.2813 | 0.2500 |
| Subject 7 | 0.3164 | 0.3047 | 0.2578 | 0.2969 |
| Subject 8 | 0.2695 | 0.2422 | 0.2227 | 0.2383 |
| Subject 9 | 0.2930 | 0.3008 | 0.2656 | 0.3125 |
| Subject 10 | 0.1172 | 0.1055 | 0.1797 | 0.1055 |

## 6   Discussion

Before classification, the independent components data for each subject was of dimensions 256 by 4 whereas the original test set started as 256 by 300,000. Hence, the temporal dimension of our data was reduced by 75,000 folds. The four independent components successfully retained a sufficient amount of information about the EEG motion artifact signals in order to successfully classify a subject's walking speed. However, it is important to take caution in interpreting the independent components. With TICA, it can be assumed that the independent components represent the unmixed cortical signals. SICA has been commonly applied to functional MRI data, where time points correspond to input dimensions and voxels are samples. In contrast, TICA for EEG assumes that sensors constitute input dimensions and time-points are samples [1]. We used SICA for EEG motion artifact signals with the assumption that sensors constitute input samples and time points are dimensions. Consequently, the EEG motion artifact signals observed at different time points are assumed to be linear sums of the source signals and maximizes spatial sparsity alone [2].

**Table 2** Model comparisons in terms of multi-class areas under the ROC (AUC)

| Methods | knn ($k = 3$) | SVM (linear kernel) | Naive Bayes | Multinomial logistic |
|---|---|---|---|---|
| *SICA with four components* | | | | |
| Subject 1 | 0.9977 | 1.0000 | 0.6174 | 0.9997 |
| Subject 2 | 0.9631 | 1.0000 | 0.8128 | 1.0000 |
| Subject 3 | 0.9472 | 0.9998 | 0.4480 | 1.0000 |
| Subject 4 | 0.8861 | 0.9974 | 0.8220 | 0.9894 |
| Subject 5 | 0.9644 | 0.9695 | 0.3556 | 0.9820 |
| Subject 6 | 0.9251 | 0.9997 | 0.4075 | 1.0000 |
| Subject 7 | 0.9914 | 0.9977 | 0.7357 | 0.9977 |
| Subject 8 | 0.9462 | 0.9896 | 0.4486 | 0.9892 |
| Subject 9 | 0.9381 | 0.9551 | 0.5486 | 0.9718 |
| Subject 10 | 0.9501 | 0.9891 | 0.6709 | 0.9902 |
| *Random sampling four time points* | | | | |
| Subject 1 | 0.4575 | 0.5503 | 0.4841 | 0.5433 |
| Subject 2 | 0.5315 | 0.5721 | 0.5243 | 0.5792 |
| Subject 3 | 0.4249 | 0.3431 | 0.4778 | 0.3463 |
| Subject 4 | 0.5166 | 0.5014 | 0.4483 | 0.5216 |
| Subject 5 | 0.5968 | 0.6533 | 0.6764 | 0.6708 |
| Subject 6 | 0.5016 | 0.4673 | 0.5232 | 0.4965 |
| Subject 7 | 0.5898 | 0.5670 | 0.5453 | 0.5549 |
| Subject 8 | 0.5502 | 0.5369 | 0.5843 | 0.5164 |
| Subject 9 | 0.5713 | 0.5727 | 0.4970 | 0.5581 |
| Subject 10 | 0.4419 | 0.3814 | 0.5056 | 0.3651 |

**Table 3** Model comparisons of simulation data with 100 repetitions in terms of average accuracy rates and AUC

| Methods | knn ($k = 3$) | SVM (linear kernel) | Naive Bayes | Multinomial logistic |
|---|---|---|---|---|
| *SICA with four components* | | | | |
| Accuracy | 0.9577(0.0081) | 0.9547(0.0120) | 0.8215(0.0360) | 0.9286(0.0204) |
| AUC | 0.9908(0.0025) | 0.9990(0.0010) | 0.4473(0.0586) | 0.9999(0.0004) |
| *Random sampling four time points* | | | | |
| Accuracy | 0.2310(0.1100) | 0.2126(0.1109) | 0.0039(0.0387) | 0.2205(0.1233) |
| AUC | 0.5267(0.0891) | 0.5342(0.1271) | 0.0069(0.0069) | 0.5382(0.1328) |

Numbers in the parenthesis are the standard deviation

It is evident that for a given subject, we are able to successfully classify walking speed with EEG motion artifact signals. The classification results (Tables 1 and 2) show that except for the Naive Bayes classifiers, $k$-nn, SVM, and multinomial logistic regression all have high classification accuracy and area under the Receiver Operating Curve (AUC). The Naive Bayes classifier assumes that every two predictors are mutually independent given the class. The classification results indicate that the statistically independent components obtained by SICA do not the class information, so that the assumption of Naive Bayes may not be satisfied by using independent components as predictors. It is also well-know that independence does not imply conditional independence generally. Future studies may use supervised ICA [24] and might be performed to create gait movement profiles across different subjects. Such that, if information existed about a group of subjects and their raw uncleaned EEG signals that includes cortical signals and motion artifact signals for a given movement, a new subject's raw uncleaned EEG signals could be used to classify the new subject's movement.

**Acknowledgement** We thank NIH for grant 1R01AG054621-01 which partially supported this study.

# References

1. Anemüller, J., Duann, J. R., Sejnowski, T. J., & Makeig, S. (2006). Spatio-temporal dynamics in fMRI recordings revealed with complex independent component analysis. *Neurocomputing, 69*, 1502–1512
2. Barua, S., & Begum, S. (2014). A review on machine learning algorithms in handling EEG artifacts. In *Proceeding of the Swedish AI Society (SAIS) Workshop (SAIS 14)* (pp. 22–23).
3. Bell, A., & Sejnowski, T. (1995). An information maximization approach to blind separation and blind deconvolution. *Advances in Neural Information Processing Systems, 7*, 1129–1159.
4. Bishop, C. M. (2006). *Pattern Recognition and Machine Learning*. Berlin: Springer.
5. Brown, G. D., Yamada, S., & Sejnowski, T. J. (2001). Independent component analysis at the neural cocktail party. *Trends in Neuroscience, 24*(1), 54–63.
6. Calhoun, V. D., Adali, T., Hansen, L. K., Larsen, J. J. & Pekar, J. J. (2003). ICA of functional MRI data: an overview. In *In Proceedings of the 4th International Symposium on Independent Component Analysis and Blind Signal Separation* (pp. 281–288).
7. Calhoun, V. D., Adali, T., Pearlson, G. D., & Pekar, J. J. (2001). Spatial and temporal independent component analysis of functional MRI data containing a pair of task-related waveforms. *Human Brain Mapping, 13*, 43–53.
8. Cortes, C., & Vapnik, V. (1995). Support-vector networks. *Machine Learning, 20*(3), 273–297.
9. Delorme, A., Palmer, J., Onton, J., Oostenveld, R., & Makeig, S. (2012). Independent EEG sources are dipolar. *PLoS One, 7*(2), e30135.
10. Enders, H., & Nigg, B. M. (2015). Measuring human locomotor control using EMG and EEG: Current knowledge, limitations and future considerations. *European Journal of Sport Science, 16*(4), 1–11.
11. Friedman, J., Hastie, T., Tibshirani, R. (2010). Regularization paths for generalized linear models via coordinate descent. *Journal of Statistical Software, 33*(1), 1–22.
12. Hand, D. J., & Till, R. J. (2001). A simple generalisation of the area under the ROC curve for multiple class classification problems. *Machine Learning, 45*(2), 171–186.
13. Hyvärinen, A., & Oja, E. (1997) A fast fixed-point algorithm for independent component analysis. *Neural Computation, 9*(7), 1483–1492.
14. Hyvärinen, A., & Oja, E. (2000) Independent component analysis: Algorithms and applications. *Neural Networks, 13*(4–5), 411–430.
15. James, G., Witten, D., Hastie, T., & Tibshirani, R. (2013). *An introduction to statistical learning*. New York: Springer.
16. Keerthi, S., & Lin, C. (2003). Asymptotic behaviors of support vector machines with Gaussian kernel. *Neural Computation, 15*(7), 1667–1689.

17. Kline, J., Huang, H., Snyder, K., & Ferris, D. (2015). Isolating gait-related movement artifacts in electroencephalography during human walking. *Journal of Neural Engineering, 12*(4), 046022.
18. Langlois, D., Chartier, S., & Gosselin, D. (2010). An introduction to independent component analysis: InfoMax and FastICA algorithms. *Tutorials in Quantitative Methods for Psychology, 6*(1), 31–38.
19. Majka, M. (2017) *naivebayes: High performance implementation of the Naive Bayes algorithm*. R package, 2017, version 0.9.1.
20. Marchini, J. L., Heaton, C., & Ripley, B. D. (2017) *Package fastICA*. R package, version 1.2-1.
21. Meyer, D., Dimiriadou, E., Hornik, K., Weingessel, A., Leisch, F., Chang, C.-C., et al. (2017) *e1071: Misc functions of the Department of Statistics, Probability Theory Group*. R package, version 1.6-8.
22. Nordin, A., Hairston, W., & Ferris, D. (2018). Dualelectrode motion artifact cancellation for mobile electroencephalography. *Journal of Neural Engineering, 15*, 056024.
23. Oja, E., & Yuan, Z. (2006). The FastICA algorithm revisited: Convergence analysis. *IEEE Transactions on Neural Networks, 17*(6), 1370–1381.
24. Sakaguchi, Y., Ozawa, S., & Kotani, M. (2002) Feature extraction using supervised independent component analysis by maximizing class distance. *IEEJ Transactions on Electronics Information and Systems, 124*(1), 2502–2506.
25. Snyder, K., Kline, J., Huang, H., & Ferris, D. (2015). Independent component analysis of gait-related movement artifact recorded using EEG electrodes during treadmill walking. *Frontiers in Human Neuroscience, 9*, 639.
26. Stone, J. (2005). Independent component analysis. *Encyclopedia of Statistics in Behavioral Science, 2*, 907–912.
27. Weston, J., & Watkins, C. (1998). *Multi-class support vector machines*. Royal Holloway University of London, 2, 907–912.
28. Yee, T. (2017). *VGAM: Vector generalized linear and additive models*. R package, version 1.0-4.

# Weighted $K$-Means Clustering with Observation Weight for Single-Cell Epigenomic Data

**Wenyu Zhang, Jiaxuan Wangwu, and Zhixiang Lin**

**Abstract** The recent advances in single-cell technologies have enabled us to profile genomic features at unprecedented resolution. Nowadays, we can measure multiple types of genomic features at single-cell resolution, including gene expression, protein-binding, methylation, and chromatin accessibility. One major goal in single-cell genomics is to identify and characterize novel cell types, and clustering methods are essential for this goal. The distinct characteristics in single-cell genomic datasets pose challenges for methodology development. In this work, we propose a weighted $K$-means algorithm. Through down-weighting cells with low sequencing depth, we show that the proposed algorithm can lead to improved detection of rare cell types in analyzing single-cell chromatin accessibility data. The weight of noisy cells is tuned adaptively. In addition, we incorporate sparsity constraints in our proposed method for simultaneous clustering and feature selection. We also evaluated our proposed methods through simulation studies.

**Keywords** Single-cell genomics · Single-cell chromatin accessibility data · Rare cell types · Weighted $K$-means clustering · Sparse weighted $K$-means clustering

## 1 Introduction

The recent advances in technologies have enabled us to profile genome-wide features at single-cell resolution [1]. A large international collaborative effort, the Human Cell Atlas Project, (see https://www.humancellatlas.org/) officially announced in 2017, aims to characterize the molecular profile of all human cell types [1]. Nowadays, we can not only measure single-cell gene expression (scRNA-Seq), but also characterize other functional genomic features at single-

W. Zhang · J. Wangwu · Z. Lin (✉)
Department of Statistics, The Chinese University of Hong Kong, Sha Tin, Hong Kong
e-mail: 1155123326@link.cuhk.edu.hk; 1155116622@link.cuhk.edu.hk;
zhixianglin@cuhk.edu.hk

© Springer Nature Switzerland AG 2020
Y. Zhao, D.-G. (Din) Chen (eds.), *Statistical Modeling in Biomedical Research*, Emerging Topics in Statistics and Biostatistics,
https://doi.org/10.1007/978-3-030-33416-1_3

cell resolution, including single-cell CHIP-seq [2], single-cell methylation [3], and single-cell chromatin accessibility [4, 5]. Different types of genomic data capture complementary information and together they provide a more complete biological picture.

Datasets arising from single-cell technologies are difficult to analyze due to the inherent sparsity and technical variability. One major goal in single-cell genomics is to identify and characterize novel cell types, and clustering methods are essential for this goal. Most clustering methods developed in single-cell genomics have been focused on single-cell gene expression data. The clustering methods are usually algorithm-based and are built upon different similarity/distance metrics between the cells. $t$-SNE + $K$-means is one common approach in practice where the $K$-means clustering algorithm is performed after dimension reduction by $t$-SNE. SNN-Cliq [6] uses shared nearest neighbor (SNN) graph based upon a subset of genes and clusters cells by identifying and merging sub-graphs; *pcaReduce* [7] integrates principal components analysis and hierarchical clustering. RaceID [8] uses an iterative $K$-means clustering algorithm based on a similarity matrix of Pearson's correlation coefficients. SC3 [9] is an ensemble clustering algorithm that combines the clustering outcomes of several other methods. CIDR [10] first imputes the gene expression profiles, calculates the dissimilarly matrix based on the imputed data matrix, performs dimension reduction by principal coordinate analysis and finally performs clustering on the first several principal coordinates. SIMLR [11] implements a kernel-based similarity learning algorithm, where RBF kernel is utilized with Euclidean distance. The "Corr" [12] method implements a new cell similarity measure based on cell-pair differentiability correlation. SAFE-clustering [13] is another ensemble clustering algorithm that uses hypergraph-based partitioning algorithms. SOUP [14] is a semi-soft clustering algorithm that first identifies the set of pure cells by exploiting the block structures in cell-cell similarity matrix, uses them to build the membership matrix, and then estimates the soft memberships for the other cells. DIMM-SC [15] is a model-based approach that builds upon a Dirichlet mixture model and is designed to cluster droplet-based single-cell transcriptomic data.

As for the analysis of single-cell epigenomic data, such as single-cell chromatin accessibility, *scABC* [16] first performs weighted $K$-medoids clustering, followed by aggregation of the reads within a cluster and cluster reassignment by the nearest neighbor. In *scABC*, the cells with low sequencing depth, which are expected to be noisier than cells with high sequencing depth, are down-weighted in the objective function. The difference between $K$-medoids and $K$-means algorithms is the choice of cluster center, where $K$-medoids uses representative data points and $K$-means uses the average of data points assigned to the same cluster. When a rare cell type is present in the dataset, it can be challenging to find a good representative cell for that particular cell type. On the other hand, averaging over similar cells help reduce the variance and can potentially lead to better estimate of the cluster center and thus may improve the detection of rare cell types. Motivated by this, we extend the weighted $K$-medoids algorithm to a weighted $K$-means algorithm. We show that the proposed algorithm can lead to improved detection of rare cell types in the analysis of single-cell chromatin accessibility data. A data adaptive tuning scheme for the weight of noisy cells is presented. In addition, we incorporate sparsity constraints in the weighted $K$-means algorithm for simultaneous clustering and feature selection. The proposed methods are also evaluated through simulation studies.

Extending the $K$-means algorithm to a weighted $K$-means algorithm is not a new idea. The majority of weighted $K$-means algorithms [17–22] aim to assign weights for the features, while ours assign weights to the observations based on prior information, i.e. the sequencing depth of single-cell data. The method that is closely related to our algorithm is the penalized and weighted $K$-means method [23]. Our weighted $K$-means objective function is a special case of the penalized and weighted $K$-means method. However, the penalized and weighted $K$-means method did not provide a systematic way to tune the weights for the observations and did not incorporate the sparsity constraint. In the Supplementary Notes of this paper, we also demonstrated the connection between our proposed method and standard $K$-means with data augmentation: our proposed method is the same as replicating some observations and then implementing the standard $K$-means algorithm.

## 2   Methodology

### 2.1   Weighted K-Means

Let $\mathbf{x}_i$ denote the vector of data for observation $i$. In $K$-means algorithm, the problem is to minimize *within-cluster sum of squares* (WCSS):

$$\text{WCSS} = \sum_{k=1}^{K} \frac{1}{n_k} \sum_{i,i' \in C_k} \|\mathbf{x}_i - \mathbf{x}_{i'}\|_2^2 = 2 \sum_{k=1}^{K} \sum_{i \in C_k} \|\mathbf{x}_i - \boldsymbol{\mu}_k\|_2^2 \qquad (1)$$

where $C_k$ represents the set of observations assigned to the $k$-th cluster, $\boldsymbol{\mu}_k = \frac{1}{n_k} \sum_{i \in C_k} \mathbf{x}_i$, and $n_k$ is the number of observations in the $k$-th cluster.

All observations are equally weighted in $K$-means clustering. In single-cell experiments, the cells have diverse sequencing depth: cells with low depth tend to be noisier compared with cells with high depth. Putting less weights on these noisy observations can potentially improve the clustering algorithm. Hence we propose the following weighted $K$-means algorithm:

$$\min_{C_1, C_2, \cdots, C_K} \left\{ \sum_{k=1}^{K} \sum_{i \in C_k} u_i \|\mathbf{x}_i - \hat{\boldsymbol{\mu}}_k\|_2^2 \right\} \qquad (2)$$

where $u_i$ is the weight for observation $\mathbf{x}_i$, and $\hat{\boldsymbol{\mu}}_k = \frac{\sum_{i \in C_k} u_i \mathbf{x}_i}{\sum_{i \in C_k} u_i}$. Here we assume that $u_i$ is known and how to choose $u_i$ is presented in Sect. 2.3. The following iterative scheme can be implemented to solve (2):

1. Initialize clusters $C_1, C_2, \ldots, C_K$.
2. Repeat the following until convergence:

   - Fix $C_1, C_2, \ldots, C_K$, update centers $\hat{\boldsymbol{\mu}}_k = \frac{\sum_{i \in C_k} u_i \mathbf{x}_i}{\sum_{i \in C_k} u_i}$, for $k = 1, 2, \ldots, K$.
   - Fix $\hat{\boldsymbol{\mu}}_k, k = 1, 2, \ldots, K$, update $C_k$ by clustering observations to the nearest centers.

Note that finding the optimal solution of the objective function is an NP-hard problem [24], and the above iterative scheme usually converges to local optima. In practice, we found that an alternative iterative scheme similar to Hartigan–Wong's algorithm [25] usually converges to a better local optimum:

1. Initialize clusters $C_1, C_2, \ldots, C_K$.
2. Repeat the following until no reallocation takes place:

   - For each observation $\mathbf{x}_i, i = 1, 2, \ldots, n$, first check if the number of observations in the cluster to which $\mathbf{x}_i$ is allocated is larger than 1. If so, then check whether the objective $Obj = \sum_{k=1}^{K} \sum_{i' \in C_k} u_{i'} \|\mathbf{x}_{i'} - \hat{\boldsymbol{\mu}}_k\|_2^2$ will decrease when $\mathbf{x}_i$ is reassigned from the current cluster to the second nearest cluster. More specifically, suppose $\mathbf{x}_i$ is currently assigned to $C_{j_1}$, and its second nearest cluster is $C_{j_2}$. It can be shown that after we reassign $x_i$ to $C_{j_2}$, the new objective minus the original objective equals $\frac{\sum_{l \in C_{j_2}} u_l}{u_i + \sum_{l \in C_{j_2}} u_l} \|\mathbf{x}_i - \hat{\boldsymbol{\mu}}_{j_2}\|_2^2 - \frac{\sum_{l \in C_{j_1}} u_l}{-u_i + \sum_{l \in C_{j_1}} u_l} \|\mathbf{x}_i - \hat{\boldsymbol{\mu}}_{j_1}\|_2^2$, where $\hat{\boldsymbol{\mu}}_{j_1}, \hat{\boldsymbol{\mu}}_{j_2}$ is the original cluster center for $C_{j_1}, C_{j_2}$. So if $\frac{\sum_{l \in C_{j_1}} u_l}{-u_i + \sum_{l \in C_{j_1}} u_l} \|\mathbf{x}_i - \hat{\boldsymbol{\mu}}_{j_1}\|_2^2 > \frac{\sum_{l \in C_{j_2}} u_l}{u_i + \sum_{l \in C_{j_2}} u_l} \|\mathbf{x}_i - \hat{\boldsymbol{\mu}}_{j_2}\|_2^2$, then we reassign $\mathbf{x}_i$ to the second nearest cluster, and update cluster centers.

The above iterative scheme is implemented with random initializations and the solution with the smallest objective is chosen as the clustering result.

## 2.2 Sparse Weighted K-Means

The *total sum of squares* (TSS) is defined as follows:

$$\text{TSS} = \frac{1}{n} \sum_{i, i' = 1}^{n} \|\mathbf{x}_i - \mathbf{x}_{i'}\|_2^2$$

where $n$ equals the total number of observations.

As TSS equals the summation of the *between-cluster sum of squares* (BCSS) and the *within-cluster sum of squares* (WCSS), given that the TSS does not depend on the cluster label, the $K$-means algorithm, which minimizes the WCSS, is equivalent to maximizing the BCSS:

$$
\begin{aligned}
\text{BCSS} &= \frac{1}{n} \sum_{i,i'=1}^{n} \|\mathbf{x}_i - \mathbf{x}_{i'}\|_2^2 - \sum_{k=1}^{K} \frac{1}{n_k} \sum_{i,i' \in C_k} \|\mathbf{x}_i - \mathbf{x}_{i'}\|_2^2 \\
&= 2 \sum_{i=1}^{n} \|\mathbf{x}_i - \boldsymbol{\mu}_0\|_2^2 - 2 \sum_{k=1}^{K} \sum_{i \in C_k} \|\mathbf{x}_i - \boldsymbol{\mu}_k\|_2^2
\end{aligned}
\tag{3}
$$

where $C_k$ represents the set of observations assigned to the $k$-th cluster, $\boldsymbol{\mu}_0 = \frac{1}{n} \sum_{i=1}^{n} \mathbf{x}_i$, $\boldsymbol{\mu}_k = \frac{1}{n_k} \sum_{i \in C_k} \mathbf{x}_i$, and $n$ is the total number of observations, $n_k$ is the number of observations in the $k$-th cluster.

Let $x_{i,j}$ denote the data for the $i$-th observation with the $j$-th feature. Based on the BCSS, the sparse $K$-means criterion [26] is as follows:

$$
\max_{C_1,C_2,\cdots,C_K,\mathbf{w}} \left\{ \sum_{j=1}^{p} w_j \left( \sum_{i=1}^{n} (x_{i,j} - \mu_{0,j})^2 - \sum_{k=1}^{K} \sum_{i \in C_k} (x_{i,j} - \mu_{k,j})^2 \right) \right\}
\tag{4}
$$

subject to $\|\mathbf{w}\|_2^2 \leq 1$, $\|\mathbf{w}\|_1 \leq s$, $w_j \geq 0$, $\forall j$

where $w_j$ represents the importance of the $j$-th feature, $\mu_{0,j} = \frac{1}{n} \sum_{i=1}^{n} x_{i,j}$, and $\mu_{k,j} = \frac{1}{n_k} \sum_{i \in C_k} x_{i,j}$, $j = 1, \ldots, p$.

Based upon the proposed weighted $K$-means algorithm, we also incorporate sparsity constraints for variable selection. In single-cell genomics, it is a common practice to remove noisy features before performing the clustering algorithms. Incorporating sparsity constraint in the clustering algorithm may help us better deal with the noisy features and select the relevant features. So we extend the objective function (4) with weights $u_i$ on each observation:

$$
\max_{C_1,C_2,\cdots,C_K,\mathbf{w}} \left\{ \sum_{j=1}^{p} w_j \left( \sum_{i=1}^{n} u_i (x_{i,j} - \hat{\mu}_{0,j})^2 - \sum_{k=1}^{K} \sum_{i \in C_k} u_i (x_{i,j} - \hat{\mu}_{k,j})^2 \right) \right\}
\tag{5}
$$

subject to $\|\mathbf{w}\|_2^2 \leq 1$, $\|\mathbf{w}\|_1 \leq s$, $w_j \geq 0$, $\forall j$

where $\hat{\mu}_{0,j} = \frac{\sum_{i=1}^{n} u_i x_{i,j}}{\sum_{i=1}^{n} u_i}$, $\hat{\mu}_{k,j} = \frac{\sum_{i \in C_k} u_i x_{i,j}}{\sum_{i \in C_k} u_i}$, $j = 1, \ldots, p$.

Similar to the sparse $K$-means algorithm, we propose an iterative scheme for (5):

1. Initialize $\boldsymbol{w}$ as $w_1 = w_2 = \cdots = w_p = \frac{1}{\sqrt{p}}$, and initialize cluster $C_1, C_2, \ldots, C_K$.
2. Iterate until convergence:

   - Fix $\boldsymbol{w}$, update $C_1, C_2, \cdots, C_K$. We need to solve the following problem

   $$\min_{C_1, C_2, \cdots, C_K} \left\{ \sum_{j=1}^{p} w_j \sum_{k=1}^{K} \sum_{i \in C_k} u_i (x_{i,j} - \hat{\mu}_{k,j})^2 \right\}.$$

   The problem can be solved by applying weighted $K$-means algorithm to $X\sqrt{W}$, where $X$ is a $n \times p$ matrix representing the original data, and $\sqrt{W}$ is a $p \times p$ diagonal matrix with elements $\sqrt{w_1}, \sqrt{w_2}, \cdots, \sqrt{w_p}$.
   - Fix $C_1, C_2, \cdots, C_K$, update $\boldsymbol{w}$ by soft-thresholding:

   $$\boldsymbol{w} = \frac{S(\boldsymbol{a}_+, \Delta)}{\|S(\boldsymbol{a}_+, \Delta)\|_2}$$

   where $S(\cdot, \cdot)$ is the soft-thresholding function, $a_j = \sum_{i=1}^{n} u_i (x_{i,j} - \hat{\mu}_{0,j})^2 - \sum_{k=1}^{K} \sum_{i \in C_k} u_i (x_{i,j} - \hat{\mu}_{k,j})^2$, $\boldsymbol{a}_+$ is the positive part of $\boldsymbol{a}$, and if $\|\boldsymbol{w}\big|_{\Delta=0}\|_1 \leq s$, then choose $\boldsymbol{w} = \boldsymbol{w}\big|_{\Delta=0}$; otherwise, pick $\Delta = \Delta_0$ s.t. $\|\boldsymbol{w}\big|_{\Delta=\Delta_0}\|_1 = s$ and let $\boldsymbol{w} = \boldsymbol{w}\big|_{\Delta=\Delta_0}$.

**Convergence of the Algorithm** When the weights and the sparsity parameter are chosen as proposed, the iterative scheme ensures the objective to be non-increasing in each step, and the objective has an obvious lower bound 0, so this method is sure to converge to a local optimum.

## 2.3 Selection of Tuning Parameter for Weighted K-Means

In weighted $K$-means algorithm, the weight vector $\mathbf{U}$ represents how much we penalize the noisy observations. Choosing $\mathbf{U}$ can be essential to the algorithm performance. To tune $\mathbf{U}$, we consider a sequence of weight vectors, $\mathbf{U}^{(1)}, \ldots, \mathbf{U}^{(Q)}$, where all observations are given the flattest weight in $\mathbf{U}^{(1)}$, and in $\mathbf{U}^{(Q)}$, the noisy observations are given the smallest weight. Details for creating the sequence of weight vectors are discussed in the simulation and real data analysis.

In order to choose the value of $\mathbf{U}$, we apply a permutation approach which is closely related to the Gap statistic [27]. The intuition for the tuning procedure is that when the weight $\mathbf{U}$ is chosen wisely, it should further decrease the objective function, compared with randomly assigning the weight.

**Algorithm to Select Tuning Parameter U for Weighted $K$-Means**

- For $\mathbf{U}^{(q)}, q = 1, \ldots, Q$, implement steps 1, 2, 3 and 4:

  1. Perform weighted $K$-means with weight $\mathbf{U}^{(q)}$ and data $\mathbf{X}$, and then compute the objective function $O(\mathbf{U}^{(q)}) = \sum_{k=1}^{K} \sum_{i \in C_k^{(q)}} u_i^{(q)} \|\mathbf{x}_i - \hat{\boldsymbol{\mu}}_k^{(q)}\|_2^2$.
  2. Obtain $\mathbf{U}_1^{(q)}, \ldots, \mathbf{U}_B^{(q)}$, by independently shuffling the elements in $\mathbf{U}^{(q)}$.
  3. For $\mathbf{U}_b^{(q)}, b = 1, \ldots, B$, perform weighted $K$-means with weight $\mathbf{U}_b^{(q)}$ and data $\mathbf{X}$, and then compute the objective function $O(\mathbf{U}_b^{(q)})$.
  4. Compute Gap$(\mathbf{U}^{(q)}) = \frac{1}{B} \sum_{b=1}^{B} \log O(\mathbf{U}_b^{(q)}) - \log O(\mathbf{U}^{(q)})$.

- Choose the smallest $q^*$ such that Gap$(\mathbf{U}^{(q^*)})$ is within one standard deviation from the largest value of Gap$(\mathbf{U}^{(q)})$.

Additionally, $K$, the number of clusters, is also a tuning parameter. Criterion for choosing $K$ is similar to tuning $U$, and details are presented in the Supplementary Notes.

## 2.4  Selection of Tuning Parameter for Sparse Weighted $K$-Means

In sparse weighted $K$-means algorithm, the weights for the samples $\mathbf{U}$ and the sparsity parameter $s$ are tuned sequentially, where we first tune $\mathbf{U}$ through weighted $K$-means without the sparsity constraint, and then tune $s$ with $\mathbf{U}$ fixed.

In order to choose $s$, a permutation approach similar to tuning the sparsity parameter in sparse $K$-means algorithm is applied.

**Algorithm to Select Tuning Parameter $s$ for Sparse Weighted $K$-Means**

1. Obtain permuted datasets $\mathbf{X}_1, \ldots, \mathbf{X}_B$ by independently permuting observations within each feature.
2. For each candidate tuning parameter value $s$:

   (a) Compute $O(s) = \sum_{j=1}^{p} w_j \left( \sum_{i=1}^{n} u_i (x_{i,j} - \hat{\mu}_{0,j})^2 - \sum_{k=1}^{K} \sum_{i \in C_k} u_i (x_{i,j} - \hat{\mu}_{k,j})^2 \right)$, the objective obtained by performing sparse weighted $K$-means with tuning parameter $s$ on the data $\mathbf{X}$.

   (b) For $b = 1, 2, \ldots, B$, compute $O_b(s)$, the objective obtained by performing sparse weighted $K$-means with tuing parameter $s$ on the data $\mathbf{X}_b$.

   (c) Calculate Gap$(s) = \log(O(s)) - \frac{1}{B} \sum_{b=1}^{B} \log(O_b(s))$.

3. Choose $s^*$ corresponding to the largest value of Gap$(s)$.

# 3  Simulation

## 3.1  Simulation 1: Multivariate Normal Distribution

The simulation setup is as follows: the total number of features $p = 1000$, the number of cluster-specific features $q = 50$, the number of classes $K = 3$, the number of observations $n = 60$ with 20 observations per class. Among the $n$ obeservations, $n_0 = 10$ noisy observations are included. We first generate $X_{ij} \sim N(\mu_{ij}, 1)$ independently, where $\mu_{ij} = \mu(1_{i \in C_1, j \leq q} - 1_{i \in C_2, j \leq q})$ and $\mu = 0.8$. Then to generate the noisy observations, we randomly select $n_0$ observations, and generate them from $N(\mu_{ij}, \sigma_0^2)$. We generated datasets with various $\sigma_0$, representing different noise levels for the noisy observations. When $\sigma_0 = 1$, all observations have the same noise level, and the larger $\sigma_0$, the larger noise level.

**Effectiveness of the Algorithm to Select the Tuning Parameter U for Weighted $K$-Means**  We fix the weight of normal observations as 1, and choose a descending sequence of candidate weights for the noisy observations to apply the method to select tuning parameter for weighted $K$-means. The results are shown in Fig. 1. When $\sigma_0$ increases, the selected weight for noisy observations tends to decrease.

**Effectiveness of the Algorithm to Select the Sparsity Parameter $s$**  We compare the number of features selected by our proposed algorithm with that selected by the sparse $K$-means method. The sparse $K$-means method was implemented with the R package sparcl. As shown in Table 1, both algorithms tend to select more features than the true number of cluster-specific features. When the noise level increases, the number of features selected by sparse $K$-means method tends to increase, deviating greatly from the true number of cluster-specific features, which is $q = 50$. The number of features selected by sparse weighted $K$-means method tend to be quite stable except when the noise level is very high ($\sigma_0 = 20$).

**Convergence of the Sparse Weighted $K$-Means Algorithm**  When the sparsity parameter and weights are chosen as proposed, we show the convergence of our proposed algorithm in Fig. 2. We generate one dataset for each noise level and plot iteration number vs objective. It is clear that the objective converges in less than 10 iterative times, which shows the sparse weighted $K$-means algorithm works effectively.

**Performance Comparison with Other Clustering Methods**  We compare the performance of our proposed approach, weighted $K$-means and sparse weighted $K$-means with that of some other approaches: standard $K$-means, sparse $K$-means, standard $K$-medoids and weighted $K$-medoids (Table 2). We use purity, which ranges from 0 to 1, to measure the clustering performance. Note that purity equals 1 if the clustering result agrees perfectly with the true label; and a small value indicates disagreement. From the table, when the noise level for the noisy observations increases, sparse weighted $K$-means outperforms the other clustering

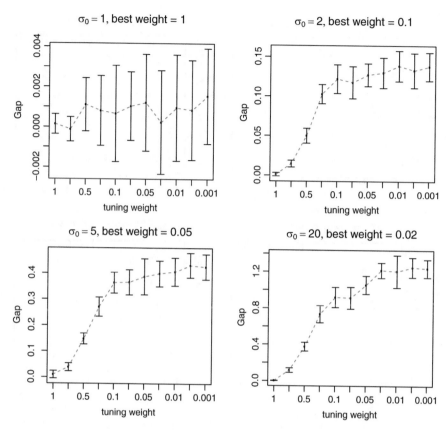

**Fig. 1** Simulation setting 1: best weight chosen by the smallest value for which Gap($\mathbf{U}$) is within one standard deviation from the largest value of Gap($\mathbf{U}$). The candidate weight sequence chosen is 1, 0.8, 0.5, 0.2, 0.1, 0.08, 0.05, 0.02, 0.01, 0.005, 0.001. The results for different noise levels are shown

**Table 1** The quantities reported are the mean and standard error (given in parentheses) of the number of features selected, i.e. features with non-zero weight in $\mathbf{w}$, over 50 runs of simulation

|  | Sparse weighted $K$-means | Sparse $K$-means |
|---|---|---|
| $\sigma_0 = 1$ | 103.02 (12.896) | 102.8 (12.269) |
| $\sigma_0 = 2$ | 100.6 (32.789) | 323.18 (370.624) |
| $\sigma_0 = 5$ | 112.9 (42.864) | 972.48 (68.234) |
| $\sigma_0 = 20$ | 712.26 (334.293) | 1000 (0) |

Recall that the true number of cluster-specific features $q = 50$. The results for simulation setting 1 is shown

methods, and weighted $K$-means is also robust against noisy observations. The other methods lead to a low purity performance when noisy observations exist.

**Effectiveness of Selecting Cluster-Specific Features** Next, we selected the sparsity parameter $s$ such that $\sim$50 or $\sim$100 features are selected in sparse $K$-means and our proposed sparse weighted $K$-means algorithm, and compared the performance

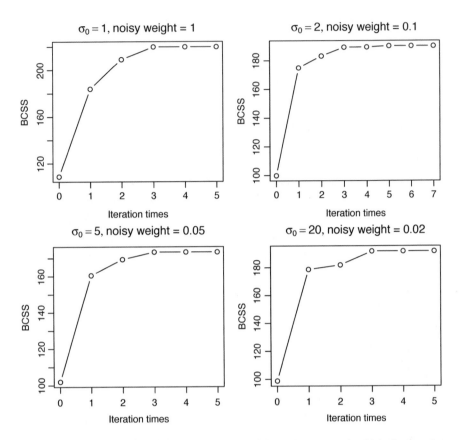

**Fig. 2** Simulation setting 1: convergence of the sparse weighted $K$-means algorithm. One iteration step includes either updating the clusters $C_1, C_2, C_3$ or updating $\boldsymbol{w}$. 0 iteration time corresponds to the initial objective. The results for different noise levels are shown

**Table 2** The quantities reported are the mean and standard error (given in parentheses) of purity[a], over 50 runs of simulation

|  | $\sigma_0 = 1$ | $\sigma_0 = 2$ | $\sigma_0 = 5$ | $\sigma_0 = 20$ |
|---|---|---|---|---|
| Weighted $K$-means | 0.836 (0.082) | 0.767 (0.081) | 0.765 (0.065) | 0.747 (0.073) |
| Sparse weighted $K$-means | 0.974 (0.034) | 0.924 (0.063) | 0.915 (0.081) | 0.815 (0.105) |
| Standard $K$-means | 0.836 (0.082) | 0.522 (0.142) | 0.376 (0.016) | 0.374 (0.015) |
| Sparse $K$-means | 0.974 (0.034) | 0.538 (0.142) | 0.376 (0.016) | 0.374 (0.015) |
| Standard $K$-medoids | 0.565 (0.073) | 0.484 (0.094) | 0.367 (0) | 0.367 (0) |
| Weighted $K$-medoids | 0.565 (0.073) | 0.542 (0.075) | 0.557 (0.075) | 0.542 (0.064) |

The results for simulation setting 1 are shown

[a]Purity [28] is given by $\frac{1}{n} \sum_{q=1}^{k} \max_{1 \leq j \leq l} \left( n_q^j \right)$, where $l$ denotes the number of original class labels, $n$ the total number of samples and $n_q^j$ the number of samples in the cluster $q$ that belong to original class $j$ $(1 \leq j \leq l)$

**Table 3** The quantities reported are the mean and standard error (given in parentheses) of the number of true cluster-specific features selected, over 50 runs of simulation

| Simulation | Noise level | Sparse weighted $K$-means | Sparse $K$-means |
|---|---|---|---|
| ~50 features selected | $\sigma_0 = 1$ | 46.72 (1.512) | 46.72 (1.565) |
| | $\sigma_0 = 2$ | 45.7 (1.689) | 37.8 (6.682) |
| | $\sigma_0 = 5$ | 44.94 (2.123) | 5.66 (6.432) |
| | $\sigma_0 = 20$ | 45.16 (1.583) | 2.76 (1.697) |
| ~100 features selected | $\sigma_0 = 1$ | 49.82 (0.438) | 49.8 (0.4949) |
| | $\sigma_0 = 2$ | 49.4 (0.881) | 43.88 (6.542) |
| | $\sigma_0 = 5$ | 49.2 (1.010) | 9.44 (9.002) |
| | $\sigma_0 = 20$ | 49.4 (0.926) | 5.36 (2.768) |

Recall that the true number of cluster-specific features $q = 50$. The results for simulation setting 1 are shown

in selecting the true cluster-specific features (Table 3). The performance of sparse weighted $K$-means algorithm is quite stable when the noise level increases and outperforms sparse $K$-means algorithm.

## 3.2 Simulation 2: Dirichlet-Multinomial Distribution

To mimic the data structure in single-cell experiments, we simulated data from the Dirichlet-multinomial distribution. Note that the Dirichlet-multinomial distribution, denoted by $DM(N, \boldsymbol{\alpha})$, has two sets of parameters: the number of trials $N$ and the concentration parameter vector $\boldsymbol{\alpha}$. The parameter $\boldsymbol{\alpha}$ is set based on a single-cell chromatin accessibility (scATAC-Seq) dataset with in silico mixture of three known cell types, K562, GM12878, and HL-60 [4], so the simulation will naturally capture the distribution and correlation in real data.

The simulation setup is as follows. We assume that the number of classes $K = 3$, the total number of observations $n = 100$, and we have $n_i$ observations for class $i$, $i = 1, 2, 3$. To incorporate as much information as possible and to reduce the computational time, the top 5000 regulatory regions ranked by total read counts over all the cells in the scATAC-Seq dataset are selected. So the total number of features $p = 5000$. Assuming that cells of the same type are generated from the same multinomial distribution, the multinomial parameter $p^{(i)}$ is calculated using the maximum likelihood estimation from the scATAC-Seq dataset. The Dirichlet-multinomial parameter vector $\boldsymbol{\alpha}^{(i)}$ is chosen as $600p^{(i)}$, and the number of trials $N = 1800$. We first generate $X_j \sim DM(N, \boldsymbol{\alpha}_j)$ independently, where $\boldsymbol{\alpha}_j = \boldsymbol{\alpha}^{(1)} 1_{\{1 \le j \le n_1\}} + \boldsymbol{\alpha}^{(2)} 1_{\{n_1+1 \le j \le n_1+n_2\}} + \boldsymbol{\alpha}^{(3)} 1_{\{n_1+n_2+1 \le j \le n\}}$. Then to generate noisy observations, we randomly pick $n_0 = 20$ observations and set 90% of their non-zero features to be 0 for each observation picked. Intuitively, this process corresponds to the fact that the sequencing depth, or the count sum, in the noisy cells is far smaller

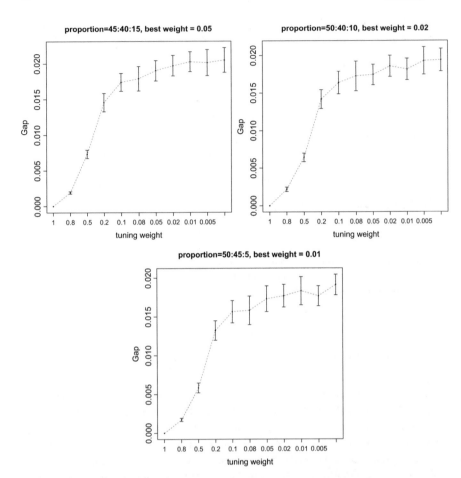

**Fig. 3** The best weight is chosen by the smallest value for which Gap(**U**) is within one standard deviation from the largest value of Gap(**U**). The candidate weights ($x$-axis) for the noisy observations are $1, 0.8, 0.5, 0.2, 0.1, 0.08, 0.05, 0.02, 0.01, 0.005, 0.001$. The results for simulation setting 2 is shown

than that in the other cells. Note that when choosing the weight, we assume that the labels for noisy observations are known, which is reasonable as the sequencing depth in single-cell experiments is known.

In this setup, we set $n_1:n_2:n_3$ to be three different proportions: 45:40:15, 50:40:10, 50:45:5. As for assigning the weight in the weighted $K$-means algorithm, we perform data preprocessing on the generated data first (details for data preprocessing are presented in the Supplementary Notes), and then choose a descending sequence of candidate weights for the noisy observations, and set the weights for the other observations to be 1. The results for tuning the weights are shown in Fig. 3.

We compare the clustering purity among different methods: $K$-means, weighted $K$-means, $K$-medoids, weighted $K$-medoids, SC3 [9], CIDR [10] and SIMLR [11].

**Table 4** Mean and standard error (given in parentheses) of purity over 50 runs of simulations, simulation setting 2

| $n_1:n_2:n_3$ | $K$-means | Weighted $K$-means | $K$-medoids | Weighted $K$-medoids | SC3 | CIDR | SIMLR |
|---|---|---|---|---|---|---|---|
| 45:40:15 | 0.793 | 0.968 | 0.819 | 0.830 | 0.853 | 0.709 | 0.860 |
| | (0.027) | (0.015) | (0.040) | (0.039) | (0.046) | (0.124) | (0.048) |
| 50:40:10 | 0.829 | 0.975 | 0.839 | 0.840 | 0.836 | 0.723 | 0.837 |
| | (0.014) | (0.012) | (0.030) | (0.030) | (0.020) | (0.152) | (0.026) |
| 50:45:5 | 0.873 | 0.972 | 0.888 | 0.883 | 0.874 | 0.783 | 0.873 |
| | (0.013) | (0.032) | (0.020) | (0.020) | (0.015) | (0.155) | (0.013) |

For $K$-means, weighted $K$-means, $K$-medoids, and weighted $K$-medoids, we first do data preprocessing and then perform clustering. For SC3, CIDR and SIMLR, we use the original data, as these methods are designed for count data. The results are shown in Table 4. We can see that under all the settings of different proportions of cells, our proposed weighted $K$-means algorithm has the best clustering result. Note that the weight in the weighted $K$-means and weighted $K$-medoids algorithm is chosen based on Fig. 3. However, it is worth mentioning that these weighted algorithms have stable clustering results as long as the weights for noisy cells are less than some threshold. Details for the stability are presented in the Supplementary Notes. Moreover, the weighted $K$-medoids algorithm tends to be more stable when the weight for noisy cell changes, while the clustering result of weighted $K$-means tends to vary when the weight changes, indicating the necessity of a good tuning scheme for the weight. Therefore, compared with weighted $K$-medoids, weighted $K$-means can suffer more from bad weighting scheme. Fortunately, we have a data adaptive tuning scheme to tune the weights for the observations.

## 3.3 Summary

To summarize, we show a schematic plot (Fig. 4) to illustrate the performance of $K$-means, weighted $K$-means, $K$-medoids and weighted $K$-medoids under different settings.

When the observations are evenly distributed and the number of observations is moderately large (Fig. 4a), all four algorithms should be able to find good centers and should perform similarly.

When observations are more spread out from the ideal cluster center (Fig. 4b), the medoid-based algorithms are less likely to find good representative centers, while by averaging over the observations, $K$-means algorithms can find better cluster centers. This corresponds to the Dirichlet-multinomial simulation setting with the absence of noisy observations.

When noise observations, i.e. cells with low sequencing depth, are present in the dataset (Fig. 4c), $K$-means is less robust, and the estimated center can deviate from

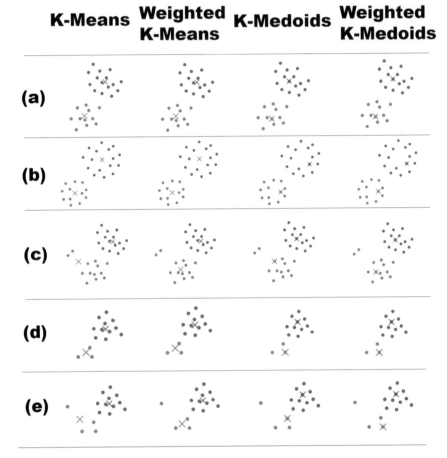

**Fig. 4** Schematic plots comparing different methods. For illustration, we assume that the true cluster labels are known (red and blue), and we compare the cluster centers estimated by different algorithms. (**a**) When observations are evenly distributed and the number of observations per cluster is moderately large, we expect that the four algorithms perform similarly: $K$-means $\approx$ weighted $K$-means $\approx$ $K$-medoids $\approx$ weighted $K$-medoids. (**b**) When observations are more spread out from the center, representing higher noise/signal ratio for all the observations, we expect that the performance of $K$-means $\approx$ weighted $K$-means $>$ $K$-medoids $\approx$ weighted $K$-medoids. The medoid-based algorithm may not find a good observation for the cluster center. (**c**) When there are noisy observations, representing cells with low sequencing depth, the performance of weighted $K$-means $\approx$ weighted $K$-medoids $\geq$ $K$-medoids $>$ $K$-means. Note that the $K$-means algorithm is sensitive to the noisy data points. (**d**) When there is a rare cell type, $K$-means $\approx$ weighted $K$-means $>$ $K$-medoids $\approx$ weighted $K$-medoids. The medoid-based algorithms are less likely to choose a good representative observation within the rare population for the cluster center. (**e**) When there are both cells with low sequencing depth and a rare cell type, the performance of weighted $K$-means $>$ weighted $K$-medoids $>$ $K$-medoids $>$ $K$-means. Weighted $K$-means has the best performance, and weighted $K$-medoids is slightly better than $K$-medoids, while $K$-means performs the worst

the ideal cluster center, while weighted $K$-means alleviates the deviation by down weighting the noisy observations. The medoid-based algorithms are also robust since the cluster centers are representative observations and not the average.

When there is a rare cell type (Fig. 4d), the medoid-based algorithms are less likely to find a good representative center for the rare cell type. $K$-means and weighted $K$-means can find a better center for the rare cell type, via averaging over the observations, which reduces the variance.

When there are both cells with low sequencing depth and a rare cell type (Fig. 4e), weighted $K$-means will outperform weighted $K$-medoids as it can find a better cluster center for the rare cell type. Weighted $K$-means will also outperform $K$-means as it is more robust to noisy observations.

We have proposed a data adaptive weighting scheme for weighted $K$-means algorithm. When the weighting scheme is able to characterize the noisy observations well, weighted $K$-means should outperform weighted $K$-medoids in principle. However, there are some other concerns include the following:

1. Implementation. The medoid-based methods are more flexible as we can use any dissimilarity metric. For the mean-based methods, we can transform the data first (as we did) and then use Euclidean distance.
2. Computation. The medoid-based methods can be faster when the number of observations is not large. The dissimilarity metric is pre-computed, so we only need to operate on the $n \times n$ dissimilarity matrix. For the mean-based methods, we need to operate on the $n \times p$ data matrix, which is large when $p \gg n$.
3. Robustness. Since medoid-based methods use less information of the data to calculate the cluster center, they can be more robust to noisy observations and misspecified weighting scheme, for example, incorrect labels for the noisy observations. For single-cell genomic data, the noise level is usually determined by the known sequencing depth.

# 4  Application to Single-Cell Chromatin Accessibility Data

Eukaryotic genomes are hierarchically packaged into chromatin, and the nature of this packaging plays a central role in gene regulation [29]. ATAC-seq maps transposase-accessible chromatin regions, and provides information for understanding this epigenetic structure of chromatin packaging and for understanding gene regulation [30]. Single-cell chromatin accessibility (scATAC-Seq) maps chromatin accessibility at single-cell resolution and provides insight on the cell-to-cell variation of gene regulation [4]. The cell types in scATAC-Seq datasets are usually not known *in priori* and need to be inferred from the data: clustering methods are essential for this goal.

Next we applied our proposed approach to a scATAC-Seq dataset. The dataset includes *in silico* mixture of three known cell types, K562, GM12878, and HL-60 [4]. We applied clustering methods to this dataset, and use the true cell type labels to evaluate the methods. The raw data matrix for this dataset is $n \times p$, where $n = 1,131$ cells is the number of observations, and $p = 68,069$ genomic regions is the number of features. The entries in this data matrix represent the read counts within each genomic region. A non-zero count suggests that the genomic region may be accessible. Some features in the dataset do not carry much information in separating the cell types: the majority of the cells have zero counts in those features, and only very few cells have non-zero counts. In the clustering algorithm, we removed the features with excessive zeros and selected the top 5000 features by sum of read counts over all the cells. Details for data preprocessing are presented in the Supplementary Notes.

In our previously proposed method based on weighted $K$-medoids algorithm [16], we implemented the following weighting scheme for cell $i$:

$$u_i = \frac{1}{1 + \exp\{-(h_i - c)/(c\lambda)\}},$$

where $h_i$ denotes a measure of relative sequencing depth for cell $i$, $c$ is chosen to be the median of $h_i$ and $\lambda$ is the tuning parameter. When $\lambda$ is large, the weight $u_i$ tends to be flat across cells with different sequencing depths. We first tune $\lambda$ based on the method proposed in Sect. 2.3. By decreasing $\lambda$, we create a sequence of weight vectors, $\mathbf{U}(\lambda=10)$, ..., $\mathbf{U}(\lambda = 0.005)$. Based on Fig. 5, the best $\lambda$ is 0.1. It is a coincidence that the tuned $\lambda$ is the same as the default $\lambda$ in our previous method.

Next, using the tuned weight $\mathbf{U}$, we compared the performance of weighted $K$-means with $K$-means, $K$-medoids, weighted $K$-medoids, SC3 [9], CIDR [10] and SIMLR [11]. Incorporating the weighting scheme in $K$-means algorithm significantly improves the clustering performance. The cluster center in $K$-means algorithm is calculated as the average of cells assigned to the same cluster. We reason that down-weighting the noisy cells in the averaging step can lead to a much better estimate of the cluster center. 17 observations are misclassified by weighted $K$-medoids, 5 by SC3, 11 by SIMLR, while only 1 misclassification given by weighted $K$-means (Table 5).

Following the discussion in Sect. 3.3, the mean-based methods may work better to detect rare cell type as averaging reduces variance and can lead to a better estimate for the cluster center. To confirm this hypothesis, we downsampled HL-60 cells to synthetically create a rare cell type in the dataset. More specifically, we picked random subsets of 100 cells from the full dataset, treating HL-60 cells as the rare population and gradually decrease the proportion of it to 15%, 10% and 5% respectively.

Our proposed weighted $K$-means algorithm achieves the best performance in detecting the rare cell type (HL-60) in all settings (Table 6). We also compared the clustering purity (Table 7). Note that when the proportion of HL-60 is 15%, weighted $K$-means performs as good as SC3. Besides, when the proportion of

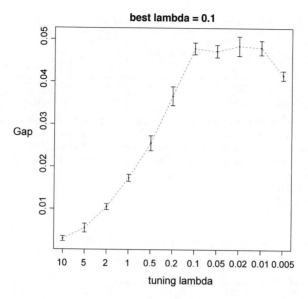

**Fig. 5** Best $\lambda$ is chosen at $\lambda = 0.1$ for the scATAC-Seq dataset

**Table 5** Clustering results comparing different methods for the scATAC-Seq dataset

| | $K$-means | | | | Weighted $K$-means | | |
|---|---|---|---|---|---|---|---|
| | K562 | GM12878 | HL60 | | K562 | GM12878 | HL60 |
| Cluster 1 | 375 | 0 | 0 | Cluster 1 | 666 | 0 | 0 |
| Cluster 2 | 0 | 361 | 85 | Cluster 2 | 0 | 372 | 0 |
| Cluster 3 | 291 | 12 | 7 | Cluster 3 | 0 | 1 | 92 |
| | $K$-medoids | | | | Weighted $K$-medoids | | |
| | K562 | GM12878 | HL60 | | K562 | GM12878 | HL60 |
| Cluster 1 | 657 | 0 | 0 | Cluster 1 | 657 | 0 | 0 |
| Cluster 2 | 2 | 372 | 7 | Cluster 2 | 2 | 372 | 7 |
| Cluster 3 | 7 | 1 | 85 | Cluster 3 | 7 | 1 | 85 |
| | SC3 | | | | CIDR | | |
| | K562 | GM12878 | HL60 | | K562 | GM12878 | HL60 |
| Cluster 1 | 666 | 2 | 3 | Cluster 1 | 391 | 244 | 70 |
| Cluster 2 | 0 | 371 | 0 | Cluster 2 | 263 | 116 | 21 |
| Cluster 3 | 0 | 0 | 89 | Cluster 3 | 12 | 13 | 1 |
| | SIMLR | | | | | | |
| | K562 | GM12878 | HL60 | | | | |
| Cluster 1 | 666 | 0 | 2 | | | | |
| Cluster 2 | 0 | 373 | 9 | | | | |
| Cluster 3 | 0 | 0 | 81 | | | | |

**Table 6** Comparing different methods for detecting[a] rare cell population, *HL-60*

| Proportion[b] | $K$-means | Weighted $K$-means | $K$-medoids | Weighted $K$-medoids | SC3 | CIDR | SIMLR |
|---|---|---|---|---|---|---|---|
| 45:40:15 | 0.12 | 1.00 | 0.24 | 0.34 | 0.92 | 0.00 | 0.68 |
| 50:40:10 | 0.00 | 0.90 | 0.12 | 0.28 | 0.62 | 0.00 | 0.42 |
| 50:45:5 | 0.00 | 0.58 | 0.00 | 0.02 | 0.06 | 0.00 | 0.04 |

The results for 50 runs of subsampling from the scATAC-Seq dataset are shown
[a]The criterion that we use for successful detection of rare cell population is as follows. Firstly, the number of observations of rare pupolation in one cluster, denoted as $n_{rare}$, should be the majority within this cluster. Secondly, $n_{rare}$ should be larger than 80% of the total number of observations in the rare pupolation. We run 50 experiments for each setting, and the proportion of success measures the ability of detection
[b]The first column denotes the proportions of three cell types (*K562:GM12878:HL-60*)

**Table 7** Mean and standard error (given in parentheses) of purity

| Proportion | $K$-means | Weighted $K$-means | $K$-medoids | Weighted $K$-medoids | SC3 | CIDR | SIMLR |
|---|---|---|---|---|---|---|---|
| 45:40:15 | 0.786 | 0.958 | 0.869 | 0.890 | 0.978 | 0.491 | 0.868 |
|  | (0.060) | (0.036) | (0.080) | (0.073) | (0.034) | (0.036) | (0.085) |
| 50:40:10 | 0.831 | 0.956 | 0.890 | 0.911 | 0.951 | 0.527 | 0.866 |
|  | (0.042) | (0.049) | (0.071) | (0.065) | (0.044) | (0.029) | (0.088) |
| 50:45:5 | 0.858 | 0.944 | 0.937 | 0.945 | 0.937 | 0.539 | 0.879 |
|  | (0.045) | (0.041) | (0.031) | (0.018) | (0.022) | (0.033) | (0.071) |

The results for 50 runs of subsampling from the scATAC-Seq dataset are shown

HL-60 is 5% (50:45:5), the purities for weighted $K$-medoids algorithm and SC3 are comparable with weighted $K$-means, but neither weighted $K$-medoids nor SC3 algorithm can detect the rare cell type.

Finally, we applied sparse weighted $K$-means. Sparse weighted $K$-means misclassifies 13 observations (Fig. 6a), the clustering result is slightly worse than weighted $K$-means with only 1 misclassification, but is comparable to $K$-medoids and weighted $K$-medoids algorithm (17 misclassified observations respectively in Table 5). After tuning the sparsity parameter $s$, all the features have non-zero weights, which may be due to the fact that we pre-selected the top 5000 features. The distribution of the weights decays exponentially, where the majority of the features have weights close to 0 (Fig. 6b). Although the weights for all features are non-zero, the weights still provide useful information on the importance of the features. We selected the top 500 features ranked by $w$ (the cutoff is plotted as the red line in Fig. 6b). It is clear that these top features differentiate the three clusters (Fig. 6c).

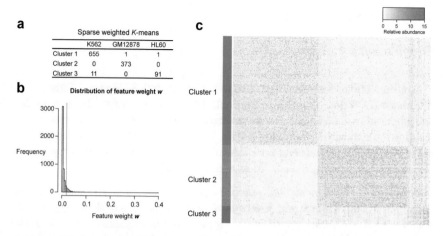

**Fig. 6** (**a**) Clustering table for sparse weighted $K$-means algorithm on scATAC-Seq data. (**b**) Distribution of the feature weights $w$. (**c**) Visualization of the top 500 features with high weight (the threshold is shown as a vertical red line in the histogram. To calculate the relative abundance, we first normalize each cell by sequencing depth $h_i$, and then normalize by the mean of each feature, to make the plot more comparable across cells and across features)

## 5 Conclusion

In this work, we have proposed a weighted $K$-means clustering algorithm and a sparse version of this algorithm. Both methods perform well on simulated datasets with different noise levels and different proportions of the cell types. On a single-cell chromatin accessibility dataset, through down-weighting cells with low sequencing depth, the proposed weighted $K$-means algorithm achieves a higher success rate of detecting rare cell types and improved clustering purity. The proposed sparse weighted $K$-means algorithm can select cluster-specific features.

Though our proposed methods work well on simulated and real data, they are based on the assumption that labels for noisy observations are known. Given a dataset without this assumption, it can be hard to select the tuning parameters. Tuning parameter selection in the unsupervised setting is known to be a difficult problem, and more work is needed in this area. In addition, weighted $K$-means algorithm can suffer more from bad weighting scheme compared with weighted $K$-medoids algorithm.

The R package SWKM is available at https://github.com/Van1yu3/SWKM.

**Acknowledgement** This work has been supported by the Chinese University of Hong Kong direct grant 2018/2019 No. 4053360.

# Supplementary Information

## *Supplementary Notes*

**The Connection Between Our Proposed Weighted $K$-Means Method and Standard $K$-Means with Data Augmentation** Here we would like to show that our proposed method is the same as replicating some observations and then implementing the standard $K$-means algorithm. The propositions below are proposed and proved in one-dimension condition. However, it can be shown that the propositions also hold in high-dimension condition, and the proof is quite similar.

**Proposition 1** *Given $n$ distinct points $\{x_1, x_2, \cdots, x_n\}$, and $s$ duplicate points $x_{01}, x_{02}, \cdots, x_{0s}$. Assume that $K$-means algorithm is applied to those $(n + s)$ data points with $K = 2$, and denote by $C_1, C_2$ the two cluster multisets. We show that to minimize the WCSS, all of these $s$ duplicate points should be in the same cluster, either $C_1$ or $C_2$. That is, if we denote by $w$ the number of duplicate points in $C_1$, then we have*

$$\min_{w \in \{0, 1, \cdots, s\}} \text{WCSS} = \min_{w \in \{0, s\}} \text{WCSS}$$

***Proof*** Define two sets $\tilde{C}_1, \tilde{C}_2$ that satisfy the following:

$$\tilde{C}_1 \subset C_1, \tilde{C}_2 \subset C_2, x_0 \notin \tilde{C}_1 \cup \tilde{C}_2, \tilde{C}_1 \cup \tilde{C}_2 = \{x_1, x_2, \cdots, x_n\}$$

Intuitively, $\tilde{C}_1, \tilde{C}_2$ is extracted from $C_1, C_2$ except the duplicate points.

Let $n_1 = \#\tilde{C}_1, n_2 = \#\tilde{C}_2$, obviously $n_1 + n_2 = n$.

$$
\begin{aligned}
\text{WCSS}(w) =& \frac{1}{n_1 + w} \sum_{i, i' \in C_1} (x_i - x_{i'})^2 + \frac{1}{n_2 + s - w} \sum_{i, i' \in C_2} (x_i - x_{i'})^2 \\
=& \frac{1}{n_1 + w} \sum_{i, i' \in \tilde{C}_1} (x_i - x_{i'})^2 + \frac{2w}{n_1 + w} \sum_{i \in \tilde{C}_1} (x_0 - x_i)^2 \\
& + \frac{1}{n_2 + s - w} \sum_{i, i' \in \tilde{C}_2} (x_i - x_{i'})^2 + \frac{2(s - w)}{n_2 + s - w} \sum_{i \in \tilde{C}_2} (x_0 - x_i)^2 \\
=& 2\{ \sum_{i \in \tilde{C}_1} x_i^2 + n_1[(x_0 - \mu_1)^2 - \mu_1^2] - \frac{n_1^2}{n_1 + w} (x_0 - \mu_1)^2 \\
& + \sum_{i \in \tilde{C}_2} x_i^2 + n_2[(x_0 - \mu_2)^2 - \mu_2^2] - \frac{n_2^2}{n_2 + s - w} (x_0 - \mu_2)^2 \}
\end{aligned}
$$

where $\mu_1 = \frac{1}{n_1} \sum_{i \in \tilde{C}_1} x_i, \mu_2 = \frac{1}{n_2} \sum_{i \in \tilde{C}_2} x_i$.

Define $a_0 \equiv -n_1^2(x_0 - \mu_1)^2$, $b_0 \equiv -n_2^2(x_0 - \mu_2)^2$. Treat $w$ as a continuous variable in $[0, s]$, then take derivative of $\frac{1}{2}\text{WCSS}(w)$:

$$\frac{1}{2}\frac{d\text{WCSS}(w)}{dw} = -\frac{a_0}{(n_1 + w)^2} + \frac{b_0}{(n_2 + s - w)^2}$$

$$= \frac{b_0(n_1 + w)^2 - a_0(n_2 + s - w)^2}{(n_1 + w)^2(n_2 + s - w)^2}$$

$$= \frac{(b_0 - a_0)w^2 + 2[n_1 b_0 + (n_2 + s)a_0]w + b_0 n_1^2 - a_0(n_2 + s)^2}{(n_1 + w)^2(n_2 + s - w)^2}$$

Let $f(w) \equiv (b_0 - a_0)w^2 + 2[n_1 b_0 + (n_2 + s)a_0]w + b_0 n_1^2 - a_0(n_2 + s)^2$. Discuss the following conditions:

- If $b_0 - a_0 \leq 0$, as $f(w)$ is a linear or quadratic function, it's easy to check that $\text{WCSS}(w)$ can either be monotonic, or firstly increase and then decrease in $[0, s]$.
- If $b_0 - a_0 > 0$, as the symmetry axis of $f(w)$ is $x = \frac{n_1 b_0 + (n_2 + s)a_0}{a_0 - b_0} > s$, easy to check that $\text{WCSS}(w)$ can either be monotonic, or firstly increase and then decrease in $[0, s]$.

Both the conditions conclude that

$$\min_{w \in \{0, 1, \cdots, s\}} \text{WCSS} = \min_{w \in \{0, s\}} \text{WCSS}$$

$\square$

**Proposition 2** *Given n data points* $x_1^{(1)}, x_1^{(2)}, \cdots, x_1^{(u_1)}, x_2^{(1)}, x_2^{(2)}, \cdots, x_2^{(u_2)}, \cdots,$ $x_s^{(1)}, x_s^{(2)}, \cdots, x_s^{(u_s)}$, *where* $x_j^{(1)} = x_j^{(2)} = \cdots = x_j^{(u_j)}$ *for* $j = 1, 2, \cdots, s$. *If standard K-means algorithm is applied to the data points ($K \leq s$), then the duplicate points must be in the same cluster.*

**Proof** Using the Proposition 1 above, this can be easily proved by contradiction.

$\square$

Here, $u_1, u_2, \cdots, u_s$ are positive integers, satisfying $\sum_{i \in \tilde{C}_k} u_i = n_k$. More generally, if $u_1, u_2, \cdots, u_s$ are real numbers representing weights of the distinct points, the proof above still holds. Hence, a weighted $K$-means algorithm could be performed with respect to the distinct points.

**Data Preprocessing for Simulated Data in Sect. 3.2 and Single-Cell Chromatin Accessibility (scATAC-Seq) Data in Sect. 4** Details for data preprocessing are similar to that in [16]. The scATAC-seq data from [4] is publicly available in the Gene Expression Omnibus (GEO) under the accession number GSE65360. We used the Kundaje pipeline (https://github.com/kundajelab/atac_dnase_pipelines) to process the raw scATAC-seq reads, aligning reads to hg19. we employed MACS2 to perform peak calling on accessibility data aggregated across all cells [31]. MACS2 generates (1) narrow peaks generally called for transcription factor binding sites and (2) broad peaks suitable for detection of functional regulatory elements such as promoters and enhancers. We utilized both narrow and broad regions, called gapped peaks, to better classify cell identities. After obtaining the data matrix for the read counts, we first take rank for each cell. For each cell, we then standardize the rank matrix to mean 0 and unit standard deviation.

Denote the data matrix as $X = (x_{ij})$. $\tilde{X}_{i,} = \frac{X_{i,}}{\sum_j X_{ij}} \times \text{median}(\sum_j X_{ij})$, where $X_{i,}$ is the $i^{th}$ row of $X$. We also applied another four methods for data preprocessing, $log(X + 1)$, $\tilde{X}$, $log(\tilde{X} + 1)$ and $z$-score. Tables S1, S2, S3 and S4 in the Supplementary Tables summarize the clustering results for these four methods respectively. Compared to these four data preprocessing methods, the normalized-rank preprocessing we employed (Table 5) offers much better performance in terms of low misclassification rate.

**Choosing Number of Clusters $K$** We make use of Gap statistics [27] with modifications similar to that in [16] to establish the following procedures to select $K$. Choice of $K$ for Simulation 2 and scATAC-Seq dataset are presented in Figs. S1 and S2 respectively.

1. Perform the weighted $K$-means clustering algorithm on the observed cell×feature data matrix $\mathbf{X}$ with tuned weight $\mathbf{U}$, varying the total number of clusters from 1 to the maximum number of clusters $N$, $K = 1, \ldots, N$, and use the weighted $K$-means optimized objective function in the last iteration as $O_K$. The objective function is the weighted within-cluster sum of squares defined in Sect. 2.1 as $\sum_{k=1}^{K} \sum_{i \in C_k} u_i \|\mathbf{x}_i - \hat{\mu}_k\|_2^2$, where $u_i$ is the weight for observation $\mathbf{x}_i$, and $\hat{\mu}_k = \frac{\sum_{i \in C_k} u_i \mathbf{x}_i}{\sum_{i \in C_k} u_i}$.

2. Generate $B$ reference data sets, by performing permutation for each feature (peak). The permutation shuffles the entries in each column of $\mathbf{X}$. Perform the weighted $K$-means clustering algorithm on the $B$ reference data sets, varying the total number of clusters, and calculate the weighted $K$-means objective $O_{Kb}^*$, for $b = 1, \ldots, B$ and $K = 1, \ldots, N$.

3. Compute the estimated gap statistics $\text{Gap}(K) = \frac{1}{B} \sum_{b=1}^{B} \log O_{Kb}^* - \log O_K$, and the standard deviation $sd(K) = \sqrt{\frac{1}{B} \sum_{b=1}^{B} (\log O_{Kb}^* - \bar{l})^2}$, where $\bar{l} = \sum_{b=1}^{B} \log O_{Kb}^* / B$. Finally we choose the number of clusters by

$$\hat{K} = \text{smallest } K \text{ s.t. } \text{Gap}(K) \geq \text{Gap}(K + 1) - sd(K + 1)$$

**Stability of the Weighted $K$-Means and Weighted $K$-Medoids Algorithm** Under the setup in Sect. 3.2, we choose a sequence of 11 candidate noisy weights. For each candidate weight, the weighted $K$-means and the weighted $K$-medoids algorithm are performed over 50 simulations, and the results of clustering purity are presented in Tables S5 and S6 in the Supplementary Tables. The results indicate that when the noisy weight is less than 0.1, the weighted $K$-means clustering becomes stable, while the threshold of the noisy weight in the weighted $K$-medoids is 0.5. Comparing these two tables, we can also draw a conclusion that weighted $K$-medoids is more robust against weights, which is reasonable as the original $K$-medoids is more robust against noisy observations naturally.

**A Simple Alternative to the Weighted $K$-Means Algorithm: A Two-Step Approach** First apply standard $K$-means to the less noisy cells (by thresholding on $h_i$ or $u_i$) and calculate the cluster centers; then use the cluster centers to cluster the noisy cells by the nearest neighbor. This simple approach does not work as well as weighted $K$-means, which implies that using the whole sample weight information is favoured. In particular, when different thresholds are chosen, the power to detect the rare cell type can be quite variable under different settings (i.e. different proportions of cell types), making it challenging to choose a good threshold in practice. The clustering results for this two-step approach under the same setting of Table 6 is shown in Table S7 in the Supplementary Tables.

## Supplementary Figures (Figs. S1 and S2)

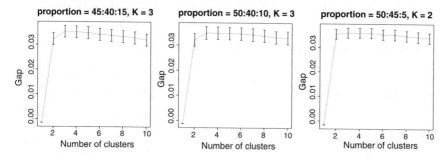

**Fig. S1** Choice of $K$ for Simulation 2 under three different proportions. The number of clusters is chosen based on large gap statistic, considering the standard error. Based on this rule, $K$ is chosen at 3, 3 and 2 for the three proportions, while the true value of $K$ is 3. When the sample size of the rare population is small (5%), the rare population may not be detected, hence $\hat{K} = 2$ is chosen. Details for the criteria of choosing $K$ are presented in the Supplementary Notes

**Fig. S2** Choice of $K$ for the scATAC-Seq dataset. $\hat{K} = 7$, while there are only 3 cell types. This may due to the heterogeneity of data, and since we have prior knowledge about the dataset, we keep $K = 3$ for the analysis

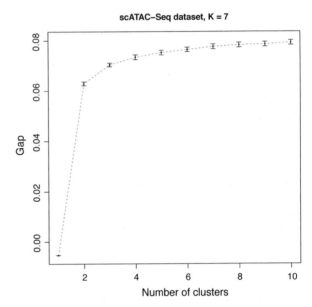

## Supplementary Tables (Tables S1, S2, S3, S4, S5, S6, and S7)

**Table S1** Clustering results using $log(X + 1)$ for the scATAC-Seq dataset

|  | *K*-means | | | | Weighted *K*-means | | |
|---|---|---|---|---|---|---|---|
|  | K562 | GM12878 | HL60 |  | K562 | GM12878 | HL60 |
| Cluster 1 | 421 | 221 | 41 | Cluster 1 | 522 | 302 | 60 |
| Cluster 2 | 227 | 107 | 42 | Cluster 2 | 138 | 28 | 26 |
| Cluster 3 | 18 | 45 | 9 | Cluster 3 | 6 | 43 | 6 |
|  | *K*-medoids | | | | Weighted *K*-medoids | | |
|  | K562 | GM12878 | HL60 |  | K562 | GM12878 | HL60 |
| Cluster 1 | 641 | 330 | 79 | Cluster 1 | 641 | 330 | 80 |
| Cluster 2 | 24 | 37 | 12 | Cluster 2 | 24 | 37 | 11 |
| Cluster 3 | 1 | 6 | 1 | Cluster 3 | 1 | 6 | 1 |

**Table S2** Clustering results using $\tilde{X}$ for the scATAC-Seq dataset

| | $K$-means | | | | Weighted $K$-means | | |
|---|---|---|---|---|---|---|---|
| | K562 | GM12878 | HL60 | | K562 | GM12878 | HL60 |
| Cluster 1 | 649 | 356 | 91 | Cluster 1 | 650 | 356 | 91 |
| Cluster 2 | 15 | 14 | 1 | Cluster 2 | 14 | 14 | 1 |
| Cluster 3 | 2 | 3 | 0 | Cluster 3 | 2 | 3 | 0 |
| | $K$-medoids | | | | Weighted $K$-medoids | | |
| | K562 | GM12878 | HL60 | | K562 | GM12878 | HL60 |
| Cluster 1 | 646 | 353 | 91 | Cluster 1 | 646 | 353 | 91 |
| Cluster 2 | 17 | 17 | 1 | Cluster 2 | 18 | 17 | 1 |
| Cluster 3 | 3 | 3 | 0 | Cluster 3 | 2 | 3 | 0 |

**Table S3** Clustering results using $log(\tilde{X}+1)$ for the scATAC-Seq dataset

| | $K$-means | | | | Weighted $K$-means | | |
|---|---|---|---|---|---|---|---|
| | K562 | GM12878 | HL60 | | K562 | GM12878 | HL60 |
| Cluster 1 | 416 | 0 | 0 | Cluster 1 | 666 | 0 | 0 |
| Cluster 2 | 0 | 311 | 83 | Cluster 2 | 0 | 372 | 0 |
| Cluster 3 | 25 | 62 | 9 | Cluster 3 | 0 | 1 | 92 |
| | $K$-medoids | | | | Weighted $K$-medoids | | |
| | K562 | GM12878 | HL60 | | K562 | GM12878 | HL60 |
| Cluster 1 | 583 | 0 | 0 | Cluster 1 | 636 | 0 | 3 |
| Cluster 2 | 14 | 230 | 55 | Cluster 2 | 28 | 373 | 89 |
| Cluster 3 | 69 | 143 | 37 | Cluster 3 | 2 | 0 | 0 |

**Table S4** Clustering results using $z$-score for the scATAC-Seq dataset

| | $K$-means | | | | Weighted $K$-means | | |
|---|---|---|---|---|---|---|---|
| | K562 | GM12878 | HL60 | | K562 | GM12878 | HL60 |
| Cluster 1 | 561 | 290 | 63 | Cluster 1 | 639 | 321 | 81 |
| Cluster 2 | 104 | 77 | 28 | Cluster 2 | 26 | 47 | 10 |
| Cluster 3 | 1 | 6 | 1 | Cluster 3 | 1 | 5 | 1 |
| | $K$-medoids | | | | Weighted $K$-medoids | | |
| | K562 | GM12878 | HL60 | | K562 | GM12878 | HL60 |
| Cluster 1 | 665 | 365 | 91 | Cluster 1 | 665 | 365 | 91 |
| Cluster 2 | 1 | 7 | 1 | Cluster 2 | 1 | 7 | 1 |
| Cluster 3 | 0 | 1 | 0 | Cluster 3 | 0 | 1 | 0 |

**Table S5** Mean and standard error (given in parentheses) of purity over 50 runs of simulation 2 for weighted $K$-means under 11 candidate noisy weights

| Noisy weight | 45:40:15 | 50:40:10 | 50:45:5 |
|---|---|---|---|
| 1 | 0.791 (0.028) | 0.826 (0.016) | 0.869 (0.013) |
| 0.8 | 0.845 (0.039) | 0.828 (0.015) | 0.869 (0.013) |
| 0.5 | 0.949 (0.028) | 0.964 (0.046) | 0.942 (0.054) |
| 0.2 | 0.964 (0.016) | 0.978 (0.019) | 0.972 (0.034) |
| 0.1 | 0.966 (0.015) | 0.980 (0.012) | 0.968 (0.039) |
| 0.08 | 0.966 (0.015) | 0.980 (0.012) | 0.971 (0.037) |
| 0.05 | 0.966 (0.015) | 0.980 (0.012) | 0.963 (0.043) |
| 0.02 | 0.965 (0.015) | 0.979 (0.019) | 0.966 (0.041) |
| 0.01 | 0.965 (0.015) | 0.980 (0.012) | 0.966 (0.043) |
| 0.005 | 0.965 (0.015) | 0.979 (0.012) | 0.962 (0.045) |
| 0.001 | 0.965 (0.015) | 0.979 (0.012) | 0.964 (0.044) |

**Table S6** Mean and standard error (given in parentheses) of purity over 50 runs of simulation 2 for weighted $K$-medoids under 11 candidate noisy weights

| Noisy weight | 45:40:15 | 50:40:10 | 50:45:5 |
|---|---|---|---|
| 1 | 0.816 (0.033) | 0.839 (0.024) | 0.882 (0.023) |
| 0.8 | 0.826 (0.031) | 0.839 (0.023) | 0.882 (0.023) |
| 0.5 | 0.820 (0.026) | 0.837 (0.022) | 0.883 (0.021) |
| 0.2 | 0.822 (0.027) | 0.838 (0.023) | 0.882 (0.021) |
| 0.1 | 0.822 (0.027) | 0.838 (0.023) | 0.883 (0.022) |
| 0.08 | 0.822 (0.026) | 0.838 (0.023) | 0.883 (0.022) |
| 0.05 | 0.822 (0.026) | 0.839 (0.023) | 0.882 (0.022) |
| 0.02 | 0.823 (0.027) | 0.839 (0.023) | 0.881 (0.021) |
| 0.01 | 0.823 (0.027) | 0.839 (0.023) | 0.881 (0.021) |
| 0.005 | 0.823 (0.027) | 0.839 (0.023) | 0.882 (0.022) |
| 0.001 | 0.823 (0.027) | 0.839 (0.023) | 0.882 (0.022) |

**Table S7** Ability of detecting rare population, mean and standard error of purity using the two-stage approach under three cell type proportions[a]

| | Proportion of success | | | Purity | | |
|---|---|---|---|---|---|---|
| Proportion | $u > 0.2$ | $u > 0.5$ | $u > 0.8$ | $u > 0.2$ | $u > 0.5$ | $u > 0.8$ |
| 45:40:15 | 0.74 | 0.92 | 0.96 | 0.907 (0.082) | 0.940 (0.063) | 0.920 (0.066) |
| 50:40:10 | 0.26 | 0.66 | 0.82 | 0.883 (0.060) | 0.926 (0.065) | 0.933 (0.055) |
| 50:45:5 | 0.00 | 0.30 | 0.48 | 0.906 (0.043) | 0.926 (0.041) | 0.935 (0.038) |

[a]Under the same setting of Table 6

# References

1. The Human Cell Atlas Participants. (2017). Science forum: The human cell atlas. *Elife, 6,* e27041.
2. Rotem, A., Ram, O., Shoresh, N., Sperling, R. A., Goren, A., Weitz, D. A., et al. (2015). Single-cell ChIP-seq reveals cell subpopulations defined by chromatin state. *Nature Biotechnology, 33*(11), 1165.
3. Smallwood, S. A., Lee, H. J., Angermueller, C., Krueger, F., Saadeh, H., Peat, J., et al. (2014). Single-cell genome-wide bisulfite sequencing for assessing epigenetic heterogeneity. *Nature Methods, 11*(8), 817.
4. Buenrostro, J. D., Wu, B., Litzenburger, U. M., Ruff, D., Gonzales, M. L., Snyder, M. P., et al. (2015). Single-cell chromatin accessibility reveals principles of regulatory variation. *Nature, 523*(7561), 486–490.
5. Cusanovich, D. A., Daza, R., Adey, A., Pliner, H. A., Christiansen, L., Gunderson, K. L., et al. (2015). Multiplex single-cell profiling of chromatin accessibility by combinatorial cellular indexing. *Science, 348*(6237), 910–914.
6. Xu, C., & Su, Z. (2015). Identification of cell types from single-cell transcriptomes using a novel clustering method. *Bioinformatics, 31*(12), 1974–1980
7. Yau, C. (2016). pcaReduce: Hierarchical clustering of single cell transcriptional profiles. *BMC Bioinformatics, 17*(1), 140.
8. Grün, D., Muraro, M. J., Boisset, J. C., Wiebrands, K., Lyubimova, A., Dharmadhikari, G., et al. (2016). De novo prediction of stem cell identity using single-cell transcriptome data. *Cell Stem Cell, 19*(2), 266–277.
9. Kiselev, V. Y., Kirschner, K., Schaub, M. T., Andrews, T., Yiu, A., Chandra, T., et al. (2017). SC3: Consensus clustering of single-cell RNA-seq data. *Nature Methods, 14*(5), 483.
10. Lin, P., Troup, M., & Ho, J. W. (2017). CIDR: Ultrafast and accurate clustering through imputation for single-cell RNA-seq data. *Genome Biology, 18*(1), 59.
11. Wang, B., Zhu, J., Pierson, E., Ramazzotti, D., & Batzoglou, S. (2017). Visualization and analysis of single-cell RNA-seq data by kernel-based similarity learning. *Nature Methods, 14*(4), 414.
12. Jiang, H., Sohn, L. L., Huang, H., & Chen, L. (2018). Single cell clustering based on cell-pair differentiability correlation and variance analysis. *Bioinformatics, 34*(21), 3684–3694.
13. Yang, Y., Huh, R., Culpepper, H. W., Lin, Y., Love, M. I., & Li, Y. (2018). SAFE-clustering: Single-cell aggregated (from Ensemble) clustering for single-cell RNA-seq data. *Bioinformatics, 35*(8), 1269–1277.
14. Zhu, L., Lei, J., Devlin, B., Roeder, K. (2019). Semi-soft clustering of single cell data. *Proceedings of the National Academy of Sciences of the United States of America, 116*(2), 466–471.
15. Sun, Z., Wang, T., Deng, K., Wang, X. F., Lafyatis, R., Ding, Y., et al. (2017). DIMM-SC: A dirichlet mixture model for clustering droplet-based single cell transcriptomic data. *Bioinformatics, 34*(1), 139–146.
16. Zamanighomi, M., Lin, Z., Daley, T., Chen, X., Duren, Z., Schep, A., et al. (2018). Unsupervised clustering and epigenetic classification of single cells. *Nature Communications, 9*(1), 2410.
17. Makarenkov, V., & Legendre, P. (2001). Optimal variable weighting for ultrametric and additive trees and $k$-means partitioning: Methods and software. *Journal of Classification, 18,* 245–271.
18. Modha, D. S., & Spangler, W. S. (2003). Feature weighting in $k$-means clustering. *Machine Learning, 52*(3), 217–237.
19. Huang, J. Z., Ng, M. K., Rong, H., & Li, Z. (2005). Automated variable weighting in $k$-means type clustering. *IEEE Transactions on Pattern Analysis and Machine Intelligence, 27,* 657–68.
20. Jing, L., Ng, M. K., & Huang, J. Z. (2007). An entropy weighting $k$-means algorithm for subspace clustering of high-dimensional sparse data. *IEEE Transactions on Knowledge and Data Engineering, 19,* 1026–1041.

21. Wu, F. X. (2008). Genetic weighted $k$-means algorithm for clustering large-scale gene expression data. *BMC Bioinformatics, 9*(Suppl. 6), S12.
22. Amorim, R., & Mirkin, B. (2012). Minkowski metric, feature weighting and anomalous cluster initializing in $k$-means clustering. *Pattern Recognition, 45*, 1061–1075.
23. Tseng, G. (2007). Penalized and weighted $k$-means for clustering with scattered objects and prior information in high-throughput biological data. *Bioinformatics (Oxford, England), 23*, 2247–55.
24. Aloise, D., Deshpande, A., Hansen, P., & Popat, P. (2009). NP-hardness of Euclidean sum-of-squares clustering. *Machine Learning, 75*,(2), 245–248.
25. Hartigan, J. A., & Wong, M. A. (1979). Algorithm as 136: A $k$-means clustering algorithm. *Journal of the Royal Statistical Society. Series C (Applied Statistics), 28*(1), 100–108.
26. Witten, D. M., & Tibshirani, R. (2010). A framework for feature selection in clustering. *Journal of the American Statistical Association, 105*(490), 713–726.
27. Tibshirani, R., Walther, G., & Hastie, T. (2001). Estimating the number of clusters in a data set via the gap statistic. *Journal of the Royal Statistical Society: Series B (Statistical Methodology), 63*(2), 411–423.
28. Park, H., & Kim, H. (2007). Sparse non-negative matrix factorizations via alternating non-negativity-constrained least squares for microarray data analysis. *Bioinformatics, 23*(12), 1495–1502.
29. Buenrostro, J. D., Giresi, P. G., Zaba, L. C., Chang, H. Y., & Greenleaf, W. J. (2013). Transposition of native chromatin for fast and sensitive epigenomic profiling of open chromatin, DNA-binding proteins and nucleosome position. *Nature Methods, 10*(12), 1213.
30. Buenrostro, J. D., Wu, B., Chang, H. Y., & Greenleaf, W. J. ATAC-seq: A method for assaying chromatin accessibility genome-wide. *Current Protocols in Molecular Biology, 109*(1), 21–29.
31. Zhang, Y., Liu, T., Meyer, C. A., Eeckhoute, J., Johnson, D. S., Bernstein, B. E., et al. (2008). Model-based analysis of chip-seq (MACS). *Genome Biology, 9*(9), R137.

# Discrete Multiple Testing in Detecting Differential Methylation Using Sequencing Data

**Guanshengrui Hao and Nan Lin**

**Abstract** DNA methylation, as one of the most important epigenetic mechanisms, is critical for deciding cell fate, and hence tightly relevant to understanding disease processes, such as cancer. We will discuss the multiple testing issue in detecting differential methylation in next generation sequencing studies. The detection requires comparing DNA methylation levels at millions of genomic loci across different genomic samples and can be viewed as a large-scale multiple testing problem. Due to low read counts at individual CpG sites, discreteness in the test statistics is nonignorable and brings up many intriguing statistical issues on proper control of false discovery rates (FDRs). Popular FDR control procedures are often underpowered in methylation sequencing data analysis due to the discreteness. We will discuss FDR control methods that accommodate such discreteness.

**Keywords** Multiple testing · Discreteness · False discovery rate · Methylation · Next generation sequencing

## 1 Introduction

### 1.1 Detecting Differential Methylation in Sequencing Data

DNA methylation typically refers to the methylation of the C-5 position of cytosine by DNA methyltransferases [23]. The methylation status of cytosines in CpGs influences protein-DNA interactions, gene expression, and chromatin structure and stability. It plays a vital role in the regulation of cellular processes, including host defense against endogenous parasitic sequences, embryonic development, transcription, X-chromosome inactivation, and genomic imprinting [6, 24, 26, 28, 31, 48, 52].

G. Hao · N. Lin (✉)
Washington University in St. Louis, St. Louis, MO, USA
e-mail: guanshengrui.hao@wustl.edu; nlin@wustl.edu

© Springer Nature Switzerland AG 2020
Y. Zhao, D.-G. (Din) Chen (eds.), *Statistical Modeling in Biomedical Research*, Emerging Topics in Statistics and Biostatistics,
https://doi.org/10.1007/978-3-030-33416-1_4

One major task of genomic methylation analysis is the detection of differentially methylated regions (DMRs). DMRs are genomic regions with different DNA methylation status across different biological conditions. They are regarded as possible functional regions involved in gene transcriptional regulation. The different biological conditions can refer to different cells or tissues within the same individual, same cell or tissue at different times, cells or tissues from different individuals, or even different alleles in the same cell [39]. The detection of DMRs can provide valuable insights into many biological fields such as cell differentiation, cancer development, epigenetic modification and gene regulation [57].

Sequencing-based DNA methylation profiling methods provide an opportunity to map complete DNA methylomes and set the basis for DMR detection. These technologies include whole-genome bisulfite sequencing (WGBS or BS-seq; [10, 29, 34]), reduced-representation bisulfite-sequencing (RRBS; [36]), enrichment-based methods (MeDIP-seq; [35, 53]), and methylation-sensitive restriction enzyme based methods (MRE-seq; [35]). These methods yield largely concordant results but differ significantly in the extent of genomic CpG coverage, resolution, quantitative accuracy, and cost [5, 21].

WGBS is by now the most comprehensive method to detect methylated cytosines in DNA and often considered as the gold standard in DMR detection. In this method, genomic DNA is treated with sodium bisulfite to convert cytosines to uracils before sequencing, providing single-base resolution of methylated cytosines in the genome [34]. Upon bisulfite treatment, unmethylated cytosines are deaminated to uracils, which are then converted to thymidines upon sequencing. Meanwhile, methylated cytosines resist deamination and are read as cytosines. Thus the location of the methylated cytosines can be determined by comparing treated and untreated sequences. WGBS data can then be summarized as counts of methylated and unmethylated reads at any given CpG site. To obtain a complete DNA methylome to cover each CpG site, this method requires essentially resequencing the entire genome multiple times for every experiment. As a result, WGBS dataset is mostly limited to only few individuals per biological condition [58].

Typically, the workflow of DMR detection involves first identifying the differentially methylated CpG sites (DMCs), and then grouping neighboring DMCs into DMRs by some distance criteria [42]. Identification of DMCs involves comparing methylation levels based on read counts at each CpG site across different biological conditions through hypothesis testing. Such a task then requires large-scale multiple testing (LSMT), where thousands or even millions of hypotheses are tested simultaneously. LSMT raised the attention of the statistical community since the 1950s, and has recently gained increased relevance with the rapid development of modern technologies and the explosive emergence of massive large-scale datasets.

Current commonly used approaches for identifying DMCs can be divided into two categories: count-based hypothesis tests and ratio-based hypothesis tests [42]. Count-based methods [1, 14, 37, 55] take short read count values as input, while ratio-based methods [20, 25, 46, 56] first convert read counts into methylation levels, i.e. the ratio of the methylated read counts out of the total read counts at a CpG site, and then compare them across different biological conditions. As read counts at a single CpG site are low, e.g. often below 15, the test statistics are in nature discretely distributed. However, many of the aforementioned methods have used asymptotic tests for identifying DMCs and ignored the discreteness in the test statistic. Consequently, standard multiple testing methods, such as the Benjamini–Hochberg method [2] and the $q$-value method [43], are used in current practice of genomewide DMC identification, which leaves the discreteness unaddressed. Recently, Dai et al. [11] demonstrated that proper treatment to the discreteness in the multiple testing step can significantly raise the detection power for DMR identification. In this chapter, we will thoroughly study current multiple testing procedures for discrete tests and provide our recommendation for the analysis of methylation sequencing data.

## 1.2 Multiple Testing and False Discovery Rate (FDR)

In a standard hypothesis testing problem, the Type-I error (false positive) rate is controlled and the Type-II error (false negative) rate is minimized to increase large detection power [30]. Likewise, in a typical LSMT problem, decisions are made based on two similar criteria:

- Control the Type-I error measurement of the multiple testing decision;
- Meanwhile, detect as many true signals (true positives) as possible.

Among several error measurements of LSMT adopted in the literature, the FDR first introduced by Benjamini and Hochberg [2], is one of the most widely used in genome-side studies.

Table 1 presents a summary on the test decision and underlying truth in an LSMT problem where $m$ hypotheses are tested. First define the false discovery proportion (FDP) as the proportion of false discoveries (rejections) in total rejections, i.e.

$$FDP = \frac{V}{\max(R, 1)},$$

(1)

which measures the accuracy of a one-time decision. For simplicity, we will use the operator $\vee$ to refer the operation of taking the maximum between two values, i.e., $R \vee 1 = \max(R, 1)$. The FDR, as the expected proportion of false rejections

**Table 1** Summary of multiple testing

| | | Decision | |
|---|---|---|---|
| | | Accept null | Reject null |
| Truth | | | |
| | True null | U | V |
| | True alternative | T | S |
| | Total | $m - R$ | R |

among all rejections, is then defined as the expectation of FDP [2]. FDR measures the accuracy of the LSMT procedure, i.e.

$$\text{FDR} = \mathbb{E}[\text{FDP}] = \mathbb{E}\left[\frac{V}{R \vee 1}\right]. \tag{2}$$

Other similar measures include the positive false discovery rate (pFDR; [43]) and the marginal false discovery rate (mFDR; [15, 47]), respectively, defined as

$$\text{pFDR} = \mathbb{E}\left(\frac{V}{R}\,\middle|\, R > 0\right), \tag{3}$$

$$\text{mFDR} = \frac{\mathbb{E}(V)}{\mathbb{E}(R)}. \tag{4}$$

The pFDR and mFDR ofter serve as approximations to the FDR when the number of tests is large. Genovese and Wasserman [15] show that under mild conditions, $\text{mFDR} = \text{FDR} + O(m^{-1/2})$. Storey [44] show that the pFDR and mFDR are equivalent when test statistics come from a two-component mixture model of null and alternative distributions. Analogously, the false non-discovery rate (FNR) is defined as

$$\text{FNR} = \mathbb{E}\left(\frac{T}{(m-R) \vee 1}\right). \tag{5}$$

The positive false non-discovery rate (pFNR) and the marginal false non-discovery rate (mFNR) is given by

$$\text{pFNR} = \mathbb{E}\left(\frac{T}{m-R}\,\middle|\, R > 0\right) \tag{6}$$

and

$$\text{mFNR} = \frac{\mathbb{E}(T)}{\mathbb{E}(m-R)}, \tag{7}$$

respectively. We call an LSMT procedure *valid* if it controls the FDR under a nominal level $\alpha$ and *optimal* if it has the smallest FNR among all valid procedures.

## 1.3 Notations

The following notations will be used throughout the remainder of this chapter, unless otherwise noted. We consider simultaneously performing $m$ hypothesis tests,

$H_1, \ldots, H_m$ at nominal FDR level $\alpha$. For each $i \in \mathbb{N}_m = \{1, \ldots, m\}$, for the $i$th test $H_i$, let $H_{i0}$ and $H_{i1}$ denote the null hypothesis and alternative hypothesis, respectively. Let $P_i$ denote the $p$-value from the $i$th test as a random variable and $p_i$ as its observed value. Let $F_{i0}$ and $F_{i1}$ be the $p$-value's cumulative distribution function (cdf) under the null and alternative hypothesis, respectively. For each test, if the null hypothesis is true, we call it a true null; otherwise, we call it a true non-null. We then call the proportion of true nulls among all tests being the null proportion and denote it by $\pi_0$. In addition, we call $\pi_1 = 1 - \pi_0$ the non-null proportion.

This chapter is organized as follows. Section 2 gives a brief overview of conventional FDR control procedures. In Sect. 3, we will address the discreteness issue arising naturally in DMR detection tasks and overview a few existing methods proposed to handle it. Such an issue could result in underpowered detection results, yet is often overlooked by conventional FDR control procedures. Simulation studies evaluating performances of existing methods are included in Sect. 4. Section 5 then discusses their advantages and limitations.

# 2 Conventional FDR Control Procedures

The Benjamini-Hochberg (BH) procedure [2] and Storey's $q$-value procedure [43] are the two most popular LSMT FDR control procedures. Many other works can be conceived as modifications or generalizations of these two. We will briefly describe the two procedures in this section.

## 2.1 The BH Step-up Procedure

Suppose $p_{(1)}, \ldots, p_{(m)}$ are the sorted observed $p$-values of each test in an ascending order and $H_{(1)}, \ldots, H_{(m)}$ are the corresponding hypotheses. The BH step-up procedure controls the FDR under the nominal level $\alpha$ as follows:

1. let $k = \max\{i : p_{(i)} \leq (i/m)\alpha\}$,
2. reject all $H_{(i)}, i \leq k$.

The BH procedure is the first FDR control procedure and provides large power gains over traditional family-wise error rate (FWER, the probability of at least one false discovery) control methods as the number of tests increases [17]. It revitalized research in multiple testing and has inspired other procedures, including the Benjamini–Liu step-down procedure [3], Sarkar's generalized step-wise procedure [41], etc.

Despite its power advantages over FWER control methods, the BH procedure is in general over-conservative. Assuming all tests are continuous Benjamini and Yekutieli [4] prove that the BH procedure controls the FDR at a level less than or equal to $\pi_0\alpha$, where $\pi_0$ is the null proportion. Furthermore, it is well known that using discrete test statistics can lead to a severe power loss even for a single test [54]. As a result, direct application of the BH procedure to discrete multiple testing will result in even more underpowered performance [17, 38].

## 2.2  Storey's q-Value Procedure

Storey [43] proposes a Bayesian LSMT framework that estimates the FDR conservatively for a given $p$-value cutoff. This framework assumes the following two-component model on the $p$-values,

$$P_i | \Delta_i \sim (1 - \Delta_i) \cdot F_0 + \Delta_i \cdot F_1, i \in \mathbb{N}_m, \tag{8}$$

where $\Delta_i$ is the indicator function which equals 0 if the $i$th null hypothesis is a true null and 1 otherwise, and $F_0$ can be viewed as the average of $F_{0i}$ overall true nulls and $F_1$ as the average of $F_{1i}$ overall all true non-nulls. Let $\Delta_i$'s be i.i.d. Bernoulli random variables with $\Pr(\Delta_i = 0) = \pi_0$ and $\Pr(\Delta_i = 1) = \pi_1$, respectively. When tests are all continuous, every $F_{0i}$ is Unif$(0, 1)$ and so is $F_0$. Storey [43] then shows that the pFDR for a given $p$-value cutoff $\lambda$ is

$$\mathrm{pFDR}(\lambda) = \frac{\pi_0 \lambda}{\pi_0 F_0(\lambda) + \pi_1 F_1(\lambda)}. \tag{9}$$

And the $q$-value corresponding to the $p$-value $p_i$ is defined as

$$q(p_i) = \inf_{\lambda \leq p_i} \{\mathrm{pFDR}(\lambda)\}. \tag{10}$$

The $q$-value $q(p_i)$ can be interpreted as the minimum pFDR level under which a hypothesis with the $p$-value of $p_i$ is rejected. For a given FDR nominal level $\alpha \in (0, 1)$, Storey's $q$-value procedure rejects the $i$th test if $q(p_i) \leq \alpha$.

For continuous tests, the $p$-value's Unif$(0, 1)$ null distribution leads to $F_0(\lambda) = \lambda$. And it is usually reasonable to assume that $F_1$ is stochastically larger than $F_0$, hence $F_1(\lambda)/\lambda$ is decreasing in $\lambda$. One can then show that $\arg\min_{\lambda \leq p_i} q(p_i) = p_i$ Storey [43]. It is then equivalent to reject the $i$th test if $p_i \leq \lambda^*(\alpha)$, where

$$\lambda^*(\alpha) = \sup\{\lambda : \mathrm{pFDR}(\lambda) \leq \alpha\}. \tag{11}$$

In practice, the null proportion $\pi_0$ and the cdfs $F_0$ and $F_1$ are usually unknown. Storey [43] proposes the following conservative estimate of the null proportion,

$$\hat{\pi}_0^S = \frac{\#\{i : p_i > c\}}{(1 - c) \cdot m} \tag{12}$$

with a suggested value of 0.5 for the threshold $c$. Furthermore, the denominator of (9), $\pi_0 F_0(\lambda) + \pi_1 F_1(\lambda)$, can be estimated by the empirical distriubtion $\frac{\#\{i:p_i \leq \lambda\}}{m}$. Therefore the $q$-values can be estimated as

$$\hat{q}(p_i) = \inf_{\lambda \leq p_i} \{\widehat{\text{pFDR}}(\lambda)\} = \frac{\hat{\pi}_0^S \cdot p_i \cdot m}{\#\{j : p_j \leq p_i\}}. \tag{13}$$

The decision is then made by rejecting all $H_i$, where $\hat{q}(p_i) \leq \alpha$.

Other procedures similar to Storey's $q$-value procedure with different estimation methods are also proposed in literature such as Liao et al. [33] and Tang et al. [49].

Storey et al. [45] showed that the BH procedure can be viewed as a special case of Storey's $q$-value procedure. Notice that the BH procedure can be stated as "rejecting all $H_i$, where $p_i \leq (\#\{j : p_j \leq p_i\}/m)\alpha$." In the $q$-value procedure, if we take $c = 0$, Eq. (12) gives $\hat{\pi}_0^S = 1$, and Eq. (13) then gives the decision rule of the $q$-value approach as $\hat{q}(p_i) = \frac{p_i \cdot m}{\#\{j:p_j \leq p_i\}} \leq \alpha$, which is equivalent to the decision rule of the BH procedure. Because of this equivalence, the two methods often yield similar performance when $\pi_0$ is close to 1.

# 3   Control the FDR in Testing Multiple Discrete Hypotheses

As introduced in Sect. 1, identifying DMCs involves testing equal methylation levels at each CpG site across biological groups, where the methylation level is usually summarized based on counts of methylated $(C)$ and unmethylated reads $(N - C)$, as illustrated in Table 2.

When there is no replicate, a typical statistical test to discern DMC is Fisher's Exact Test (FET; [34]), which is commonly used to examine the significance of association between two conditions (in this case it examines that of methylation levels across biological groups). When replicates are available in each biological group, the FET is criticized for ignoring variation among biological replicates [14]. Current available methods include the $t$-test approach by Hansen et al. [20] and other methods based on the beta-binomial model [14, 37, 55]. The beta-binomial model assumes that, conditional on the methylation proportion at a particular CpG site, the read counts are binomial distributed, while the methylation proportion itself can vary across replicates and biological groups, according to a beta distribution [40]. However, these methods all rely on asymptotic theory to develop tests at each CpG site and the accuracy of the asymptotic approximation can be hard to justify with limited replicates.

**Table 2** Data structure in identifying DMC for the $i$th site

|  | $C$ | $N - C$ | Total |
|---|---|---|---|
| Group 1 | $c_{1i}$ | $n_{1i} - c_{1i}$ | $n_{1i}$ |
| Group 2 | $c_{2i}$ | $n_{2i} - c_{2i}$ | $n_{2i}$ |

Besides the limited number of replicates, prevalence of small read counts in methylation sequencing data, e.g. WGBS data, makes it more urgent to concern about the accuracy of asymptotic approaches. As read counts in methylation sequencing data are summarized from reads covering a single CpG site, they tend to be much smaller than those in other next generation sequencing experiments, such as RNA-seq where read counts are collected over a much wider region of a gene.

Discreteness arising from small read counts and limited replicates in DMR detection brings new challenges to the LSMT problems. It has been shown that ill-conducted FDR control procedures without properly addressing the discreteness issue led to underpowered performance [17, 38]. To develop better FDR control procedures for the discrete paradigm, three major approaches can be taken: (1) modify the step-up sequence in the BH procedure according to the achievable significance level of a discrete $p$-value distribution Gilbert [17] and Heyse [22]; (2) use randomized $p$-values [11, 19]; (3) propose less upwardly biased estimators of the proportion $\pi_0$ of true null hypotheses and use them to induce more powerful adaptive FDR procedures [9, 32]. Next, we will describe methods under these categories in more details.

## 3.1 Modify the Step-Up Sequence

### 3.1.1 Gilbert's Method

Consider an LSMT problem consisting $m$ tests, and denote the number of true null hypotheses by $m_0$. Benjamini and Yekutieli [4] point out that for independent test statistics, the BH procedure in Sect. 2.1 conducted at significance level $\alpha$ controls the FDR at exactly $(m_0/m)\alpha$ for continuous test statistics, and at level less than or equal to $(m_0/m)\alpha$ for general test statistics. The equality holds for continuous test statistics because the $m$ $p$-values $P_i$'s are uniformly distributed under the null hypotheses, which implies that $\Pr(P_i \leq (k/m)\alpha) = (k/m)\alpha$ for all $i, k \in \mathbb{N}_m$. Yet for discrete statistics, $\Pr(P_i \leq (k/m)\alpha)$ may be less than $(k/m)\alpha$. Gilbert [17] sees the opportunity to improve the performance by filling the gap. We will refer the method proposed in Gilbert [17] as Gilbert's method hereafter.

Gilbert's method consists of two main steps. The first step borrows the idea from Tarone [50]. Note that for the discrete tests not all significance levels can be achieved exactly. Let $\alpha_i^*$ be the minimum achievable significance level for the $i$th test. For each $k \in \mathbb{N}_m$, the first step defines a set of indices $R_k$ as all tests satisfying $\alpha_i^* < \alpha/k$, and denotes $m(k)$ as the number of tests included in $R_k$. It then specifies $K$ to be the smallest $k$ that satisfies $m(k) \leq k$, with corresponding set of indices $R_K$ and its size $m(K)$. It then moves on to the second step and performs the BH procedure at level $\alpha$ on the subset of tests $R_K$. That is, sort all the observed $p$-values $p_{(1)}, \ldots, p_{(m(K))}$ of tests from $R_K$, find the threshold $p$-value $p_I$, where $I = \max\{i : p_{(i)} \leq i/m(K)\alpha\}$, and reject all tests with $p$-values $p_i \leq p_I$ for all $i \in \mathbb{N}_m$.

Gilbert's method improves the performance of the BH procedure by restricting onto a subset of tests $R_K$ when finding the threshold $p$-value. By doing so all tests in $R_K$ can be legitimately brought into the BH procedure, as the minimum achievable significance level

$$\alpha_i^* < \alpha/K \leq \alpha/m(K), \tag{14}$$

where the last term is used to compare with the smallest observed $p$-value in the BH procedure. Besides, by choosing $K$ as the smallest $k$ such that $m(k) \leq k$, it can include as many tests as possible into the subset without violating the inequality (14).

Gilbert [17] also pointed out that the performance can be further improved since the BH procedure only controls the FDR at $(m_0/m)\alpha < \alpha$. In particular Gilbert [17], shows that when Gilbert's method is carried out at level $\alpha$, the FDR is bounded above by

$$\sum_{i=1}^{m(K)} \sum_{k=1}^{m(K)} \frac{1}{k} \eta_{ik} \omega_{ik}, \tag{15}$$

where $\eta_{ik}$ is the largest achievable significance level that is less than or equal to $(k/m(K))\alpha$ for each $i$ in $R_K$ and each $k = 1, \ldots, m(K)$, and $\{\omega_{ik}\}$ are weights satisfying $\sum_{k=1}^{m(K)} \omega_{ik} = 1$. This bound can be approximated by setting $\omega_{ik} = \mathbb{1}(k = m(K))$, which places all weight on the largest $\eta_{ik}$ (i.e., $\eta_{im(K)}$) for each $i$. Under this approximation, the FDR is bounded by

$$\text{FDR}^* = \frac{1}{m(K)} \sum_{i=1}^{m(K)} \eta_{im(K)}, \tag{16}$$

and the bound FDR$^*$ may be substantially less than $\alpha$. Gilbert [17] proposes a grid search procedure that conducts Gilbert's method for a grid of $\alpha^+ \geq \alpha$ for which FDR$^* \leq \alpha$, and keeps the results from the iteration for which FDR$^*$ is as close as possible to $\alpha$ without exceeding it.

### 3.1.2 The BHH Procedure

Instead of restricting the BH procedure onto a proper subset of tests to find the threshold $p$-value, Heyse [22] proposes to utilize an average related to the minimal achievable significant levels of individual $p$-values and modify the original critical values of BH procedure, thereby referred to as the BHH procedure. The original BHH procedure could be reduced to the following easier-to-handle procedure as stated in [9]. Let $F_{0i}$ denote the cdf of the $i$th $p$-value under null, and define

$$\bar{F}_0(t) = \frac{1}{m} \sum_{i=1}^{m} F_{i0}(t), \quad t \in [0, 1]. \tag{17}$$

Then the critical values $\lambda_k$ can be calculated by inverting $\bar{F}_0$ at the $\alpha k/m$ for all $k \in \mathbb{N}_m$

$$\lambda_k = \bar{F}_0^{-1}(\alpha k/m). \tag{18}$$

Take the threshold $p$-value $\lambda^* = \lambda_{k^*}$, where $k^* = \max\{k \in \mathbb{N}_m : p_{(k)} \leq \lambda_k\}$. With the threshold $p$-value identified, the procedure can thus reject all tests with $p$-values smaller or equal to $\lambda^*$. We refer to this method as the Benjamini-Hochberg-Heyse (BHH) procedure due to its close relationship with the BH procedure.

The BHH method reduces to the standard BH procedure if there is no discreteness issue, because the $F_{i0}$'s are then Unif(0, 1). The BH procedure essentially compares ordered $p$-values with critical values defined by inverting the CDF of Unif(0, 1) and then evaluating at $\alpha k/m$, $k \in \mathbb{N}_m$. With the commonly assumed condition that $F_{i0}(t) \leq t$, for all $t \in [0, 1]$ and $i \in \mathbb{N}_m$, the BHH method also has $\bar{F}_0(t) \leq t$, for all $t \in [0, 1]$ and $i \in \mathbb{N}_m$. Thus the smaller the $\bar{F}_0$ values, the larger the critical values, which yields more rejections than the BH procedure.

### 3.1.3 The HSU and AHSU Procedure

Although the BHH procedure tends to be more powerful than the BH procedure for discrete tests Döhler et al. [12], point out that the BHH procedure is not correctly calibrated for a rigorous FDR control and provide concrete counterexample. Döhler et al. [12] propose a heterogeneous step-up (HSU) procedure, which corrects the BHH procedure. Döhler et al. [12] also introduce an adaptive version of HSU (AHSU) procedure, which further improves its performance.

To start with Döhler et al. [12], assume that $\{P_i, i \in I_0\}$ consists of independent random variables and is independent of $\{P_i, i \in I_1\}$, where $I_0$ and $I_1$ are the sets of true null hypotheses and true non-null hypotheses, respectively. Let $\mathscr{A}_i$ be the support of $P_i$. In our discrete context $\mathscr{A}_i$ is some finite set. Let $\mathscr{A} = \cup_{i=1}^{m} \mathscr{A}_i$ be the overall $p$-value support. The authors then define the corrected version of critical values

$$\lambda_m = \max \left\{ t \in \mathscr{A} : \frac{1}{m} \sum_{i=1}^{m} \frac{F_{i0}(t)}{1 - F_{i0}(t)} \leq \alpha \right\}, \tag{19}$$

$$\lambda_k = \max \left\{ t \in \mathscr{A} : t \leq \lambda_m, \frac{1}{m} \sum_{i=1}^{m} \frac{F_{i0}(t)}{1 - F_{i0}(\lambda_m)} \leq \alpha k/m \right\}, \quad k \in \mathbb{N}_{m-1}, \tag{20}$$

corresponding to the ones defined in BHH procedure as in (18). The correction term in the critical values (20) lies in the additional denominator $1 - F_{i0}(\lambda_m)$. Similar to the decision rule of the BHH procedure, the HSU procedure takes the threshold $p$-value $\lambda^* = \lambda_{k^*}$, where $k^* = \max\{k \in \mathbb{N}_m : p_{(k)} \le \lambda_k\}$, and reject all tests with $p$-values smaller than or equal to $\lambda^*$.

One consequence of the correction is that the HSU procedure can sometimes be more conservative than the BH procedure. To improve its performance, the authors introduce the adaptive version, the AHSU procedure. The critical value $\lambda_m$ is defined the same way as in (19), while for $k \in \mathbb{N}_{m-1}$, the critical values are defined as

$$\lambda_k = \max\left\{t \in \mathscr{A} : t \le \lambda_m, \left(\frac{F(t)}{1-F(\lambda_m)}\right)_{(1)} + \cdots + \left(\frac{F(t)}{1-F(\lambda_m)}\right)_{(m-k+1)} \le \alpha k\right\},$$

(21)

where each $\left(\frac{F(t)}{1-F(\lambda_m)}\right)_{(i)}$ denotes the $i$th largest element of the range of values $\left\{\frac{F(t)}{1-F(\lambda_m)}, i \in \mathbb{N}_m\right\}$. The decision rule is the same as that in the HSU procedure. Notice that the critical values of AHSU is clearly larger than or equal to those of its non-adaptive counterparts in HSU, which indicates that AHSU mostly yields more rejections.

Besides the HSU and AHSU procedures Döhler et al. [12], also analogously propose the heterogeneous step-down (HSD) procedure and its adaptive version AHSD. Readers may refer to the original reference for details. Another major contribution of [12] is that it provides the unified FDR bounds for general step-up and step-down FDR control procedures under the assumption of independence between $p$-values. The authors use the bounds to show that HSU, AHSU, HSD, AHSD procedures all control the FDR at level $\alpha$ in the independent setup.

## 3.2   Use Randomized Tests

### 3.2.1   Habiger's Method

To reduce the conservativeness caused by the discrete raw $p$-values Habiger [18], suggests utilizing the randomized $p$-values instead. Let us start with the single discrete test scenario. Tocher [51] shows that a single discrete test may not be able to achieve an exact significance level for that its raw $p$-value is not continuously distributed. He further suggests using an efficient randomized test strategy as a remedy. Specifically, consider a right-tailed test with discrete test statistic $T$, whose observed value is denoted by $t$. Let $P$ denote the raw $p$-value of this test, and let the observed value be $p = P(t) = \mathrm{Pro}_0(T \ge t)$ calculated under the null distribution of $T$. When considering the sampling variation, the $p$-value is then a random variable. Since $T$ has a discrete support, the support of $P$ is also discrete. Thus the test can not obtain certain significance $\alpha$ exactly. This difficulty can be solved by introducing randomized tests. Given observed test statistics $t$, the randomized $p$-value is defined as $\tilde{P}(t) = \mathrm{Pro}_0(T > t) + U \cdot \mathrm{Pro}_0(T = t)$ for $U \sim \mathrm{Unif}(0, 1)$ and independent with

$T$. The randomizer $U$ can be interpreted as a need for an extra Bernoulli experiment with the probability of rejection $(\alpha - \mathrm{Pr}_0(T > t))/\mathrm{Pr}_0(T = t)$ at $T = t$. Given $p$, let $p^- = \mathrm{Pr}(T > t)$ be the largest possible value less than $p$ in the support of the raw $p$-value [16], then

$$\tilde{P}|P = p \sim \mathrm{Unif}(p^-, p). \tag{22}$$

Marginally, when integrating out $P$, $\tilde{P}$ follows the $\mathrm{Unif}(0, 1)$ distribution under the null hypothesis, and the exact level-$\alpha$ test can be achieved.

To generalize the idea of randomized tests to LSMT, consider testing $m$ hypotheses with discrete test statistics, and let $P_1, \ldots, P_m$ be their corresponding raw $p$-values and $\tilde{P}_1, \ldots, \tilde{P}_m$ be their randomized $p$-values. Assuming that unconditionally, $\tilde{P}_i$, $i \in \mathbb{N}_m$, independently follow the two-component mixture model,

$$\tilde{P}_i|\Delta_i \sim (1 - \Delta_i) \cdot \mathrm{Unif}(0, 1) + \Delta_i \cdot F_1, \text{ with } F_1 = m^{-1} \sum_{i=1}^{m} F_{1i}, \tag{23}$$

where $\Delta_i$ is the indicator function that equals 0 if the $i$th null hypothesis is true (true null) and equals 1 if it is false (true non-null), and $F_{1i}$ is the alternative distribution of $\tilde{P}_i$. Under the mixture model (23), following Storey [43] similar as in (9), the pFDR corresponding to a threshold $\lambda$ on the randomized $p$-values is

$$\mathrm{pFDR}(\lambda) = \frac{\pi_0 \lambda}{\pi_0 F_0(\lambda) + \pi_1 F_1(\lambda)}. \tag{24}$$

Given a nominal FDR level $\alpha \in (0, 1)$ Habiger [18], defines

$$\lambda^*(\alpha) = \sup \left\{ \lambda : \mathrm{pFDR}_\infty(\lambda) \le \alpha \right\}, \tag{25}$$

and suggests rejecting the $i$th tests if $\tilde{P}_i \le \lambda^*(\alpha)$. We will refer this method as Habiger's method hereafter and denote $\lambda^*(\alpha)$ as $\lambda^*$ with no confusion. The conservativeness of the Habiger's method follows as a corollary of Theorem 3 in [45].

### 3.2.2    MCF-Based Procedure

Although enjoying nice theoretical properties, Habiger's method is likely to be undesirable in practice due to its instability in terms of the variance of its FDP and true discovery proportion [7, 9], caused by the usage of randomized tests. In order to resolve this Dai et al. [11], consider making decisions on the expected results instead of the random experiment, and aligning the proportion of rejections according to the expected proportion from Habiger's method to keep its advantage.

First let us consider the *marginal critical function* (MCF) of a single randomized test [27] defined as follows.

**Definition 1** Suppose that $p$ is the observed $p$-value from a discrete test and $p^-$ is the largest possible value less than $p$ in the support of $p$-value as before. If no such $p^-$ exists, let it be 0. For a given threshold $\lambda \in (0, 1)$, the MCF of a randomized test is defined as

$$
r(p, \lambda) = \begin{cases} 1, & \text{if } p < \lambda \\[2mm] \dfrac{\lambda - p^-}{p - p^-}, & \text{if } p^- < \lambda \leq p, \\[2mm] 0, & \text{if } \lambda \leq p^-. \end{cases}
$$

Following the two-component model (23), the conditional distribution of $\tilde{P}$ in (22) leads to $r(p_i, \lambda^*) = \Pr(\tilde{P}_i < \lambda^* | p_i) = \mathbb{E}(X_i), i \in \mathbb{N}_m$, where $X_i = \mathbb{1}\{\tilde{P}_i \leq \lambda^* | p_i\}$. For simplicity, the authors use $r_i$ to refer to $r(p_i, \lambda^*)$ conditional on $p_i$. Habiger's method rejects the $i$th test if $X_i = 1$, and the MCF $r_i$ represents the conditional probability being rejected by Habiger's method. Therefore, the tests with larger MCF values are more likely to be true non-null and should be rejected. To avoid the random decisions in Habiger's method caused by the random variable $X_i$'s, the authors make decisions based on the expected value of each $X_i$, $\mathbb{E}(X_i | p_i) = r_i$, which is fixed given the observed $p_i$.

To ensure the FDR is controlled exactly under the nominal level Dai et al. [11], make the same proportion of rejections as in Habiger's method. Specifically, following the two-component model (23), given threshold $\lambda^*$ corresponding to the nominal level $\alpha$, the expected proportion of rejections by Habiger's method is

$$
\mu^* = \frac{1}{m} \sum_{i=1}^{m} \Pr(\tilde{P}_i < \lambda^*) = \pi_0 \lambda^* + \pi_1 F_1(\lambda^*). \tag{26}
$$

The decision rule is to reject the $i$-th test if $r_i > Q(1 - \mu^*)$, where $Q(1 - \mu^*)$ is the $(1 - \mu^*)$-th quantile of the pooled MCF's $\{r_1, \ldots, r_m\}$.

## 3.3 Use a Less Upwardly Biased Estimator of $\pi_0$

The third approach aims at proposing a less conservative estimator of $\pi_0$. Let us consider Storey's $\pi_0$ estimator in (12). Its expected bias $\mathbb{E}(\hat{\pi}_0^S - \pi_0)$ is the sum of $\frac{1}{m(1-c)}$ and

$$
b_0 = \frac{1}{m(1-c)} \sum_{i \in I_0} [c - F_{0i}(c)], \tag{27}
$$

$$
b_1 = \frac{1}{m(1-c)} \sum_{i \in I_1} [1 - F_{1i}(c)], \tag{28}
$$

where $I_0$ is the set of true null hypotheses and $I_1$ is the set of true non-nulls; $F_{0i}$ and $F_{i1}$ are the CDFs of the $p$-value $P_i$ when the $i$th test is a true null and true non-null, respectively. The bias $b_0$ is associated with null $p$-values, and is zero when the null $p$-values are continuous. However, $b_0$ is usually positive when $p$-values have discrete distributions with different supports. On the other hand, the bias associated with the alternative $p$-values, $b_1$, is always positive regardless of whether the $p$-value is continuously distributed or not [9]. Due to positive of $b_0$ and $b_1$, Storey's estimator of $\pi_0$ tends to be upwardly biased, which leads the associated FDR control procedure conservative. Thus reducing the bias in estimating $\pi_0$ in general helps to improve the detection power. While $b_1$ usually cannot be reduced unless more information is available, most of the time $b_0$ could be reduced by choosing the tuning parameter $c$ carefully when the $p$-values have discrete distributions.

### 3.3.1 The aBH and aBHH Procedure

As explained at the end of Sect. 2.2, the BH procedure can be viewed as a special case of the $q$-value method using an estimate of $\hat{\pi}_0 = 1$. But this overestimate of $\pi_0$ also results in conservativeness in the BH procedure.

In testing multiple discrete hypotheses Chen et al. [9], proposed using a refined estimator of $\pi_0$ that accommodates the discreteness in the support of $p$-values. Combining this improved estimator with the BH and BHH method, they proposed two adaptive FDR control procedures called the aBH and aBHH methods, respectively.

Let $F_i$ denote the CDF of the $p$-value $P_i$ of the $i$th test. The authors make two basic assumptions:

- Each $F_i$ has a non-empty support $S_i = \{t \in \mathbb{R} : F_i(t) - F_i(t^-) > 0\}$;
- Under null, the $p$-value $P_i$ stochastically dominates Unif$(0, 1)$, i.e. $F_{i0}(t) \leq t$ for all $t \in [0, 1]$.

Let $t_i = \inf\{t : t \in S_i\}$ for each $i \in \mathbb{N}_m$, and let $\gamma = \max\{t_i : i \in \mathbb{N}_m\}$. Pick a sequence of $n$ increasing, equally spaced "guiding values" $\{\tau_j\}_{j=1}^n$ such that $\tau_0 \leq \tau_1 \leq \ldots \leq \tau_n < 1$, for which $\tau_0 = \max\{t_i : t_i < 1\}$ if $\gamma = 1$, or $\tau_0 = \gamma$ if $\gamma < 1$. Further consider the set of indices $C = \{i \in \mathbb{N}_m : t_i = 1\}$, and for each $i \in \mathbb{N}_m \setminus C$ and $j \in \mathbb{N}_n$, set $\lambda_{ij} = \sup\{\lambda \in S_i : \lambda \leq \tau_j\}$. Chen et al. [9] define a "trial estimator" for each $j \in \mathbb{N}_n$,

$$\beta(\tau_j) = \frac{1}{(1 - \tau_j)m} + \frac{1}{m} \sum_{i \in \mathbb{N}_m \setminus C} \frac{\mathbb{1}\{P_i > \lambda_{ij}\}}{1 - \lambda_{ij}} + \frac{1}{m}|C|, \tag{29}$$

where $|C|$ is the cardinality of the set $C$. After truncating $\beta(\tau_j)$ at 1 when it is greater than 1, it then delivers the estimator of $\pi_0$ as

$$\hat{\pi}_0^G = \frac{1}{n} \sum_{j=1}^n \beta(\tau_j). \tag{30}$$

It is clear that for each $j \in \mathbb{N}_n$, the expected bias for the trial estimator $\beta(\tau_j)$ is

$$\delta_j = \mathbb{E}(\beta(\tau_j) - \pi_0) = \frac{1}{(1-\tau_j)m} + \frac{1}{m} \sum_{i \in I_1 \setminus C} \frac{1 - F_{1i}(\lambda_{ij})}{1 - \lambda_{ij}}, \tag{31}$$

and therefore the expected bias of $\pi_0^G$ is $\delta = \frac{1}{n}\sum_{j=1}^n \delta_j$. The authors prove that for each $j \in \mathbb{N}_n$, $\delta_j \geq 0$. Therefore $\delta \geq 0$ and $\hat{\pi}_0^G$ is upwardly biased to $\pi_0$. It is undetermined which estimator, $\hat{\pi}_0^S$ or $\hat{\pi}_0^G$, is less conservative without information on the cdf's $F_i$ of the alternative $p$-values.

But Chen et al. [9] prove that the induced BH procedure at the new nominal FDR level $\alpha/\hat{\pi}_0^G$ is conservative. An induced BHH procedure is also proposed by applying the BHH procedure in Sect. 3.1.2 at the FDR level $\alpha/\hat{\pi}_0^G$ analogously. The authors show by simulation studies that the induced BHH procedure yields good results, but provide no theoretical guarantee for conservativeness. We will refer to the BH procedure and BHH procedure induced by $\hat{\pi}_0^G$ as the aBH (adaptive BH) procedure and aBHH (adaptive BHH) procedure hereafter.

Based on the estimator (30) of $\pi_0$ Chen et al. [7], further propose a weighted FDR procedure with a grouping algorithm. Chen et al. [7] first define a metric

$$d(F, G) = \eta(S_F \Delta S_G) + \|F - G\|_\infty, \tag{32}$$

where $F$ and $G$ are two cdfs with finitely many discontinuities, with $S_F$ and $S_G$ being their support, respectively; $\eta$ is the counting measure and $\Delta$ is the symmetric difference operator between two sets; $\|\cdot\|_\infty$ is the supremum norm for functions. The procedure first group the null cdfs $\{F_{i0}\}_{i=1}^m$ using the metric $d$ into $K$ groups $G_k, k = 1, \ldots, K$. Then for each $k$, it estimates the null proportion of $G_k$, $\pi_{k0}$, as $\hat{\pi}_{k0}^G$ using (30), and therefore estimates the overall null proportion $\pi_0$ as

$$\hat{\pi}_0^* = m^{-1} \sum_{k=1}^K \hat{\pi}_{k0}|G_k|, \tag{33}$$

where $|A|$ is the cardinality of set $A$. Next, it sets the weight for group $G_k$ as

$$w_k = \hat{\pi}_{k0}(1 - \hat{\pi}_{k0})^{-1}\mathbb{1}\{\hat{\pi}_{k0} \neq 1\} + \infty \cdot \mathbb{1}\{\hat{\pi}_{k0} = 1\}, \tag{34}$$

and weighs the $p$-value $p_i$, $i \in G_k$ into $\tilde{p}_i = w_k p_i$. And finally, for a given FDR level $\alpha$, it rejects the $i$th null hypothesis whenever $\tilde{p}_i \leq t_\alpha$, where the rejection threshold is

$$t_\alpha = \mathbb{1}\{\hat{\pi}_0^* < 1\} \sup\left\{t \geq 0 : \widetilde{\mathrm{FDR}}(t) \leq \alpha\right\} \tag{35}$$

and

$$\widetilde{\text{FDR}}(t) = \min\left\{1, \frac{(1 - \hat{\pi}_0^*)t}{m^{-1}\max\{R(t), 1\}}\right\}, \tag{36}$$

and $R(t) = \sum_{i=1}^{m} \mathbb{1}\{\tilde{p}_i < t\}$. The intuition behind the grouping algorithm is that similar $p$-value distributions could represent statistical evidence of similar strength against the null hypothesis, as explained in [7]. However, this algorithm is time consuming when a large number of tests are tested for that it needs to evaluate pairwise distances for all the tests. We will refer this procedure as the grouping algorithm hereafter.

### 3.3.2 Liang's Discrete Right-Boundary Procedure

Liang [32] considers a special case where all $p$-values across $m$ discrete tests share the identical discrete support $S = \{t_1, \ldots, t_s, t_{s+1}\}$, with $0 < t_1 < \cdots < t_s < t_{s+1} \equiv 1$, and the true null distributions satisfy that $F_{0i}(t) = t$ only at $t \in S$. Such a scenario often arises when simultaneously testing many mean differences between two groups using permutation tests. Without loss of generality, suppose large values of test statistics provide evidence against the null hypothesis, then the $p$-value is $p = \frac{1}{B}\sum_{i=1}^{B}\mathbb{1}\{T^i \geq T^*\}$, where $B$ is the number of all possible permutations of group labels, $T^i$ is the test statistic computed for the $i$th permutation, and $T^*$ is the observed test statistic. The permutation $p$-values computed in this way clearly satisfy the assumption and the support is thus $S = \{\frac{1}{B}, \frac{2}{B}, \ldots, \frac{B-1}{B}, 1\}$.

Liang's method is based on the framework of Storey et al. [45], but uses a different estimator of $\pi_0$. Storey et al. [45] estimate $\pi_0$ using a constant value for the tuning parameter $c$ (0.5 by default) in (12), whereas Liang [32] proposes an adaptive procedure that chooses $c$ according to the distribution of the $p$-values. Let $\mathscr{C} = \{c_1, \ldots, c_n\}$ be a candidate set for $c$ of size $n$ such that $\mathscr{C}$ is an ordered positive subset of $\mathscr{L} = \{t_0 = 0, t_1, \ldots, t_s\}$. Then the value of $c$ is chosen as $c_I$ where $I = \min\{n, \min\{1 \leq i \leq n - 1 : \hat{\pi}_0(c_i) \geq \hat{\pi}_0(c_{i-1})\}\}$ with $\hat{\pi}_0^L(c_i) = \frac{1 + \#\{p > c_i\}}{m(1 - c_i)}$ following Storey's $\pi_0$ estimator except the value of tuning parameter $c_i$.

We can consider this procedure from another perspective. The set $\mathscr{C}$ divides the interval $(0, 1]$ into $n + 1$ bins such that the $i$th bin is $(c_{i-1}, c_i]$ for $i \in \mathbb{N}_{n+1}$. Let $b_i = \#\{p : p \in (c_{i-1}, c_i]\}$ be the number of $p$-values in the $i$th bin, i.e. the $i$th bin count. If the spacings between $c_i$'s are equal, then the procedure is equivalent to selecting the right boundary of the first bin whose bin count is no larger than the average of the bin counts to its right. Therefore, we would refer this procedure as Liang's discrete right-boundary procedure, or Liang's method for short.

The intuition behind Liang's method is to expand the range of $p$-values used to estimate $\pi_0$ as large as possible. For continuous tests, Storey's method estimates the null proportion $\pi_0$ relying on the intuition that almost all large $p$-values are from true nulls. Using tuning parameter $c = 0.5$, Storey's method essentially assumes $p$-values from the right half (those larger than 0.5) are all from true nulls. Then based on the two-component model, the null proportion $\pi_0$, as the mixing proportion of the

$U(0, 1)$ component, can be easily estimated from the empirical distribution of the large $p$-values. For the discrete testing scenario considered in this section, the null distributions of $p$-values are no longer all $U(0, 1)$ but different discrete distributions on the same support $S$. Although the same idea can be applied, it requires individual adjustment on $c_i$ for each test to precisely estimate $\pi_0$.

Liang's method involves a candidate set $\mathscr{C}$, which needs to be specified beforehand. Liang [32] recommends to start from 11 equally-spaced bins with dividers being $\{0.05, 0.1, \dots, 0.45, 0.5\}$, and then let $\mathscr{C}$ be the set of unique nonzero elements in $\mathscr{L}$ that are closest to each of the dividers. In this setup, the last divider only goes up to 0.5 to ensure that roughly at least half of the true null $p$-values are utilized to estimate $\pi_0$.

## 3.4 Software Availability

The BH procedure, BHH method, aBH method, aBHH method, grouping algorithm and Habiger's method are implemented in the package **fdrDiscreteNull** [8], while the HSU and AHSU methods are implemented in the package **DiscreteFDR** [13]. For the purpose of boosting computational speed as well as avoiding rounding errors, we extract the core code from the packages, slightly modify and regroup together. The rest of the aforementioned methods are also implemented. All source code is put in a public GitHub repository with demos. Please see https://github.com/ghao89/gary_research_projects for details.

## 4   Simulation Study

In this section, we compare the performance of the aforementioned methods through simulation under different scenarios.[1] Let $j = 1, 2$ denote the two groups under comparison. Consider testing $m = 10{,}000$ hypotheses between the two groups. Each hypothesis $i$ is to discern if the success probabilities $q_{ji}$ between two groups are the same. Such success probabilities resemble the methylation levels in real DMR detection problems. We set the null proportion at three different levels ($\pi_0 = 0.3, 0.6$ or $0.9$), and evaluate the performance of each method under different signal (true non-null) abundance. Let $L$ denote the number of samples in each group. We set $L$ to be either 2 or 5, which reflects the fact that the number of replicates is often limited in real DMR detection problems. We conduct a FET for each test $i$. The

---

[1] We only include the aBHH method out of the aBH and the aBHH methods, and the AHSU method out of the HSU and the AHSU methods, as those two have been shown yielding better performance than their non-adaptive counterparts in their original references. Besides, due to high computational cost, we do not include the grouping algorithm in our simulation study.

**Table 3** Contingency table
for a FET

|                        | $C$      | $N - C$              | Total    |
| ---------------------- | -------- | -------------------- | -------- |
| Binomial $(n_{1i}, q_{1i})$ | $c_{1i}$ | $n_{1i} - c_{1i}$ | $n_{1i}$ |
| Binomial $(n_{2i}, q_{2i})$ | $c_{2i}$ | $n_{2i} - c_{2i}$ | $n_{2i}$ |

FET is built on a $2 \times 2$ contingency table, which consists of the counts $(C, N - C)$ from two Binomial distributions, Binomial$(n_{1i}, q_{1i})$ and Binomial$(n_{2i}, q_{2i})$. Table 3 shows the contingency table.

For simplicity, we condense the counts within each group for each test.[2] The data are generated as follows:

1. Randomly choose $\pi_0 \cdot m$ tests (true nulls), and for each test $i$ from this set, generate the common success probability $q_{1i} = q_{2i}$ from Unif$(0, 1)$.
2. For each test $i$ from the other $(1 - \pi_0) \cdot m$ tests, generate $q_{1i} = 0.5\mu_i$, $q_{2i} = q_{1i} + \delta_i$, where $\mu_i \sim$ Unif$(0, 1)$ and $\delta_i \sim$ Unif$(0.2, 0.5)$.
3. For each replicate $l \in \mathbb{N}_L$ of each test $i \in \mathbb{N}_m$ in each group $j = 1, 2$, generate the number of trials $n_{jil} \sim$ Poisson$(20)$. Then draw the count $c_{jil}$ from Binomial$(n_{jil}, q_{ji})$.
4. For each test $i$, condense the counts as $c_{ji} = \sum_{l=1}^{L} c_{jil}$ and $n_{ji} = \sum_{l=1}^{L} n_{jil}$, $j = 1, 2$ to prepare the contingency table.

With the data generated, we can then apply FET to test $H_{0i} : q_{1i} = q_{2i}$ v.s. $H_{1i} : q_{1i} \neq q_{2i}$, for each $i \in \mathbb{N}_m$, and control the FDR using each method discussed in Sect. 3, with the exception being Liang's method. Liang's method assumes that all $m$ tests share the identical discrete support. To meet its assumption, we use a permutation test instead, as suggested in [32], and define a test statistic $T = \frac{1}{L} \left| \sum_{l=1}^{L} \frac{c_{1il}}{n_{1il}} - \sum_{l=1}^{L} \frac{c_{2il}}{n_{2il}} \right|$. The $p$-values are calculated based on the permutation tests and Liang's method can thus be applied to deliver the estimator $\hat{\pi}_0^L$ of $\pi_0$. The rejections are made using Storey's method [45] by substituting $\hat{\pi}_0^S$ with $\hat{\pi}_0^L$. Note that the performance of Liang's method depends on which test statistic $T$ is used. We have followed the example in the original reference [32] by obtaining $T$ as the absolute group mean difference.

For each combination of $\pi_0$ and $L$, we run 500 Monte Carlo simulations to investigate the average performance of each method. To make sure that the repetitions are identical and independent, for each combination of $\pi_0$ and $L$, across 500 repetitions, we fix the indices of true nulls and true non-nulls, the success probabilities $q_{ji}$, and the number of trials $n_{jil}$, for all $i, j, l$. The realized FDRs and statistical power are evaluated using the simulation truth at different nominal FDR level $\alpha$, where the statistical power is defined as the ratio between the number

---

[2] When multiple samples are available in each group, other approaches like those based on $t$-test or the beta-binomial model may also be used, as discussed in Sect. 3. Our focus is not to address how to model the replicates, but using the FET to demonstrate the performance of various methods in the context of multiple testing of discrete hypotheses.

of correct rejections and the number of true non-null hypotheses. Those for the BH procedure and Storey's $q$-value method are plotted in Figs. 1 and 2, while those for the remaining methods are plotted in Figs. 3 and 4. For each figure, the left column plots the cases where $L = 2$, while the right column plots those where $L = 5$; The first, second and third row correspond to the cases where the null proportion $\pi_0 = 0.3, 0.6$ and $0.9$, respectively.

From the figures, we can see that the two conventional methods control the FDR over-conservatively comparing to other methods. Such over-conservativeness leads to a loss of statistical power, especially when there are lack of replicates and the null proportion is high. Yet it is often what the real situations are. The BH procedure performs better as the null proportion increases, but never exceeds that of the Storey's method, since the BH procedure actually controls the FDR at level $\pi_0\alpha$ [4]. The two methods perform equally when $\pi_0 = 0.9$, which illustrates empirically that the BH procedure is equivalent to a special case of the Storey's method, as we point out at the end of Sect. 2.2.

For the realized FDR, according to Fig. 3, all methods control it under the nominal level $\alpha$. Gilbert's method controls the FDR at $\pi_0\alpha$, but it performs better than the BH procedure, when compared to Fig. 1.[3] Liang's method is not sensitive to the null proportion $\pi_0$, and yields better performance when $L = 5$, as the $p$-values calculated based on permutation lead to a more accurate estimation of $\pi_0$ with more replicates. Overall, Habiger's method controls the FDR closest to the nominal level, closely followed by the aBHH method and MCF method.

As for the statistical power, according to Fig. 4, we can see that the aBHH method always performs the best. When the null proportion is not high, the MCF method and Habiger's method perform nearly as good as the aBHH method. When the null proportion is high, the difference among those methods are marginal, except for Liang's method when $L = 2$. Again this is because that the permutation with only 2 replicates in each group cannot accurately estimate $\pi_0$.

In practice, due to high cost of methylation sequencing experiments, there are either no or just a small number, e.g. 2 or 3, of biological replicates available. The simulation results show that, for every method, the statistical power under more replicates is clearly higher than that under fewer replicates. However, it is worth noting that we have simply aggregated the read counts across different replicates and ignored the biological variations. For practical data, a more thorough treatment is needed to model the biological variation. We consider the replicates in the simulation study, mainly to include Liang's method, which requires replicates to perform the permutation test.

---

[3] As mentioned in Sect. 3.1.1 Gilbert [17], recognized this issue and proposed a grid search method. However, the grid search method is computationally too costly to be included in the simulation study.

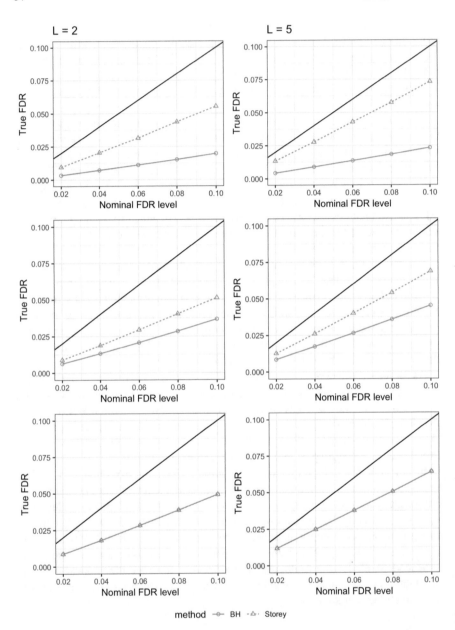

**Fig. 1** The realized FDR for the BH procedure and Storey's $q$-value method when $m = 10,000$. The first column plots the results for the cases where $L = 2$, while the second column for $L = 5$. The first, second and third row correspond to the cases where $\pi_0 = 0.3$, 0.6 and 0.9, respectively. The black solid line plots the nominal FDR as reference

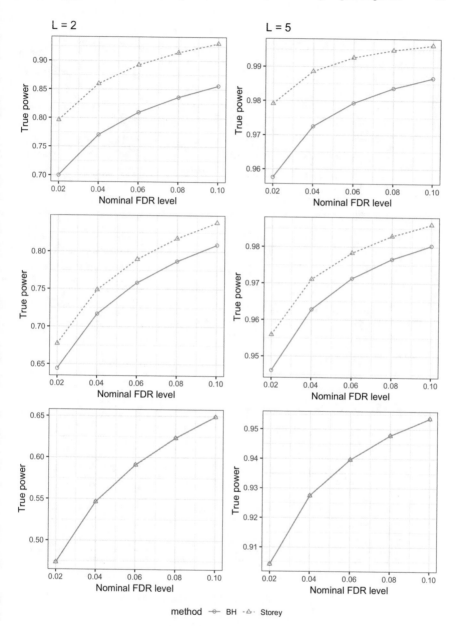

**Fig. 2** The statistical power for the BH method and Storey's $q$-value method when $m = 10,000$. The first column plots the results for the cases where $L = 2$, while the second column for $L = 5$. The first, second and third row correspond to the cases where $\pi_0 = 0.3, 0.6$ and $0.9$, respectively

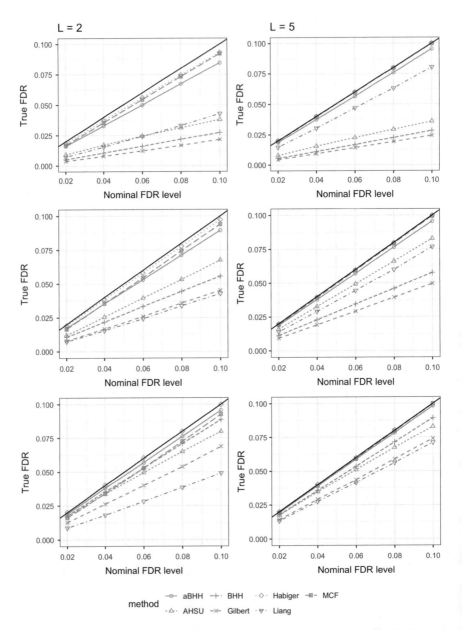

**Fig. 3** Comparisons for the resulted FDR across different methods when $m = 10,000$. The first column plots the results for the cases where $L = 2$, while the second column for $L = 5$. The first, second and third row correspond to the cases where $\pi_0 = 0.3, 0.6$ and $0.9$, respectively. The black solid line plots the nominal FDR as reference

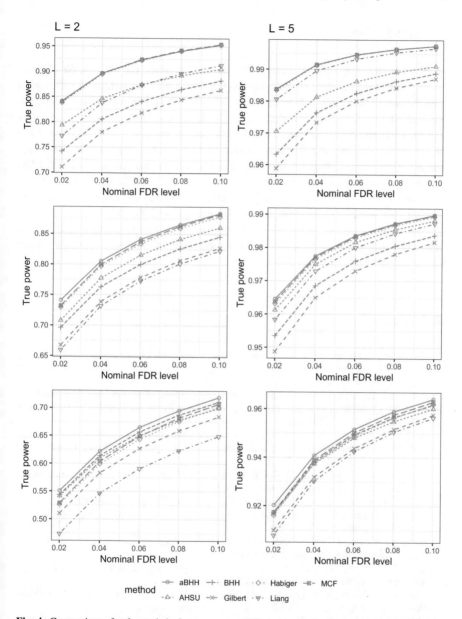

**Fig. 4** Comparisons for the statistical power across different methods when $m = 10,000$. The first column plots the results for the cases where $L = 2$, while the second column for $L = 5$. The first, second and third row correspond to the cases where $\pi_0 = 0.3$, 0.6 and 0.9, respectively

# 5 Conclusion

In this chapter, we study various FDR control methods for large-scale discrete multiple testing problems often appearing in the context of detecting differential methylation in sequencing data. Simulation studies show the necessity of adjusting for discreteness. Conventional procedures like the BH method and Storey's $q$-value method often result in over-conservative FDR control and thus lead to underpowered performance. Among our discussed methods that address the discreteness issue, the MCF method, Habiger's method, and the aBHH method control the FDR closest to the nominal level and yield the highest detection power in most cases. However, Habiger's method is practically undesirable due to its random decisions. Overall, we would recommend the aBHH method and the MCF method based on our comparison, whereas the MCF method's asymptotic control of the FDR is theoretically established while that for the aBHH method still requires further theoretical contributions.

# References

1. Akalin, A., Kormaksson, M., Li, S., Garrett-Bakelman, F. E., Figueroa, M. E., Melnick, A., et al. (2012). methylKit: A comprehensive R package for the analysis of genome-wide DNA methylation profiles. *Genome Biology, 13*(10), R87.
2. Benjamini, Y., & Hochberg, Y. (1995). Controlling the false discovery rate: A practical and powerful approach to multiple testing. *Journal of the Royal Statistical Society. Series B (Methodological), 57*, 289–300.
3. Benjamini, Y., & Liu, W. (1999). A step-down multiple hypotheses testing procedure that controls the false discovery rate under independence. *Journal of Statistical Planning and Inference, 82*, 163–170.
4. Benjamini, Y., & Yekutieli, D. (2001). The control of the false discovery rate in multiple testing under dependency. *Annals of Statistics, 29*, 1165–1188.
5. Bock, C., Tomazou, E. M., Brinkman, A. B., Müller, F., Simmer, F., Gu, H., Jäger, N., et al. (2010). Quantitative comparison of genome-wide DNA methylation mapping technologies. *Nature Biotechnology, 28*(10), 1106–1114.
6. Boyes, J., & Bird, A. (1991). DNA methylation inhibits transcription indirectly via a methyl-CpG binding protein. *Cell, 64*(6), 1123–1134.
7. Chen, X., & Doerge, R. W. (2015). A weighted FDR procedure under discrete and heterogeneous null distributions. Preprint. arXiv:1502.00973.
8. Chen, X., & Doerge, R. W. (2018). *fdrDiscreteNull: False Discovery Rate Procedures Under Discrete and Heterogeneous Null Distributions*. R package version 1.3.
9. Chen, X., Doerge, R. W., & Heyse, J. F. (2018). Multiple testing with discrete data: Proportion of true null hypotheses and two adaptive FDR procedures. *Biometrical Journal, 60*(4), 761–779.
10. Cokus, S. J., Feng, S., Zhang, X., Chen, Z., Merriman, B., Haudenschild, C. D., et al. (2008). Shotgun bisulphite sequencing of the Arabidopsis genome reveals DNA methylation patterning. *Nature, 452*, 215–219.
11. Dai, X., Lin, N., Li, D., & Wang, T. (2019). A non-randomized procedure for large-scale heterogeneous multiple discrete testing based on randomized tests. *Biometrics, 75*(2), 638–649.

12. Döhler, S., Durand, G., & Roquain, E. (2018). New FDR bounds for discrete and heterogeneous tests. *Electronic Journal of Statistics, 12*(1), 1867–1900.
13. Durand, G., & Junge, F. (2019). *DiscreteFDR: Multiple Testing Procedures with Adaptation for Discrete Tests*. R package version 1.2.
14. Feng, H., Conneely, K. N., & Wu, H. (2014). A Bayesian hierarchical model to detect differentially methylated loci from single nucleotide resolution sequencing data. *Nucleic Acids Research, 42*(8), e69.
15. Genovese, C., & Wasserman, L. (2002). Operating characteristics and extensions of the false discovery rate procedure. *Journal of the Royal Statistical Society: Series B (Statistical Methodology), 64*(3), 499–517.
16. Geyer, C. J., & Meeden, G. D. (2005). Fuzzy and randomized confidence intervals and *p*-values. *Statistical Science, 20*, 358–366.
17. Gilbert, P. B. (2005). A modified false discovery rate multiple-comparisons procedure for discrete data, applied to human immunodeficiency virus genetics. *Journal of the Royal Statistical Society: Series C (Applied Statistics), 54*(1), 143–158.
18. Habiger, J. D. (2015). Multiple test functions and adjusted *p*-values for test statistics with discrete distributions. *Journal of Statistical Planning and Inference, 167*, 1–13.
19. Habiger, J. D., & Pena, E. A. (2011). Randomised *P*-values and nonparametric procedures in multiple testing. *Journal of Nonparametric Statistics, 23*(3), 583–604.
20. Hansen, K. D., Langmead, B., & Irizarry, R. A. (2012). BSmooth: From whole genome bisulfite sequencing reads to differentially methylated regions. *Genome Biology, 13*(10), R83.
21. Harris, R. A., Wang, T., Coarfa, C., Nagarajan, R. P., Hong, C., Downey, S. L., et al. (2010). Comparison of sequencing-based methods to profile DNA methylation and identification of monoallelic epigenetic modifications. *Nature Biotechnology, 28*(10), 1097–1105.
22. Heyse, J. F. (2011). A false discovery rate procedure for categorical data. In *Recent advances in biostatistics: False discovery rates, survival analysis, and related topics* (pp. 43–58). Singapore: World Scientific.
23. Jin, B., Li, Y., & Robertson, K. D. (2011). DNA methylation: Superior or subordinate in the epigenetic hierarchy? *Genes & Cancer, 2*(6), 607–617.
24. Jones, P. A. (2012). Functions of DNA methylation: Islands, start sites, gene bodies and beyond. *Nature Reviews Genetics, 13*(7), 484–492.
25. Jühling, F., Kretzmer, H., Bernhart, S. H., Otto, C., Stadler, P. F., & Hoffmann, S. (2016). Metilene: Fast and sensitive calling of differentially methylated regions from bisulfite sequencing data. *Genome Research, 26*(2), 256–262.
26. Khulan, B., Thompson, R. F., Ye, K., Fazzari, M. J., Suzuki, M., Stasiek, E., et al. (2006). Comparative isoschizomer profiling of cytosine methylation: The HELP assay. *Genome Research, 16*(8), 1046–1055.
27. Kulinskaya, E., & Lewin, A. (2009). On fuzzy familywise error rate and false discovery rate procedures for discrete distributions. *Biometrika, 96*(1), 201–211.
28. Laird, P. W. (2010). Principles and challenges of genome-wide DNA methylation analysis. *Nature Reviews Genetics, 11*(3), 191–203.
29. Laurent, L., Wong, E., Li, G., Huynh, T., Tsirigos, A., Ong, C. T., et al. (2010). Dynamic changes in the human methylome during differentiation. *Genome Research, 20*, 320–331.
30. Lehmann, E. L., & Romano, J. P. (2006). *Testing statistical hypotheses*. Berlin: Springer.
31. Levenson, J. M., & Sweatt, J. D. (2005). Epigenetic mechanisms in memory formation. *Nature Reviews Neuroscience, 6*(2), 108–118.
32. Liang, K. (2016). False discovery rate estimation for large-scale homogeneous discrete *p*-values. *Biometrics, 72*(2), 639–648.
33. Liao, J., Lin, Y., Selvanayagam, Z. E., & Shih, W. J. (2004). A mixture model for estimating the local false discovery rate in DNA microarray analysis. *Bioinformatics, 20*(16), 2694–2701.
34. Lister, R., Pelizzola, M., Dowen, R. H., Hawkins, R. D., Hon, G., Tonti-Filippini, J., et al. (2009). Human DNA methylomes at base resolution show widespread epigenomic differences. *Nature, 462*, 315–322.

35. Maunakea, A. K., Nagarajan, R. P., Bilenky, M., Ballinger, T. J., D'souza, C., Fouse, S. D., et al. (2010). Conserved role of intragenic DNA methylation in regulating alternative promoters. *Nature, 466*(7303), 253–257.
36. Meissner, A., Mikkelsen, T. S., Gu, H., Wernig, M., Hanna, J., Sivachenko, A., et al. (2008). Genome-scale DNA methylation maps of pluripotent and differentiated cells. *Nature, 454*(7205), 766–770.
37. Park, Y., Figueroa, M. E., Rozek, L. S., & Sartor, M. A. (2014). MethylSig: A whole genome DNA methylation analysis pipeline. *Bioinformatics, 30*(17), 2414–2422.
38. Pounds, S., & Cheng, C. (2006). Robust estimation of the false discovery rate. *Bioinformatics, 22*(16), 1979–1987.
39. Rakyan, V. K., Down, T. A., Balding, D. J., & Beck, S. (2011). Epigenome-wide association studies for common human diseases. *Nature Reviews Genetics, 12*(8), 529–541.
40. Robinson, M. D., Kahraman, A., Law, C. W., Lindsay, H., Nowicka, M., Weber, L. M., & Zhou, X. (2014). Statistical methods for detecting differentially methylated loci and regions. *Frontiers in Genetics, 5*, 324.
41. Sarkar, S. K. (2002). Some results on false discovery rate in stepwise multiple testing procedures. *Annals of Statistics, 30*, 239–257.
42. Shafi, A., Mitrea, C., Nguyen, T., & Draghici, S. (2017). A survey of the approaches for identifying differential methylation using bisulfite sequencing data. *Briefings in Bioinformatics, 19*, 737–753.
43. Storey, J. D. (2002). A direct approach to false discovery rates. *Journal of the Royal Statistical Society: Series B (Statistical Methodology), 64*(3), 479–498.
44. Storey, J. D. (2003). The positive false discovery rate: A Bayesian interpretation and the $q$-value. *The Annals of Statistics, 31*, 2013–2035.
45. Storey, J. D., Taylor, J. E., & Siegmund, D. (2004). Strong control, conservative point estimation and simultaneous conservative consistency of false discovery rates: A unified approach. *Journal of the Royal Statistical Society: Series B (Statistical Methodology), 66*(1), 187–205.
46. Sun, S., & Yu, X. (2016). HMM-Fisher: Identifying differential methylation using a hidden Markov model and Fisher's exact test. *Statistical Applications in Genetics and Molecular Biology, 15*(1), 55–67.
47. Sun, W., & Cai, T. T. (2007). Oracle and adaptive compound decision rules for false discovery rate control. *Journal of the American Statistical Association, 102*(479), 901–912.
48. Suzuki, M. M., & Bird, A. (2008). DNA methylation landscapes: Provocative insights from epigenomics. *Nature Reviews Genetics, 9*(6), 465–476.
49. Tang, Y., Ghosal, S., & Roy, A. (2007). Nonparametric Bayesian estimation of positive false discovery rates. *Biometrics, 63*(4), 1126–1134.
50. Tarone, R. (1990). A modified Bonferroni method for discrete data. *Biometrics, 46*, 515–522.
51. Tocher, K. (1950). Extension of the Neyman-Pearson theory of tests to discontinuous variates. *Biometrika, 37*, 130–144.
52. Watt, F., & Molloy, P. L. (1988). Cytosine methylation prevents binding to DNA of a HeLa cell transcription factor required for optimal expression of the adenovirus major late promoter. *Genes and Development, 2*(9), 1136–1143.
53. Weber, M., Davies, J. J., Wittig, D., Oakeley, E. J., Haase, M., Lam, W. L., et al. (2005). Chromosome-wide and promoter-specific analyses identify sites of differential DNA methylation in normal and transformed human cells. *Nature Genetics, 37*(8), 853–862.
54. Westfall, P. H., & Wolfinger, R. D. (1997). Multiple tests with discrete distributions. *The American Statistician, 51*(1), 3–8.
55. Wu, H., Xu, T., Feng, H., Chen, L., Li, B., Yao, B., et al. (2015). Detection of differentially methylated regions from whole-genome bisulfite sequencing data without replicates. *Nucleic Acids Research, 43*(21), e141.
56. Yu, X., & Sun, S. (2016). HMM-DM: Identifying differentially methylated regions using a hidden Markov model. *Statistical Applications in Genetics and Molecular Biology, 15*(1), 69–81.

57. Zhang, Y., Liu, H., Lv, J., Xiao, X., Zhu, J., Liu, X., et al. (2011). QDMR: A quantitative method for identification of differentially methylated regions by entropy. *Nucleic Acids Research, 39*(9), e58.
58. Ziller, M. J., Hansen, K. D., Meissner, A., & Aryee, M. J. (2014). Coverage recommendations for methylation analysis by whole-genome bisulfite sequencing. *Nature Methods, 12*(3), 230–232.

# Part II
# Deep Learning, Precision Medicine and Applications

# Prediction of Functional Markers of Mass Cytometry Data via Deep Learning

**Claudia Solís-Lemus, Xin Ma, Maxwell Hostetter II, Suprateek Kundu, Peng Qiu, and Daniel Pimentel-Alarcón**

**Abstract** Recently, there has been an increasing interest in the analysis of flow cytometry data, which involves measurements of a set of surface and functional markers across hundreds and thousands of cells. These measurements can often be used to differentiate various cell types and there has been a rapid development of analytic approaches for achieving this. However, in spite of the fact that measurements are available on such a large number of cells, there have been very limited advances in deep learning approaches for the analysis of flow cytometry data. Some preliminary work has focused on using deep learning techniques to classify cell types based on the cell protein measurements. In a first of its kind study, we propose a novel deep learning architecture for predicting functional markers in the cells given data on surface markers. Such an approach is expected to automate the measurement of functional markers across cell samples, provided data on the surface markers are available, that has important practical advantages. We validate and compare our approach with competing machine learning methods using a real flow cytometry dataset, and showcase the improved prediction performance of the deep learning architecture.

**Keywords** Single-cell genomics · Single-cell chromatin accessibility data · Rare cell types · Weighted $K$-means clustering · Sparse weighted $K$-means clustering

C. Solís-Lemus · X. Ma · S. Kundu (✉)
Emory University, Atlanta, GA, USA
e-mail: csolisl@emory.edu; xin.ma@emory.edu; suprateek.kundu@emory.edu

M. Hostetter II · D. Pimentel-Alarcón
Georgia State University, Atlanta, GA, USA
e-mail: mhostetter1@student.gsu.edu; pimentel@gsu.edu

P. Qiu
Georgia Institute of Technology and Emory University, Atlanta, GA, USA
e-mail: peng.qiu@bme.gatech.edu

© Springer Nature Switzerland AG 2020
Y. Zhao, D.-G. (Din) Chen (eds.), *Statistical Modeling in Biomedical Research*, Emerging Topics in Statistics and Biostatistics,
https://doi.org/10.1007/978-3-030-33416-1_5

# 1 Introduction

Multiparametric single-cell analysis has advanced our understanding of diverse biological and pathological processes, providing insights into cellular differentiation, intracellular signaling cascades and clinical immunophenotyping. Modern flow cytometers typically provide simultaneous single-cell measurements of up to 12 fluorescent parameters in routine cases, and analysis of up to 30 protein parameters has been recently made commercially available. In addition, a next-generation mass cytometry platform (CyTOF) has become commercially available, which allows routine measurement of 50 or more protein markers.

Despite the technological advances in acquiring an increasing number of parameters per single cell, approaches for analyzing such complex data lag behind. The existing approaches are often subjective and labor-intensive. For example, the widely used gating approach identifies cell types by user-defined sequences of nested 2-D plots. There have been efforts to develop clustering algorithms (e.g., flowMeans [1], flowSOM [2], X-shift [3]), and dimension reduction algorithms (e.g., SPADE [4], tSNE [5], Scaffold [6]). However, there is still huge space for developing new methods to ask new questions in this field.

Recently, deep learning models are revolutionizing the fields of precision medicine, data mining, astronomy, human-computer interactions, among many others, by becoming a major discovery force in science due to the unprecedented accuracy in prediction. However, deep learning approaches showing accurate performance on genomics and biomedical applications [7–13], the CyTOF community has not fully adopted these methods yet. In fact, it turns out that CyTOF data is perfectly suited for deep learning methods. On one side, identify markers define a cell type (e.g., B cell, T cell, monocytes, MSC), and on the other side, expressions of functional markers identify the cell's activity (e.g., quiescent, secreting cytokines, proliferating, apoptosis). Since CyTOF technology allows for the simultaneous measurement of a large number of protein markers, most CyTOF studies measure both identity markers and functional markers, providing data for supervised learning tools, like neural networks. In addition, each CyTOF run typically collects data on $10^6$ cells, creating an ideal large dataset in which the number of samples (cells) is orders of magnitude larger than the number of variables (markers). Deep learning methods are particularly suited for this type of big data.

In terms of motivation, there are two main reasons to predict the functional markers from surface markers in CyTOF data: (1) monetary and time cost, and (2) technical limit of the total number of markers CyTOF can measure, which is currently around 50 protein markers. That is, if we can accurately predict some functional markers based on surface markers, there is no longer the need to include those functional markers in the staining panel (experimental design), and thereby freeing up channels to measure more surface markers or additional functional markers that cannot be predicted.

Here, we present the first work to explore neural network models to predict functional markers (internal phosphoproteins) with identify markers (cell surface proteins). We compare the performance of neural networks in terms of accuracy and speed to other standard statistical approaches like regression, and random forests. We show that neural networks improve prediction of functional markers, making them a powerful alternative to the usual regression techniques, thus, providing quantitive evidence that deep learning methods can enrich the existing research landscape of CyTOF big data.

## 2 Data

### 2.1 Pre-processing

The CyTOF dataset has been previously published in [4, 14]. It contains single-cell data for 5 bone marrow samples from healthy donors. The data for each sample contains measurements for 31 protein markers for individual cells, including 13 cell surface markers which are conventionally used to define cell types, as well as 18 functional markers which reflect the signaling activities of cells. The number of cells per sample is roughly 250,000, and the total number of cells across all 5 samples is 1,223,228. Thus, the data can be expressed in a $1,223,228 \times 31$ matrix.

The data was transformed with inverse hyperbolic sine function ($arcsinh$ with co-factor of 5), which is the standard transformation for CyTOF data [14].

### 2.2 Exploratory Analysis

We will compare the performance of different methods (explained next section) to predict the functional markers with the surface markers. The data is highly complex and correlated, violating some of the fundamental assumptions of standard statistical approaches (like regression). For example, the data is highly skewed and the pattern between response and predictor is not linear (see Fig. 1).

## 3 Materials and Methods

### 3.1 Background on Neural Networks

A neural network model is formed by several *neurons*. Each neuron receives an input vector $x$, then weights its components according to the neuron's weight vector $w$, adds a *bias* constant $b$, and passes the result through a non-linear *activation function* $\sigma$. This way, the output of a neuron is given by $\sigma(w^T x + b)$. There are several options for the activation function $\sigma$. Common choices include the *sigmoid*

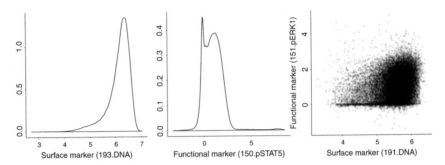

**Fig. 1** Exploratory plots of surface and functional markers. The histograms show a biased pattern, and the scatterplot shows non linearity, both violations of crucial assumptions in standard regression models

function $\sigma(z) = \frac{1}{1+e^{-z}}$ or the *rectified linear unit* (ReLU) $\sigma(z) = \max(0, z)$. For the CyTOF data, we use the hyperbolic tangent as activation function, as it showed better performance than the sigmoid or ReLU functions (more details on the specific neural network fit in Sect. 3.2).

The final output of the network is given by $\hat{f}(x)$ with parameters $\mathbf{W}_1, \cdots, \mathbf{W}_L$ for the weight matrices and $b_1, \cdots, b_L$ for the bias vectors for each layer.

The estimation of the parameters is done through the following optimization

$$\min_{\{W_l, b_l\}_{l=1}^{L}} \sum_{i=1}^{n} \| y_i - \hat{f}(x_i) \|^2. \tag{1}$$

The most widely used technique to solve this optimization is through stochastic gradient descent (SGD) and back-propagation, but we discovered that Adam [15], an algorithm for first-order gradient-based optimization of stochastic objective functions, based on adaptive estimates of lower-order moments had better performance for our data (more details in Sect. 3.2).

## 3.2 Methods Comparison

We fit a neural network model to predict functional markers from surface markers, and compare its performance to three classical statistical methods: (1) linear regression (unpenalized and penalized), (2) decision trees, and (3) random trees. Due to computational time constraints, we could not fit a support vector regression (SVR) model (more in Discussion). We compared the performance of the four approaches by computing the mean square error (MSE) of the predicted responses.

To fit the models, we divided the data into training set, and testing set. The training set was used to perform a tenfold cross validation scheme to choose the best model fit for each method. We chose the model fit with the smallest average MSE. Then, we used all the training samples to estimate the final model for each method (e.g. model and tuning parameters), and reported the prediction MSE of each method based on the testing samples.

The complete data consisted of 1,223,228 cells in 18 functional markers (responses) and 15 surface markers (predictors), which we divided as follows: 1,000,000 rows as training set, and 223,228 rows as testing set.

We used two separate measure of performance: a vector MSE (Eq. (2)) and individual MSE (Eq. (3)), one per predictor (so, 18 in total).

The vector MSE is defined as

$$MSE_{vec} = \frac{1}{2n} \sum_{i=1}^{n} ||\hat{Y}_i - Y_i||_2^2 \qquad (2)$$

where $\hat{Y}_i \in \mathbf{R}^{18}$ is the predicted vector of responses for individual $i$, and $Y_i \in \mathbf{R}^{18}$ is the observed vector of responses for individual $i$.

The individual MSE for predictor $k$ is defined as

$$MSE_{(k)} = \frac{1}{2n} \sum_{i=1}^{n} (\hat{Y}_{k,i} - Y_{k,i})^2 \qquad (3)$$

where $\hat{Y}_{k,i} \in \mathbf{R}$ is the $k^{th}$ predicted response ($k = 1, \cdots, 18$) for individual $i$, and $Y_{k,i} \in \mathbf{R}$ is the $k^{th}$ observed response for individual $i$.

**Neural Network Model** We tested different network architectures, activation functions, regularization coefficients, solver methods, momentum policies, and learning rates with 50,000 maximum epochs. The best network has four layers (see Fig. 2) with 90, 90, 45 and 45 nodes. The network uses hyperbolic tangent as activation function, regularization coefficient of 0.0001, momentum policy fixed at 0.8, inverse-decay learning rate policy with base learning rate, gamma and power

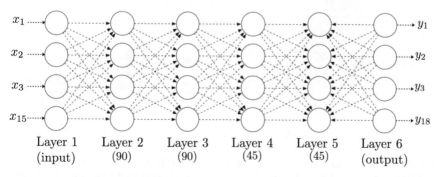

**Fig. 2** Neural network for predicting functional markers (18 responses) from surface markers (15 predictors) with 4 hidden layers with 90, 90, 45 and 45 nodes each

parameters at 0.01, 0.0001, 0.75. We used Adam solver [15], an algorithm for first-order gradient-based optimization of stochastic objective functions, based on adaptive estimates of lower-order moments, instead of Stochastic Gradient Descent (SGD) as the former showed increased accuracy. All networks were trained using the julia package Mocha [16, 17].

**Linear Regression (Unpenalized/Penalized)** We fit standard linear regression, as well as the penalized version with LASSO penalty under different penalization parameters. We used the ScikitLearn [18] Julia Wrapper, with default settings. We noted that the penalized version performed worse than the unpenalized version for all the predictors (regardless of penalty parameter), so we only present results below for the unpenalized linear regression model.

**Decision Tree and Random Forest Regressions** We fit one decision tree regression per response with ScikitLearn julia wrapper, with default settings. We compared the performance of the "mse" criterion and the Friedman's improvement score, deciding on the former ("mse") which is the default setting. We did not constraint the maximum depth of the tree, and set as 2 the minimum number of samples required to split an internal node. In addition, we did not constraint the maximum number of features to consider when looking for the best split. Later, we fit 20 trees into a random forest regression. We could not explore more than 20 trees due to computational time constraints.

## 4   Results

Figure 3 (left) shows the vector MSE (Eq. (2)) across all four different methods, being decision tree the least accurate and neural network the most accurate. Figure 3 (right) shows a comparison on computation time (in seconds) among the four

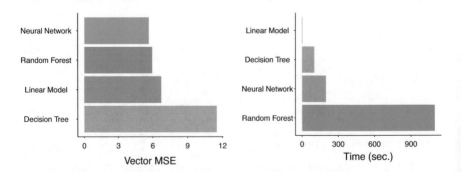

**Fig. 3** Left: Vector MSE (Eq. (2)) for all four methods sorted from most accurate (neural network) to least accurate (decision tree). Right: Running time (in seconds) for the training and validation sets (sample 750,000 rows) for all four methods, sorted from fastest (linear regression) to slowest (random forest)

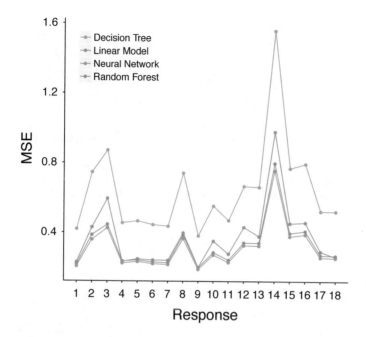

**Fig. 4** Individual MSE (Eq. (3)) for each 18 responses. The neural network outperforms all other methods across all responses. Lines are drawn simply for visual effect

methods, being linear regression the fastest and random forest the slowest. To sum up, the neural network approach outperforms the other three methods in terms of prediction accuracy, without sacrificing too much computational speed.

Figure 4 shows the individual MSE (Eq. (3)) per response (18 responses in $x$-axis) for each of the four methods. Again, the prediction accuracy of neural network is better than the other three methods for all the 18 predictors.

The MSE performance varies across responses. For example, the first response (functional marker 141.pPLCgamma2) has an overall MSE lower than other responses like the third (functional marker 152.Ki67), the 8th (functional marker 159.pSTAT3) or the 14th (functional marker 171.pBtk.Itk).

Figure 5 (left) shows the violin plots for these 4 functional markers. We observe that the 14th response has a wider range and heavier tails than the other responses, which is confirmed in the scatterplots on the center and right (Fig. 5). It appears that the wider spread and higher variability of the 14th response (functional marker 171.pBtk.Itk) causes the lower prediction accuracy compared to other responses, like the first one (functional marker 141.pPLCgamma2).

Finally, we present selected scatterplots of surface markers as predictors for the responses 1, 3, 8 and 14 (Fig. 6). We can appreciate in these plots the non-linear relationship between the predictors and responses, which justifies the use of a neural network approach.

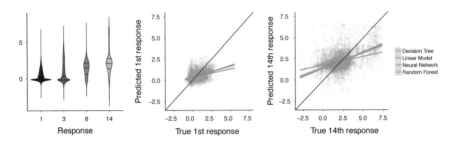

**Fig. 5** Left: Violin plot for four functional markers (responses). Horizontal lines represent the 25th quantile, median and 75th quantile. Center: Predicted vs observed responses on the first functional marker (141.pPLCgamma2) across all four methods. Left: Predicted vs observed responses on the 14th functional marker (171.pBtk.Itk) across all four methods. The closer the slope to 1 (black line), the better

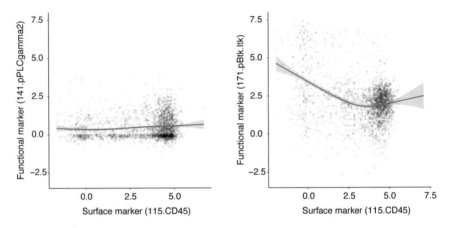

**Fig. 6** Scatterplot of selected surface markers (predictors) and selected functional markers (responses). Left: the first response (functional marker 141.pPLCgamma2) shows a linear relationship to the predictor (surface marker 115.CD45), which partially explains the better MSE in Fig. 4. Right: the 14th response (functional marker 171.pBtk.Itk) shows a non-linear relationship to the predictor (surface marker 115.CD45), which partially explains the worse MSE in Fig. 4

## 5 Discussion

To the best of our knowledge, our work presents the first neural network model for the prediction of functionality in CyTOF big data. In this work, we showed that a neural network model outperforms standard statistical approaches like linear regression and random forest in the prediction of functional markers from surface markers for CyTOF data. Neural networks were also faster and more efficient than random forests, which make them a more viable choice for big datasets.

The improved prediction accuracy of neural networks can be explained by their flexibility to account for non-linearity or skewness. Unlike regression models, neural networks do not have linearity or normality assumptions, and they take advantage of the correlation structure among responses by fitting a network for the whole response vector. It is important to note that the while the neural network model shows better performance than the other methods, this edge is still quite modest. Random forest models also represent a suitable choice for prediction under non-linear assumptions. However, we show here that when scalability also matters, the neural network model outperforms random forests (in computation time), while providing more accurate predictions. We claim that neural networks are better suited for big CyTOF data than random forests, but more work is needed to corroborate this claims.

As mentioned already, CyTOF data is perfectly suited for deep learning methods given the simultaneous measurement of a large number of protein markers, including both identity markers and functional markers. Both measurements allow for the implementation of highly accurate supervised methods, like neural networks. In addition, the structure of CyTOF data is ideal for deep learning: number of samples orders of magnitude greater than the number of variables.

The accuracy in the prediction of functional markers from surface markers has economic and computational advantages, for example, considering the limitation to the total number of markers CyTOF can measure, which is currently around 50 protein markers. Being able to predict functional markers from surface markers could allow for different types of staining panels which could measure more surface markers, or focus on functional markers not so easily predicted.

Initially, we were surprised by the lack of scalability of SVR models. However, given the non-linearity and optimization complexity [19, 20], it appeared that our dataset was too large for the computation of the kernel matrix, which is $n \times n$ where $n$ is the number of samples (more than 1 million in our case). More work is needed to assess the performance of SVR under smaller datasets to assess the accuracy of such models and the limits in scalability.

For future work, we can include an extended version of the dataset [4, 14] that includes 24 healthy sample of bone marrow treated by 24 different drugs. In this setting, we are interested in predicting the functional markers under different drug scenarios, using information at baseline (no treatment) and surface markers at different treatment levels. Furthermore, based on the trained deep learning model, we are interested in the question of whether we can identify cell clusters, and whether these cell clusters agree with well-accepted cell types in literature. Finally, if we focus on cells belonging to the same known cell type, and examine the distribution of functional markers and the correlation with the subtle variations of the identity markers among cells of this type, we can explore whether there is evidence that the specific cell type could be further divided into subtypes.

**Acknowledgement** We thank the editor as well as two anonymous reviewers whose suggestions greatly improved the manuscript.

**Data Sharing** The data is publicly available through the original publications [4, 14] in the following website: http://reports.cytobank.org/1/v1.

# References

1. Aghaeepour, N., Nikolic, R., Hoos, H. H., & Brinkman, R. R. (2010). Rapid cell population identification in flow cytometry data. *Cytometry Part A, 79A*(1), 6–13.
2. Van Gassen, S., Callebaut, B., Van Helden, M. J., Lambrecht, B. N., Demeester, P., Dhaene, T., et al. (2015). FlowSOM: Using self-organizing maps for visualization and interpretation of cytometry data. *Cytometry Part A, 87*(7), 636–645.
3. Samusik, N., Good, Z., Spitzer, M. H., Davis, K. L., & Nolan, G. P. (2016). Nolan. Automated mapping of phenotype space with single-cell data. *Nature Methods, 13*, 493.
4. Qiu, P., Simonds, E. F., Bendall, S. C., Gibbs Jr, K. D., Bruggner, R. V., Linderman, M. D., et al. (2011). Extracting a cellular hierarchy from high-dimensional cytometry data with SPADE. *Nature Biotechnology, 29*, 886.
5. Maaten, L. V. D., & Hinton, G. (2008). Visualizing Data using t-SNE. *Journal of Machine Learning Research, 9*, 2579–2605.
6. Spitzer, M. H., Gherardini, P. F., Fragiadakis, G. K., Bhattacharya, N., Yuan, R. T., Hotson, A. N., et al. (2015). An interactive reference framework for modeling a dynamic immune system. *Science, 349*(6244), 2015.
7. Cire_san, D., Giusti, A., Gambardella, L., & Schmidhuber, J. (2013). Mitosis detection in breast cancer histology images with deep neural networks. In Mori, K.Sakuma, I, Sato, Y., Barillot, C., & Navab, N. (Eds.), *Medical image computing and computer-assisted intervention*. Berlin: Springer.
8. O. Denas, O., & J. Taylor (2013). Deep modeling of gene expression regulation in an Erythropoiesis model. In *Representation Learning, ICML Workshop* New York: ACM.
9. Fakoor, R., Ladhak, F., Nazi, A., & Huber, M. (2013). Using deep learning to enhance cancer diagnosis and classification. In *Proceedings of the 30th International Conference on Machine Learning (ICML)*. New York: ACM.
10. Leung, M. K., Xiong, H. Y., Lee, L. J., & Frey, B. J. (2014). Deep learning of the tissue-regulated splicing code. *Bioinformatics, 30*(12), i121–i129.
11. Cruz-Roa, A., Basavanhally, A., González, F., Gilmore, H., Feldman, M., Ganesan, S., .et al. (2014). Automatic detection of invasive ductal carcinoma in whole slide images with convolutional neural networks. In *SPIE Medical Imaging* (Vol. 9041, pp. 904103).
12. Li, H., Shaham, U., Stanton, K. P., Yao, Y., Montgomery, R. R., & Kluger, Y. (2017). Gating mass cytometry data by deep learning. *Bioinformatics, 33*(21), 3423–3430.
13. Mobadersany, P., Yousefi, S., Amgad, M., Gutman, D. A., Barnholtz-Sloan, J. S., Vega, J. E. V., et al. (2018). Predicting cancer outcomes from histology and genomics using convolutional networks. *Proceedings of the National Academy of Sciences, 115*(13), E2970–E2979
14. Bendall, S. C., Simonds, E. F., Qiu, P., El-ad, D. A., Krutzik, P. O., Finck, R., et al. (2011). Single-cell mass cytometry of differential immune and drug responses across a human hematopoietic continuum. *Science, 332*(6030), 687–696.
15. Kingma, D. P., & Ba, J. (2014). Adam: A method for stochastic optimization. Preprint. arXiv:1412.6980.
16. Bezanson, J., Edelman, A., Karpinski, S., & Shah, V. (2017). Julia: A Fresh Approach to Numerical Computing. *SIAM Review, 59*(1), 65–98.
17. Mocha: Julia package. https://mochajl.readthedocs.io/en/latest/. Retrieved October 22, 2018.
18. ScikitLearn: Julia package. https://scikitlearnjl.readthedocs.io/en/latest/. Retrieved October 22, 2018.
19. Smola, A., & Schölkopf, B. (2004). A tutorial on support vector regression. *Statistics and Computing, 14*(3), 199–222.
20. Welling, M. (2004). Support vector regression. *Tech. Rep., Department of Computer Science, Univ. of Toronto*.

# Building Health Application Recommender System Using Partially Penalized Regression

Eun Jeong Oh, Min Qian, Ken Cheung, and David C. Mohr

**Abstract** Behavioral intervention technologies through mobile applications have a great potential to enhance patient care by improving efficacy. One approach to optimize the utility of mobile health applications is through an individualized health application recommender system. We formalize such a recommender system as a policy that maps individual subject information to a recommended app. We propose to estimate the optimal policy which maximizes the expected utility by partial regularization via orthogonality using the adaptive Lasso (PRO-aLasso). We also derive the convergence rate of the expected outcome of the estimated policy to that of the true optimal policy. The PRO-aLasso estimators are shown to enjoy the same oracle properties as the adaptive Lasso. Simulations studies show that the PRO-aLasso yields simple, more stable policies with better results as compared to the adaptive Lasso and other competing methods. The performance of our method is demonstrated through an illustrative example using IntelliCare mobile health applications.

**Keywords** Mobile health · Application recommender system · Partial regularization via orthogonality (PRO) · Adaptive lasso · Optimal policy

## 1 Introduction

With increasing utilization of mobile devices, there is a great potential for behavioral intervention technologies via mobile applications to be included in a portfolio of available resources [7], and to be a viable option for delivering psychological

E. J. Oh (✉) · M. Qian · K. Cheung
Columbia University, New York, NY, USA
e-mail: eo2366@cumc.columbia.edu; mq2158@cumc.columbia.edu; yc632@cumc.columbia.edu

D. C. Mohr
Northwestern University, Evanston, IL, USA
e-mail: d-mohr@northwestern.edu

© Springer Nature Switzerland AG 2020
Y. Zhao, D.-G. (Din) Chen (eds.), *Statistical Modeling in Biomedical Research*, Emerging Topics in Statistics and Biostatistics,
https://doi.org/10.1007/978-3-030-33416-1_6

treatments to mental health patients who will otherwise not have access to traditional treatments [13]. With more than 165,000 mobile health applications estimated to be available [16], it is crucial to create a recommender system for health applications, so as to increase user engagement and adherence and ultimately lead to health benefits [2]. Our goal is to develop an individualized recommender system for health applications. Specifically, we consider building a recommender system for apps in the IntelliCare ecosystem, which is a suite of health apps for users with depression and anxiety disorders [1, 9]. Briefly, IntelliCare consists of 12 apps each implementing a psychological therapy with simple interactional elements. A Hub app is used to organize the user's experience with IntelliCare, with a specific function of pushing recommendations for other IntelliCare apps. Description of the IntelliCare apps and the effectiveness of the Hub recommendation can be found in [9]. Cheung et al. [1] showed that the Hub recommendation is effective at increasing user engagement, and the current version of Hub makes recommendations for up to 2 apps randomly at weekly intervals. However, it is conceivable that we can further improve performance of the Hub by tailoring recommendations based on each individual's past interaction with the apps and the system's recommendation history.

One way to operationalize this type of recommender system is through a policy that takes individual information as an input and returns an action (e.g., recommendation) as an output. Our goal is to construct a high quality policy that, when implemented, will maximize the value associated with the outcome of interest. Various methods have been developed to estimate this optimal policy. Gunter et al. [6] proposed ranking techniques designed to differentiate variables that are included merely to facilitate estimation and variables involved in the decision rules. Zhang et al. [23, 24] developed an approach for estimating policy using doubly robust augmented inverse probability weighted estimator over a restricted class of regimes. Zhao et al. [28, 29], Zhang et al. [22], and Zhang and Zhang [25] proposed a statistical learning procedure, which reformulates the optimal policy estimation as a weighted classification problem. There is also a vast literature on the estimation of optimal policy based on tree-based methods [4, 8, 11, 18]. Zhang et al. [26, 27] and Rudin and Ertekin [17] also proposed list-based methods which are special cases of tree-based rules.

A main challenge in developing optimal policy in our example, however, is the high-dimensionality of the covariate space and the action space. For the IntelliCare Hub, with up to 2 recommendations among 13 apps (including Hub's self-recommendation), there are 92 possible actions. Furthermore, as in most policy development, it is imperative to consider interactions between the actions and the covariates; and this will result in a very large model that is prone to overfitting and aggravate the "curse of dimensionality". To address this challenge, researchers have applied regularization and variable selection techniques to correctly select a subset of relevant variables from the huge set of candidates. Recent developments in high-dimensional variable selection approaches include shrinkage regression methods, such as least absolute shrinkage and selection operator (Lasso) [20], smoothly clipped absolute deviation method [3], elastic net [31], adaptive Lasso

[30], nonnegative garrote [21], and many others. Penalized regression methods for estimating optimal policy were proposed by Qian and Murphy [15] and Lu et al. [12].

The foregoing variable selection methods are completely data-driven. However, there are at least two reasons for including human decisions in building a predictive model. First, investigators may have strong prior evidence that certain variables contribute much information to the response, and should be kept regardless of the data. For example, Chueng et al. [1] demonstrated significant main effects of the Hub's recommendation; that is, users receiving a recommendation of a given app will more likely engage with the app. Keeping those *known* main effects in the model will intuitively improve precision in variable selection and estimation. Second, even when there is no evidence that a variable has a strong effect, the variable may be included if it facilitates interpretation of a model. We emphasize that the contribution of human expert goes beyond the identification of which variables to penalize or not to penalize in the model; it is the integration of domain knowledge into the model building and validation process.

We propose to incorporate expert knowledge in a Lasso-type variable selection procedure by performing regularization only for a pre-specified partial set of variables. Specifically, we will achieve partial regularization via an orthogonalization (PRO) technique, and apply it in conjunction with the adaptive Lasso. The remainder of the paper is organized as follows. In Sect. 2, we provide a general framework for estimating an optimal policy using the adaptive Lasso (aLasso) and applying the proposed PRO technique, and we also present the asymptotic behavior of our estimators and the rate of convergence for the value of the estimated policy. In Sect. 3, we compare the proposed method with some existing alternatives through extensive simulation studies. In Sect. 4, we apply the PRO-aLasso to the IntelliCare data to estimate the optimal recommender algorithm after 6 weeks of use. Discussion and conclusions are presented in Sect. 5. Proofs of theorems are included in the Appendix.

## 2  Partial Regularization via Orthogonality Using the Adaptive Lasso

Suppose we observe data from $n$ individuals. For each individual, the data is of the form $\{O, A, Y\}$, where $O$ is the vector of individual covariates, $A$ denotes recommended actions, and $Y$ is the outcome of interest with large values desired. For instance, in terms of the IntelliCare data, $O$ is the baseline number of app usage (i.e., count), $A$ is the recommendation action by the Hub, and $Y$ is the count on log scale, observed the week after the recommendation. We assume $A$ is a categorical variable (i.e., discrete actions). If there are more than two possible actions, $A$ is coded as a vector of dummy variables. In this context, a policy $\pi$, is a mapping from the space of observations, $\mathcal{O}$, to the action space, $\mathcal{A}$. The *value* of the policy, denoted as $V(\pi)$, is the expected outcome that would be obtained if the policy were to be implemented in the population of interest. The goal is to estimate the optimal policy, $\pi_0$, that would maximize the expected outcome if implemented:

$$\pi_0 = \arg\max_\pi V(\pi).$$

Define the $Q$-function $Q(\boldsymbol{O}, \boldsymbol{A}) = E(Y|\boldsymbol{O}, \boldsymbol{A})$ so that $Q(o, a)$ measures the quality of assigning action $\boldsymbol{A} = \boldsymbol{a}$ to an individual with $\boldsymbol{O} = \boldsymbol{o}$ [14, 15]. Then, the optimal policy is the best action for each individual; i.e., $\pi_0(\boldsymbol{O}) = \arg\max_a Q(\boldsymbol{O}, \boldsymbol{a})$. We construct the optimal policy by estimating the $Q$-function. We assume

$$Q(\boldsymbol{O}, \boldsymbol{A}) = \Phi(\boldsymbol{O}, \boldsymbol{A})^T \boldsymbol{\gamma}_0, \tag{1}$$

where $\Phi(\boldsymbol{O}, \boldsymbol{A})$ is a vector summary of $(\boldsymbol{O}, \boldsymbol{A})$. It may contain linear or higher order terms of $\boldsymbol{O}$, $\boldsymbol{A}$, and their interactions; thus, it could be high-dimensional. We separate $\Phi(\boldsymbol{O}, \boldsymbol{A})$ into two parts: those need to be penalized, denoted by $\boldsymbol{X} \in \mathbb{R}^{p_1}$, and those left unpenalized, denoted by $\boldsymbol{Z} \in \mathbb{R}^{p_2}$. Usually $\boldsymbol{Z}$ is low-dimensional and only includes several key variables. For instance, we could let $\boldsymbol{X} = (\boldsymbol{O}, \boldsymbol{OA})$ and $\boldsymbol{Z} = (1, \boldsymbol{A})$ if the main effect of action is desired to remain in the model along with the unpenalized intercept. Thus, model (1) can be re-written as

$$Q(\boldsymbol{O}, \boldsymbol{A}) = \boldsymbol{X}^T \boldsymbol{\beta}_0 + \boldsymbol{Z}^T \boldsymbol{\alpha}_0, \tag{2}$$

where $\boldsymbol{\alpha}_0$ and $\boldsymbol{\beta}_0$ are the vectors of true parameters.

Although the model is high-dimensional, we expect only a few terms in $\boldsymbol{X}$ are active. It is well-known that the adaptive Lasso possesses the so-called oracle property so that the set of non-zero coefficients is correctly identified with probability converging to one, and the estimated coefficients within this set are asymptotically normal [30]. In what follows, we describe the PRO-aLasso algorithm that imposes an adaptive Lasso penalty only on $\boldsymbol{X}$ but not on $\boldsymbol{Z}$, and will show that the oracle properties are preserved.

Let $E_n$ denote the sample average. The PRO-aLasso aims to find $(\hat{\boldsymbol{\alpha}}_n, \hat{\boldsymbol{\beta}}_n)$ that minimizes the following objective function

$$L_n(\boldsymbol{\alpha}, \boldsymbol{\beta}) = nE_n \left( Y - \boldsymbol{X}^T \boldsymbol{\beta} - \boldsymbol{Z}^T \boldsymbol{\alpha} \right)^2 + \lambda_n \sum_{j=1}^{p_1} w_j |\beta_j|, \tag{3}$$

and the estimated policy is the action which maximizes the estimated $Q$-function

$$\hat{\pi}(\boldsymbol{O}) \in \arg\max_{a \in A} (\boldsymbol{X}^T \hat{\boldsymbol{\beta}}_n + \boldsymbol{Z}^T \hat{\boldsymbol{\alpha}}_n).$$

Note that $\lambda_n$ in (3) is a tuning parameter which controls the model complexity of $X$, and $w = (w_1, \ldots, w_{p_1})$ is a vector of weights that are used to adjust a level of penalization on individual variables. Ideally, large penalties are suitable for zero coefficients (inactive covariates) and small penalties for non-zero coefficients (active covariates). This can be achieved by defining the weight vector as $\hat{w} = |\bar{\beta}|^{-\delta}$ for some $\delta > 0$ with $\bar{\beta}$ being a root-$(n/p_1)$-consistent estimator. That is, heavier penalties are put on the coefficients with smaller $\bar{\beta}$ estimates and thus smaller true parameters. In practice, we propose to set $\bar{\beta}$ as perturbed elastic net estimates, following Zou and Zhang [32], and fivefold cross-validation can be used to select an optimal pair of $(\delta, \lambda_n)$.

The PRO-aLasso algorithm is given below. It implies that $\hat{\beta}_n$ is the adaptive Lasso estimator obtained based on the new response vector $\tilde{Y} = Y - Z^T \hat{v}_n$ and the new predictor matrix $\tilde{X} = X - Z^T \hat{\Gamma}_n$, where $\tilde{Y}$ is the residuals of $Y$ on a direction orthogonal to $Z$ (or simply $Y$ adjusted for $Z$) and $\tilde{X}$ is the residuals of $X$ on a direction orthogonal to $Z$ (or simply $X$ adjusted for $Z$). The adaptive Lasso estimates can be obtained using a coordinate descent algorithm with the R package glmnet [5], which is integrated in the PRO-aLasso algorithm.

---

**PRO-aLasso algorithm**

---

**Input:** data $(O, A, Y)$
**Output:** policy $\hat{\pi}$
1: Formulate $X$ and $Z$ as a function of $O$ and $A$ in order to impose an adaptive Lasso penalty on $X$ but not on $Z$
2: $\hat{v}_n \leftarrow \arg\min_v E_n \left( Y - Z^T v \right)^2$
3: **for** $j = 1, \ldots, p_1$ **do**
4: $\quad \hat{\gamma}_{nj} \leftarrow \arg\min_{\gamma_j} E_n \left( X_j - Z^T \gamma_j \right)^2$
5: **end for**
6: $\hat{\Gamma}_n \leftarrow (\hat{\gamma}_{n1}, \ldots, \hat{\gamma}_{np_1})$
7: Construct $\hat{w} = |\bar{\beta}|^{-\delta}$ for some $\delta > 0$ with $\bar{\beta}$ being a root-$(n/p_1)$-consistent estimator, which is obtained from the response $Y - Z^T \hat{v}_n$ and the predictor matrix $X - Z^T \hat{\Gamma}_n$
8: Define $(X - Z^T \hat{\Gamma}_n)^* = (X - Z^T \hat{\Gamma}_n)/\hat{w}$
9: Solve the lasso problem for all $\lambda_n$,

$$\hat{\beta}_n^* \leftarrow \arg\min_\beta n E_n \left( Y - Z^T \hat{v}_n - ((X - Z^T \hat{\Gamma}_n)^*)^T \beta \right)^2 + \lambda_n \sum_{j=1}^{p_1} |\beta_j|$$

10: $\hat{\beta}_n \leftarrow \hat{\beta}_n^*/\hat{w}$
11: $\hat{\alpha}_n \leftarrow \hat{v}_n - \hat{\Gamma}_n \hat{\beta}_n$
12: $\hat{\pi}(O) \in \arg\max_a \hat{Q}(O, a) = \arg\max_a (X^T \hat{\beta}_n + Z^T \hat{\alpha}_n)$

---

To study the properties of the PRO-aLasso estimator, we introduce some additional notation. Let $\mathcal{J} = \{j : \beta_{0j} \neq 0, j = 1, \ldots, p_1\}$ be the true active set of variables in $X$, and assume that $|\mathcal{J}| = r < p_1$. Denote the estimated active set of variables by $\hat{\mathcal{J}}_n = \left\{ j : \hat{\beta}_{nj} \neq 0, j = 1, \ldots, p_1 \right\}$. Let $\boldsymbol{\beta}_{0\mathcal{J}} = \{\beta_{0j} : j \in \mathcal{J}\}$ and $\hat{\boldsymbol{\beta}}_{n\mathcal{J}} = \{\hat{\beta}_j : j \in \mathcal{J}\}$. Denote $\boldsymbol{\theta} = (\boldsymbol{\alpha}^T, \boldsymbol{\beta}^T)^T$ for any $\boldsymbol{\alpha} \in \mathbb{R}^{p_2}, \boldsymbol{\beta} \in \mathbb{R}^{p_1}$. Then $\mathcal{S} = \{1, 2, \ldots, p_2\} \cup \{s : \theta_{0s} \neq 0, s = p_2 + 1, \ldots, p\}$ is the true active set of variables in $(\boldsymbol{Z}, \boldsymbol{X})$, and thus $\mathcal{J}$ is always the subset of $\mathcal{S}$. Denote

$$\boldsymbol{\Sigma} = E \begin{pmatrix} \boldsymbol{Z}\boldsymbol{Z}^T & \boldsymbol{Z}\boldsymbol{X}^T \\ \boldsymbol{X}\boldsymbol{Z}^T & \boldsymbol{X}\boldsymbol{X}^T \end{pmatrix}, \quad \boldsymbol{\Sigma}_{\mathcal{S}} = E \begin{pmatrix} \boldsymbol{Z}\boldsymbol{Z}^T & \boldsymbol{Z}\boldsymbol{X}_{\mathcal{J}}^T \\ \boldsymbol{X}_{\mathcal{J}}\boldsymbol{Z}^T & \boldsymbol{X}_{\mathcal{J}}\boldsymbol{X}_{\mathcal{J}}^T \end{pmatrix},$$

where $\boldsymbol{\Sigma} \in \mathbb{R}^{p \times p}$ and $\boldsymbol{\Sigma}_{\mathcal{S}} \in \mathbb{R}^{(p_2+r) \times (p_2+r)}$.

Theorem 1 below shows that the PRO-aLasso estimator enjoys variable selection consistency and asymptotic normality even when the number of parameters diverges.

**Theorem 1** *Suppose assumptions (A1)–(A6) in the Appendix hold. Under model (2), the PRO-aLasso estimator possesses the following properties:*

*(i) (variable selection consistency)* $\lim_n P(\hat{\mathcal{J}}_n = \mathcal{J}) = 1,$
*(ii) (joint asymptotic normality)*

$$\sqrt{n} \boldsymbol{\psi}^T \boldsymbol{\Sigma}_{\mathcal{S}}^{1/2} \begin{pmatrix} \hat{\boldsymbol{\alpha}}_n - \boldsymbol{\alpha}_0 \\ \hat{\boldsymbol{\beta}}_{n\mathcal{J}} - \boldsymbol{\beta}_{0\mathcal{J}} \end{pmatrix} \to_d N(0, \sigma^2),$$

*where $\boldsymbol{\psi}$ is a vector of norm 1.*

In the Theorem below, we provide a rate of convergence for the value of the estimated policy to that of the optimal policy. Theorem 2 advocates the approach of minimizing the estimated prediction error to estimate $Q_0$ and maximizing $\hat{Q}$ over $\boldsymbol{a} \in A$ to obtain an policy.

**Theorem 2** *Let $p(A|\boldsymbol{O})$ denote the conditional distribution of action assignment given $\boldsymbol{O}$ in the training data. Suppose all assumptions in Theorem 1 hold, and $p(\boldsymbol{a}|\boldsymbol{o}) \geq S^{-1}$ for a positive constant S for all $(\boldsymbol{o}, \boldsymbol{a})$ pairs. Assume that there exist some constants $C > 0$ and $\eta \geq 0$ such that*

$$P \left( \max_{a \in A} Q_0(\boldsymbol{O}, a) - \max_{a \in A / \arg\max_{a \in A} Q_0(\boldsymbol{O}, a)} Q_0(\boldsymbol{O}, a) \leq \epsilon \right) \leq C\epsilon^{\eta} \qquad (4)$$

*for all positive $\epsilon$. Then*

$$V(\pi_0) - V(\hat{\pi}) \leq O_P \left[ \left( \frac{p_2 + r}{n} \right)^{(1+\eta)/(2+\eta)} \right].$$

*Remark* Condition (4) is a "margin" type condition. It measures the difference in mean outcomes between the optimal action(s) and the best suboptimal action(s) at

$O$. For $C = 1, \eta = 0$, condition (4) always holds for all $\epsilon > 0$. See Qian and Murphy [15] for discussion of this condition.

## 3 Simulation Experiments

We conduct a set of numerical studies to assess the performance of each method. The simulated data are generated from the model

$$
Y = (1, \boldsymbol{O})^T \underbrace{\begin{pmatrix} \alpha_1 \\ \boldsymbol{\beta}_1 \end{pmatrix}}_{\text{main effects}} + (A, \boldsymbol{OA})^T \underbrace{\begin{pmatrix} \alpha_2 \\ \boldsymbol{\beta}_2 \end{pmatrix}}_{\text{trt effects}} + \epsilon,
$$

where $\epsilon \sim N(0, \sigma^2)$. In our simulation, we set $\sigma = 1$. Covariates $\boldsymbol{O} \in \mathbb{R}^q$ are generated from $N(0, \hat{\Omega}_{q \times q})$ where $\hat{\Omega}_{q \times q}$ is a sample correlation matrix of the real data. The following is the minimum, mean, and maximum of absolute value of the correlations in $\hat{\Omega}_{q \times q}$: (0.000, 0.076, 0.933). Policy action $A$ is randomly generated from $\{-1, 1\}$ with equal probability 0.5. A number of scenarios are considered based on the generating model that differs by the number of observations $n$, the number of predictors $p = 2(q + 1)$, the effect size ($es$), and the following two cases:

1. Weak dense: $\alpha_1 = 1$, $\boldsymbol{\beta}_1 = \{1.25_{q/2}, 0_{q/2}\}$, $\boldsymbol{\beta}_2 = 4.5 \cdot |es - 0.3| \cdot \boldsymbol{\beta}_1$,

$$
\alpha_2 = \frac{es \cdot \sqrt{\boldsymbol{\beta}_1^T \Omega \boldsymbol{\beta}_1 + \boldsymbol{\beta}_2^T \Omega \boldsymbol{\beta}_2 + \sigma^2}}{2};
$$

2. Sparse signal: $\alpha_1 = 1$, $\boldsymbol{\beta}_1 = \{seq(.1q + .5, 1.5), rep(0, .9q)\}$, $\boldsymbol{\beta}_2 = 4.5 \cdot |es - 0.3| \cdot \boldsymbol{\beta}_1$,

$$
\alpha_2 = \frac{es \cdot \sqrt{\boldsymbol{\beta}_1^T \Omega \boldsymbol{\beta}_1 + \boldsymbol{\beta}_2^T \Omega \boldsymbol{\beta}_2 + \sigma^2}}{2}.
$$

In settings with the weak dense scenario, half of the $\boldsymbol{\beta}_1$ components are zero. However, in the sparse signal case, nine-tenths of $\boldsymbol{\beta}_1$ are zero; e.g., if $q = 10$, $\boldsymbol{\beta}_1 = (1.5, 0, 0, \ldots, 0)$, and if $q = 40$, $\boldsymbol{\beta}_1 = (4.5, 3.5, 2.5, 1.5, 0, 0, \ldots, 0)$. In both cases, $\boldsymbol{\beta}_2$ has the same structure to $\boldsymbol{\beta}_1$ with a different magnitude. In each scenario, we generate $n = 50$ and $n = 200$ samples with $p = 82$ (i.e., $q = 40$) and $es$ ranging over 0, 0.2, 0.5, 0.8. The performances of the methods are assessed by the following three aspects. The first is to evaluate the variable selection performance in $\boldsymbol{\beta}_2$ using (C, IC), where C is the number of correctly identified active variables and IC is the number of zero variables incorrectly selected in the final model, since the size of $\boldsymbol{\beta}_2$ indicates the number of tailoring variables to construct the optimal policy,

$\hat{\pi}(\boldsymbol{O}) = \left| \hat{\alpha}_2 + \boldsymbol{O}^T \hat{\boldsymbol{\beta}}_2 \right|$. The second is to assess the value function by the estimated optimal policy using an independent test dataset with sample size of 5000. The third is to estimate the root-mean-squared error (RMSE), $\sqrt{E_n (Y - \boldsymbol{X}^T \hat{\boldsymbol{\beta}}_n - \boldsymbol{Z}^T \hat{\boldsymbol{\alpha}}_n)^2}$. The simulation results are summarized in Table 1.

In the weak dense case, as the sample size increases, all the methods tend to correctly identify the active variables. However, the PRO-aLasso selects less number of true zero variables which are incorrectly set to non-zero, compared to other competing methods. It is worth noting that good variable selection results lead to the value estimates closer to the optimal value. In the sparse signal case, the PRO-aLasso outperforms its counterparts in almost all simulation settings in terms of better variable selection performance, higher value function estimate, and smaller prediction error. In particular, our proposed method produces the estimated values nearly close to the optimal value, as the sample size grows. Not surprisingly, the forward variable selection shows a lower performance than other methods since it is highly likely to miss the ultimate model by the one-at-a-time nature of adding variables. The ridge regression performs competitively in the weak dense case but not in the sparse signal case. Based on the overall comparison between the PRO-aLasso and the adaptive Lasso (aLasso), the PRO technique seems to be a better idea in both cases.

## 4   Real Data Application

In this section, we apply our proposed method to the IntelliCare data introduced earlier. The data consists of use patterns of the 13 apps (including Hub) and the recommendation records by the Hub at 1–16 weeks after first download in 2508 Hub users. For illustration purposes, we apply the proposed method to estimate the optimal 6-week recommendation based on the use history in the week prior to recommendations. We considered the number of meaningful app use session ("count", $O$) on each app. With 13 apps including the Hub, we therefore have $\boldsymbol{O} = (O_1, \ldots, O_{13})$ from each user as the baseline covariates. We recoded each of the count variables to be 3 if greater than or equal to 3 to minimize the effect of fairly large counts. Using the notation developed above, we also let $\boldsymbol{A} = (A_1, \ldots, A_{13})$ indicate the recommendation action by the Hub. The primary outcome $\boldsymbol{Y} = (Y_1, \ldots, Y_{13})$ is the count on log scale, observed the week after the recommendation; precisely, we added one before taking the log transformation to handle zero counts.

We applied various regularization and variable selection methods to build the model for each individual app use. For the model for app $j$, we postulate

$$E(Y_j | \boldsymbol{O}, \boldsymbol{A}) = (1, A_j, A_j O_j)^T \boldsymbol{\alpha}_j + (A_1, \ldots, A_{j-1}, A_{j+1}, \ldots, A_{13},$$

$$O_1, \ldots, O_{13}, A_j O_1, \ldots, A_j O_{j-1}, A_j O_{j+1}, \ldots, A_j O_{13})^T \boldsymbol{\beta}_j,$$

**Table 1** Simulation results based on 1000 replications

| es | Method | n = 50 | | | | n = 200 | | | |
|---|---|---|---|---|---|---|---|---|---|
| | | C | IC | Value | RMSE | C | IC | Value | RMSE |
| *(a) Weak dense case* | | | | | | | | | |
| 0 | Truth | 20 | 0 | 7.19 | | 20 | 0 | 7.19 | |
| | PRO-aLasso | 7 (2.97) | 1 (1.48) | 5.26 (1.14) | **7.23 (1.26)** | 20 (0) | 1 (1.48) | **7.18 (0.01)** | **0.69 (0.16)** |
| | ALasso | 4 (4.45) | 0 (0) | 4.21 (1.87) | 8.14 (1.32) | 20 (0) | 6 (4.45) | 7.17 (0.01) | 0.75 (0.13) |
| | Ridge | 20 (0) | 20 (0) | **5.72 (0.34)** | 9.39 (0.5) | 20 (0) | 20 (0) | 7.14 (0.01) | 1.38 (0.21) |
| | Forward | 13 (1.48) | 11 (1.48) | 1.62 (1.43) | 13.6 (2.41) | 20 (0) | 4 (1.48) | 6.6 (0.38) | 5.04 (1.04) |
| 0.2 | Truth | 20 | 0 | 3.13 | | 20 | 0 | 3.13 | |
| | PRO-aLasso | 3 (1.48) | 1 (1.48) | 2.01 (0.44) | **4.44 (0.62)** | 18 (1.48) | 2 (1.48) | **3.08 (0.02)** | **0.75 (0.12)** |
| | ALasso | 1 (1.48) | 0 (0) | 1.64 (0.52) | 5.01 (0.8) | 19 (1.48) | 3 (2.97) | 3.07 (0.02) | 0.79 (0.14) |
| | Ridge | 20 (0) | 20 (0) | **2.05 (0.46)** | 6.21 (0.31) | 20 (0) | 20 (0) | 3.06 (0.02) | 1.11 (0.14) |
| | Forward | 12 (1.48) | 11 (1.48) | 1.49 (0.44) | 8.04 (1.77) | 20 (0) | 5 (2.97) | 2.76 (0.18) | 3.33 (0.5) |
| 0.5 | Truth | 20 | 0 | 5.5 | | 20 | 0 | 5.5 | |
| | PRO-aLasso | 5 (2.97) | 1 (1.48) | 4.17 (0.58) | **5.81 (0.99)** | 20 (0) | 2 (1.48) | **5.48 (0.01)** | **0.69 (0.13)** |
| | ALasso | 3 (2.97) | 0 (0) | 3.22 (1.31) | 6.65 (1.12) | 20(0) | 4 (4.45) | **5.48 (0.01)** | 0.72 (0.13) |
| | Ridge | 20 (0) | 20 (0) | **4.19 (0.38)** | 7.72 (0.39) | 20 (0) | 20 (0) | 5.46 (0.01) | 1.17 (0.16) |
| | Forward | 13 (1.48) | 11 (1.48) | 2.38 (1.11) | 10.69 (2.15) | 20 (0) | 5 (2.97) | 5.14 (0.21) | 3.63 (0.76) |
| 0.8 | Truth | 20 | 0 | 12 | | 20 | 0 | 12 | |
| | PRO-aLasso | 9 (2.97) | 1 (1.48) | **10 (0.83)** | **9.46 (1.39)** | 20 (0) | 0 (0) | **11.99 (0.01)** | 0.91 (0.32) |
| | ALasso | 6 (2.97) | 0 (0) | 8.65 (2.15) | 11.01 (1.88) | 20 (0) | 3 (2.97) | **11.99 (0.01)** | **0.82 (0.24)** |
| | Ridge | 20 (0) | 20 (0) | 9.41 (0.56) | 14.29 (0.7) | 20(0) | 20(0) | 11.95 (0.02) | 1.94 (0.28) |
| | Forward | 14 (1.48) | 11 (1.48) | 5.27 (2.38) | 19.97 (2.98) | 20(0) | 4 (1.48) | 10.75 (0.44) | 11.9 (1.06) |

*(b) Sparse signal case*

| | | C | IC | Value | RMSE | C | IC | Value | RMSE |
|---|---|---|---|---|---|---|---|---|---|
| 0 | Truth | 4 | 0 | 7.48 | | 4 | 0 | 7.48 | |
| | PRO-aLasso | 3 (1.48) | 0 (0) | **7.25 (0.48)** | **2.66 (1.33)** | 4 (0) | 0 (0) | **7.48 (0.00)** | **0.39 (0.11)** |
| | ALasso | 1 (1.48) | 0 (0) | 4.34 (1.84) | 8.78 (1.37) | 4 (0) | 3 (1.48) | 7.28 (0.63) | 1.61 (1.93) |
| | Ridge | 4 (0) | 36 (0) | 4.92 (0.49) | 10.26 (0.22) | 4 (0) | 36 (0) | 7.44 (0.02) | 1.65 (0.27) |
| | Forward | 4 (0) | 20 (2.97) | 1.01 (0.32) | 11.3 (0.71) | 4 (0) | 7 (2.97) | 1.38 (2.43) | 9.95 (0.79) |
| 0.2 | Truth | 4 | 0 | 3.36 | | 4 | 0 | 3.36 | |
| | PRO-aLasso | 2 (0) | 0 (0) | **3.11 (0.32)** | **1.76 (0.71)** | 4 (0) | 0(0) | **3.35 (0.01)** | **0.33 (0.08)** |
| | ALasso | 1 (1.48) | 0 (0) | 2.2 (0.64) | 3.75 (1.6) | 4 (0) | 2 (2.97) | 3.19 (0.28) | 0.89 (0.67) |
| | Ridge | 4 (0) | 36 (0) | 1.91 (0.37) | 6.63 (0.15) | 4 (0) | 36 (0) | 3.29 (0.02) | 1.25 (0.16) |
| | Forward | 4 (0) | 19.5 (2.22) | 1.83 (0.11) | 6.26 (0.75) | 4 (0) | 6 (2.97) | 1.84 (0.01) | 5.46 (0.26) |
| 0.5 | Truth | 4 | 0 | 5.63 | | 4 | 0 | 5.63 | |
| | PRO-aLasso | 3 (1.48) | 0 (0) | **5.47 (0.21)** | **2.02 (0.96)** | 4 (0) | 0 (0) | **5.63 (0.00)** | **0.35 (0.09)** |
| | ALasso | 2 (1.48) | 0 (0) | 4.02 (0.76) | 4.91 (1.37) | 4 (0) | 2 (2.97) | 5.29 (0.57) | 1.47 (1.61) |
| | Ridge | 4 (0) | 36 (0) | 3.55 (0.42) | 8.18 (0.19) | 4 (0) | 36 (0) | 5.59 (0.02) | 1.32 (0.2) |
| | Forward | 4 (0) | 20 (2.97) | 3.02 (0.47) | 7.9 (0.93) | 4 (0) | 6 (2.97) | 3.17 (0.14) | 6.96 (0.55) |
| 0.8 | Truth | 4 | 0 | 13.07 | | 4 | 0 | 13.07 | |
| | PRO-aLasso | 4 (0) | 0 (0) | **12.89 (0.21)** | **3.56 (1.44)** | 4 (0) | 0 (0) | **13.06 (0.00)** | **0.56 (0.3)** |
| | ALasso | 3 (1.48) | 0 (0) | 8.53 (2.35) | 12.26 (2.79) | 4 (0) | 2 (1.48) | 12.3 (1.36) | 3.67 (3.75) |
| | Ridge | 4 (0) | 36 (0) | 8.97 (0.83) | 16.23 (0.41) | 4 (0) | 36 (0) | 13.02 (0.02) | 2.44 (0.36) |
| | Forward | 4 (0) | 20 (1.48) | 7.12 (0.08) | 17.02 (0.69) | 4 (0) | 6 (2.97) | 7.14 (0.15) | 16.4 (0.78) |

The median number of correctly identified active variables in $\beta_2$, denoted by C, and the median number of zero variables in $\beta_2$ incorrectly selected in the final model, denoted by IC, are recorded along with the mean absolute deviation in parentheses. The mean of values and the root-mean-squared error (RMSE) are also reported with the standard deviation in parentheses. The best results are highlighted in boldface where $\boldsymbol{\alpha}_j \in \mathbb{R}^3$ and $\boldsymbol{\beta}_j \in \mathbb{R}^{37}$. This model allows for the possibility that the use history of other apps *may* have an effect on the use of app $j$; however, regularization will be applied to avoid overfitting when we build the prediction model and the recommendation algorithm. On the other hand, because we expect the recommendation of app $j$ will have a direct effect on the use pattern of app $j$, and are interested in estimating this effect, the PRO-aLasso does not place a penalty on the intercept, $A_j$, and $A_j O_j$ (which we call concordant interaction). That is, $\boldsymbol{Z} = (1, A_j, A_j O_j)$.

We also considered maximizing the total usage as an outcome, for which we postulate

$$E(\sum_{j=1}^{13} Y_j | \boldsymbol{O}, \boldsymbol{A}) = (1, A_1, \ldots, A_{13}, A_1 O_1, \ldots, A_{13} O_{13})^T \boldsymbol{\alpha}$$

$$+ (O_1, \ldots, O_{13}, A_1 O_2, A_1 O_3, \ldots, A_{13} O_{12})^T \boldsymbol{\beta},$$

where $\boldsymbol{\alpha} \in \mathbb{R}^{27}$ and $\boldsymbol{\beta} \in \mathbb{R}^{169}$. Like the individual app models, the PRO-aLasso does not place a penalty on the intercept, the direct main effects $\{A_j, j = 1, \ldots, 13\}$, and the concordant interactions $\{A_j O_j, j = 1, \ldots, 13\}$.

The data is randomly split so that three-fourths of data is used to estimate the optimal policy, and the remaining is used to estimate the value of the policies. In addition to the PRO-aLasso, we analyzed the data using the adaptive Lasso and the ridge regression, both of which placed penalties on all coefficients. We also ran the forward variable selection by the Akaike information criterion (AIC).

To illustrate the results of the PRO-aLasso and other methods, we examine the optimal recommender algorithm in terms of improving the usage of Daily Feats (app $j = 4$). According to the analysis results of the PRO-aLasso, the optimal decision is always to push a recommendation of Daily Feats. In contrast, the adaptive Lasso shrank all coefficients to 0 (including that of $A_4$) and the ridge regression yielded coefficients all very close to 0. As a result, these methods were not able to provide any policy. This indicates a pragmatic reason for avoiding penalizing the main effects.

For maximizing the total usage, the PRO-aLasso would mostly recommend the combination of Boost Me and Worry Knot in about 90.5% of the users in our data, followed by Boost Me and Day to Day (1.2%) and Boost Me and My Mantra (1.0%). The forward variable selection would recommend the combination of Thought Challenger and Worry Knot in 87.2% of the users in the data, and Hub and Worry Knot in 5.1%. The ridge regression would recommend the combination of Boost Me and Worry Knot in 68.9% and Boost Me and My Mantra in 20.7% of the users. Again, the adaptive Lasso could not provide any policy for the mobile health application recommendation.

To compare the performance of the various methods, Table 2 reports the estimated value and the size of the policy. The size of the policy is equivalent to the total number of non-zero coefficients except for the intercept and that of the baseline

**Table 2** Estimated value and size of the policy (in parentheses) for maximizing the app use count on log scale

|  | PRO-aLasso | aLasso | Ridge | Forward | Observed |
|---|---|---|---|---|---|
| *Individual app use* | | | | | |
| Aspire | **0.15** (2) | **0.15** (1) | **0.15** (26) | 0.07 (16) | 0.05 |
| Boost Me | 0.07 (2) | 0.04 (4) | 0.06 (26) | **0.11** (13) | 0.02 |
| Hub | **1.20** (14) | 0.78 (12) | 0.78 (26) | 0.34 (17) | 0.33 |
| Daily Feats | **0.08** (2) | 0.03 (0) | 0.03 (26) | 0.07 (11) | 0.03 |
| iCope | **0.05** (2) | **0.05** (1) | 0.04 (26) | **0.05** (19) | **0.05** |
| My Mantra | 0.02 (2) | **0.07** (0) | 0.02 (26) | **0.07** (16) | **0.07** |
| Day to Day | 0.06 (2) | 0.06 (2) | **0.12** (26) | 0.11 (19) | 0.09 |
| MoveMe | **0.11** (2) | **0.11** (1) | 0.05 (26) | 0.04 (12) | 0.04 |
| Purple Chill | **0.09** (3) | **0.09** (1) | **0.09** (26) | 0.05 (14) | 0.04 |
| Slumber Time | **0.07** (2) | 0.03 (0) | 0.03 (26) | **0.07** (10) | 0.03 |
| Social Force | **0.18** (2) | **0.18** (1) | 0.07 (26) | **0.18** (17) | 0.04 |
| Thought Challenger | 0.08 (2) | 0.07 (4) | **0.09** (26) | 0.06 (14) | 0.05 |
| Worry Knot | **0.17** (2) | **0.17** (2) | **0.17** (26) | 0.14 (19) | 0.04 |
| Total usage | **4.65** (31) | 0.89 (0) | 4.12 (182) | 2.27 (108) | 0.89 |

The size of the policy is the total number of non-zero coefficients except the intercept and baseline covariates. Numbers associated with the highest value are in boldface

covariates. It is called the size of the policy because it indicates the number of input variables required to operate the policy. The last column of the tables reports the observed outcome in the data set, which reflects the properties of the Hub built-in recommender system. The PRO-aLasso yielded policies with the highest values for 9 apps including ties, and this was achieved with generally small policy size. The adaptive Lasso tended to over-shrink, whereas the forward variable selection tended to overfit. Table 2 also compares the performance of the various methods when the objective is to maximize the total usage. The PRO-aLasso produced the policy with the highest value. Using the algorithm by PRO-aLasso would increase the sum of log-transformed number of app use sessions by 4.65 in a week on average, whereas the other methods did not appear to make a significant increase. By examining the size of the policy, the PRO-aLasso seems to strike the right balance between over shrinkage (cf. aLasso) and overfitting (cf. forward variable selection).

# 5 Conclusion

In this paper, we propose a PRO-aLasso algorithm that can be used to develop a recommender system for mobile health applications. Since the PRO involves orthogonalization, which is a linear operation, the computational cost of the PRO-aLasso is only marginally higher than that of the adaptive Lasso. The PRO technique is also versatile and can be applied with other regularization methods, although we opted to use the adaptive Lasso for its oracle property. However, it is well-known that the oracle property provides little value in finite samples (see the series of papers by Potscher and Leeb among others).

For the purpose of illustrating the PRO technique, we have developed the PRO-aLasso algorithm to construct one-stage policy, and applied it to the IntelliCare data for a one-off recommendation at week 6 by the Hub. We chose week 6 as the decision time, because the users would have established certain app use habits so that the weekly use data (covariate) would be relatively representative of general patterns. While the choice of week 6 is pragmatic, the Hub by design gives recommendations on a regular basis. Therefore, a realistic recommender system should provide sequential decision rules that adapt over time, and ideally account for additional personal information such as demographic variables. The versatility and computational efficiency of the PRO allow for a straightforward and feasible extension to build multi-stage policy by incorporating the PRO to reinforcement methods, such as $Q$-learning [19]. As we have demonstrated that the PRO-aLasso is superior to some common existing methods in producing one-stage recommender algorithm for the simplified setting, the PRO technique is set to be a promising tool for the multi-stage setting.

## Appendix

The proof of Theorems 1 and 2 relies on the following assumptions and lemmas.

### Assumptions

(A1) $\epsilon \triangleq Y - Z^T\alpha_0 - X^T\beta_0$ has mean zero and finite variance $\sigma^2$, and is independent of $(Z, X)$ with $E(|\epsilon|^{2+\kappa}) < \infty$ for some $\kappa > 0$.

(A2) $(Z^T, X^T)^T$ is uniformly bounded.

(A3) There exist positive constants $b$ and $B$ such that $b \le \lambda_{\min}(\Sigma) \le \lambda_{\max}(\Sigma) \le B$, where $\lambda_{\min}(\Sigma)$ and $\lambda_{\max}(\Sigma)$ are the smallest and the largest eigenvalues of $\Sigma$, respectively.

(A4) $\left\| \hat{\Sigma} - \Sigma \right\|_F \to_p 0$, where $\|\cdot\|_F$ stands for the Frobenius norm.

(A5) $\frac{\log p}{\log n} \to \nu$ for some $0 \le \nu < 1$.

(A6) $\lambda_n = o(\sqrt{n})$,   $\frac{\lambda_n}{\sqrt{n}} n^{((1-\nu)(1+\delta)-1)/2} \to \infty$.

*Remark* Assumptions (A1) and (A2) are employed in the proof of the asymptotic results which are regular requirements. Assumption (A3) implies that the matrix $\Sigma$ has a reasonably good behavior. Assumption (A4) is needed for the random design case. Also, note that the convergence in Frobenius norm implies the convergence in operator norm, which further guarantees the consistency of the sample eigenvalues. When $p^2/n \to 0$, this assumption is usually satisfied, see, e.g., the proof of Lemma 3.1 in Ledoit and Wolf [10] for more details. Assumptions (A5) and (A6) are needed for the rate of convergence and oracle properties. Following Zou and Zhang [32], we can fix $\delta = \left\lceil \frac{2v}{1-v} \right\rceil + 1$ to avoid the tuning on $\delta$, and the oracle properties hold as long as $\delta > \frac{2v}{1-v}$.

**Lemma 1** *Suppose assumptions (A1)–(A6) hold. Then under model (2), we have*

$$\left\| \begin{pmatrix} \hat{\boldsymbol{\alpha}}_n - \boldsymbol{\alpha}_0 \\ \hat{\boldsymbol{\beta}}_n - \boldsymbol{\beta}_0 \end{pmatrix} \right\|_2^2 = O_P\left(\frac{p}{n}\right).$$

We derive the excess loss bound of the PRO-aLasso estimator in Lemma 1, which helps to prove the oracle properties. Under the regularity conditions, Lemma 1 also tells us that the PRO-aLasso estimator is a root-$(n/p)$-consistent estimator.

**Lemma 2** *Let us write $(\boldsymbol{\alpha}_0, \boldsymbol{\beta}_0) = (\boldsymbol{\alpha}_0, \boldsymbol{\beta}_{0\mathcal{J}}, 0)$ and define*

$$(\tilde{\boldsymbol{\alpha}}_n, \tilde{\boldsymbol{\beta}}_{n\mathcal{J}}) = \arg\min_{(\boldsymbol{\alpha},\boldsymbol{\beta})} nE_n\left(Y - (\boldsymbol{Z}, \boldsymbol{X}_{\mathcal{J}})^T(\boldsymbol{\alpha}^T, \boldsymbol{\beta}^T)^T\right)^2 + \lambda_n \sum_{j\in\mathcal{J}} \hat{w}_j |\beta_j|.$$

*Then with probability tending to 1, $(\tilde{\boldsymbol{\alpha}}_n, \tilde{\boldsymbol{\beta}}_{n\mathcal{J}}, 0)$ is the solution to (3).*

Lemma 2 provides an asymptotic characterization for solving the PRO-aLasso criterion. Lemma 2 also shows that the PRO-aLasso estimator possesses oracle properties in Theorem 1.

***Proof of Theorem 1*** Denote $\boldsymbol{\theta} = (\boldsymbol{\alpha}^T, \boldsymbol{\beta}^T)^T$ for any $\boldsymbol{\alpha} \in \mathbb{R}^{p_2}$, $\boldsymbol{\beta} \in \mathbb{R}^{p_1}$, $\hat{\boldsymbol{\theta}}_n = (\hat{\boldsymbol{\alpha}}_n^T, \hat{\boldsymbol{\beta}}_n^T)^T$, and $\boldsymbol{\theta}_0 = (\boldsymbol{\alpha}_0^T, \boldsymbol{\beta}_0^T)^T$. Let $\boldsymbol{\Phi} = (\boldsymbol{Z}, \boldsymbol{X}) \in \mathbb{R}^{p \times p}$, where $p_1 + p_2 = p$. We first prove the model selection consistency part. Lemma 2 shows that the estimator minimizing the objective function (3) is equivalent to $(\tilde{\boldsymbol{\theta}}_{n\mathcal{S}}, 0)$. Thus, it suffices to show that $\Pr(\min_{s\in\mathcal{S}} |\tilde{\theta}_{ns}| > 0) \to 1$. Let $\eta = \min_{s\in\mathcal{S}} |\theta_{0s}|$. Note that

$$\min_{s\in\mathcal{S}} |\tilde{\theta}_{ns}| > \min_{s\in\mathcal{S}} |\theta_{0s}| - \left\| \tilde{\boldsymbol{\theta}}_{n\mathcal{S}} - \boldsymbol{\theta}_{0\mathcal{S}} \right\|_2.$$

By Lemma 1, it is straightforward that

$$\left\| \tilde{\boldsymbol{\theta}}_{n\mathcal{S}} - \boldsymbol{\theta}_{0\mathcal{S}} \right\|_2^2 = O_P\left(\frac{p_2 + r}{n}\right).$$

Therefore it follows that

$$\min_{s\in\mathcal{S}} |\tilde{\theta}_{ns}| > \eta - \sqrt{\frac{p_2 + r}{n}} O_P(1)$$

and finally $\Pr(\min_{s\in\mathcal{S}} |\tilde{\theta}_{ns}| > 0) \to 1$.

Now we show the asymptotic normality part. Note that from Lemma 2 the estimator $\tilde{\boldsymbol{\theta}}_{n\mathcal{S}}$ satisfies the following first order equation:

$$-2nE_n\left[\phi_s(Y-\boldsymbol{\Phi}_{\mathcal{S}}^T\tilde{\boldsymbol{\theta}}_{n\mathcal{S}})\right]+\lambda_n\hat{w}_s\,\mathrm{sgn}(\tilde{\theta}_{ns})I\,(s\in\mathcal{S}\backslash\{1,\dots,p_2\})=0\quad\text{for }s\in\mathcal{S}.$$

Since $\theta_{0s}=0$ for $\forall s\in\mathcal{S}^c$ and $\epsilon=Y-\boldsymbol{\Phi}_{\mathcal{S}}^T\boldsymbol{\theta}_{0\mathcal{S}}$, this equation can be written

$$-2nE_n\left[\phi_s\boldsymbol{\Phi}_{\mathcal{S}}^T(\boldsymbol{\theta}_{0\mathcal{S}}-\tilde{\boldsymbol{\theta}}_{n\mathcal{S}})\right]-2nE_n(\phi_s\epsilon)$$
$$+\lambda_n\hat{w}_s\,\mathrm{sgn}(\tilde{\theta}_{ns})I\,(s\in\mathcal{S}\backslash\{1,\dots,p_2\})=0\quad\text{for }s\in\mathcal{S}.$$

Therefore, we have

$$\sqrt{n}\boldsymbol{\Sigma}_{\mathcal{S}}(\tilde{\boldsymbol{\theta}}_{n\mathcal{S}}-\boldsymbol{\theta}_{0\mathcal{S}})=\sqrt{n}E_n(\boldsymbol{\Phi}_{\mathcal{S}}\epsilon)-\frac{\lambda_n}{2\sqrt{n}}\hat{w}_{\mathcal{S}}\,\mathrm{sgn}(\tilde{\boldsymbol{\theta}}_{n\mathcal{S}})I_{\mathcal{S}}+\sqrt{n}(\boldsymbol{\Sigma}_{\mathcal{S}}-\hat{\boldsymbol{\Sigma}}_{\mathcal{S}})(\tilde{\boldsymbol{\theta}}_{n\mathcal{S}}-\boldsymbol{\theta}_{0\mathcal{S}})$$

where $I_{\mathcal{S}}=(0_1\dots,0_{p_2},1_{p_2+1},\dots,1_{p_2+r})^T$.

Let $D_n=\sqrt{n}\psi^T\boldsymbol{\Sigma}_{\mathcal{S}}^{1/2}(\tilde{\boldsymbol{\theta}}_{n\mathcal{S}}-\boldsymbol{\theta}_{0\mathcal{S}})$. Then $D_n=T_1+T_2+T_3$, where

$$T_1=\sqrt{n}\psi^T\boldsymbol{\Sigma}_{\mathcal{S}}^{-1/2}E_n(\boldsymbol{\Phi}_{\mathcal{S}}\epsilon),$$
$$T_2=-\frac{\lambda_n}{2\sqrt{n}}\psi^T\boldsymbol{\Sigma}_{\mathcal{S}}^{-1/2}\hat{w}_{\mathcal{S}}\,\mathrm{sgn}(\tilde{\boldsymbol{\theta}}_{n\mathcal{S}})I_{\mathcal{S}},$$
$$T_3=\sqrt{n}\psi^T\boldsymbol{\Sigma}_{\mathcal{S}}^{-1/2}(\boldsymbol{\Sigma}_{\mathcal{S}}-\hat{\boldsymbol{\Sigma}}_{\mathcal{S}})(\tilde{\boldsymbol{\theta}}_{n\mathcal{S}}-\boldsymbol{\theta}_{0\mathcal{S}}).$$

Using similar techniques as in the proof of Zou and Zhang [32], we obtain $D_n\to_d N(0,\sigma^2)$. The result follows from Lemma 2 that with probability tending to 1, $\sqrt{n}\psi^T\boldsymbol{\Sigma}_{\mathcal{S}}^{1/2}(\hat{\boldsymbol{\theta}}_{n\mathcal{S}}-\boldsymbol{\theta}_{0\mathcal{S}})=D_n\to_d N(0,\sigma^2)$.

**Proof of Theorem 2** We show the convergence rate of the value function of the estimated policy. Observe that

$$E[\boldsymbol{\Phi}^T(\hat{\boldsymbol{\theta}}_n-\boldsymbol{\theta}_0)]^2=E[\boldsymbol{\Phi}_{\mathcal{S}}^T(\hat{\boldsymbol{\theta}}_{n\mathcal{S}}-\boldsymbol{\theta}_{0\mathcal{S}})+\boldsymbol{\Phi}_{\mathcal{S}^c}^T(\hat{\boldsymbol{\theta}}_{n\mathcal{S}^c}-\boldsymbol{\theta}_{0\mathcal{S}^c})]^2$$
$$\leq 2(\hat{\boldsymbol{\theta}}_{n\mathcal{S}}-\boldsymbol{\theta}_{0\mathcal{S}})^T E\left[\boldsymbol{\Phi}_{\mathcal{S}}\boldsymbol{\Phi}_{\mathcal{S}}^T\right](\hat{\boldsymbol{\theta}}_{n\mathcal{S}}-\boldsymbol{\theta}_{0\mathcal{S}})$$
$$+2E(\hat{\boldsymbol{\theta}}_{n\mathcal{S}^c}-\boldsymbol{\theta}_{0\mathcal{S}^c})^T E\left[\boldsymbol{\Phi}_{\mathcal{S}^c}\boldsymbol{\Phi}_{\mathcal{S}^c}^T\right](\hat{\boldsymbol{\theta}}_{n\mathcal{S}^c}-\boldsymbol{\theta}_{0\mathcal{S}^c})$$
$$\leq 2B\left\|\hat{\boldsymbol{\theta}}_{n\mathcal{S}}-\boldsymbol{\theta}_{0\mathcal{S}}\right\|_2^2+2B\left\|\hat{\boldsymbol{\theta}}_{n\mathcal{S}^c}-\boldsymbol{\theta}_{0\mathcal{S}^c}\right\|_2^2.$$

By Theorem 1, it is true that for any $a_n$

$$P\left(a_n^{-1}\left\|\hat{\boldsymbol{\theta}}_{n\mathcal{S}^c} - \boldsymbol{\theta}_{0\mathcal{S}^c}\right\|_2^2 > \epsilon\right) \le P(\exists s \in \mathcal{S}^c, \hat{\theta}_s \ne 0) \to 0,$$

and since $\left\|\hat{\boldsymbol{\theta}}_{n\mathcal{S}} - \boldsymbol{\theta}_{0\mathcal{S}}\right\|_2^2 = O_P(\frac{p_2+r}{n})$, we have

$$E[\boldsymbol{\Phi}^T(\hat{\boldsymbol{\theta}}_n - \boldsymbol{\theta}_0)]^2 \le O_P\left(\frac{p_2+r}{n}\right) + o_P(1)$$

$$= O_P\left(\frac{p_2+r}{n}\right).$$

Hence, using Theorem 1 of Qian and Murphy [15], we obtain

$$V(\pi_0) - V(\hat{\pi}) \le E[\boldsymbol{\Phi}^T(\hat{\boldsymbol{\theta}}_n - \boldsymbol{\theta}_0)]^2$$

$$\le O_P\left[\left(\frac{p_2+r}{n}\right)^{(1+\eta)/(2+\eta)}\right].$$

**Proof of Lemma 1** The PRO-aLasso estimator minimizing the objective function (3) can be re-written as

$$\hat{\boldsymbol{\theta}}_n(\lambda_n) = \arg\min_{\boldsymbol{\theta}} nE_n(Y - \boldsymbol{\Phi}^T\boldsymbol{\theta})^2 + \lambda_n \sum_{s=p_2+1}^{p} \hat{w}_s|\theta_s|.$$

We know that for $s \in \{1\ldots, p\}$, the estimator $\hat{\boldsymbol{\theta}}_n(\lambda_n)$ satisfies the first order equation: $-2nE_n\left[\phi_s(Y - \boldsymbol{\Phi}^T\hat{\boldsymbol{\theta}}_n(\lambda_n))\right] + \lambda_n\hat{w}_s\text{sgn}(\hat{\theta}_{ns}(\lambda_n))I(s \in \{p_2+1, \ldots, p\}) = 0$, where $\text{sgn}(\theta_s) = 1$ if $\theta_s > 0$, $\text{sgn}(\theta_s) = -1$ if $\theta_s < 0$, and $\text{sgn}(\theta_s) \in [-1, 1]$ if $\theta_s = 0$ for any $\theta_s \in \mathbb{R}$. This implies

$$-2nE_n\left[\boldsymbol{\Phi}(Y - \boldsymbol{\Phi}^T\hat{\boldsymbol{\theta}}_n(\lambda_n))\right] + \lambda_n\hat{\boldsymbol{w}}\,\text{sgn}(\hat{\boldsymbol{\theta}}_n(\lambda_n))\boldsymbol{I} = 0,$$

where $\boldsymbol{I} = (0_1, \ldots, 0_{p_2}, 1_{p_2+1}, \ldots, 1_p)^T$. Note that assumption (A4) implies $\lambda_{\min}(\hat{\boldsymbol{\Sigma}} - \boldsymbol{\Sigma}) \le \lambda_{\max}(\hat{\boldsymbol{\Sigma}} - \boldsymbol{\Sigma}) \to_p 0$. Then by the Courant-Fischer min-max Theorem, we have $\lambda_{\min}(\boldsymbol{\Sigma}) + \lambda_{\min}(\hat{\boldsymbol{\Sigma}} - \boldsymbol{\Sigma}) \le \lambda_{\min}(\hat{\boldsymbol{\Sigma}})$ and $\lambda_{\max}(\hat{\boldsymbol{\Sigma}}) \le \lambda_{\max}(\boldsymbol{\Sigma}) + \lambda_{\max}(\hat{\boldsymbol{\Sigma}} - \boldsymbol{\Sigma})$. This implies $\lambda_{\min}(\hat{\boldsymbol{\Sigma}}) \to_p b$ and $\lambda_{\max}(\hat{\boldsymbol{\Sigma}}) \to_p B$, respectively, by assumption (A3). Also, note that the estimator $\hat{\boldsymbol{\theta}}_n(0)$ satisfies $-2nE_n\left[\boldsymbol{\Phi}(Y - \boldsymbol{\Phi}^T\hat{\boldsymbol{\theta}}_n(0))\right] = 0$. Therefore,

$$E_n\boldsymbol{\Phi}\boldsymbol{\Phi}^T(\hat{\boldsymbol{\theta}}_n(\lambda_n) - \hat{\boldsymbol{\theta}}_n(0)) = \frac{\lambda_n\hat{\boldsymbol{w}}\,\text{sgn}(\hat{\boldsymbol{\theta}}_n(\lambda_n))\boldsymbol{I}}{2n},$$

which yields

$$\left\|\hat{\boldsymbol{\theta}}_n(0) - \hat{\boldsymbol{\theta}}_n(\lambda_n)\right\|_2^2 \le \frac{\lambda_n^2(\sum_{s=p_2+1}^{p} \hat{w}_s^2)}{4n^2(\lambda_{\min}(\hat{\boldsymbol{\Sigma}}))^2},$$

since $(\operatorname{sgn}(\theta_s))^2 \le 1$ for any $\theta_s \in \mathbb{R}$. Also, note that $\hat{\boldsymbol{\theta}}_n(\lambda_n) - \boldsymbol{\theta}_0 = (\hat{\boldsymbol{\theta}}_n(\lambda_n) - \hat{\boldsymbol{\theta}}_n(0)) + \hat{\boldsymbol{\Sigma}}^{-1} E_n \boldsymbol{\Phi} \epsilon$. Then it follows that

$$\left\|\hat{\boldsymbol{\theta}}_n(\lambda_n) - \boldsymbol{\theta}_0\right\|_2^2 \le 2 \left\|\hat{\boldsymbol{\theta}}_n(\lambda_n) - \hat{\boldsymbol{\theta}}_n(0)\right\|_2^2 + 2\frac{\|E_n \boldsymbol{\Phi} \epsilon\|_2^2}{(\lambda_{\min}(\hat{\boldsymbol{\Sigma}}))^2}$$

$$\le 2\frac{\lambda_n^2(\sum_{s=p_2+1}^{p} \hat{w}_s^2) + n^2 \|E_n \boldsymbol{\Phi} \epsilon\|_2^2}{n^2(\lambda_{\min}(\hat{\boldsymbol{\Sigma}}))^2},$$

$$\le 2\frac{\lambda_n^2 p_1 + \|n E_n \boldsymbol{\Phi} \epsilon\|_2^2}{n^2(\lambda_{\min}(\hat{\boldsymbol{\Sigma}}))^2},$$

where we set $\hat{w}_s = 1$ for all $s \in \{p_2 + 1, \ldots, p\}$ in the last inequality. Note that $E \|n E_n \boldsymbol{\Phi} \epsilon\|_2^2 = E(\sum_{i=1}^{n} \boldsymbol{\Phi}_i \epsilon_i)^2 = n\sigma^2 E(\boldsymbol{\Phi}^T \boldsymbol{\Phi}) = n\sigma^2 \operatorname{Tr}(E(\boldsymbol{\Phi}^T \boldsymbol{\Phi})) = n\sigma^2 \operatorname{Tr}(\boldsymbol{\Sigma}) \le n\sigma^2 p\lambda_{\max}(\boldsymbol{\Sigma})$. Thus, $\left\|\hat{\boldsymbol{\theta}}_n(\lambda_n) - \boldsymbol{\theta}_0\right\|_2^2 = O_P(p/n)$.

**Proof of Lemma 2** Denote $\tilde{\boldsymbol{\theta}}_{n\mathcal{S}} = (\tilde{\boldsymbol{\alpha}}_n^T, \tilde{\boldsymbol{\beta}}_{n\mathcal{J}}^T)^T$. We show that $(\tilde{\boldsymbol{\theta}}_{n\mathcal{S}}, 0)$ satisfies the KKT condition of (3) with probability tending to 1. It suffices to show that

$$\Pr(\exists s \in \mathcal{S}^c \mid -2n E_n \phi_s(Y - \boldsymbol{\Phi}_{\mathcal{S}}^T \tilde{\boldsymbol{\theta}}_{n\mathcal{S}})| > \lambda_n \hat{w}_s) \to 0. \tag{5}$$

Note that (5) can be regarded as the adaptive elastic-net problem when the $L_2$ penalty is eliminated, and thus the proof follows Zou and Zhang [32].

# References

1. Cheung, K., Ling, W., Karr, C., Weingardt, K., Schueller, S., & Mohr, D. (2018). Evaluation of a recommender app for apps for the treatment of depression and anxiety: An analysis of longitudinal user engagement. *Journal of the American Medical Informatics Association, 25*(8), 955–962.
2. Christensen, H., Griffiths, K., & Farrer, L. (2009). Adherence in internet interventions for anxiety and depression. *Journal of Medical Internet Research, 11*(2), e13.
3. Fan, J., & Li, R. (2001). Variable selection via nonconcave penalized likelihood and its oracle properties. *Journal of the American Statistical Association, 96*(456), 1348–1360.
4. Foster, J., Taylor, J., & Ruberg, S. (2011). Subgroup identification from randomized clinical trial data. *Statistics in Medicine, 30*(24), 2867–2880.
5. Friedman, J., Hastie, J.,& Tibshirani, R. (2010). Regularization paths for generalized linear models via coordinate descent. *Journal of Statistical Software, 33*(1), 1–22.

6. Gunter, L., Zhu, J., & Murphy, S. (2011). Variable selection for qualitative interactions. *Statistical Methodology, 8* (1), 42–55.
7. Kazdin, A. & Blase, S. (2011). Rebooting psychotherapy research and practice to reduce the burden of mental illness. *Perspectives on Psychological Science, 6*(1), 21–37.
8. Laber, E., & Zhao, Y. (2015). Tree-based methods for individualized treatment regimes. *Biometrika, 102*(3), 501–514.
9. Lattie, E., Schueller, S., Sargent, E., Stiles-Shields, C., Tomasino, K., Corden, M., et al. (2016). Uptake and usage of intellicare: A publicly available suite of mental health and well-being apps. *Internet Interventions, 4*(2), 152–158.
10. Ledoit, O., & Wolf, M. (2004). A well-conditioned estimator for large-dimensional covariance matrices. *Journal of Multivariate Analysis, 88*(2), 365–411.
11. Lipkovich, I., Dmitrienko, A., Denne, J., & Enas, G. (2011). Subgroup identification based on differential effect search: A recursive partitioning method for establishing response to treatment in patient subpopulations. *Statistics in Medicine,30*(21), 2601–2621.
12. Lu, W., Zhang, H., & Zeng, D. (2013). Variable selection for optimal treatment decision. *Statistical Methods in Medical Research, 22*(5), 493–504.
13. Mohr, D., Schueller, S., Montague, E., Burns, M., & Rashidi, P. (2014). The behavioral intervention technology model: An integrated conceptual and technological framework for ehealth and mhealth interventions. *Journal of Medical Internet Research, 16*(6), e146.
14. Murphy, S. (2005). A generalization error for Q-learning. *Journal of Machine Learning Research, 6,* 1073–1097.
15. Qian, M., & Murphy, S. (2011). Performance guarantees for individualized treatment rules. *Annals of Statistics, 39*(2), 1180–1210.
16. Research 2 Guidance. (2013). Mobile health market report 2013–2017: The commercialization of mhealth application (Vol. 3). Berlin: Research 2 Guidance.
17. Rudin, C., & Ertekin, Ş. (2018). Learning customized and optimized lists of rules with mathematical programming. *Mathematical Programming Computation, 10*(4), 659–702.
18. Su, X., Zhou, T., Yan, X., & Fan, J. (2008). Interaction trees with censored survival data. *International Journal of Biostatistics, 4*(1), 1–26.
19. Sutton, R., & Barto, A. (2017). *Reinforcement learning: An introduction* (2nd edn.). Cambridge, MA: MIT Press.
20. Tibshirani, Tibshirani, R. (1996). Regression shrinkage and selection via the lasso. *Journal of the Royal Statistical Society: Series B, 58*(1), 267–288.
21. Yuan, M., & Lin, Y. (2007). On the non-negative garrotte estimator. *Journal of the Royal Statistical Society: Series B, 69*(2), 143–161.
22. Zhang, B., Tsiatis, A., Davidian, M., Zhang, M., & Laber, E. (2012). Estimating optimal treatment regimes from a classification perspective. *Stat, 1*(1), 103–114.
23. Zhang, B., Tsiatis, A., Laber, E., & Davidian, M. (2012). A robust method for estimating optimal treatment regimes. *Biometrics, 68*(4), 1010–1018.
24. Zhang, B., Tsiatis, A., Laber, E., & Davidian, M. (2013). Robust estimation of optimal dynamic treatment regimes for sequential treatment decisions. *Biometrika, 100*(3), 681–694.
25. Zhang, B., & Zhang, M. (2018). C-learning: A new classification framework to estimate optimal dynamic treatment regimes. *Biometrics, 74*(3), 891–899.
26. Zhang, Y., Laber, E., Davidian, M., & Tsiatis, A. (2018). Estimation of optimal treatment regimes using lists. *Journal of the American Statistical Association, 71*(4), 895–904.
27. Zhang, Y., Laber, E., Tsiatis, A., & Davidian, M. (2015). Using decision lists to construct interpretable and parsimonious treatment regimes. *Biometrics, 71*(4), 895–904.
28. Zhao, Y., Zeng, D., Laber, E., & Korosok, M. (2015). New statistical learning methods for estimating optimal dynamic treatment regimes. *Journal of the American Statistical Association, 110*(510), 583–598.
29. Zhao, Y., Zeng, D., Rush, A., & Korosok, M. (2012). Estimating individualized treatment rules using outcome weighted learning. *Journal of the American Statistical Association, 107*(449), 11061118.

30. Zou, H. (2006). The adaptive lasso and its oracle properties. *Journal of the American Statistical Association, 101*(476), 1418–1429.
31. Zou, H., & Hastie, T. (2005). Regularization and variable selection via the elastic net. *Journal of the Royal Statistical Society: Series B, 67*(2), 301–320.
32. Zou, H., & Zhang, H. (2009). On the adaptive elastic-net with a diverging number of parameters. *Annals of Statistics, 37*(4), 1733–1751.

# Hierarchical Continuous Time Hidden Markov Model, with Application in Zero-Inflated Accelerometer Data

**Zekun Xu, Eric B. Laber, and Ana-Maria Staicu**

**Abstract** Wearable devices including accelerometers are increasingly being used to collect high-frequency human activity data in situ. There is tremendous potential to use such data to inform medical decision making and public health policies. However, modeling such data is challenging as they are high-dimensional, heterogeneous, and subject to informative missingness, e.g., zero readings when the device is removed by the participant. We propose a flexible and extensible continuous-time hidden Markov model to extract meaningful activity patterns from human accelerometer data. To facilitate estimation with massive data we derive an efficient learning algorithm that exploits the hierarchical structure of the parameters indexing the proposed model. We also propose a bootstrap procedure for interval estimation. The proposed methods are illustrated using data from the 2003–2004 and 2005–2006 National Health and Nutrition Examination Survey.

**Keywords** Continuous-time hidden Markov model · Consensus optimization · Accelerometer data

## 1 Introduction

The development of the wearable technology has given rise to a variety of sensing devices and modalities. Some of these devices, e.g., Fitbit or Apple Watch, can be worn continuously and thereby produce huge volumes of high-frequency human activity data. Because these data present little burden on the wearer to collect and

**Electronic Supplementary Material** The online version of this chapter (https://doi.org/10.1007/978-3-030-33416-1_7) contains supplementary material, which is available to authorized users.

Z. Xu (✉) · E. B. Laber · A.-M. Staicu
Department of Statistics, North Carolina State University, Raleigh, NC, USA
e-mail: zxu13@ncsu.edu; elaber@ncsu.edu; astaicu@ncsu.edu

© Springer Nature Switzerland AG 2020
Y. Zhao, D.-G. (Din) Chen (eds.), *Statistical Modeling in Biomedical Research*, Emerging Topics in Statistics and Biostatistics, https://doi.org/10.1007/978-3-030-33416-1_7

provide rich information on the in situ behavior of the wearer, they have tremendous potential to inform decision making in healthcare. Examples of remote sensing data in healthcare include elder care, remote monitoring of chronic disease, and addition management [3, 12, 18]. Accelerometers are among the most commonly used and most widely studied types of wearable devices, they have been used both in randomized clinical trials to evaluate treatment effect on activity-related impairment [15, 21] and in observational studies to characterize activity patterns in a free-living environment [12, 20, 36]. However, despite rapidly growing interest and investment in wearable devices for the study of human activity data, a general and extensible class of models for analysis of the resulting data is lacking.

We propose a continuous-time hidden Markov model for the modeling human accelerometer data that aligns with scientific (conceptual) models of human activity data; in the proposed model, latent states correspond to latent (unobserved) activities, e.g., resting, running, jumping, etc., that are shared across the population yet the accelerometer signatures within these activities are allowed to vary across subjects. Furthermore, differences across subgroups, e.g., defined by sex, age, or the presence-absence of a comorbid condition, can be identified by aggregating individual-level effects across these groups. This work is motivated in part by the physical activity data set from the 2003–2004 National Health and Nutrition Examination Survey (NHANES). In this study, human activity patterns were measured at one-minute intervals for up to 7 days using the ActiGraph Model 7164 accelerometer [19, 29, 33]. Activity for each minute was recorded as an integer-valued intensity-level commonly referred to as an activity count. In the study, subjects were instructed to remove the device during sleep or while washing (to keep it dry). Therefore, the observed data comprise high-frequency, integer-valued activity counts for each subject with intervals of missing values corresponding to when the device was removed.

The goal of paper is to use the observed data to characterize activity patterns of each subject, subjects within pre-defined subgroups, and the population as a whole. This is important because the estimated physical activity model can potentially serve the following three purposes. On the subject level, the estimated activity model can be used both for the prediction of future activities and the imputation of missing activity readings. On the subgroup level, the estimated activity patterns provide useful insights into clustering people based on their activity profiles. On the population level, public policies can be designed based on the estimated activity model so as to encourage everyday exercise and healthy life style.

Prior work on modeling activity counts has focused on aggregation and other smoothing techniques. One common approach is to average the activity counts over time for each subject and then compare the group means using two-sample $t$-tests [33], analysis of covariance [12], or linear mixed effects models [7]. However, in these approaches, averaging focuses on overall activity levels and may obscure trends in activity type, activity duration, and transitions between activities. Another approach is to use functional data analysis methods wherein the integer activity counts are first log-transformed to fix the right-skewedness in the distribution and the transformed activity modeled as a function of time of day and other covariates [11, 20, 36]. These approaches are best-suited for the identification of smooth, cyclical patterns in the data whereas the observed accelerometer data are characterized by abrupt (i.e., non-smooth) changes in activity levels.

Discrete-time hidden Markov models are another common approach to the analysis of mobility data measured by wearable devices [13, 22, 28, 35]. In these models, activity is partitioned into different latent behavioral states and the observed activity count is dependent on the unobserved latent activity. The latent states evolve according to a discrete-time Markov process and a primary goal is the correct classification of the latent activity. To construct and validate these models requires training data that are labeled by latent activity. However, the NHANES data, like many accelerometer studies, are not labeled by activity. Furthermore, our goal is to identify the dynamics of a patients evolution through these latent activities including activity duration, activity intensity, and transitions between activities. Discrete-time hidden Markov models have been used to model latent health states and subsequently conduct inference for activity patterns within each state [2, 30, 32], but the time scales in these applications are rather coarse (daily or weekly). By contrast, the physical activity in the NHANES data is measured for each minute; this results in a much larger data volume and the ability to provide are more complete picture of activity dynamics.

A technical limitation of the discrete-time approach, is that it assumes that the observations are equally spaced in time. Continuous-time hidden Markov models (CTHMM) have been used to analyze the irregularly-sampled temporal measurements [17, 23, 34]. The flexibility of the CTHMM comes at the expense of increased computational cost, which makes it infeasible for large datasets without modification. Liu et al. [17] developed an efficient learning algorithm for parameter estimation in the CTHMMs. However, this algorithm is only suitable for either the completely pooled or unpooled cases wherein all subjects are assumed to be either completely homogeneous so that they share the same parameters, or completely heterogeneous so that all parameters are subject-specific. Moreover, the algorithm cannot estimate the effects of subject covariates and environmental factors on activity counts.

We propose to model minute-by-minute accelerometer data using a hierarchical continuous-time hidden Markov model (HCTHMM). This model is aligned with scientific models of activity as the latent states represent different types of unobserved physical activities. The continuous-time Markov process for the latent states evolution avoids having to perform imputation for missing yet allows for the possibility that the temporal measurements are irregularly spaced. Furthermore, the proposed model can incorporate both baseline subject covariates and time-varying environmental factors. The proposed model is hierarchical in that it is parameterized by: (1) subject-specific parameters to account for variability between subjects; (2) subgroup-specific parameters parameters to account for similarity in activity patterns within groups; (3) population parameters that are common across all subjects. This specification allows us to pool information on some parameters while retaining between-group and between-subject variability. We proposed an estimator of these parameters that is based on consensus optimization using the alternating direction method of multipliers (ADMM). There is a vast literature on the convergence properties of ADMM [4, 14, 31] which can be readily ported to the proposed algorithm. Finally, we use the nonparametric bootstrap [9] to estimate the sampling distributions of parameter estimators and to conduct statistical inference.

## 2 Model Framework

We assume that the observed data are of the form $\{\mathbf{W}_i, Y_i(\mathbf{T}_i), \mathbf{X}_i(\mathbf{T}_i)\}_{i=1}^n$, which comprise $n$ independent copies of the trajectory $\{\mathbf{W}, Y(\mathbf{T}), \mathbf{X}(\mathbf{T})\}$, where: $\mathbf{W} \in \mathbb{R}^p$ are baseline subject characteristics; $Y(\mathbf{T}) = \{Y(T_1), \ldots, Y(T_K)\}$ are the non-negative integer activity counts at times $\mathbf{T} = (T_1, \ldots, T_K) \in [0, 1]^K$; and $\mathbf{X}(\mathbf{T}) = \{\mathbf{X}(T_1), \ldots, \mathbf{X}(T_K)\}$ are concurrent environmental factors such that $\mathbf{X}(\cdot) \in \mathbb{R}^q$. Both $\mathbf{T}$ and $K$ are treated as random variables as the number and timing of observations vary across subjects. We model the evolution of the observed data using a hierarchical continuous-time hidden Markov model (HCTHMM), which we will develop over the remainder of this section.

Let $S_i(t) \in \{1, \ldots, M\}$ denote the unobserved latent state for subject $i = 1, \ldots, n$ at time $t \in [0, 1]$. The latent state evolves according to a Markov process indexed by: (1) an initial state distribution $\pi_i(m) \triangleq P\{S_i(0) = m)\}$ for $m = 1, \ldots, M$ such that $\sum_{m=1}^M \pi_i(m) = 1$; (2) a transition rate matrix $\mathbf{Q}_i = \{q_i(m, \ell)\}_{m,\ell=1,\ldots,M}$ such that $q_i(m, m) = -\sum_{\ell \neq m} q_i(m, \ell)$. The transition rate matrix, also known as the infinitesimal generator matrix, describes the rate of movements between states in a continuous-time Markov chain [1, 24, 25]; the transition probabilities are derived from the transition rates through a matrix exponential operation such that for $k = 1, \ldots, K - 1$ and $t > u$, $P_i^{t-u}(m, \ell) \triangleq P\{S_i(t) = \ell | S_i(u) = m\} = \{e^{(t-u)\mathbf{Q}_i}\}_{m,\ell}$.

We assume that the conditional distribution of the activity counts is homogeneous in time given the current latent state and environmental factors (to streamline notation, we include baseline characteristics in the time-varying environmental factors). For $i = 1, \ldots, n$ and $m = 1, \ldots, M$ define $g_{i,m}(y; \mathbf{x}) \triangleq P\{Y_i(t) = y | S_i(t) = m, \mathbf{X}_i(t) = \mathbf{x}\}$. Because longitudinal activity count data are zero-inflated, we set $g_{i,1}(y; \mathbf{x})$ to be the probability mass function for a zero-inflated Poisson distribution with structural zero proportion $\delta_i$ and mean $\lambda_{i,1}$ for state 1 such that

$$g_{i,1}(y; \mathbf{x}) = \delta_i(\mathbf{x})1_{y=0} + \{1 - \delta_i(\mathbf{x})\} \frac{\{\lambda_{i,1}(\mathbf{x})\}^y \exp\{\lambda_{i,1}(\mathbf{x})\}}{y!}.$$

For $m = 2, \ldots, M$ we model the activity counts using a Poisson regression model so that

$$g_{i,m}(y; \mathbf{x}) = \frac{\{\lambda_{i,m}(\mathbf{x})\}^y \exp\{\lambda_{i,m}(\mathbf{x})\}}{y!}.$$

For each subject $i$, and latent state $m$, we assume that functions $\delta_i(\mathbf{x})$ and $\lambda_{i,m}(\mathbf{x})$ are of the form

$$\log\left\{\frac{\delta_i(\mathbf{x})}{1-\delta_i(\mathbf{x})}\right\} = b_{i,0,0} + \mathbf{x}'\mathbf{b}_{i,0,1},$$

$$\log\left\{\lambda_{i,m}(\mathbf{x})\right\} = b_{i,m,0} + \mathbf{x}'\mathbf{b}_{i,m,1},$$

where $b_{i,0,0}, \ldots, b_{i,M,0}$ and $\mathbf{b}_{i,0,1}, \ldots, \mathbf{b}_{i,M,1}$ are unknown coefficients.

In the foregoing model description, all parameters are subject-specific so that each subject's trajectory can be modeled separately. However, in the HCTHMM, some of the parameters are shared among pre-defined subgroups of the subjects. We assume that subjects are partitioned into $J$ such subgroups based on their baseline characteristics $\mathbf{W}$. For example, these groups might be determined by age and sex. Subjects within the same group are though to behave more similarly to each other than across groups. Let $G_i \in \{1, \ldots, J\}$ be the subgroup to which subject $i$ belongs, and let $n_j$ denote the number of subjects in group $j = 1, \ldots, J$.

The HCTHMM is a flexible multilevel model in that it allows for three levels of of parameters: (1) subject-specific, (2) subgroup-specific, (3) population-level. For example, one might let the intercepts in the generalized linear models for state-dependent parameters be subject-specific to account for the between-subject variability; let the initial state probabilities and the transition rate parameters depend on group-membership, i.e. $\pi_{i_1} = \pi_{i_2}$ and $\mathbf{Q}_{i_1} = \mathbf{Q}_{i_2}$ for all $i_1, i_2$ such that $G_{i_1} = G_{i_2}$; and let the slope parameters in the generalized linear models for state-dependent parameters be common across all subjects.

If all the observed time points are equally spaced and all the parameters are subject-specific, the HCTHMM reduces to the subject-specific zero-inflated Poisson hidden Markov model. If there are no covariates and all parameters are common for all subjects, the HCTHMM reduces to a zero-inflated variant of the continuous-time hidden Markov model [17]. The extension from the previous models to the HCTHMM better matches the scientific goals associated with analyzing the NHANES data but also requires new methods for estimation. Because of the hierarchical structure in the parameters, joint parameter estimation is no longer embarrassingly parallelizable as it would be in the case of its completely pooled or unpooled counterparts.

# 3 Parameter Estimation

## 3.1 Forward-Backward Algorithm

For subject $i = 1, \ldots, n$, let $\mathbf{a}_i \in \mathbb{R}^{M-1}$ be the $M-1$ free parameters in the initial probabilities $\pi_i$, and let $\mathbf{c}_i \in \mathbb{R}^{M(M-1)}$ be the $M(M-1)$ free parameters in the transition matrix $\mathbf{Q}_i$. To simplify notation, write $\mathbf{b}_{i,0} \triangleq [b_{i,0,0}, \ldots, b_{i,M,0}] \in \mathbb{R}^{M+1}$

and $\mathbf{b}_{i,1} \triangleq [\mathbf{b}'_{i,0,1}, \ldots, \mathbf{b}'_{i,M,1}] \in \mathbb{R}^{q(M+1)}$ to denote the parameters indexing the generalized linear models for the activity counts in each state. Define the entire vector of parameters for subject $i$ to be $\boldsymbol{\theta}_i \triangleq [\mathbf{a}'_i, \mathbf{c}'_i, \mathbf{b}'_{i,0}, \mathbf{b}'_{i,1}] \in \mathbb{R}^{(M+1)(M+q)}$. The likelihood function for subject $i$ is computed using the forward-backward algorithm [26] as follows. For subject $i = 1, \ldots, n$, define the forward variables for $k = 1, \ldots, K - 1$, and $m = 1, \ldots, M$,

$$
\alpha_i^{T_k}(m; \boldsymbol{\theta}_i) \triangleq P_{\boldsymbol{\theta}_i} \left\{ Y_i(T_1), \ldots, Y_i(T_k), S_i(T_k) = m \Big| X_i(T_1) = \mathbf{x}_{T_1}, \right.
$$

$$
\left. \ldots, X_i(T_k) = \mathbf{x}_{T_k} \right\}.
$$

The initialization and recursion formulas are defined as

$$
\alpha_i^{T_1}(m; \boldsymbol{\theta}_i) = \pi_i(m; \boldsymbol{\theta}_i) g_{i,m}\{Y_i(T_1); \mathbf{x}_{T_1}, \boldsymbol{\theta}_i\},
$$

$$
\alpha_i^{T_{k+1}}(m; \boldsymbol{\theta}_i) = \left[ \sum_{\ell=1}^{M} \alpha_i^{T_k}(\ell; \boldsymbol{\theta}_i) \{e^{(T_{k+1} - T_k)\mathbf{Q}_i}\}_{\ell,m} \right] g_{i,m}\{Y_i(T_{k+1});
$$

$$
\mathbf{x}_{T_{k+1}}, \boldsymbol{\theta}_i\},
$$

where $m = 1, \ldots, M$ and $k = 1, \ldots, K - 1$. The negative log-likelihood for $\boldsymbol{\theta}_i$ is therefore $f_i(\boldsymbol{\theta}_i) = -log\left\{\sum_{m=1}^{M} \alpha_i^{T_K}(m; \boldsymbol{\theta}_i)\right\}$. Define the joint likelihood for $\boldsymbol{\theta} = (\boldsymbol{\theta}_1, \ldots, \boldsymbol{\theta}_n)$ to be $f(\boldsymbol{\theta}) = \sum_{i=1}^{n} f_i(\boldsymbol{\theta}_i)$.

To compute the conditional state probabilities in the HCTHMM, we need to generate a set of auxiliary backward variables analogous to the forward variables defined previously. For subject $i = 1, \ldots, n$, define the backward variables for $k = 1, \ldots, K$, and $m = 1, \ldots, M$,

$$
\beta_i^{T_k}(m; \boldsymbol{\theta}_i) \triangleq P_{\boldsymbol{\theta}_i} \left\{ Y_i(T_{k+1}), \ldots, Y_i(T_K) \Big| S_i(T_k) = m, \right.
$$

$$
\left. X_i(T_{k+1}) = \mathbf{x}_{T_{k+1}}, \ldots, X_i(T_K) = \mathbf{x}_{T_K} \right\}.
$$

The initialization and recursion formulas are

$$
\beta_i^{T_K}(m; \boldsymbol{\theta}_i) = 1,
$$

$$
\beta_i^{T_k}(m; \boldsymbol{\theta}_i) = \sum_{\ell=1}^{M} \{e^{(T_{k+1} - T_k)\mathbf{Q}_i}\}_{m,\ell} \, g_{i,\ell}\{Y_i(T_{k+1}); \mathbf{x}_{T_{k+1}}, \boldsymbol{\theta}_i\}
$$

$$
\beta_i^{T_{k+1}}(\ell; \boldsymbol{\theta}_i),
$$

where $m = 1, \ldots, M$. The probability of state $m$ for subject $i$ at time $t$ is

$$\gamma_i^t(m; \boldsymbol{\theta}_i) \triangleq P_{\boldsymbol{\theta}_i}\{S_i(t) = m | Y_i(T_1), \ldots, Y_i(T_K)\}$$

$$= \frac{\alpha_i^t(m; \boldsymbol{\theta}_i)\beta_i^t(m; \boldsymbol{\theta}_i)}{\sum_{m=1}^M \alpha_i^t(m; \boldsymbol{\theta}_i)\beta_i^t(m; \boldsymbol{\theta}_i)},$$

where $t = T_1, \ldots, T_k$, $m = 1, \ldots, M$, and $i = 1, \ldots, n$. The mean probability of state $m$ among subjects in group $j$ is thus

$$\phi_j(m; \boldsymbol{\theta}) = \frac{1}{n_j} \sum_{\{i:G_i=j\}} \eta_i(m; \boldsymbol{\theta}_i), \quad j = 1, \ldots, J,$$

$$\text{where } \eta_i(m; \boldsymbol{\theta}_i) = \frac{1}{K} \sum_{k=1}^K \gamma_i^{T_k}(m; \boldsymbol{\theta}_i), \quad m = 1, \ldots, M.$$

The mean state probabilities $\phi_j(m; \boldsymbol{\theta})$ can be interpreted as the mean proportion of time spent in latent state $m$ for subjects in group $j$, whereas $\eta_i(m; \boldsymbol{\theta}_i)$ represents the mean proportion of time spent in state $m$ for subject $i$.

## 3.2 Consensus Optimization

If all sets of parameters are subject-specific, then the maximum likelihood estimates for the parameters can be obtained by minimizing $f(\boldsymbol{\theta})$ using the gradient-based methods which can be parallelized across subjects. However, in the general setting where parameters are shared across subgroups of subjects, such paralellization is no longer possible. Instead, we use the consensus optimization approach to obtain the maximum likelihood estimates in the HCTHMM, which is performed via the alternating direction method of multipliers (ADMM) [4]. We use the Bayesian Information Criterion (BIC) to select the number of latent states $M$.

Let $\mathbf{D}$ denote a contrast matrix such that $\mathbf{D}\boldsymbol{\theta} = 0$ corresponds to equality of subgroup-specific parameters within each subgroup and equality of all population-level parameters across all subjects. The maximum likelihood estimator solves

$$\min_{\boldsymbol{\theta}} f(\boldsymbol{\theta}) \quad s.t. \quad \mathbf{D}\boldsymbol{\theta} = 0.$$

For the purpose of illustration, suppose that: (1) the intercepts in the generalized linear models for state-dependent parameters are subject-specific; (2) the initial state probabilities and the transition rate parameters are subgroup-specific; (3) the slope parameters in the generalized linear models for state-dependent parameters are common across all subjects. Then $\mathbf{D}\boldsymbol{\theta} = 0$ is the same as restricting (1) $\mathbf{a}_{i_1} = \mathbf{a}_{i_2}$ for all $G_{i_1} = G_{i_2}$; (2) $\mathbf{c}_{i_1} = \mathbf{c}_{i_2}$ for all $G_{i_1} = G_{i_2}$; (3) $\mathbf{b}_{i,1} = \mathbf{b}_1$.

In our illustrative example, the maximum likelihood estimator solves

$$\min_{\theta, z} f(\theta)$$

$$s.t.\ \mathbf{A}_i \theta_i = \mathbf{B}_i z,\ i = 1, \ldots, n,$$

where $z$ represents the set of all subgroup-specific and common parameters in $\theta$ so the linear constraint $\mathbf{A}_i \theta_i = \mathbf{B}_i z$ is equivalent to $\mathbf{D}\theta = 0$. The corresponding augmented Lagrangian is

$$L_\rho(\theta, z, \xi) = f(\theta) + \xi^T (\mathbf{A}\theta - \mathbf{B}z) + \frac{\rho}{2} \|\mathbf{A}\theta - \mathbf{B}z\|_2^2$$

$$= \sum_{i=1}^{n} \{ f_i(\theta_i) + \xi_i^T (\mathbf{A}_i \theta_i - \mathbf{B}_i z) + \frac{\rho}{2} \|\mathbf{A}_i \theta_i - \mathbf{B}_i z\|_2^2 \},$$

where $\xi = [\xi_1', \ldots, \xi_n']$,

$$\mathbf{A} = \begin{bmatrix} \mathbf{A}_1 & 0 & \cdots & 0 \\ 0 & \mathbf{A}_2 & \cdots & 0 \\ \vdots & & \ddots & 0 \\ 0 & 0 & \cdots & \mathbf{A}_n \end{bmatrix}, \mathbf{B} = \begin{bmatrix} \mathbf{B}_1 \\ \mathbf{B}_2 \\ \vdots \\ \mathbf{B}_n \end{bmatrix}.$$

Here $\xi$ are the Lagrange multipliers and $\rho$ is a pre-specified positive penalty parameter. Let $\tilde{\theta}_n^{(v)}, \tilde{z}_n^{(v)}, \tilde{\xi}_n^{(v)}$ be the $v^{th}$ iterates of $\theta, z, \xi$. Then, at the iteration $v + 1$, the ADMM algorithm updates are

$$\theta - \text{update} : \nabla f(\tilde{\theta}_n^{(v+1)}) + \mathbf{A}^T \tilde{\xi}_n^{(v)} + \rho \mathbf{A}^T (\mathbf{A}\tilde{\theta}_n^{(v+1)} - \mathbf{B}\tilde{z}_n^{(v+1)}) = 0,$$

$$z - \text{update} : \mathbf{B}^T \tilde{\xi}_n^{(v)} + \rho \mathbf{B}^T (\mathbf{A}\tilde{\theta}_n^{(v+1)} - \mathbf{B}\tilde{z}_n^{(v)}) = 0,$$

$$\xi - \text{update} : \tilde{\xi}_n^{(v+1)} - \tilde{\xi}_n^{(v)} - \rho(\mathbf{A}\tilde{\theta}_n^{(v+1)} - \mathbf{B}\tilde{z}_n^{(v+1)}) = 0,$$

where the most computationally expensive $\theta$-update can be programmed in parallel across each $i = 1, \ldots, n$ as

$$\theta_i - \text{update} : \nabla f_i(\tilde{\theta}_{i,n}^{(v+1)}) + \mathbf{A}_i^T \tilde{\xi}_{i,n}^{(v)} + \rho \mathbf{A}_i^T (\mathbf{A}_i \tilde{\theta}_i^{(v+1)} - \mathbf{B}_i \tilde{z}_n^{(v)}) = 0.$$

The gradients $\nabla f_i(\cdot)$ for subject $i$'s HMM parameters can be computed using Fisher's identity [5] based on the efficient EM algorithm proposed in [17]. The details are included in Supplementary Materials. The use of gradients is needed in our model both due to the ADMM update and the covariate structure. Even when there are no covariates and all parameters are shared across subjects, the gradient method is still faster than the EM algorithm because M-step is expensive in the zero-inflated Poisson distribution.

## 3.3  Theoretical Properties

Define $\hat{\theta}_n$ to be the maximum likelihood estimator for $\theta$ and let $\theta^\star$ denote its population-level analog. The following are the sufficient conditions to ensure: (1) almost sure convergence of $\hat{\theta}_n$ to $\theta^\star$ as $n \to \infty$, and (2) numerical convergence of $\tilde{\theta}_n^{(v)}$ to $\hat{\theta}_n$ as $v \to \infty$.

(A0)  The true parameter vector $\theta^\star$ for the unconstrained optimization problem $\min_{\theta} f(\theta)$ is an interior point of $\Theta$, where $\Theta$ is a compact subset of $\mathbb{R}^{\dim \theta}$.

(A1)  The constraint set $\mathcal{C} \triangleq \{\theta \in \Theta; \mathbf{D}\theta = 0\}$ is nonempty and for some $r \in \mathbb{R}$, the set $\{\theta \in \mathcal{C}; f(\theta) \le r\}$ is nonempty and compact.

(A2)  The observed time process $(T_k : k \in \mathbb{N})$ is independent of the generative hidden Markov process: the likelihood for the observed times do not share parameters with $\theta$.

(A3)  There exist positive real numbers $0 < \kappa^- \le \kappa^+ < 1$ such that for all subjects $i = 1, \ldots, n$, $\kappa^- \le P_i^{T_{k+1}-T_k}(m, \ell) \le \kappa^+$ for $k = 1, \ldots, K - 1$ and $m, \ell = 1, \ldots, M$, almost surely and $g_{i,m}(y; \mathbf{x}) > 0$ for all $y \in \operatorname{supp} Y$ for some $m = 1, \ldots, M$.

(A4)  For each $\theta \in \Theta$, the transition kernel indexed by $\theta$ is Harris recurrent and aperiodic. The transition kernel is continuous in $\theta$ in an open neighborhood of $\theta^\star$.

(A5)  The hidden Markov model is identifiable up to label switching of the latent states.

(A6)  Denote by $e_{\min}(\theta)$ and $e_{\max}(\theta)$ to be the smallest and largest eigenvalues of $\nabla^2 f(\theta)$. There exist positive real numbers $\epsilon$ and $\varrho_- \le \varrho_+$ such that $\inf_{\theta: \|\theta-\theta^\star\|_2 < \epsilon} e_{\min}(\theta) \ge \varrho_- > 0$ and $\sup_{\theta: \|\theta-\theta^\star\|_2 < \epsilon} e_{\max}(\theta) \le \varrho_+ < \infty$.

Assumption (A0)–(A2) are mild regularity conditions whereas (A3)–(A5) are standard in hidden Markov models [8]; together they ensures that the model is well-defined. Assumption (A4) avoids non-standard asymptotic behavior associated with non-smooth functionals. Assumption (A6) states that the smallest and largest eigenvalues for the Hessian of the negative log likelihood function are bounded away from 0 and infinity in an open neighborhood of the true parameter values, indicating the local Lipschitz differentiability and convexity, which are used in [31] to establish the numerical convergence in the ADMM algorithm.

**Theorem 3.1**  *Under assumptions (A0)–(A5), as $T_i \to \infty$ for $i = 1, \ldots, n$,*

*(i) $\hat{\theta}_n$ converges to $\theta^\star$ almost surely as $n \to \infty$,*

(ii) *suppose (A6) also holds, then $\tilde{\boldsymbol{\theta}}_n^{(v)}$ converges numerically to $\hat{\boldsymbol{\theta}}_n$ in an open neighborhood of $\boldsymbol{\theta}^\star$ as $v \to \infty$.*

The first part of Theorem 3.1 states the almost sure convergence of the constrained maximum likelihood estimator $\hat{\boldsymbol{\theta}}_n$ to the true parameter value $\boldsymbol{\theta}^\star$. This can be shown using the uniform convergence results of the log likelihood [8] for each subject-specific hidden Markov model, along with the feasibility assumption (A1) and identifiability assumption (A5). The second part of Theorem states the numerical convergence of the ADMM algorithm. This is anticipated by [4] which identifies general conditions for the numerical convergence of the residual, the dual variable, and the objective function. [31] extended the convergence to the primal variable by adding the Lipschitz continuity and convexity assumptions. The details for those assumptions, as well as the proof for Theorem 3.1, are included in Supplementary Materials.

For $i = 1, \ldots, n$, define the estimator for the mean proportion of time in state $m$ in group $k$ as $\hat{\phi}_{j,n}(m)$, $j = 1, \ldots, J, m = 1, \ldots, M$, and the estimator for the mean proportion of time in state $m$ as $\hat{\eta}_{i,k_i}$ where $k_i$ is the number of observed time points for subject $i$. The following result characterizes the limiting behavior of the estimated time in each state.

**Theorem 3.2** *Under (A0)–(A5), as $k_i \to \infty$ for $i = 1, \ldots, n$, $n_j \to \infty$ for $j = 1, \ldots, J$,*

(i) *$\hat{\phi}_{j,n}(m; \hat{\boldsymbol{\theta}}_n)$ converges to $\mu_j(m; \boldsymbol{\theta}^\star)$ almost surely,*

(ii) *$\frac{\hat{\phi}_{j,n}(m;\hat{\boldsymbol{\theta}}_n)-\mu_j(m;\hat{\boldsymbol{\theta}}_n)}{\sqrt{\sigma_j^2(m;\hat{\boldsymbol{\theta}}_n)/n_j}}$ converges in distribution to a standard normal random variable, where $\mu_j(m; \hat{\boldsymbol{\theta}}_n) = E[\hat{\eta}_{i,k_i}(m; \hat{\boldsymbol{\theta}}_n)]$, $\sigma_j^2(m; \hat{\boldsymbol{\theta}}_n) = Var[\hat{\eta}_{i,k_i}(m; \hat{\boldsymbol{\theta}}_n)]$ for all $i$ such that $G_i = j$.*

A proof of the preceding result is given in the Supplementary Materials, which follows from the almost sure convergence of a bounded continuous function and the central limit theorem. In principle, $\mu_j(m; \hat{\boldsymbol{\theta}}_n)$ can be obtained from the limiting distribution of a stationary continuous-time Markov chain, which is determined by the transition as a function of $\hat{\boldsymbol{\theta}}_n$. However, it is generally not easy to compute the standard error analytically for the estimated mean state probabilities. Instead, we use a stratified nonparametric bootstrap [9] in which we resample subjects with replacement from each subgroup.

## 4 Simulation Experiments

We study the finite sample performance of the proposed estimator for the state probabilities using a suite of simulation experiments. We simulate minute-by-minute activity counts of length $T \sim \text{Uniform}(500, 2500)$ for $n = 20$ and $n = 200$ subjects, where half of the subjects are male (Group 1) and the other half female

(Group 2). The intervals between consecutive time points are independently drawn from $\{1, 2, \ldots, 10\}$ with equal probabilities. For each subject, we assume 2/5 of the observations are from weekends and 3/5 of the observations are from weekdays.

The activity counts are generated using a three state continuous-time zero-inflated Poisson hidden Markov model. We assume that during the weekend the log mean activity decreases by 10%, 20%, 30% in states 1, 2, 3 respectively, while the log odds of zero in state 1 increases by 10%, so that

$$\log\left\{\frac{\delta_i(\mathbf{x})}{1-\delta_i(\mathbf{x})}\right\} = b_{i,0,0} + 0.1 \times \mathbf{I}\{\text{Weekend}\}_i^t,$$

$$\log\left\{\lambda_{i,1}(\mathbf{x})\right\} = b_{i,1,0} - 0.1 \times \mathbf{I}\{\text{Weekend}\}_i^t,$$

$$\log\left\{\lambda_{i,2}(\mathbf{x})\right\} = b_{i,2,0} - 0.2 \times \mathbf{I}\{\text{Weekend}\}_i^t,$$

$$\log\left\{\lambda_{i,3}(\mathbf{x})\right\} = b_{i,3,0} - 0.3 \times \mathbf{I}\{\text{Weekend}\}_i^t,$$

where $b_{i,0,0} \overset{iid}{\sim} N(-1, 0.1^2)$, $b_{i,1,0} \overset{iid}{\sim} N\left\{\log(50), 0.1^2\right\}$, $b_{i,2,0} \overset{iid}{\sim} N\{\log(300),$ $0.1^2\}$, $b_{i,3,0} \overset{iid}{\sim} N\left\{\log(700), 0.1^2\right\}$ are subject-specific intercepts; the weekend effect is assumed to be common across all subjects.

The initial probabilities for male are $(U_1, U_2, 1 - U_1 - U_2)$, where $U_1, U_2 \overset{iid}{\sim} \text{Uniform}(0.2, 0.4)$; for female, the initial probabilities are $(U_3, U_4, 1 - U_3 - U_4)$, where $U_3 \overset{iid}{\sim} \text{Uniform}(0.6, 0.8)$, $U_4 \overset{iid}{\sim} \text{Uniform}(0.1, 0.2)$. The transition rate matrix for male is

$$\begin{bmatrix} -U_5 - U_6 & U_5 & U_6 \\ U_7 & -U_7 - U_8 & U_8 \\ U_9 & U_{10} & -U_9 - U_{10} \end{bmatrix},$$

where $U_5, \ldots, U_{10} \overset{iid}{\sim} \text{Uniform}(0.05, 0.15)$; for female, the transition rate matrix is

$$\begin{bmatrix} -U_{11} - U_{12} & U_{11} & U_{12} \\ U_{13} & -U_{13} - U_{14} & U_{14} \\ U_{15} & U_{16} & -U_{15} - U_{16} \end{bmatrix},$$

where $U_{11}, U_{12} \overset{iid}{\sim} \text{Uniform}(0.05, 0.1)$, $U_{13}, U_{15} \overset{iid}{\sim} \text{Uniform}(0.3, 0.4)$, and $U_{14}, U_{16} \overset{iid}{\sim} \text{Uniform}(0.1, 0.2)$.

Table 1 shows the bias and standard error of the estimators for different hierarchies of parameters in the HCTHMM via 500 simulations. In both cases, the biases are small due to the fact that the length of each individual series is large. As the sample size increases, the standard errors become smaller which is expected. Figure 1 shows the average runtime (s) for each ADMM iteration scales linearly with the number of subjects. It generally takes some 30–100 iterations for the algorithm to converge. Table 2 compares the mean coverage probability of the

**Table 1** The bias and standard error for the estimated population and subgroup-specific parameters in HCTHMM

| Parameter | $n = 20$<br>Bias (s.e.) | $n = 200$<br>Bias (s.e.) |
|---|---|---|
| *Population parameters* | | |
| Slope for State 1 zero odds | 0.0021 (0.0422) | 0.0032 (0.0134) |
| Slope for State 1 Poisson mean | 0.0001 (0.0034) | 0.0001 (0.0011) |
| Slope for State 2 Poisson mean | 0.0016 (0.0053) | 0.0019 (0.0018) |
| Slope for State 3 Poisson mean | 0.0036 (0.0120) | 0.0046 (0.0044) |
| *Subgroup-specific parameters* | | |
| Initial probabilities (Male) | 0.0169 (0.0022) | 0.0165 (0.0008) |
| Initial probabilities (Female) | 0.0152 (0.0069) | 0.0284 (0.0038) |
| Transition rates (Male) | 0.0038 (0.0029) | 0.0011 (0.0006) |
| Transition rates (Female) | 0.0099 (0.0089) | 0.0016 (0.0012) |

The metric is Euclidean norm for population parameters, and Frobenius norm for subgroup-specific parameter vectors

**Fig. 1** Average runtime (s) using eight cores on a Unix cluster for each ADMM iteration in different configurations (number of subjects, length of each series)

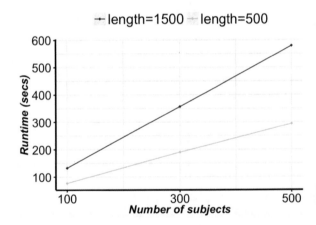

**Table 2** Comparisons on the mean coverage probability for the 95% and 99% bootstrap confidence intervals for the mean proportion of time in each latent state between subject-specific HMM and HCTHMM ($n = 200$)

| State | Subject-specific HMM | | HCTHMM | |
|---|---|---|---|---|
| | Male | Female | Male | Female |
| 95% C.I. | | | | |
| 1 | 0.942 | 0.942 | 0.942 | 0.950 |
| 2 | 0.944 | 0.938 | 0.950 | 0.960 |
| 3 | 0.946 | 0.936 | 0.960 | 0.944 |
| 99% C.I. | | | | |
| 1 | 0.982 | 0.988 | 0.986 | 0.994 |
| 2 | 0.986 | 0.984 | 0.986 | 0.988 |
| 3 | 0.978 | 0.980 | 0.994 | 0.992 |

95% and 99% bootstrap confidence intervals for the mean proportion of time in each latent state between a baseline subject-specific HMM and the proposed HCTHMM when the sample size is 200. As we can see, the baseline subject-specific HMM suffers undercoverage (coverage probability smaller than nominal level), while the proposed HCTHMM recovers the nominal level on average in both the 95% and 99% cases.

## 5  Application

The motivating application is a human physical activity data set from the 2003–2004 National Health and Nutrition Examination Survey (NHANES), which is publicly available at the National Center for Disease Control (CDC) website https://wwwn. cdc.gov/Nchs/Nhanes/2003-2004/PAXRAW_C.htm. There are 7176 participants in the study, and for each participant we have minute-by-minute activity counts for up to seven days. As the subjects were supposed to remove the accelerometer when washing, there are prolonged intervals during the day when accelerometer readings are zeros. We further impose the following two inclusion/exclusion criteria,

- Subjects whose age is between 20 and 60 are included.
- Subjects with very few measurements are excluded.

The first criterion specifies the scope of inference. The second criterion exclude subjects with very few non-missing data available ($<500$ min out of 7 days). There are 2467 subjects who satisfy both conditions, which constitute more than 95% of those whose age is between 20 and 60. Further, we split those subjects by their baseline characteristics (gender, age) into 4 subgroups. Subgroup 1 consists of 608 male subjects with age from 20 to 40; subgroup 2 consists of 557 male subjects with age from 40 to 60; subgroup 3 consists of 712 female subjects with age from 20 to 40; and subroup 4 consists of 590 female subjects with age from 40 to 60.

Table 3 summarizes the related work on the length of an extended period of zero activity counts to be defined as missingness. In this paper, we choose to define missingness as a sustained interval of greater than or equal to 20 consecutive zero activity counts, which is the most commonly used criterion in the literature. Most

**Table 3** The definition of missing interval in terms of consecutive minutes of zeros in the literature on human activity

| Literature | Definition of missing |
| --- | --- |
| [7] | 30 min |
| [6] | 20 min |
| [33] | 60 min |
| [27] | 20 min |
| [10] | 20 min |
| [29] | 60 min |
| [16] | 20 min |

missingness occurs between 10 pm to 8 am, which is the sleep time for most of the subjects. There is still sporadic missingness during other periods of time in the day, which may correspond to activities like swimming or bathing. The missingness periods are removed during the data preprocessing. The average proportion of zeros after removing the missingness is around 25%, so that zero-inflation is still an issue to be considered in the modeling. In the data preprocessing, activity counts greater than 1500 (<5%) are truncated at 1500 to ensure the numeric stability of the fitting algorithm.

To apply the HCTHMM model on the activity counts data, we need to select the number of latent states as well as the hierarchy for different sets of the parameters. The weekend effect is adjusted for in the Poisson and zero-inflated Poisson regression on the activity counts in each latent state. By the minimum BIC criterion as shown in Table 4, we select the type IV HCTHMM with six latent states, where the intercepts in the state-dependent generalized linear models for logit zero proportion in state 1 and log Poisson means in the all states are subject-specific, while the initial probabilities, transition rates, and the slopes in the state-dependent generalized linear models are subgroup-specific. This final model indicates the baseline zero proportion and mean activity counts in each latent state vary across subjects. For all the other parameters, the between-subgroup variability is more prominent than the within-subgroup variability. Figure 2 shows the 99% confidence interval for the estimated proportion of time spent in latent activity states for each subgroup in 03–04 NHANES. There are several interesting findings. First, younger men spend less time in the low intensity activity states (state 1, 2) than older men and women. Second, men spend less time than women in the medium intensity activity states (state 3, 4). Third, men spend more time than women in the high intensity activity states (state 5, 6). To validate the results, we apply the HCTHMM methodology to 05–06 NHANES, which has the same study setup and data structure as the 03–04 NHANES. Figure 3 shows the 99% confidence interval for the estimated proportion of time spent in latent activity states for each subgroup in 05–06 NHANES, which has a similar pattern as seen in 03–04 NHANES.

**Table 4** Summary of BIC from model selection

| Model specifications | BIC |
|---|---|
| 5 states, type I | 248,009,082 |
| 6 states, type I | 202,804,081 |
| 7 states, type I | 203,261,150 |
| 6 states, type II | 200,457,217 |
| 6 states, type III | 198,808,738 |
| 6 states, type IV | 198,807,080 |

In type I models, all parameters are subject-specific. In type II models, all parameters are subject-specific except the slopes, which are population parameters. In type III models, the intercepts are subject-specific; the slopes are population; the initial probabilities and transitions are subgroup-specific. In type IV models, all parameters are subgroup-specific except the intercepts, which are subject-specific

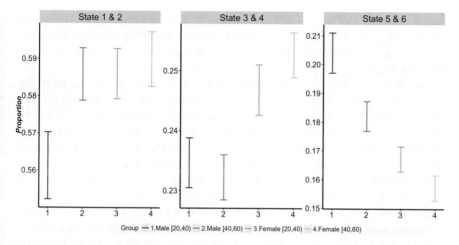

**Fig. 2** The 99% bootstrap confidence intervals for the estimated proportion of time spent in latent activity states by subgroup in 03–04 NHANES

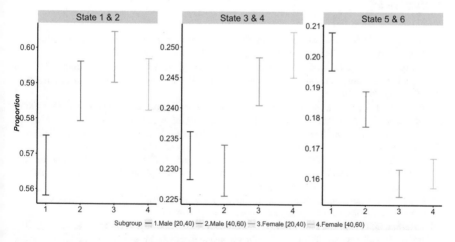

**Fig. 3** The 99% bootstrap confidence intervals for the estimated proportion of time spent in latent activity states for each subgroup in 05–06 NHANES

## 6 Conclusions

We propose HCTHMM to be valid inference strategy for the longitudinal activity data. Within this framework, we can estimate the mean state probabilities for different subgroups of subjects as well as quantify the uncertainty. Our findings are consistent with previous literature on human physical activity [12, 19, 33, 36], which indicated that the physical activity can be classified into different categories by intensity, and that the activity level decreases as a result of aging. Moreover, women tend to spend more time in lighter intensity activity, whereas younger men tend to have periods of higher intensity activities.

In the future, this HCTHMM framework can be extended to the controlled clinical studies to estimate certain treatment effects in a specific cohort of patients. We can also allow for time-varying covariates in the transition rates. Moreover, when some model parameters are truly subject-specific or subgroup-specific, it may be more powerful to model them as random so that tests based on variance components can be constructed to test their effects. Another modification is to extend the latent continuous-time Markov process to a semi-Markov process. This will be scientifically interesting because it is reasonable to assume that the current latent state not only depends on the most recent past state but also on the history of the state trajectory. However, all these changes are computationally expensive, especially on such large-scale high-frequency data. Corresponding estimation methods have to be developed before the application becomes feasible.

# References

1. Albert, A. (1962). Estimating the infinitesimal generator of a continuous time, finite state Markov process. *The Annals of Mathematical Statistics, 33*(2), 727–753.
2. Altman, R. M. (2007). Mixed hidden Markov models: An extension of the hidden Markov model to the longitudinal data setting. *Journal of the American Statistical Association, 102*(477), 201–210.
3. Bartalesi, R., Lorussi, F., Tesconi, M., Tognetti, A., Zupone, G., & De Rossi, D. (2005). Wearable kinesthetic system for capturing and classifying upper limb gesture. In *Eurohaptics Conference, 2005 and Symposium on Haptic Interfaces for Virtual Environment and Teleoperator Systems, 2005. World Haptics 2005. First Joint* (pp. 535–536). New York: IEEE.
4. Boyd, S., Parikh, N., Chu, E., Peleato, B., & Eckstein, J. (2011). Distributed optimization and statistical learning via the alternating direction method of multipliers. *Foundations and Trends® in Machine Learning, 3*(1), 1–122.
5. Cappé, O., Moulines, E., & Rydén, T. (2005). *Inference in hidden Markov models. Springer series in statistics.* Basel: Springer Nature Switzerland AG
6. Catellier, D. J., Hannan, P. J., Murray, D. M., Addy, C. L., Conway, T. L., Yang, S., et al. (2005). Imputation of missing data when measuring physical activity by accelerometry. *Medicine and Science in Sports and Exercise, 37*(11 suppl.), S555.
7. Cradock, A. L., Wiecha, J. L., Peterson, K. E., Sobol, A. M., Colditz, G. A., & Gortmaker, S. L. (2004). Youth recall and tritrac accelerometer estimates of physical activity levels. *Medicine and Science in Sports and Exercise, 36*(3), 525–532.
8. Douc, R., Moulines, E., & Rydén, T. (2004). Asymptotic properties of the maximum likelihood estimator in autoregressive models with Markov regime. *The Annals of Statistics, 32*(5), 2254–2304.
9. Efron, B. (1992). Bootstrap methods: another look at the jackknife. In *Breakthroughs in statistics* (pp. 569–593). New York: Springer.
10. Evenson, K. R. (2011). Towards an understanding of change in physical activity from pregnancy through postpartum. *Psychology of Sport and Exercise, 12*(1), 36–45.

11. Gruen, M. E., Alfaro-Córdoba, M., Thomson, A. E., Worth, A. C. , Staicu, A.-M. , & Lascelles, B. D. X. (2017). The use of functional data analysis to evaluate activity in a spontaneous model of degenerative joint disease associated pain in cats. PLoS One, 12(1), e0169576.

12. Hansen, B. H., Kolle, E., Dyrstad, S. M., Holme, I., & Anderssen, S. A. (2012). Accelerometer-determined physical activity in adults and older people. *Medicine and Science in Sports and Exercise, 44*(2), 266–272.

13. He, J., Li, H., & Tan, J. (2007). Real-time daily activity classification with wireless sensor networks using hidden Markov model. In *Engineering in Medicine and Biology Society, 2007. EMBS 2007. 29th Annual International Conference of the IEEE* (pp. 3192–3195). New York: IEEE.

14. Hong, M., & Luo, Z.-Q. (2017). On the linear convergence of the alternating direction method of multipliers. *Mathematical Programming, 162*(1–2), 165–199.

15. Kanai, M., Izawa, K. P., Kobayashi, M., Onishi, A., Kubo, H., Nozoe, M., et al. (2018). Effect of accelerometer-based feedback on physical activity in hospitalized patients with ischemic stroke: A randomized controlled trial. *Clinical Rehabilitation.* https://doi.org/10.1177/0269215518755841

16. Lee, J. A., & Gill, J. (2016). Missing value imputation for physical activity data measured by accelerometer. *Statistical Methods in Medical Research.* https://doi.org/10.1177/0962280216633248

17. Liu, Y.-Y., Li, S., Li, F., Song, L., & Rehg, J. M. (2015). Efficient learning of continuous-time hidden Markov models for disease progression. In *Advances in Neural Information Processing Systems* (pp. 3600–3608).

18. Marshall, A., Medvedev, O., & Markarian, G. (2007). Self management of chronic disease using mobile devices and bluetooth monitors. In *Proceedings of the ICST 2nd International Conference on Body Area Networks* (pp. 22). ICST (Institute for Computer Sciences, Social-Informatics and Telecommunications Engineering).

19. Metzger, J. S., Catellier, D. J., Evenson, K. R., Treuth, M. S., Rosamond, W. D., & Siega-Riz, A. M. (2008). Patterns of objectively measured physical activity in the United States. *Medicine and Science in Sports and Exercise, 40*(4), 630–638.

20. Morris, J. S., Arroyo, C., Coull, B. A., Ryan, L. M., Herrick, R., & Gortmaker, S. L. (2006). Using wavelet-based functional mixed models to characterize population heterogeneity in accelerometer profiles: a case study. *Journal of the American Statistical Association, 101*(476), 1352–1364.

21. Napolitano, M. A., Borradaile, K. E., Lewis, B. A., Whiteley, J. A., Longval, J. L., Parisi, A. F., et al. (2010). Accelerometer use in a physical activity intervention trial. *Contemporary Clinical Trials, 31*(6), 514–523.

22. Nickel, C., Busch, C., Rangarajan, S., & Möbius, M. (2011). Using hidden Markov models for accelerometer-based biometric gait recognition. In *2011 IEEE 7th International Colloquium on Signal Processing and its Applications (CSPA)* (pp. 58–63). New York: IEEE.

23. Nodelman, U., Shelton, C. R., & Koller, D. (2012). Expectation maximization and complex duration distributions for continuous time Bayesian networks. Preprint. arXiv:1207.1402.

24. Pyke, R. (1961a). Markov renewal processes: Definitions and preliminary properties. *The Annals of Mathematical Statistics, 32*, 1231–1242.

25. Pyke, R. (1961b). Markov renewal processes with finitely many states. *The Annals of Mathematical Statistics, 32*, 1243–1259.

26. Rabiner, L. R. (1989). A tutorial on hidden Markov models and selected applications in speech recognition. *Proceedings of the IEEE, 77*(2), 257–286.

27. Robertson, W., Stewart-Brown, S., Wilcock, E., Oldfield, M., & Thorogood, M. (2010). Utility of accelerometers to measure physical activity in children attending an obesity treatment intervention. *Journal of Obesity 2011.* http://dx.doi.org/10.1155/2011/398918

28. Ronao, C. A., & Cho, S.-B. (2014). Human activity recognition using smartphone sensors with two-stage continuous hidden Markov models. In *2014 10th International Conference on Natural Computation (ICNC)* (pp. 681–686). New York: IEEE.

29. Schmid, D., Ricci, C., & Leitzmann, M. F. (2015). Associations of objectively assessed physical activity and sedentary time with all-cause mortality in us adults: The NHANES study. *PLoS One, 10*(3), e0119591.
30. Scott, S. L., James, G. M., & Sugar, C. A. (2005). Hidden Markov models for longitudinal comparisons. *Journal of the American Statistical Association, 100*(470), 359–369.
31. Shi, W., Ling, Q., Yuan, K., Wu, G., & Yin, W. (2014). On the linear convergence of the admm in decentralized consensus optimization. *IEEE Transactions on Signal Processing* 62(7), 1750–1761.
32. Shirley, K. E., Small, D. S., Lynch, K. G., Maisto, S. A., & Oslin, D. W. (2010). Hidden Markov models for alcoholism treatment trial data. *The Annals of Applied Statistics, 4*, 366–395.
33. Troiano, R. P., Berrigan, D., Dodd, K. W., Mâsse, L. C., Tilert, T., McDowell, M., et al. (2008). Physical activity in the United States measured by accelerometer. *Medicine and Science in Sports and Exercise, 40*(1), 181.
34. Wang, X., Sontag, D., & Wang, F. (2014). Unsupervised learning of disease progression models. In *Proceedings of the 20th ACM SIGKDD International Conference on Knowledge Discovery and Data Mining* (pp. 85–94). New York: ACM.
35. Witowski, V., Foraita, R., Pitsiladis, Y., Pigeot, I., & N. Wirsik (2014). Using hidden Markov models to improve quantifying physical activity in accelerometer data—A simulation study. *PLoS One, 9*(12), e114089.
36. Xiao, L., Huang, L., Schrack, J. A., Ferrucci, L., Zipunnikov, V., & Crainiceanu, C. M. (2014). Quantifying the lifetime circadian rhythm of physical activity: A covariate-dependent functional approach. Biostatistics, 16(2), 352–367.

# Part III
# Large Scale Data Analysis and Its Applications

# Privacy Preserving Feature Selection via Voted Wrapper Method for Horizontally Distributed Medical Data

**Yunmei Lu and Yanqing Zhang**

**Abstract** Feature selection plays a crucial step for data mining algorithms via eliminating the curse of dimensionality. Many feature selection approaches are developed for analyzing centralized data on the same location. In recent years, multi-source biomedical data mining methods have been developed to analyze different distributed databases at different locations such as different hospitals. However, a major concern is privacy of sensitive personal medical records in different hospitals. Therefore, as the needs for new privacy preserving distributed data mining algorithms increase, it is necessary to develop new privacy preserving feature selection algorithms for biomedical data mining. In this paper, a privacy preserving feature selection method named "Privacy Preserving Feature Selection algorithm via Voted Wrapper methods (PPFSVW)" is developed. This method was tested on six benchmark datasets under two testing scenarios. Our experimental results indicate that the proposed algorithm workflow can work effectively to improve the classification performance regarding accuracy via selecting informative features and genes. Besides, the proposed method can make the classifier achieve higher or same level classification accuracy with fewer features compared with those sophisticated methods, such as SVM-RFE, RSVM and SVM-t. More importantly, the individual private information can be protected during the whole feature selection process.

**Keywords** Privacy preserving · Horizontally distributed data mining · Support vector machine · SVM · Feature selection · PAN-SVM

## 1 Introduction

Data mining approaches have been widely used to analyze the massive amount of data in lots of fields such as medical data, consumer purchase data and census data,

Y. Lu · Y. Zhang (✉)
Department of Computer Science, Georgia State University, Atlanta, GA, USA
e-mail: yzhang@gsu.edu

© Springer Nature Switzerland AG 2020
Y. Zhao, D.-G. (Din) Chen (eds.), *Statistical Modeling in Biomedical Research*, Emerging Topics in Statistics and Biostatistics,
https://doi.org/10.1007/978-3-030-33416-1_8

and they have become increasingly important tools to discover useful knowledge. However, the potential divulged sensitive information during the data mining process has been raised as a private issue and the high dimension of data attributes often makes a curse to data mining tasks, thus data mining tasks have been encountering more and more challenges as new concerns and applications emerge. Many approaches and techniques have been developed to address the two issues separately; novel approaches that could integrate solutions for these two issues are also in high demand.

One of the sources for emerged concerns for privacy during data mining process is its application in distributed scenario. Recently, assembling datasets maintained by different sources have become increasingly common, and applying data mining techniques on the aggregated datasets may build more reliable prediction models and attain useful patterns, which benefits for medical research, improving customer service and homeland security, and so forth. However, this multi-data source system might divulge sensitive information about individuals. It thus leads to increasing concerns about privacy during the process of data mining, which in turn prevents different parties from sharing information. For examples, the Centers for Disease Control (CDC) may want to identify the trends of some disease to understand its progression via data mining techniques but has no relevant data. Insurance companies that have considerable data are unwilling to share these data due to patient privacy concerns.

A number of state-of-the-art techniques of privacy preserving data mining have been developed to leverage the privacy and mining issue. Among these methods, the most popular ones are randomization [1], k-anonymity [2] and l-diversity [3]. Methods based on such technologies usually employ data transformation techniques or add some noise to protect privacy and sensitive data. The granularity of representation of data is usually reduced after transformation to mitigate the risk of divulging privacy, which results in the loss of information or effectiveness of data management and data mining algorithms. However, it is inevitable and usually a trade-off between privacy and information loss.

Privacy Preserving Distributed Data Mining (PPDDM) provides another way to address the privacy issue without accessing the actual data values to avoid the disclosure of information beyond the final results at the era of more and more available datasets on multi-site. In such case, a variety of cryptographic protocols usually needed to communicate with different parties. Secure Multiparty Computation (SMC) is a possible way to make it possible of distributed data mining without divulging sensitive information. The problem PPDDM overlaps closely with the field of cryptography for determining the secure multiple computation, which aims to design secure protocols to make sure those different parties, can perform joint computation by providing inputs without actual disclosure or sharing the individual inputs. In this paper, a SMC method was employed to protect data, details will be expressed in the *Method* section.

High dimension of attributes is another issue for data mining. The huge number of data attributes or dimensions often makes a curse to data mining tasks. Feature selection techniques address the issue of dimensionality reduction by selecting some available subset of features via predetermined selecting criteria to decrease the complexity of data mining tasks and thus improve the performances (such as classification accuracy) of data mining algorithms. Take the classification problem into consideration, by doing feature selection, irrelevant and redundant features are usually eliminated. Thus the computational complexity of classification procedure is reduced, and a better classifier with generalization ability will be constructed, and the risk of over-fitting is also be reduced. Therefore, feature selection plays a vital role in optimizing classification procedure.

Feature selection methods can be grouped into two categories according to their searching directions: *forward selection* and *backward selection*. Forward selection usually starts searching relevant features from an empty subset and adds one or several ones at each step until a stop criterion is met. On contrast, the backward selection methods usually start searching for the whole feature space and eliminate or remove one or some at each step, until some the predetermined stop criteria are reached. Besides, feature selection algorithms can also be classified into two categories based on the relationship of features: *feature ranking* and *subset selection*. In the ranking list, the importance of each gene is unequal. Usually the most top one is supposed to be the most important one, and so forth; while in the subset selection, each feature is equal, they work together making the classifier obtain the best performance.

Moreover, feature selection methods can also be classified into three main groups: *filter, wrapper* and *embedded approaches* [4] according to different selecting strategies and procedures of algorithms. The filter methods usually take account of the statistical properties of features and rank them according to some criteria of relevant information. This step is always before the classification step and is entirely independent of data mining algorithms; they are usually fast. Just as the name implies, the wrapper methods often wrapped the feature selection step in the process of mining algorithms. Compared with the filter methods, wrapper methods have the advantages of taking account into the performance of mining algorithms or tasks. Thus a better classification model will be built with high performance, says high classification accuracy. However, it needs to repeatedly train and test the data and build classification model at each step when a subset of features are selected; the computational complexity thus increased sharply. In recent years, many approaches of wrapper feature selections are developed [5–9]. The third kind of feature selection approaches is named embedded method, which performs feature selection in the process of the building data mining model by adding or modifying the optimizing process of classification [10, 11]. Different from the wrapper methods, the embedded methods could better use of the available data without splitting the dataset into training and validation set, and thus convers faster by reaching a solution. However, the embedded methods are usually specific to given learning approaches, while the wrapper methods usually take the learning machine as a black box and thus are remarked as universal and simple. Therefore, a general framework by employing SMC for privacy issue and wrapper methods for feature selection was proposed in this paper, which could be applied in a general scenario. This paper only focuses experiments on medical data.

The feature selection methods mentioned above [4–11] are developed for centered data, however, assembling datasets and sharing information from multiple locations such as health relevant organizations have become increasingly common in recent years [12–14]. It is not only to reduce cost, but also to dig much more useful knowledge from a wider picture by applying data mining techniques on the aggregated datasets and build much more reliable prediction. As the needs for privacy preserving distributed data mining algorithms increase, the needs for privacy preserving feature selection algorithms also grow rapidly, and the privacy concerns of sharing data by distributed parties also brings significant challenges to feature selection. Data can be distributed among multiple sites by horizontally or by vertically. For horizontally partitioned data, the individual records are distributed across multiple parties, and each of them has the data with all the same attributes; while for vertically partitioned data, each party has the same set of entries, but the individual entries may contain different attributes. In the current work, data are distributed horizontally.

In the current work, a Privacy Preserving Feature Selection algorithm via Voted Wrapper methods (PPFSVW) [15] is proposed. PPFSVW is based on our previous work PAN-SVM [16] to protect individual privacy. Compared with traditional centered feature selection methods, it could be applied to distributed scenario, especially with the ability of protecting sensitive information from being divulged. Besides, PPFSVW inherits the advantages of other three popular feature selection methods to avoid overfitting and outliers. It was tested on six benchmark datasets, including gene expression datasets by partitioned horizontally. The experimental results demonstrated that the proposed method could achieve higher classification accuracy, with less number of selected features. Details about PPFSVW are described in *Methods* section, and the experimental results are shown in the *Results and Discussion* section, followed by the *Conclusion* at last.

# 2 Methods

## 2.1 Definition of Privacy

It is important to define privacy before measuring it and protect its confidentiality. However, this could be the hardest part, since it is inevitable to get totally different answers from different individuals when asking what privacy is. Privacy can mean different things to different audience, at different environments, in various contexts; and across different cultures. Fortunately, no matter how different the boundaries and content of privacy are among various groups and cultures, the common principles should be the same. It is most common that individuals consider something inherently special or sensitive as privacy, like HIV disease. First of all, privacy is not security, even though the domain of privacy partially overlaps security, which could include the appropriate use and how to protect the individual information.

According to the view of Ruth Gavison [17], the privacy can be defined in the term of access that others have to us, as well as our information. A general definition of privacy must to be one which is measurable of values and actionable. The common definition [18] of privacy in the community of cryptography limits the information that is leaked by the distributed computation function, while information learned from the output regards as no-privacy leakage, since it is inevitable and designed by the secure computation function. For example, if two millionaires would like to know who is richer without telling the other his/her net worth. A secure computation function must return the result without revealing private information. Suppose one has $10,000,000 net worth, and he knows that he is richer from the function output. Therefore, he can learn that the net worth of the other one is less than $10,000,000, and this information leakage is inevitable.

In addition, privacy preserving is not only in the interest of individual but also to the public. On the other hand, privacy preserving is for the sake of both people and the society. Nowadays, many laws are issued to protect privacy, and various techniques are developed to prevent privacy from disclosure when using personal or public databases.

## 2.2 Secure Multiparty Computation

Secure Multiparty Computation (SMC) is derived from Yao's Millionaires' problem [19], which states that two millionaires would like to know who is richer without telling each other their net worth. There are two basic adversarial models in SMC, and one is named *Semi-Honest*. In this model, the participants will follow the secure protocol, but keep curious and may attempt to dig some sensitive information from the received data from the other parties during the execution of the protocol. The other one is *Malicious model*, in which case, the participants may do anything to learn sensitive information, such as abort the protocol at any time, send sophisticated inputs to others, or send spurious messages and collude with other malicious parties.

The semi-honest model may seem questionable for preserving privacy if a party can be trusted to follow the secure protocol, why don't we trust them with the data? The following example can explain this. Consider the situation that several credit card companies would like to detect fraud via jointly building data mining models, and every business has been authorized to access that data. Once the data processing is completed, the data are supposed to be removed, since storing data brings the companies responsibility and cost to save the data. If there is a way that can build data mining models across distributed parties without actually accessing the original data, then they can save the responsibility and cost to protect the data from other parties other than their own.

However, no matter how secure the computation is, it is inevitable to leak some information. Still take the two millionaires as an example; once one party knows another party is richer or poorer, it can learn the upper bound or the lower bound of their net worth. In general, two kinds of information will leak, the information leaks from the secure computation function, and the information leaks from the computation process. Whatever is leaked from the former case, it is unavoidable as long as the function has to be computed. The latter case of information leakage during secure computation is provable prevented. Another key point is how to demonstrate that the security of the secure protocol used in the privacy preserving distributed data mining. It is common to restrict the secure against polynomial time adversary. According to the SMC literature, the composition theorem [20] is a very useful theorem.

> Composition Theorem for the semi-honest model: Suppose that g is privately reducible to f and that there exists a protocol for privately computing f. Then there exists a protocol for privately computing g.

The composition theorem states that if the sub-protocols are proved secure, then the entire protocol is secure. Therefore, if algorithms can be efficiently implemented on the sub-protocols, it can significantly improve the overall efficiency. Thus a lot of privacy preserving distributed data mining algorithms can be developed following the sub-protocols. These sub-protocols can be described using *homomorphic encryption* techniques [21]. Homomorphic encryption techniques allow operations such as search, comparison on encrypted data and obtain the same results as those based on plaintext data. Decryption becomes unnecessary during the whole computing process. Thus data and computation do not need put in a third party, the risk of revealing information to other can be deduced. The following protocols only use homomorphic encryption, and all of them are secure in the semi-honest model with no collusion. According to the composition theorem, they can be combined to produce new privacy-preserving algorithms.

**Secure Sum Protocol** In this secure protocol, the sum of values from each site will be securely calculated. Let $v$ denote the sum and be represented as: $v = \sum_{i=1}^{s} v_i$, where $v$ is known in the range $[0 \ldots n]$. In this secure sum protocol [22], one site will be assumed as a master site, numbered 1, and $2 \ldots s$ for the left sites. Normally, site 1 will uniformly generate a random number R in $[0 \ldots n]$, adds it to its local value $v_1$, and then sends the sum of $R + v_1 \mod n$ to site 2. Since R is chosen uniformly from $[0 \ldots n]$, and then $R + v_1 \mod n$ also distributes uniformly in this region. Thus site 2 learns nothing from this value. Site 2 receives this sum from site 1, and sends $S + v_2 \mod n$ to site 3, where S is the sum received from site 1, and $v_2$ is its local value. In general, the site $l$ receives: $v = R + \sum_{i=1}^{l-1} v_i \mod n$. Since $v$ is uniformly distributed, site $l$ learns nothing from another site. It then computes the sum and passes it to next site by $v = R + \sum_{i=1}^{l} v_i \mod n$.

The last site $s$ also performs the above steps and sends the sum to site 1, since only site 1 knows the value of R, and then it can subtract R from this sum value to get the actual result. The details of how this method operates are introduced in [22]. This protocol is proved secure for the semi-honest model but faces a clear problem of leakage information if collusion exists. For example, if the site $l - 1$ and $l + 1$ collude, and tell each other the values they sent/received, they can determine the value at the site $l$. Different from the randomization, k-anonymity and l-diversity methods, which usually employ data transformation techniques or add some noise to protect privacy and sensitive data, and the granularity of representation of data is usually reduced after transformation to mitigate the risk of divulging privacy; the Secure Sum Protocol has potential information leakage if collusion between parities exists, otherwise, information will be protected. Therefore, we do not add measurement to assess the privacy preservation ability in the experiment section.

## 2.3  PAN-SVM Classifier

The present proposed method is classified into a wrapper feature selection category, and as mentioned above, wrapper methods usually integrate feature selection step in the process of mining algorithms. When applied to a classification problem, methods used for selecting features are closely related to classifiers. In the current work, one of our previous works, Privacy-Aware Non-linear SVM (PAN-SVM) [16] is used to be as the classifier, which guarantees the private information to be protected during the whole mining process. The framework of PAN-SVM for distributed data sources is shown as in Fig. 1.

PAN-SVM contains three layers to finish corresponding functions. The bottom layer protects private individual data information and makes data invisible to other parties through the encrypting protocol of *Secure Sum Protocol* (SSP) [22]. Data will be encrypted by SSP before being sent to the remote miner. The SSP works like this: assume that there are three or more data sources numbered from 1 to S and no collusion, site 1 is designed as the master site. Site 1 randomly generates a number $X \sim uniform[1,N]$ and adds it to its local sum value $V_1$, and sends the sum $X + V_1$ mod N to site 2. Since $X$ is uniformly selected from $1 \sim N$, $X + V_1$ mod N is also uniformly distributed in the range of $1 \sim N$. Therefore, site 2 knows nothing about the local value of site 1. Site 2 receives the sum and adds it to its local sum of $V_2$ mod $N$, and then passes the new sum to the next site without disclosing its local values, and so on, until to the first site. Since the sum is always uniformly distributed in $1 \sim N$, each site cannot learn the private information from the previous sites. Details about this protocol could be found from [22]. The protocol works for an honest majority and assumes no collusion between sites.

The master site grabs the encrypted data from the other sites and builds a global classification model in the Medium layer. Since kernel matrix calculation is one of the most time consuming parts during the whole process of SVM, sophisticated apporaches that could alleviate the computation burden should be employed to accelerate the whole training process. In the proposed framework, the low-rank Nystrom method [23] is used to approximate the kernel matrix.

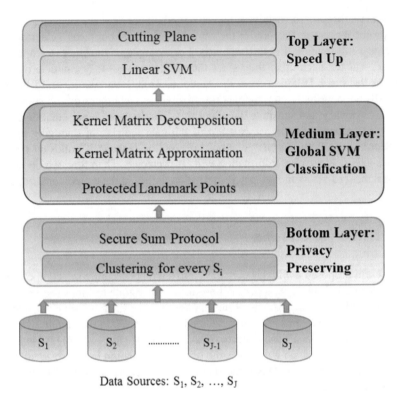

Data Sources: $S_1, S_2, \ldots, S_J$

**Fig. 1** Proposed framework of PAN-SVM

The Nystrom method randomly picks $l$ global landmark points, named a set of $L$, from all data sources, and then infers the kernel value of $K(x_i, x_j)$ implicitly from the relations of $x_i$ and $x_j$ and with these landmarks. Let $R_i$ be a $1 \times l$ vector that contains kernel values between $x_i$ and $L$ respectively: $R_i = [K(x_i, L_1), K(x_i, L_2), \ldots, K(x_i, L_l)]$ and similarly, $R_j = [K(x_j, L_1), K(x_j, L_2), \ldots, K(x_j, L_l)]$; finally, let A be the $l \times l$ kernel matrix between any pair of $l$ andmarks. Then, $K(x_i, x_j)$ can be approximated by Eq. (1).

$$K(x_i, x_j) = R_i A^{-1} R_j^T \tag{1}$$

By approximation using the Nystrom method, the kernel values between any pair of samples can by replaced by Eq. (1). However, the quality of Nystrom approximation highly depends on landmarks (sampled data); many sampling schemes [23–26] have been proposed to select the best landmarks. Among those state-of-the-art sampling approaches, [24] shows that the k-means clustering method can achieve significant performance and provide a low approximation error bound; helpfully, the k-means clustering algorithm is also simple to implement. Therefore, the k-means algorithm is adopted to select landmarks in the system and the data centers that are selected by k-means at each single site are treated as landmarks, which are used in the medium layer.

In the medium layer, the computation cost of kernel matrix can be further reduced via eigenvalue decomposition method. Zhang et al. in [27] show that the kernel matrix $K$ can be decomposed into the form of $K = FF^T$. If a kernel matrix of $n$ samples can be decomposed into $FF^T$, where F is a $n \times m$ matrix, then F can be treated as *virtual inputs* for a linear SVM model by mapping X from the original higher $p$-dimensional space into a much lower $m$-dimensional space, p $\gg$ m. Equation (1) can be rewritten in a general form as in Eq. (2).

$$K = RA^{-1}R^T = R\left(U\Lambda U^T\right)^{-1}R^T = R\left(U^T\Lambda^{-1}U\right)R^T \tag{2}$$

Here "A" is an $l \times l$ symmetric and positive semi-definite matrix; thus Eigen-decomposition of A can be expressed as A = $U\Lambda U^T$, where U and $\Lambda$ are the eigenvectors and eigenvalues of A, respectively. If K is decomposed into a K = $FF^T$ form, it is obvious that F can be approximated as in Eq. (3):

$$F = RU\Lambda^{-1/2} \tag{3}$$

It is interesting to note in Eq. (3) that it is not necessary to calculate any pair of the kernel values $K(x_i, x_j)$ across data sources at all. Only the kernel value between each data point and the chosen landmarks need to be calculated, which can then be mapped on to the eigenvectors of the landmarks. Since approximating all pairs of $(x_i, x_j)$ that are located at different locations requires a large amount of communication among data sources, which does not scale well when the number of data or data sources is significant. Since only small sizes of samples are used to approximate the kernel matrix, a large number of complex communication and computation cost are avoided.

Moreover, the non-linear SVM is converted into a linear one by the Nystrom approximation and matrix decomposition techniques with the kernel matrix $K = FF^T$, where F can be regarded as virtual points. Thus the global "*linear*" classification model has been constructed with virtual points of $F = RU\Lambda^{-1/2}$. The representations of all data in the non-linear space will be converted into virtual points in the final linear space, thus a linear SVM model is built in the medium layer.

To further improve the efficiency of the proposed model, the linear search and cutting-plane techniques introduced in [28] are employed in the top layer. The proposed framework provides a good solution to preserve sensitive information via secure sum protocol. It can also be applied to large datasets very efficiently since data size is reduced by sampling. Although the classification accuracy of PAN-SVM sacrifices slightly because of sampling when compared with the traditional SVM, such as LIBSVM with RBF kernel, the training process is speeded up when compared with other distributed classification methods; especially the individual private information is preserved. Details can be found from [16].

## 2.4 *Wrapper Methods*

### 2.4.1 SVM-RFE

Just as the name implies, the wrapper methods often wrapped the feature selection step in the process of mining algorithms. Compared with the filter methods, wrapper methods have the advantages of taking account into the performance of mining algorithms or tasks; thus a better classification model will be built with high performance, says high classification accuracy. However, it needs to repeatedly train and test the data and build classification model at each step when a subset of features are selected; the computational complexity thus increased sharply. In recent years, many approaches of wrapper feature selections are developed [5–9]. Among these methods, the Recursive Feature Elimination (RFE-SVM) proposed by Guyon [5] is very popular. RFE-SVM employs Support Vector Machine as a classifier and aims to find the best subset with $r$ features by ranking the whole feature set according to a criterion of $w^2$, which is formulated in Eq. (4):

$$\omega_i = \sum_i^m \alpha_i y_i x_i \tag{4}$$

where $\omega$ is the weighted vector of SVM classifier, $\alpha_i$ is nonzero if $x_i$ is support vector, otherwise, $\alpha_i$ equals to zero. Therefore, this criterion can also be explained as the weighted sum of support vectors, which tries to achieve high performance by maximization the separation margin in SVM. The elimination procedure can be described by three steps:

- *Step 1*: Train SVM classifier.
- *Step 2*: Calculate the ranking scores $\omega^2$ for all features according to equation.
- *Step 3*: Eliminate the feature (features) which has (have) the smallest ranking scores.

The elimination procedure iterates the above steps until all features are eliminated and ranked, top features that make the classifier attain highest accuracy performance will be selected. However, over-fitting is an important issue in machine learning study, since SVM-RFE is aiming to find the features that maximum the separation margin, over-fitting also exists.

### 2.4.2 RSVM

SVM-RFE works very well for many problems but data with outliers. To improve the robustness to noise and outliers, another Recursive Support Vector Machine (RSVM) is proposed in [7]. RSVM shares the same iterative procedures with SVM-RFE, but different ranking criterion, which is formulated by Eq. (5). RSVM also starts from the whole feature set and backwardly eliminates the feature with the least ranking score.

$$\text{ranking score} = \omega_j m_j^+ m_j^- \tag{5}$$

where $\omega_j$ represents the weight of the $j^{\text{th}}$ feature, $m_j^+$ and $m_j^-$ denote the means of $j^{th}$ feature in the positive and negative class, respectively. Unlike SVM-RFE, this method of RSVM takes account into the classification information via weight, as well as the data itself by calculating the means of each class. By this recursive iteration step, a feature subset with smaller and smaller size will be selected, and the classification can also be performed on the selected features at each step. Top features with high selected-frequency will be chosen as the final selection results. However, this method is greatly affected by the class label, since the class means are used to calculate the ranking criterion, which makes the selection method unstable.

### 2.4.3 SVM-t

To conquer the disadvantages of RSVM and develop a stable selection method, Tsai et al. [9] proposed another wrapped feature selection method named SVM-t. It also follows the workflow of SVM-RFE and RSVM to eliminate least important features through backward selection procedure but employs t-statistics to be as the ranking criterion, as denotes in the Eq. (6).

$$|t_j| = \frac{\mu_j^+ - \mu_j^-}{\sqrt{\left(\left(s_j^+\right)^2/n^+\right) + \left(\left(s_j^-\right)^2/n^-\right)}} \tag{6}$$

where $n^+$ and $n^-$ denotes the number of support vectors for the positive class $(+)$ and negative class $(-)$, respectively. $\mu_j^+$ and $\mu_j^-$ indicate the means of the $j^{th}$ feature in class$+$ and class$-$; $s_j^+$ and $s_j^-$ represent the standard deviations of the $j^{th}$ feature in class$+$ and class$-$, respectively. SVM-t just uses the most important subset of data, says support vectors, to evaluate the importance of each feature and construct the ranking criterion. It works well when data have significant statistical differences.

## 2.5 Workflow of PPFSVW

The above mentioned three feature selection methods employ the wrapper strategy and use SVM as the classifier. SVM-RFE directly chooses the weight vector as a ranking criterion, but it does not consider class information and has a high risk of over-fitting. RSVM outperforms SVM-RFE in the way of improving its robustness to noise and outliers, but unstable to class label assignment. SVM-t uses only the support vectors information and outperforms other two methods when considering distinct variance between informative and non-informative genes, but it is only suitable for linear support vector machine. Although any of the three methods are not perfect or suitable to every scenario, they share some common of returning a ranking list of features, and thus users could choose different subsets of top ranked features according to their contributions to classification accuracy. Besides, the iteration process is simple and easy to implement.

The current work proposed a feature selection framework aiming to inheriting the advantages of the above three methods via voting in the form of classification accuracies returned by the three methods. In the meanwhile protect individual privacy via employing the privacy preserving framework of PAN-SVM. PPFSVW [15] shares the common workflow with SVM-RFE, RSVM, and SVM-t, but has two main differences from them in the way of choosing eliminating feature at each step. First, PPFSVW employs PAN-SVM as classifier, which can guarantee the privacy to be preserved; second, it calculates the ranking scores for each feature according to Eqs. (4), (5) and (6), respectively, and then eliminate the least important one via voting by the three measurements. The workflow of PPFSVW is described as following and presented in Fig. 2.

- *Step 1*: Train PAN-SVM, privacy preserved classifier.
- *Step 2*: Calculate ranking scores using the criteria of SVM-RFE, RSVM, and SVM-t according to Eqs. (4), (5) and (6),
- *Step 3*: Rank features according to three measuring scores obtained from step 2, and obtain three ranking lists, respectively.
- *Step 4*: Choose one feature that needed to be eliminated at this iteration according to the following way:
- *Step 4.1*: Select one least important feature from each list obtained from Step 3 waiting for eliminating as following:
- *Step 4.2a)*: If two of the selected three least important features are the same, then this feature win this votes, and will be selected at this step. Selected feature at this step will be removed from the feature list and put in the head of another ranking list of features. The program here will go to step 1 until all features are ranked; otherwise, go to step 4.2b);
- *Step 4.2b)*: if the selected three least important features from Step 4.1 are different from each other, calculating the classification accuracy by fivefold cross validation for classifiers, which with the three selected features eliminated, respectively. Feature that has highest negative affection to the classifier will be selected and removed. Once selected, the program will go to step 1 until all features are ranked.
- *Step 5*: Return a ranked list of removed features at each step, with most top features with highest importance.

In step 3, three feature ranking lists will be generated according to the three ranking criteria formulated in Eqs. (4), (5) and (6), and the least important feature in each ranking list will be voted in step 4 to decide which one should be eliminated finally at this iteration. If the three temporally selected features are different from each other, PPFSVW will train three classifiers, which have one of the three features removed respectively. For example, features 1, 2, and 3 are three temporally selected

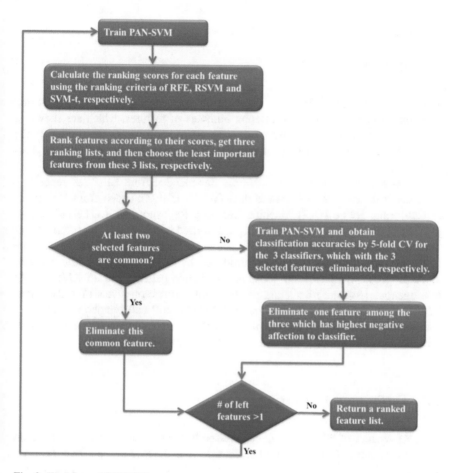

**Fig. 2** Workflow of PPFSVW

features waiting for eliminating, PPFSVW will train classifier number one with feature 1 being removed and get the classification accuracy of 90%, classifier number two with feature 2 being eliminated and get accuracy of 93%, and classifier number three with feature 3 being eliminated and get accuracy of 92%. Number two classifier obtains the highest accuracy by eliminating feature 2, so feature 2 makes the highest negative affection to classifier. In other word, it is the least important one among the three temporally selected features; therefore, PPFSVW will eliminate feature 2 at this iteration and restore features 1 and 3. The eliminated feature will be put at the head in the queue of the ranking list. This procedure will repeat until all features are eliminated and ranked, with the most important feature at the top and least important one at the bottom (the tail in the queue).

## 3  Experiment Results and Discussions

### 3.1  Datasets

The performance of PPFSVW is assessed on six benchmark datasets, including three microarray datasets with different numbers of features, which are shown in Table 1. C and $\gamma$ are the penalty parameter for SVM and a free parameter for Radial Basis Function kernel (RBF) used in SVM. They are generated by fivefold cross validation.

The *Diabetes* and *Ionosphere* data are downloaded from LIBSVM repository [29], the Wisconsin Breast Cancer data (WBC) is downloaded from University of California, Irvine (UCI) Machine Learning Repository [30]. The *colon data* [31–33] contain 62 samples including 22 normal samples and 40 colon cancer samples. Each sample is described by the expression levels of 2000 genes. The *Leukemia data* [31, 33], originally introduced by Golub et al., in 1999, contains 47 ALL (Acute lymphoblastic leukemia) leukemia patients and 25 AML (Acute myelogenous leukemia) leukemia patients with expression levels of 7129 genes. *DLBCL data* [34], the distinct types of diffuse large B-cell lymphoma (DLBCL) with expression levels of 4026 genes, contains 47 samples, 24 of them are from "germinal center B-like" group and 23 are "activated B-like" group.

### 3.2  Performance Assessing

The performance of PPFSVW will be assessed by the measurement of classification accuracy, which is formulated by the Eq. (7), Where *TP* represents *True Positive*, *TN* denotes *True Negative*, *FP* means *False Positive* and *FN* states *False Negative*.

$$\text{Accuracy} = \frac{TP + TN}{TP + FP + TN + FN} \tag{7}$$

The Cross Validation (CV) method is often used to assess the performance of classifier due to lack of data that can be utilized as separate testing samples

**Table 1** Details about datasets used for PPFSVM

| Dataset | # of samples | # of features | C | $\gamma$ |
|---------|--------------|---------------|-----|----------|
| Diabetes (DIA) | 768 | 8 | 512.0 | 0.0078125 |
| Ionosphere | 351 | 34 | 8.0 | 0.5 |
| Colon | 62 | 2000 | 32.0 | 0.0078125 |
| Leukemia | 72 | 7129 | 128.0 | 0.0001220703125 |
| Lymphoma (DLBCL) | 47 | 4026 | 2.0 | 0.0078125 |
| Breast Cancer (WBC) | 569 | 30 | 128.0 | 8.0 |

(like fivefold cross validation, Leave One Out method). During the cross-validation process, data will be randomly split into $k$ ($k$-fold) subsets, and at each training round, $k-1$ subsets are used as training data, and the left $1$ subset is used as testing set. However, as pointed by [7], the feature selection results may vary due to even a single difference in the training set, especially for small datasets. Many feature selection methods are done with all samples, and the cross-validation step is only done during the classification process, which makes the feature selection external to the cross-validation procedures, and leads to 'information leak' in the feature selection step. It calls this kind of error made by cross-validation as a CV1 error [35–37]. Also points out that CV1 error may severely bias the evaluation of feature selection. The work in [7] also demonstrates the existing of the bias via simulation data and suggests another error evaluation method, named CV2. Under the CV2 scenario, a separate dataset is used as test samples and leaves out of training set before any feature selection step. In the current work, PPFSVW will be tested and evaluated under the two testing schemes. We use '*Whole*' to denote the experiment is conducted under CV1, which means the whole dataset is involved in the training and feature selection process, and '*Separate*' to denote that the testing is conducted under CV2, which means testing data are separate from the training one. fivefold cross-validation is used to generated the classification accuracy at each selection iteration, the classification accuracies in the following sections are average value of 10-times running.

## 3.3  Feasibility and Effectiveness

The effectiveness and feasibility of the proposed method is assessed via conducting experiments on PAN-SVM, as well as a popular regular SVM package of LIBSVM [29, 38]. The experiments are conducted under both CV1 and CV2 testing scenario, and the results are presented in Tables 2 and 3, respectively. We use '*Voted*' to denote the classification accuracy which is obtained after applying the proposed algorithm and '*NoSelection*' denotes the accuracy that is obtained without a feature selection procedure. For LIBSVM, it follows the proposed workflow and selection strategies, only uses LIBSVM instead of PAN-SVM as the classifier.

From the results shown in Tables 2 and 3, we can observe that the classification accuracy for most of the classifiers that conduct by LIBSVM, as well as PAN-SVM, are improved after being applied the proposed feature selection methods PPFSVW when assessed under both testing scenarios, which indicates that the proposed feature selection is feasiable and works well. If summate all of the improvements together, they are 26.76% versus 39.99% for LIBSVM and PAN-SVM under CV1 scenario, and 36.32% versus 41.82% under CV2 scenario, respectively. Moreover, the results also show that PAN-SVM works better than LIBSVM, especially under CV1 testing scenario, the classification accuracies in sum have been improved 39.99% (PAN-SVM) v.s 26.76% (LIBSVM). The reason is probably because LIBSVM can achieve slight higher prediction accuracy under

**Table 2** Classification accuracy (%) before and after feature selection under CV1 scenario

| CV1 | LIBSVM | | | PAN-SVM | | |
|---|---|---|---|---|---|---|
| Datasets | Voted | NoSelection | Improvement | Voted | NoSelection | Improvement |
| DIA | 77.91 | 76.54 | 1.37 | 80.13 | 76.76 | 3.37 |
| Ionosphere | 97.50 | 93.78 | 3.72 | 96.29 | 93.03 | 3.27 |
| Colon | 100.00 | 82.30 | 17.70 | 100.00 | 82.00 | 18.00 |
| Leukemia | 94.29 | 93.10 | 1.19 | 94.29 | 89.65 | 4.64 |
| WBC | 98.23 | 96.10 | 2.13 | 96.46 | 96.69 | −0.23 |
| DLBCL | 91.11 | 90.46 | 0.65 | 100.00 | 89.05 | 10.95 |
| SUM | 559.04 | 532.28 | 26.76 | 567.17 | 527.17 | 39.99 |

**Table 3** Classification accuracy (%) before and after feature selection under CV2 scenario

| CV2 | LIBSVM | | | PAN-SVM | | |
|---|---|---|---|---|---|---|
| Datasets | Voted | NoSelection | Improvement | Voted | NoSelection | Improvement |
| DIA | 75.95 | 75.63 | 0.32 | 79.35 | 76.48 | 2.86 |
| Ionosphere | 97.50 | 93.04 | 4.47 | 96.86 | 93.94 | 2.91 |
| Colon | 100.00 | 82.79 | 17.21 | 100.00 | 81.92 | 18.08 |
| Leukemia | 92.86 | 90.00 | 2.86 | 92.86 | 87.14 | 5.72 |
| WBC | 98.41 | 93.54 | 4.87 | 96.64 | 96.64 | 0.00 |
| DLBCL | 95.56 | 88.95 | 6.61 | 100.00 | 87.76 | 12.24 |
| SUM | 560.27 | 523.94 | 36.32 | 565.70 | 523.88 | 41.82 |

CV1 than that under CV2 before applying the proposed feature selection procedure; thus the improvement in sum reduced, which probably indicates that LIBSVM has the problem of over-fitting, whereas, the accuracy imporvement achieved by PAN-SVM under CV1 and CV2 has no significant difference; therefore it may say that PAN-SVM can reduce or avoid the risk of over-fitting when compared with regular SVM.

The experimental results are also represented in bar charts in Figs. 3 and 4 to show the effectiveness of PPFSVW via classification accuracy improvements achieved by PAN-SVM and regular SVM of LIBSVM. "*Whole*" denotes that experiment is conducted under CV1 scenario, means the whole dataset was involved in the feature selection procedure; while "*Separate*" represents the experiment was conducted under CV2 test scenario with separate dataset as testing samples. PAN-SVM is shown as '*PrivacySVM*', aiming to emphasize its difference from the regular SVM at the aspect of privacy preserving property, and '*RegularSVM*' denotes LIBSVM.

Figure 3 shows the results conducted by PAN-SVM. The classification accuracy has been significantly improved, especially for the *Colon, DLBCL* and *Leukemia* microarray data, and improvements are 18.08%, 12.24% and 5.72% under CV2 testing scenario, and 18%, 10.95% and 4.64% under CV1 testing situation. The classification accuracy is also improved for datasets *DIA* and *Ionosphere*, and they are 2.86% and 2.91%, 3.37% and 3.27% for CV2 and CV1, respectively. There is

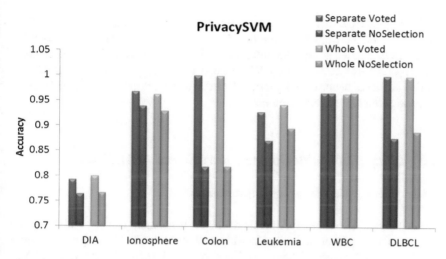

**Fig. 3** Performance improvement achieved after feature selection by PAN-SVM

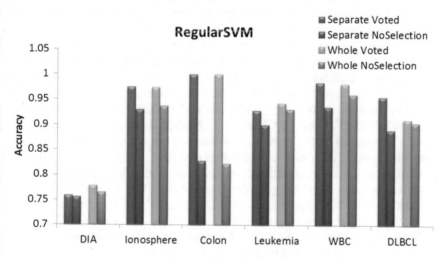

**Fig. 4** Performance improvement achieved after feature selection by LIBSVM

no improvement for *WBC* datasets under CV2 and a slight sacrifice under CV1. Besides, from Fig. 3 we can also observe that the classification accuracy can be improved slightly higher by PAN-SVM under CV2 test situation than that under CV1 test scenario, when compared with the total improvements added from each dataset, but there is no significant difference (41.82% vs. 39.99% in total) between the improvements obtained under CV1 and CV2.

Figure 4 shows the results conducted by the regular SVM of LIBSVM. Similar to the results obtained by executing PAN-SVM, the classification accuracy has been significantly improved after executing the proposed feature selection procedure for

*Colon* and *DLBCL* microarray dataset under CV2 test situation, they are 17.21% and 6.61%, respectively. However, the "*Voted*"classification accuracy of LIB-SVM for *DLBCL* dataset is only 95.56%, which is 100% for PAN-SVM under CV2, and 91.11% verus 100% under CV1, respectively. These results may indicate that PPFSVW works better for microarray datasets, which always include small sample size and much higher gene number.

## 3.4  Comparison with Other Feature Selection Methods

### 3.4.1  Classification Accuracy Improvement

We firstly conducted our experiments on the six benchmark datasets and compared some of the results obtained by the proposed algorithm in this paper with those obtained by other state-of-the-art methods, such as Fisher-SVM, FSV, RFE-SVM and KP-SVM [5, 39]. The accuracies obtained from these four methods shown in Table 4 are cited from [39]. *DIA, WBC,* and *Colon* are three common datasets which are used as the benchmark datasets in paper [39] and in the current work.

There is no privacy preserving issue or testing scheme in [39], therefore, we can compared our experimental results conducted via regular SVM under CV1 test situation, which are shown in the last column in Table 4, from which we can observe that the proposed method of PPFSVW outperforms the other methods for all of the three datasets *DIA, WBC, and Colon*. Besides, experimental results obtained by LIBSVM under CV2 and by PAN-SVM are also listed in Table 4 for a better comparison, and the results show that the proposed algorithm in this paper outperforms all the other four state-of-the-art methods.

Furthermore, we also conduct our experiments on the six benchmark datasets described in Table 1 and compare the results obtained by PPFSVW with those obtained by SVM-RFE, RSVM, and SVM-t. The classification accuracies achieved by different methods under two test scenarios are shown as in Figs. 5, 6, 7, and 8 in the form of bar charts and the results of accuracy improvement achieved by these four methods are shown in Tables 5, 6, 7, and 8, respectively.

From Fig. 5 and Table 5, we can observe that all of the four methods, SVM-RFE, RSVM, SVM-t, as well as the proposed method of PPFSVM in this paper can significantly improve the classifier predicting performance after executing the

**Table 4** Classification accuracy after feature selection achieved by different methods

| Datasets | Fisher-SVM | FSV | RFE-SVM | KP-SVM | Privacy SVM (CV2) | Privacy SVM (CV1) | Regular SVM (CV2) | Regular SVM (CV1) |
|---|---|---|---|---|---|---|---|---|
| DIA | 76.42 | 76.58 | 76.56 | 76.74 | 79.35 | 80.13 | 75.95 | 77.91 |
| WBC | 94.7 | 95.23 | 95.25 | 97.55 | 96.64 | 96.46 | 98.41 | 98.23 |
| Colon | 87.46 | 92.03 | 92.52 | 96.57 | 1.00 | 1.00 | 1.00 | 1.00 |

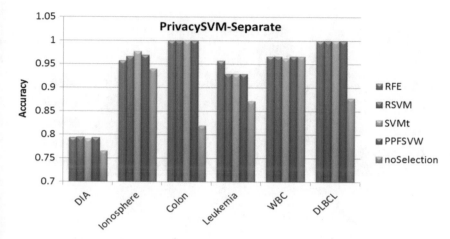

**Fig. 5** Comparison of classification accuracy achieved by PAN-SVM under CV2

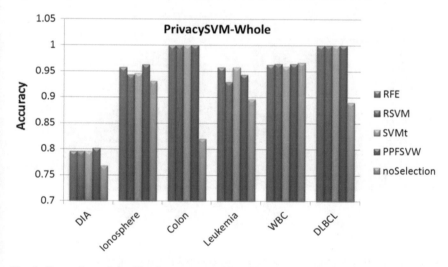

**Fig. 6** Comparison of classification accuracy achieved by PAN-SVM under CV1

feature selection procedure for most datasets except the WBC dataset. However, different methods have different behaviors when working with various datasets. For example, the method of SVM-t works better on *Ionosphere* dataset, but achieves worse classification results when compared with the other three methods on the microarray datasets, which contain much more features, and fails to improve the classifier's predicting performance for *WBC* datasets. RFE, RSVM, and PPFSVW can achieve almost the same level accuracy improvement for *DIA, Colon, WBC* and *DLBCL* datasets, but slightly lower for *Ionosphere* dataset and higher on *Leukemia* data. Compared with the total sum improvement on all datasets, RFE-SVM defeats

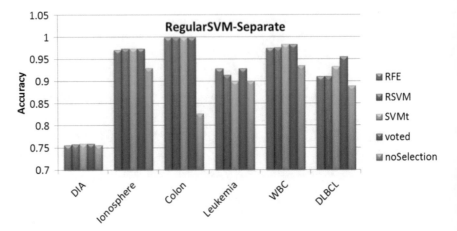

**Fig. 7** Comparison of classification accuracy achieved by LIBSVM under CV2

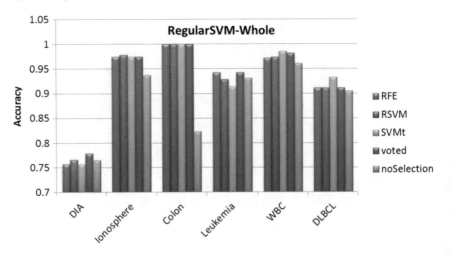

**Fig. 8** Comparison of classification accuracy achieved by LIBSVM under CV1

**Table 5** Accuracy improvement achieved by different methods via PAN-SVM under CV2

|            | SVM-RFE (%) | RSVM (%) | SVM-t (%) | PPFSVW (%) |
|------------|-------------|----------|-----------|------------|
| DIA        | 2.86        | 2.99     | 2.60      | 2.86       |
| Ionosphere | 1.77        | 2.63     | 3.77      | 2.91       |
| Colon      | 18.08       | 18.08    | 18.08     | 18.08      |
| Leukemia   | 8.57        | 5.72     | 5.72      | 5.72       |
| WBC        | 0.00        | 0.00     | −0.35     | 0.00       |
| DLBCL      | 12.24       | 12.24    | 12.24     | 12.24      |
| Sum        | 43.53       | 41.66    | 42.06     | 41.82      |

**Table 6** Accuracy improvement achieved by different methods via PAN-SVM under CV1

|            | RFE (%) | RSVM (%) | SVM-t (%) | PPFSVW (%) |
|------------|---------|----------|-----------|------------|
| DIA        | 2.71    | 2.71     | 2.71      | 3.37       |
| Ionosphere | 2.69    | 1.27     | 1.55      | 3.27       |
| Colon      | 18.00   | 18.00    | 18.00     | 18.00      |
| Leukemia   | 6.06    | 3.21     | 6.06      | 4.64       |
| WBC        | −0.41   | −0.23    | −0.76     | −0.23      |
| DLBCL      | 10.95   | 10.95    | 10.95     | 10.95      |
| Sum        | 40.01   | 35.91    | 38.52     | 39.99      |

**Table 7** Accuracy improvement achieved by different methods via LIBSVM under CV2

|            | RFE (%) | RSVM (%) | SVM-t (%) | PPFSVW (%) |
|------------|---------|----------|-----------|------------|
| DIA        | 0.05    | 0.18     | 0.32      | 0.32       |
| Ionosphere | 4.11    | 4.47     | 4.47      | 4.47       |
| Colon      | 17.21   | 17.21    | 17.21     | 17.21      |
| Leukemia   | 2.86    | 1.43     | 0.00      | 2.86       |
| WBC        | 3.99    | 4.16     | 4.87      | 4.87       |
| DLBCL      | 2.16    | 2.16     | 4.38      | 6.61       |
| Sum        | 30.37   | 29.61    | 31.24     | 36.32      |

**Table 8** Accuracy improvement achieved by different methods via LIBSVM under CV1

|            | RFE (%) | RSVM (%) | SVM-t (%) | PPFSVW (%) |
|------------|---------|----------|-----------|------------|
| DIA        | −0.85   | 0.07     | −0.85     | 1.37       |
| Ionosphere | 3.72    | 4.08     | 3.72      | 3.72       |
| Colon      | 17.70   | 17.70    | 17.70     | 17.70      |
| Leukemia   | 1.19    | −0.24    | −1.67     | 1.19       |
| WBC        | 1.07    | 1.25     | 2.49      | 2.13       |
| DLBCL      | 0.65    | 0.65     | 2.87      | 0.65       |
| Sum        | 23.47   | 23.50    | 24.26     | 26.76      |

all other three feature selection methods benefiting from its higher improvement on the *Leukemia* data.

The results in Fig. 6 and Table 6 show the classification performance and comparison of classification accuracy improvements that have been achieved by SVM-RFE, RSVM, SVM-t and PPFSVM under CV1 test situation using a separate testing sample set. These results indicate a similar pattern made by these four feature selection methods via PAN-SVM under CV1 to that under CV2. All of these four methods can improve the classifier's ability to predict unknown samples, for *DIA, Ionosphere, Colon, Leukemia* and *DLBCL* datasets, and achieve a significant improvement for microarray datasets. The performance improvement has no significant difference among these four methods.

Figures 7 and 8 show the comparison of classification accuracies by using LIB-SVM as the classifier for SVM-RFE, RSVM, SVM-t and the proposed algorithm workflow in this paper. Tables 7 and 8 show accuracy improvements achieved by these four different methods via employing LIBSVM. Each method is tested under CV1, and CV2 testing mode and the accuracies at each iteration step are obtained by fivefold cross-validation, as well as the final accuracy using the series of selected features.

From Figs. 7 and 8, Tables 7 and 8, we can observe that all of these four methods perform better under CV2 testing environment, which is similar to PAN-SVM. However, the overall improvement achieved by LIBSVM under CV2 is much higher than that under CV1 when summarizing all of the improvements together (as shown in the last line in Tables 7 and 8) than PAN-SVM, the reason is probably there exists overfitting for LIBSVM under CV1, and the regular SVM cannot achieve higher or same level of predicting accuracy for separating testing samples under CV2 scenario. Besides, when compared all the overall improvements achieved by these four different methods, we can observe that the proposed workflow can make the classifier achieve higher classification accuracy than the other three methods and have significant improvements, no matter under CV1 or CV2 test environment. In other word, the proposed workflow in this paper works better for regular SVM and can preserve individual privacy when employing PAN-SVM as the classifier.

### 3.4.2   Number of Selected Features

We also compare the selected number of features by these four methods on datasets *DIA, Ionosphere, Colon, Leukemia, WBC* and *DLBCL*, and only show the results achieved by PAN-SVM under CV2 test situation. The results are represented as curves in Fig. 9 and the detail descriptions are shown in Table 9, from which we can observe that PPFSVW can make the classifier achieve the highest predicting accuracy for *DIA* dataset by the top five features (with accuracy 79.35%), which is the same as SVM-RFE and is fewer than 7 (79.48%) and 8 (79.09%) for RSVM and SVM-t, respectively. For the *Colon* data, the classifier can achieve the best classification performance with top 53 features (with accuracy 100%) after conducting PPFSVW algorithms, but 63 (accuracy 100%), 61 (accuracy 100%) and 617 (accuracy 100%) for RFE-SVM, RSVM, and SVM-t, respectively.

For *WBC* data, the number of best-selected feature subset is 11 (accuracy 96.64%), which is fewer than 18 (accuracy 96.64%), 17 (accuracy 96.64%) and 21 (accuracy 96.28%) for SVM-RFE, RSVM, and SVM-t, respectively. For the three datasets of *DIA, Colon,* and *WBC*, PPFSVW can not only select fewer features but also keep the classifier with higher or almost same level of classification accuracy. For the *Ionosphere* data, although PPFSVW selects a subset of features with a larger number than other methods, it makes the classifier achieve the highest classification performance. For the *Leukemia* and *DLBCL* data, PPFSVW is defeated by SVM-RFE but still works better than RSVM and SVM-t with fewer features but the same level of accuracy.

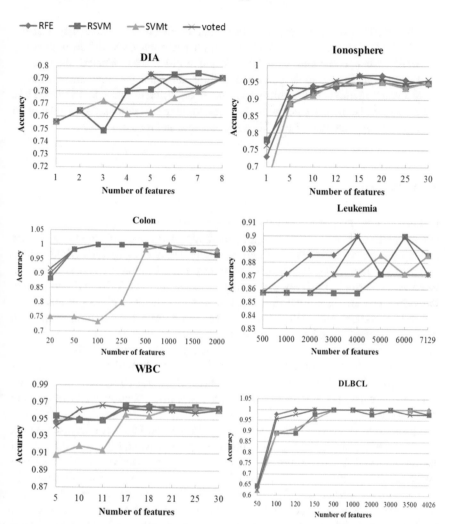

**Fig. 9** Comparison of accuracy as the number of selected features increases

**Table 9** Selected feature number by different methods

|        | DIA        | Ionosphere  | Colon      | Leukemia      | WBC        | DLBCL     |
|--------|------------|-------------|------------|---------------|------------|-----------|
| RFE    | 5 (79.35)  | 12 (95.71)  | 63 (100)   | 4565 (95.71)  | 18 (96.64) | 114 (100) |
| RSVM   | 7 (79.48)  | 12 (96.57)  | 61 (100)   | 6380 (92.86)  | 17 (96.64) | 147 (100) |
| SVM-t  | 8 (79.09)  | 10 (97.71)  | 617 (100)  | 5420 (92.86)  | 21 (96.28) | 166 (100) |
| PPFSVW | 5 (79.35)  | 17 (96.86)  | 53 (100)   | 4826 (92.86)  | 11 (96.64) | 121 (100) |

From these results, we can conclude that PPFSVW can make the classifier achieve higher or same level of classification performance with fewer features, especially when compared with RSVM and SVM-t. The selected six datasets are different at their sample sizes and feature numbers; the other three existing sophisticated methods outperforms each other on different datasets, but PPFSVW can always make the classifier achieve competitive results compared with the other three, which indicate that PPFSVW is much stable and robust.

## 4 Conclusions

In this paper, we proposed a privacy preserving feature selection method (PPFSVW) via integrating three popular wrapper methods in the way of voting at feature eliminating phase. PPFSVW is based on our previous work of PAN-SVM, which is a privacy preserving framework for binary classification on SVM; therefore, PPFSVM inherits the privacy preserving property of PAN-SVM and can protect individual privacy during the procedure of feature selection. PPFSVW shares the common workflow with RFE-SVM, RSVM, and SVM-t, but different from them at the step of choosing to be eliminated feature at each iteration. It combines the three criteria used by these three methods, and votes to be eliminated one. If eliminating feature cannot be decided by voting, PPFSVW will construct classifiers and compare the negative affection to classifiers which caused by those temporarily selected three features, and the one with highest negative affection will be eliminated at this iteration.

The feasibility and performance of the proposed workflow are assessed on six benchmark datasets, including three microarray datasets, and they are different at sample size and feature numbers. The experiments are also conducted under two different testing situations, CV1 and CV2. Our experimental results indicate that the proposed algorithm workflow can work effectively to improve the classification performance regarding accuracy via selecting informative features and genes, for both PAN-SVM with privacy preserving consideration and LIBSVM without privacy consideration under CV1 and CV2. Besides, PPFSVW outperforms other state-of-the-art feature selection methods of Fisher-SVM, FSV, RFE-SVM and KP-SVM [5, 39] for *DIA, Ionosphere* and *Colon* datasets. Furthermore, we also conducted the proposed workflow on PAN-SVM and LIBSVM and compared their classification accuracies with those obtained from SVM-RFE, RSVM, and SVM-t. The experimental results show that PPFSVW has no significant difference from these three methods when employing PAN-SVM, but works better when conducting on LIBSVM. The reason for this is because of the stability and ability of PAN-SVM to reduce the risk of over-fitting. In addition, our experimental results also show that PPFSVM can make the classifier achieve higher or same level classification accuracy with fewer features when compared with SVM-RFE, RSVM and SVM-t.

**Acknowledgements** This work is part of the Ph.D. dissertation of Yunmei Lu, who would like to express her great gratitude to all of her committee members, Prof. Yanqing Zhang, Prof. Yi Pan, Prof. Rajshekhar Sunderraman and Prof. Yichuan Zhao, for their guidance and support. This work would have not been possible without their guidance and support. The authors also would like to thank the reviewers of this paper for their constructive comments and suggestions. Yunmei Lu is grateful to the continued financial support from the Department of Computer Science and the Molecular Basis of Disease (MBD) fellowship at GSU.

# References

1. Agrawal, R., & Srikant, R. (2000). Privacy-preserving data mining. *ACM Sigmod Record, 29,* 439–450.
2. Bayardo, R. J., & Agrawal, R. (2005). Data privacy through optimal k-anonymization. In *Data engineering, 2005. ICDE 2005. Proceedings 21st international conference on* (pp. 217–228). Piscataway, NJ: IEEE.
3. Machanavajjhala, A., Kifer, D., Gehrke, J., & Venkitasubramaniam, M. (2007). l-diversity: Privacy beyond k-anonymity. *ACM Transactions on Knowledge Discovery from Data, 1,* 3.
4. Guyon, I., & Elisseeff, A. (2003). An introduction to variable and feature selection. *Journal of Machine Learning Research, 3,* 1157–1182.
5. Guyon, I., Weston, J., Barnhill, S., & Vapnik, V. (2002). Gene selection for cancer classification using support vector machines. *Machine Learning, 46,* 389–422.
6. Díaz-Uriarte, R., & Alvarez de Andrés, S. (2006). Gene selection and classification of microarray data using random forest. *BMC Bioinformatics, 7,* 3.
7. Zhang, X., Lu, X., Shi, Q., Xu, X.-Q., Hon-chiu, E. L., Harris, L. N., et al. (2006). Recursive SVM feature selection and sample classification for mass-spectrometry and microarray data. *BMC Bioinformatics, 7,* 197.
8. Sharma, A., Imoto, S., & Miyano, S. (2012). A top-r feature selection algorithm for microarray gene expression data. *IEEE/ACM Transactions on Computational Biology and Bioinformatics, 9,* 754–764.
9. Chen-An Tsai, C.-H. H., Chang, C.-W., & Chen, C.-H. (2012). Recursive feature selection with significant variables of support vectors. *Computational and Mathematical Methods in Medicine, 2012,* 12.
10. Miranda, J., Montoya, R., & Weber, R. (2005). Linear penalization support vector Machines for Feature Selection. In S. K. Pal, S. Bandyopadhyay, & S. Biswas (Eds.), *Proceedings of the pattern recognition and machine intelligence: First international conference, PReMI 2005,* Kolkata, India, December 20–22, 2005 (pp. 188–192). Berlin: Springer.
11. Bradley, P. S., & Mangasarian, O. L. (1998). Feature selection via concave minimization and support vector machines. In *Proceedings of the fifteenth international conference on machine learning.* San Francisco, CA: M. Kaufmann Publishers.
12. Kholod, I., Kuprianov, M., & Petukhov, I. (2016). Distributed data mining based on actors for internet of things. In *2016 5th Mediterranean Conference on Embedded Computing (MECO)* (pp. 480–484). Piscataway, NJ: IEEE.
13. Bendechache, M., & Kechadi, M. T. (2015). Distributed clustering algorithm for spatial data mining. In *Spatial Data Mining and Geographical Knowledge Services (ICSDM), 2015 2nd IEEE international conference on* (pp. 60–65). Piscataway, NJ: IEEE.
14. Parmar, K., Vaghela, D., & Sharma, P. (2015). Performance prediction of students using distributed data mining. In *Innovations in Information, Embedded and Communication Systems (ICIIECS), 2015 international conference on* (pp. 1–5). Piscataway, NJ: IEEE.
15. Lu, Y., & Zhang, Y. (2017). Privacy preserving feature selection on horizontally distributed datasets. In *2017 5th International Conference on Bioinformatics and Computational Biology (ICBCB 2017) (Accepted).* Hong Kong, China: ACM.

16. Lu, Y., Phoungphol, P., & Zhang, Y. (2014). Privacy aware non-linear support vector machine for multi-source big data. In *2014 IEEE 13th international conference on trust, security and privacy in computing and communications* (pp. 783–789). Piscataway, NJ: IEEE.
17. Gavison, R., & Gavison, R. (1984). *Privacy and the limits of law philosophical dimensions of privacy*. New York: Cambridge University Press.
18. Pinkas, B. (2002). Cryptographic techniques for privacy-preserving data mining. *ACM Sigkdd Explorations Newsletter, 4*, 12–19.
19. Yao, A. C.-C. (1986). How to generate and exchange secrets. In *Foundations of Computer Science, 1986, 27th Annual Symposium on* (pp. 162–167). Piscataway, NJ: IEEE.
20. Goldreich, O. (2004). *Foundations of cryptography: Volume 2, basic applications*. New York: Cambridge University Press.
21. Paillier, P. (1999). Public-key cryptosystems based on composite degree residuosity classes. In *Proceedings of the 17th international conference on theory and application of cryptographic techniques*. Prague, Czech Republic: Springer.
22. Clifton, C., Kantarcioglu, M., Vaidya, J., Lin, X., & Zhu, M. Y. (2002). Tools for privacy preserving distributed data mining. *ACM Sigkdd Explorations Newsletter, 4*, 28–34.
23. Drineas, P., & Mahoney, M. W. (2005). On the Nystrom method for approximating a gram matrix for improved kernel-based learning. *Journal of Machine Learning Research, 6*, 2153–2175.
24. Zhang, K., Tsang, I. W., & Kwok, J. T. (2008). Improved Nystrom low rank approximation and error analysis. In *Presented at the Proceedings of the 25th international conference on Machine learning*. Helsinki, Finland: ACM.
25. Kumar, S., Mohri, M., & Talwalkar, A. (2012). Sampling methods for the Nyström method. *Journal of Machine Learning Research, 13*, 981–1006.
26. Harbrecht, H., Peters, M., & Schneider, R. (2012). On the low-rank approximation by the pivoted Cholesky decomposition. *Applied Numerical Mathematics, 62*, 428–440.
27. Zhang, K., Lan, L., Wang, Z., & Moerchen, F. (2012). Scaling up kernel SVM on limited resources: A low-rank linearization approach. *International Conference on Artificial Intelligence and Statistics (AISTATS), 22*, 1425–1434.
28. Franc, V., & Sonnenburg, S. (2009). Optimized cutting plane algorithm for large-scale risk minimization. *Journal of Machine Learning Research, 10*, 2157–2192.
29. LIBSVM. (2016). *LIBSVM data*. Retrieved from http://www.csie.ntu.edu.tw/~cjlin/libsvmtools/datasets/
30. Bache, K., & Lichman, M. (2013). *UCI machine learning repository*. Retrieved from http://archive.ics.uci.edu/ml
31. Golub, T. R., Slonim, D. K., Tamayo, P., Huard, C., Gaasenbeek, M., Mesirov, J. P., et al. (1999). Molecular classification of cancer: Class discovery and class prediction by gene expression monitoring. *Science, 286*, 531–537.
32. Alon, U., Barkai, N., Notterman, D. A., Gish, K., Ybarra, S., Mack, D., et al. (1999). Broad patterns of gene expression revealed by clustering analysis of tumor and normal colon tissues probed by oligonucleotide arrays. *Proceedings of the National Academy of Sciences of the United States of America, 96*, 6745–6750.
33. Zhu, Z., Ong, Y. S., & Dash, M. (2007). Markov blanket-embedded genetic algorithm for gene selection. *Pattern Recognition, 49*, 3236–3248.
34. Alizadeh, A. A., Eisen, M. B., Davis, R. E., Ma, C., Lossos, I. S., Rosenwald, A., et al. (2000). Distinct types of diffuse large B-cell lymphoma identified by gene expression profiling. *Nature, 403*, 503–511.
35. Ambroise, C., & McLachlan, G. J. (2002). Selection bias in gene extraction on the basis of microarray gene-expression data. *Proceedings of the National Academy of Sciences of the United States of America, 99*, 6562–6566.
36. Amir Ben-Dor, L. B., Friedman, N., Nachman, I., Schummer, M., & Yakhini, Z. (2000, April). Tissue classification with gene expression profiles. *Journal of Computational Biology, 7*, 559–583.

37. Ben-Dor, L. B. A., Friedman, N., Nachman, I., Schummer, M., & Yakhini, Z. (2007). *Journal of Computational Biology, 7*, 559–583.
38. Furlanello, C., Serafini, M., Merler, S., & Jurman, G. (2003). Entropy-based gene ranking without selection bias for the predictive classification of microarray data. *BMC Bioinformatics, 4*, 54.
39. Chang, C.-C., & Lin, C.-J. (2011). LIBSVM: A library for support vector machines. *ACM Transactions on Intelligent Systems and Technology, 2*, 1–27.
40. Maldonado, S., Weber, R., & Basak, J. (2011). Simultaneous feature selection and classification using kernel-penalized support vector machines. *Information Sciences, 181*, 115–128.

# Improving Maize Trait through Modifying Combination of Genes

Duolin Wang, Juexin Wang, Yu Chen, Sean Yang, Qin Zeng, Jingdong Liu, and Dong Xu

**Abstract** In molecular breeding, trait improvement has been focused on exploring genetic variations of single genes. To explore the potential of modifying multiple genes simultaneously for trait improvement, we developed a systematic computational method aiming at detecting complex traits associated with gene interactions using a combination of gene expression and trait data across a set of maize hybrids. This method represents changes of expression patterns in a gene pair in uniform statistics and employs network topology to describe the inherent genotype-phenotype associations at the systems level. We applied and evaluated our method on several phenotypic traits measured on a set of maize hybrids across 2 years (2013 and 2014) and achieved consistent and biologically meaningful results. Our results provide a subset of candidate gene pairs that have the potential to improve several specific traits by gene expression enhancement or silence. Our

Duolin Wang and Juexin Wang contributed equally with all other contributors.

**Electronic supplementary material** The online version of this chapter (https://doi.org/10.1007/978-3-030-33416-1_9) contains supplementary material, which is available to authorized users.

D. Wang · J. Wang · D. Xu (✉)
Department of Electric Engineering and Computer Science, and Christopher S. Bond Life Sciences Center, University of Missouri, Columbia, MO, USA
e-mail: wangdu@missouri.edu; wangjue@missouri.edu; xudong@missouri.edu

Y. Chen
Bayer U.S. Crop Science, Monsanto Legal Entity, Chesterfield, MO, USA

Current address: Eli Lilly and Company, Lilly Corporate Center, Indianapolis, IN, USA
e-mail: yu.chen@lilly.com

S. Yang · Q. Zeng · J. Liu (✉)
Bayer U.S. Crop Science, Monsanto Legal Entity, Chesterfield, MO, USA
e-mail: sean.yang@bayer.com; qin.zeng@bayer.com; jingdong.liu@bayer.com

© Springer Nature Switzerland AG 2020
Y. Zhao, D.-G. (Din) Chen (eds.), *Statistical Modeling in Biomedical Research*, Emerging Topics in Statistics and Biostatistics,
https://doi.org/10.1007/978-3-030-33416-1_9

work partially addresses the "missing heritability" problem in complex traits and offers an alternative way for improving crop traits via modifying a combination of multiple loci.

**Keywords** Maize · Complex trait · Yield improvement · Gene expression data analysis · Network biomarker

# 1  Introduction

Continuously advancing crop yield is a long-term task and a formidable challenge for crop breeders given the growing population and climate change. It is estimated that 60% more food will be required by 2050 (compared to 2005) to meet human nutrition needs [1]. Crop yield is a complex plant phenotype that is synthetically impacted by different physiological and molecular traits varying with environment and genetics. Under an identical controlled environment, the ideal trait for genetic improvement of crop yield is one that is heritable and correlated to yield. After these targeted traits have been identified, the next task is to determine how genetic variations (i.e. genes) impact these traits. This type of investigation offers opportunities to improve the traits by modifying the relevant genes via breeding or transgenic approaches. For example, biomarkers can be developed based on the gene information to assist in the selection of a relevant exchange of genetic materials in breeding, or alternatively, gene candidates can be manipulated with altered expression or coding sequences by transgenic or gene editing, especially using the clustered regularly interspaced short palindromic repeats (CRISPR) technique to achieve better trait efficacies. A significant yield improvement work has been done for maize [2–4], which is one of the most important crops in the world since its domestication in Central Mexico at least 9000 years ago [5].

While the traditional strategy assuming that genes are independent has approached its limit [6], gene-gene interaction has attracted more and more interest in genotype-phenotype relationship analysis in recent years. For example, in the field of complex human diseases' research, dysfunctional gene-gene interactions or even dysfunctional regulatory networks have been identified [7, 8]. In genetics, the interaction between genetic variations is also referred as "epistasis," which indicates that the effect of a specific genetic variant on a trait depends on the genotype of another variant. Detecting epistasis also partly addresses the phenomenon of "missing heritability" in a genome wide association study (GWAS) analyses [9, 10]. There are various computational tools for calculating the epistasis effects, such as PLINK, a toolset for whole-genome association and population-based linkage analysis [11], the Bayesian method (BEAM) [12], and multifactor-dimensionality reduction (MDR) [13]. In our previous work, a Bayesian high-order interaction toolkit (BHIT) was developed to detect associations between trait and genetic epistasis in GWAS [14]. However, epistasis identified in GWAS may not be actionable for trait improvement and trait-dependent gene expression analysis may help address the problem. The levels of gene expression in different crop lines reflect inherited or genetic differences among these individuals, which can serve as the basis for predicting gene combinations to be used in trait improvement. However, few studies have been applied to breeding practices for detecting trait-dependent interacting genes at the expression level.

Our primary objective is to detect interactions between genes that are associated with phenotypic traits in maize and to identify a subset of gene pairs as candidates for modifying the traits. Based on gene expression data, trait-dependent interacting gene pairs are typically represented by the patterns of "shift," "cross," and "rewiring" [15]. "Shift" represents changes in the mean gene expression value; "cross" represents changes in the rotation angle of correlation; and "rewiring" represents changes from having no correlation to having a significant correlation between a gene pair or *vice versa*. These gene interaction expression patterns may not be detected by any single gene testing approach, since neither of the two genes alone necessarily has a strong association with the phenotype (technically referred to as marginal effects).

To address this problem, a Bayesian-based method implemented in our previously developed R package Bayes factor for differential co-expression analysis (BFDCA) [16] was applied to infer trait-dependent interacting genes and gene modules based on gene expression data across a set of maize hybrids. By using the Bayes factor as a score to distinguish trait-dependent interacting genes from the noisy background, our method can identify "shift," "cross," and "rewiring," as well as their complex combinations with or without high marginal effects. The effectiveness of BFDCA in identifying differentially expressed interacting gene pairs was demonstrated by comparing it with several existing methods on simulation data, and BFDCA was the only method that could correctly identify interacting patterns of "shift," "cross," and "rewiring" consistently across these gene pairs.

In BFDCA, by making use of gene-gene interactions, subnetworks are constructed by integrating information of trait-dependency gene pairs with information on topological similarity. Then, each gene within a subnetwork module is assigned a weight according to the topological structure to indicate its importance within the module. Finally, taking the edge and node information together from the subnetworks, a subset of gene pairs is selected, which serves as candidates to modify the traits by expression enhancement or silence. In this work, both the trait-associated genes, gene-gene interactions selected in this work, and their associations with traits were demonstrated with some degree of consistency on two independent maize data sets cross 2 years. Notably, compared with the traditional single-gene-based method, the edge-based markers can achieve higher prediction accuracy, especially for trait grain moisture, with an accuracy of more than 90%. The functional analyses such as gene ontology (GO) enrichment and pathway analysis for trait-dependent gene modules provided several potential biological explanations. Our study offers a method that potentially addresses the "missing heritability" problem in complex traits, as well as alternative means for improving crop traits via modifying multiple loci genetically.

## 2  Materials and Methods

This section includes two subsections. Section 2.1 describes the data materials we used, including the germplasm selection, the phenotyping, the RNA-seq profiling and how we processed these materials to fit our method. Section 2.2 describes the details of the analysis method.

### 2.1  Materials

#### 2.1.1  Data Description

A panel of 57 lines that represents genetic diversities of the Monsanto maize germplasm was created using 34,000 homozygous marker genotype data on 4458 lines. The panel consisted of commercial and elite male and female lines spanning 95–115 days relative maturity range (6 early, 17 medium and 34 late maturity group lines). Hybrids were made by crossing each of the 57 inbred lines described above into one pool of six inbred lines, not among the 57, within the same maturity group and from the opposite-gender heterotic group.

  Flowering time within a plot was measured as the number of accumulated growing degree units (GDUs) between planting and when 50% of plants within a plot reached anthesis (P50) and silking (S50). Plant height (PHT) was measured for five plants per plot from the soil to the ligule of the uppermost fully expanded leaf. Grain yield, moisture and test weight (YLD, MST and TWT) were determined by harvesting two rows of the eight-row plot where no previous sampling had occurred, and no impact was observed on other destructive samplings in one row bordering land used for combine harvest.

  Top leaf tissue samples were collected from corn plants at the V8 stage. Total RNA was isolated from three biological replicates for each tissue using TRIzol (Invitrogen) according to the manufacturer's protocol. The RNA quantity was determined with the Thermo Scientific NanoDrop 8000 spectrophotometer (Thermo Scientific, Wilmington, DE, USA) and the integrity was assessed by a bioanalyzer assay with RIN greater than 6. 2 µg of total RNA was used for sequencing library preparation with Illumina TruSeq RNA Sample Prep Kit V2 (RS-122-2001, Illumina Inc., San Diego, CA, USA) following manufacturer's protocol. qPCR (SYBR PCR Master Mix, Applied Biosystems, Foster City, CA, USA) was utilized to quantify sequencing libraries. Sequencing was performed with HiSeq2000 sequencing using 50 base pair reads.

  RNA-Seq data was normalized by RPKM (reads per kilobase per million) mapped reads [17]. The normalized reads were subsequently converted to log2 scale by $\log(1 + c)$, where c is the normalized read value. Reads with extremely low expression values in all samples with $\log2(1 + c)$ less than 1 were removed. The resulting 19,319 common genes between 2013 and 2014 experiments that mapped to GRAMME IDs (http://www.gramene.org/) were used for subsequent analyses.

### 2.1.2 Data Preprocessing

The resulting 19,319 genes were further filtered. Following the process in [18], genes with median absolute deviation (MAD) smaller than 0.5 were removed from each dataset (each year), except for transcription factors (TFs), which may have major causal regulatory effects in biological processes. Then the union genes between the two datasets (in 2 years) were kept, resulting in 4312 genes in total.

Because all the traits involved in our work were continuous data, we had to convert them into discrete data to fit our method. For each trait, maize hybrids were classified into binary-level trait groups partitioned by the mean value of the trait. Hybrids with trait values smaller than the mean value were classified as a low-level trait group and given an assigned designation of Label 1, while hybrids with trait values larger than the mean value were classified as the high-level trait group and given an assigned designation of Label 2.

## 2.2 Methods

Figure 1 summarizes our method. The major part and some additional details are described as follows. For other details refer to our previous paper [16]. The crucial component of the method is the Bayes factor, which is used as a score to distinguish trait-dependent interacting genes from the null background. The Bayes factor is a ratio of marginal likelihood of the data between two models, the null model under the null hypothesis and the alternative model under the alternative hypothesis. In this application, the alternative hypothesis is that the gene pair under the test had differential (non-random) interacting patterns under different trait levels. The null hypothesis describes the complementary scenarios to the alternative hypothesis, where either gene pair has no interaction or has an identical pattern among different trait levels. All the gene pairs were tested, and a Bayes factor for each gene pair was calculated. After filtering out the insignificant gene pairs by a permutation procedure, the remaining interacting gene pairs were further analyzed and ranked by a network topology method. Finally, a subset of interacting genes was selected according to their end-node importance and the module assignment.

### 2.2.1 Calculation of Bayes Factor

For each gene pair $G$, the Bayes factor is defined as:

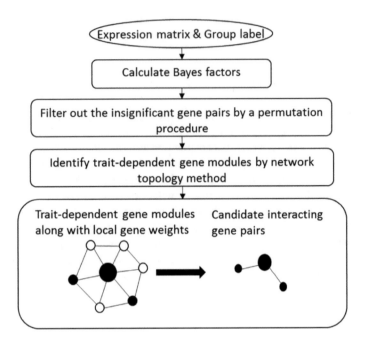

**Fig. 1** Overview of the method

$$BF = \ln \frac{P_A\,(C1_G, C2_G)}{P_0\,(C1_G, C2_G)}$$

$$= \ln \frac{P_{join}\,(C1_G) \cdot P_{join}\,(C2_G) + P_{join}\,(C1_G) \cdot P_{ind}\,(C2_G) + P_{ind}\,(C1_G) \cdot P_{join}\,(C2_G)}{P_{join}\,(C1_G, C2_G) + P_{ind}\,(C1_G, C2_G) + P_{ind}\,(C1_G) \cdot P_{ind}\,(C2_G)} \tag{1}$$

where $C1_G$ and $C2_G$ denote the lines for $G$ partitioned into two different trait groups ($C1$, $C2$). $P_A(C1_G, C2_G)$ denotes the marginal likelihood of the alternative model under the alternative hypothesis, and $P_0(C1_G, C2_G)$ denotes the marginal likelihood of the null model under the null hypothesis. They contain different combinations of two distributions: $P_{join}(X)$ and $P_{ind}(X)$, where $X$ represents the two-dimensional vector of gene expression of $G$. $P_{join}(X)$ assumes a joint distribution of $X$ and is modeled as a bivariate normal distribution whose marginal likelihood is formulated in Eq. (4), while $P_{ind}(X)$ assumes that genes in $X$ are independent and modeled as multiplying two independent normal distributions according to the expression of each gene whose marginal likelihood is formulated in Eq. (7). Under the alternative hypothesis, we assume that the gene pairs in $G$ follow a bivariate normal distribution in at least one trait group with different expression profile correlations in different trait groups. Therefore, $P_A(C1_G, C2_G)$ is modeled considering the following three scenarios:

1. The two genes in $G$ interact in group $C1$ and group $C2$, and their gene expression profile relationships are different in these two groups. It can be described by $P_{join}(C1_G)P_{join}(C2_G)$ representing a joint distribution of two independent bivariate normal distributions.
2. The two genes in G only interact in group $C1$ but not in group $C2$. It can be described by $P_{join}(C1_G)P_{ind}(C2_G)$, representing a joint distribution of one bivariate normal distribution and one product of two independent normal distributions.
3. The two genes in $G$ only interact in group $C2$ but not in group $C1$. It can be described by $P_{ind}(C1_G)P_{join}(C2_G)$, representing a joint distribution of one product of two independent normal distributions and one bivariate normal distribution.

The null hypothesis needs to cover all of the above complementary scenarios to the alternative hypotheses; therefore, $P_0(C1_G, C2_G)$ is modeled by combinations of identical distributions of gene expression profiles in different trait groups, as in $P_{join}(C1_G, C2_G)$ and $P_{ind}(C1_G, C2_G)$, except that the last term $P_{ind}(C1_G)P_{ind}(C2_G)$ is used as a constraint when two genes in the gene pair $G$ are generated from independent distributions, which cannot be counted as an interacting gene pair. The bigger the Bayes factor, the stronger the evidence, which supports the conclusion that interaction of the gene pair impacts the specific trait.

Let $X = (X_1, \ldots, X_N)$ be the data. $N$ is the number of samples in each condition (number of samples are the same for all the genes), and $d = 2$ is the gene dimension for each $Xi$ in our case.

$P_{join}(X)$ is modeled as a bivariate normal distribution ($X \sim N(\mu, \Sigma)$) with a normal-inverse-Wishart (NIW) conjugate prior on mean vector ($\mu$) and covariance matrix ($\Sigma$). The likelihood can be written in the following form:

$$P_{join}\left(X | \mu, \Sigma\right) = \frac{1}{(2\pi)^{Nd/2}|\Sigma|^{N/2}} \exp\left(-\sum_{i=1}^{N} (X_i - \mu) \Sigma^{-1} (X_i - \mu)/2\right)$$

(2)

The normal-inverse-Wishart prior is:

$$p(\mu, \Sigma) = NIW(\mu_0, k_0, \Lambda_0, \nu_0) = \frac{1}{Z}|\Sigma|^{-\left(\frac{\nu_0+d}{2}+1\right)} \exp\left(-\frac{1}{2}tr\left(\Lambda_0 \Sigma^{-1}\right)\right.$$
$$\left. -\frac{k_0}{2}(\mu - \mu_0)^T \Sigma^{-1} (\mu - \mu_0)\right)$$

(3)

and

$$Z = \frac{2^{\nu_0 d/2}\Gamma_d(\nu_0/2)(2\pi/k_0)^{d/2}}{|\Lambda_0|^{\nu_0/2}}$$

where $\mu_0$, $k_0$, $\nu_0$, and $\Lambda_0$ are hyper-parameters selected according to [2], where $\mu_0$ is the mean of the data, $k_0$ is 0.01, $\nu_0$ is 4, and $\Lambda_0$ is the empirical covariance matrix. By integrating $\mu$ and $\Sigma$, we get:

$$p_{join}(X) = \frac{1}{\pi^{Nd/2}} \frac{\Gamma_d(\nu_N/2)}{\Gamma_d(\nu_0/2)} \frac{|\Lambda_0|^{\nu_0/2}}{|\Lambda_N|^{\nu_N/2}} \left(\frac{k_0}{k_N}\right)^{d/2} \tag{4}$$

and

$$k_N = k_0 + N$$
$$\nu_N = \nu_0 + N$$
$$\Lambda_N = \Lambda_0 + S + \frac{k_0 N}{k_0+N}(\bar{x} - \mu_0)(\bar{x} - \mu_0)^T$$
$$S = \sum_{i=1}^{N}(x_i - \bar{x})(x_i - \bar{x})^T$$

$P_{ind}(X)$ is modeled as the product of two independent normal distributions () $\left(X_g \sim N\left(\mu_g, \sigma_g^2\right), g \in \{1, \ldots, d\}\right)$ with the normal-inverse-chi-squared conjugate priors on mean $(\mu_g)$ and variance $\left(\sigma_g^2\right)$. The likelihood can be written as the following form:

$$P_{ind}\left(X|\mu_g, \sigma_g\right) = \prod_{g=1}^{d}\left(2\pi\sigma_g^2\right)^{-\frac{N}{2}} \exp\left(-\frac{1}{2\sigma_g^2}\sum_{i=1}^{N}\left(X_{ig} - \mu_g\right)^2\right) \tag{5}$$

The normal-inverse-chi-squared prior is:

$$p\left(\mu_g, \sigma_g\right) = NI\chi^2\left(\mu_0 \kappa_0 \nu_0 | \sigma_0^2\right) = N\left(\mu_g | \mu_0, \sigma_g^2/k_0\right) \times \chi^{-2}\left(\sigma_g^2 | \nu_0, \sigma_0^2\right) \tag{6}$$

Here, $\mu_0$, $k_0$, $\nu_0$, and $\sigma_0^2$ are hyper-parameters selected according to [19], where $\mu_0$ is the mean of data, $k_0$ is 0.01, $\nu_0$ is 3, and $\sigma_0^2$ is the empirical covariance matrix. By integrating $\mu_g$ and $\sigma_g^2$, we get:

$$P_{ind}(X) = \prod_{g=1}^{d}\frac{1}{\pi^{\frac{N}{2}}}\sqrt{\frac{\kappa_0}{\kappa_{N,g}}}\frac{\Gamma\left(\frac{\nu_{N,g}}{2}\right)}{\Gamma\left(\frac{\nu_0}{2}\right)}\frac{\left(\nu_0 \sigma_0^2\right)^{\frac{\nu_0}{2}}}{\left(\nu_{N,g}\sigma_{N,g}^2\right)^{\frac{\nu_{N,g}}{2}}} \tag{7}$$

and

$$k_{N,g} = k_0 + N$$

$$\nu_{N,g} = \nu_0 + N$$

$$\sigma^2_{N,g} = \frac{1}{\nu_{N,g}} \left( \nu_0 \sigma_0 + \sum_i \left( x_{ig} - \overline{X}_g \right)^2 + \frac{N k_0}{k_0 + N} \left( \mu_0 - \overline{X}_g \right)^2 \right)$$

### 2.2.2 Permutation Procedure

We extended the previous BFDCA method with a permutation test to estimate the significance of observing the calculated Bayes factor scores. Only gene pairs with significantly high Bayes factor scores were provided to the subsequent analysis. In the permutation procedure, the samples are permuted $N$ times across different trait conditions to simulate a null background of the Bayes factor $BF\_null$ for each gene pair independently and the permutation $P$-value of gene pair $G$ is calculated by $\left\{ 1 + \sum_{i=1}^N I \left( BF_{null i} \geq BF_G \right) \right\}$, where $I$ is an indicator function and is equal to 1 only when $BF\_null_i \geq BF_G$. By default, $N$ is set as 100 to reduce the computational burden. Out of the ranked list of gene pairs, we discarded gene pairs with $P$-values higher than 0.01 (i.e., more than one occurrence out of 100 permutations).

### 2.2.3 Identifying Trait-Dependent Gene Modules and Estimating the Importance of Genes Interacting with Traits

To identify trait-dependent gene modules, we followed a similar approach in weighted correlation network analysis (WGCNA) [20]. First, we generated an adjacency matrix by using the normalized Bayes factors calculated for all the selected gene pairs from the previous filtering procedures, defined as $a_{ij}$ in Eq. (8). Second, we considered the topological overlap between each gene and calculated a dissimilarity matrix from the adjacency matrix; then, we applied a hierarchical clustering method for the dissimilarity matrix to cluster genes into different modules.

$$A : a_{ij} = \left( \frac{\log \left( BF_{ij} \right) - \min}{\max - \min} \right)^{\beta} \tag{8}$$

In Eq. (8), the max and min are the maximum and minimum values of $log(BF)$, respectively. $\beta$ is a tuning parameter in WGCNA, which is used in our case to reduce the noise of the Bayes factors in the adjacency matrix. Following the instruction of the WGCNA, we set $\beta$ to 6 by default to maintain the scale-free network property.

To estimate the importance of the inner-module genes associated with the specific trait quantitatively, we calculated a weight for each gene proportional to their differential connectivity with all the other genes within the module. The weight assignment was the same as in [21]. All we had to do was to simply replace their gene correlation matrix with our adjacency matrix, which is formulated as:

$$w_i = \sum_{j \neq i} w_j a_{ij}^m, \quad 1 \leq i \leq n \tag{9}$$

Here, $n$ represents the number of genes in module $m$, $a_{ij}^m$ represents the element of the submatrix of matrix $A$ in Eq. (8), whose edges are presented in module $m$. This problem is equivalent to solving eigenvector $w$ in the matrix form, shown as:

$$\left(A^m - I\right) w = w \tag{10}$$

Because matrix $A^m$ is a non-negative, irreducible, and symmetric, it can be solved equivalently by Eq. (11). The unique solution for Equation (11) is $w = v^*$, where $v^*$ is the positive eigenvector corresponding to the largest real eigenvalue $\lambda^*$ of $A^m$.

$$\frac{1}{\lambda^*-1} \left(A^m - I\right) w = w, \; \lambda^* \neq 1 \tag{11}$$

After this procedure, we obtained submodules of fully connected genes (no connections between modules), where each gene had a weight representing its importance associated with a specific trait. All the genes within each module were assumed to function together but had different degrees of contributions to the specific trait.

### 2.2.4 Extraction of Candidates of Interacting Gene Pairs

We extracted the candidates of interacting gene pairs for each specific trait by considering both end-node importance and the module assignment. For the remaining gene pairs, $w_1$ and $w_2$ indicated the two end-node weights that comprised the gene pair, and $BF_{ij}$ indicated the original Bayes factor, a score evaluating the importance of this pair was calculated by $\sqrt{w_1 \cdot w_2} \cdot BF_{ij}$. For each trait-dependent gene module generated in the former procedure, a union of the first and second minimum spanning trees (MST2) was constructed with the distance between gene pairs calculated by (1- $a_{ij}$), where $a_{ij}$ was the normalized Bayes factor. Gene pairs that were not represented in the MST2 were removed; in this way, a subset of gene pairs was selected and assigned with scores. These gene pairs capture the main skeleton of the network associated with a specific trait, but they were still too large for downstream analyses. So we applied the generalized sequential forward selection algorithm [22] to further constrain the candidate gene pairs into an acceptable size. Gene pairs were sorted in decreasing order in terms of their scores; moreover, gene pairs assigned to the same module were kept together. In other words, gene pairs assigned to the same module were grouped together and were ranked by their scores within each group. Starting from an empty set, the next $m$ gene pairs were added to the set iteratively. The tradeoff for maximizing the accuracy and minimizing the number of gene pairs was made according to the cross-validation accuracy curve to select the final candidate gene pairs, which could be used in a future field test.

## 2.2.5 Classification Models

To demonstrate that the candidate interacting gene pairs identified by our method were associated with a specific trait level, we designed a classification model to test whether the binary-condition trait samples can be classified correctly by the candidate interacting gene pairs. The idea of this classification model was similar to the Naive Bayes classifier [23], but instead of manipulating single genes, the classifier worked on gene pairs. Our assumption was that gene pairs followed one of the three mutual exclusive distributions as described in the alternative models of Bayes factors in Equation (1). One was represented by $P_{join}(D_G) \cdot P_{join}(U_G)$, indicating that the gene pairs from the case and control groups followed two different joint distributions. The second was represented by $P_{join}(D_G) \cdot P_{ind}(U_G)$, indicating that the gene pairs from the case group followed joint distributions but were independent when they were from the control group. The third mutually exclusive distribution was represented by $P_{ind}(D_G) \cdot P_{join}(U_G)$, which was opposite to the second distribution. The representing model for each gene pair had to be determined first; then, the parameters of the model were estimated. For each gene pair, the representing model with the maximum marginal likelihood was selected, while for the determined model, the parameters were estimated by the *maximum a posterior* probability (MAP). Two distinct distributions were involved in the three representing models, where one was the bivariate normal distribution as in $P_{join}(X)$, and the other was the univariate normal distribution as in $P_{ind}(X)$. The parameters of the two distributions were estimated as follows:

For the bivariate normal distribution:

$$MAP(\mu) = \overline{x} \tag{12}$$

$$MAP(\Sigma) = \frac{\Lambda_0 + \frac{k_0 N}{k_0 + N}(\overline{x} - \mu_0)(\overline{x} - \mu_0)^T + S}{v_0 + N + d + 2} \tag{13}$$

For the univariate normal distribution:

$$MAP(\mu) = \overline{x} \tag{14}$$

$$MAP(\sigma^2) = \frac{v_0 \sigma_0 + \sum_i (x_i - \overline{x})^2 + \frac{k_0 N}{k_0 + N}(\overline{x} - \mu_0)^2}{v_0 + N - 1} \tag{15}$$

Here, all the other parameters were the same as in calculating the Bayes factor. The training and testing followed the standard method of the Naive Bayes classifier.

#### 2.2.6 Significant Estimation of Overlapping Genes and Gene Pairs Across 2 Years

We estimated the repeatability of our method in identifying genes and gene pairs across 2 years by *p-value*. We assumed that the number of overlapping genes or gene pairs followed the hypergeometric distribution. If $x$ represents the number of overlapping genes/gene pairs, $n$ represents the number of genes/gene pairs in the 2013 dataset, $D$ represents the number of genes in the 2014 dataset, $N$ represents the total number of genes, according to the hypergeometric distribution; thus, the probability of $x$ overlapping genes/gene pairs was calculated as follows:

$$P(x) = \frac{C\,(D, x)\,C\,(N - D, n - x)}{C\,(N, n)} \qquad (16)$$

The probability of finding $x$ or more genes/gene pairs, *i.e. p-value*, was formulated as follows:

$$P\,(i \geq x) = 1 - \sum_{i=0}^{x-1} P(x) \qquad (17)$$

## 3  Results

### 3.1  Analyze the Trait-Dependent Gene Modules in Maize

We conducted a comprehensive investigation of gene expression data from 57 genetically diverse commercial maize hybrids across 2 years (2013 and 2014) to identify different expression patterns associated with specific agronomic traits. The traits we focused on are listed in Table 1. For each trait, we identified a number of mutually exclusive gene modules associated with the specific trait based on the trait-dependent interacting genes.

The numbers of modules and genes in the whole gene interacting network are listed in Table 2. Along with the module assignment, each gene was assigned a weight representing its contribution to the trait in the gene interacting network. Figure 2 shows an example of Module 13 generated for trait MST, with pathways

**Table 1** Information of trait

| Trait name | Units |
|---|---|
| MST | Grain moisture (%) |
| P50 | Days to 50% pollen shed |
| PHTR3 | Plant height (cm) |
| TWT | Test weight (lb/bu)3 |
| YLD | Yield (t/ha) |

**Table 2** Number of modules and corresponding genes

| # of modules/# of genes | P50 | MST | PHTR3 | TWT | YLD |
|---|---|---|---|---|---|
| 2013 dataset | 19/1285 | 20/1058 | 22/1113 | 23/1734 | 17/1081 |
| 2014 dataset | 21/1323 | 15/941 | 13/967 | 23/1364 | 21/1443 |

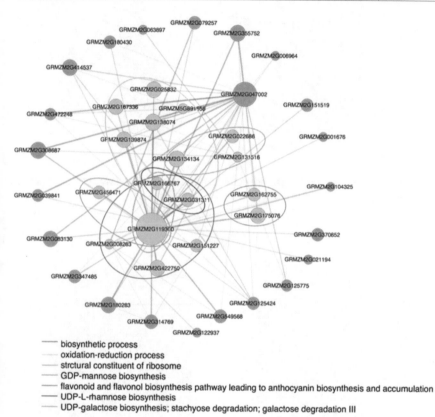

— biosynthetic process
— oxidation-reduction process
— strctural constituent of ribosome
— GDP-mannose biosynthesis
— flavonoid and flavonol biosynthesis pathway leading to anthocyanin biosynthesis and accumulation
— UDP-L-rhamnose biosynthesis
— UDP-galactose biosynthesis; stachyose degradation; galactose degradation III

**Fig. 2** An example of Module 13 of trait MST. Nodes represent genes and edges represent gene-gene interactions. Some enriched pathways and GO terms with their over-represented genes are shown within circles of different colors. The size of each gene and the width of each edge are shown according to gene weight and value of Bayes factor, respectively. To make the display clear, only edges with significantly high Bayes factors are shown

and gene oncology (GO) terms, and some common genes shared by different clusters; in particular, GRMZM2G119300 is shared with nearly half of all clusters with high weights, indicating its key role in trait MST.

We analyzed the overlapping trait-dependent genes across 2 years, as shown in a Venn plot in Fig. 3, where different traits shared many trait-dependent genes. It shows which patterns were consistent across 2 years (2013 and 2014). Figure 4 shows heat maps representing the proportion of overlapping modules between pairwise traits across both years. Overlapping modules are defined as modules from

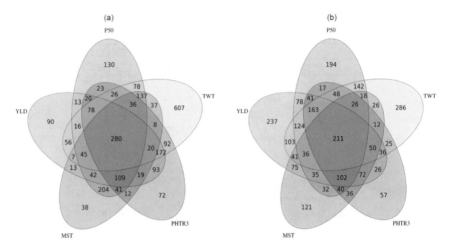

**Fig. 3** Venn plot of overlapping trait-dependent genes for traits P50, TWT, PHTR3, MST and YLD across 2 years: (**a**) the 2013 dataset and (**b**) the 2014 dataset

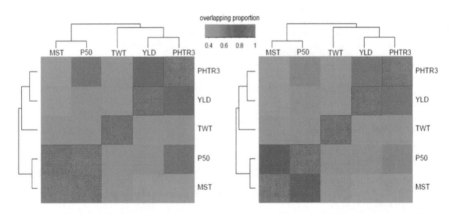

**Fig. 4** Heat maps represent the proportion of overlapping modules between pair-wise traits across 2 years (left, the 2013 dataset and right, the 2014 dataset). Two modules belonging to two different traits are counted as an overlapping module between these two traits when the overlapping numbers of genes within these modules are significant ($p$-value $\leq 0.01$). The proportion of overlapping modules for the pair of traits under comparison was calculated by dividing by the minimum module number of these two traits as presented in these heat maps

different traits sharing a significant number of overlapping genes ($p$-value $\leq 0.01$). The proportion of overlapping modules was calculated by dividing the number of overlapping modules by the minimum module number of the comparing traits. Figure 4 shows that traits YLD and PHTR3, as well as traits MST and P50 were consistently clustered together across the 2 years. At the gene expression level, we can see PHT was much more relevant to yield than any other traits, and MST had many more underlying gene modules overlapping with trait pollen shed.

## 3.2 Functional Enrichment Analysis on Trait-Dependent Gene Modules

We applied pathway enrichment analysis and gene-ontology enrichment analysis to explore the biological explanations of the identified gene modules. Pathway enrichment analysis was performed based on the MaizeCyc database (http://maizecyc.maizegdb.org/) [24]. Gene ontology enrichment analysis was conducted using the AgriGO database (http://bioinfo.cau.edu.cn/agriGO/) [25].

Trait YLD was the most interesting trait in this study. The functional analysis result of Module 1 is presented in Table 3. The basic functionality of the genes in Module 1 is glycolysis [26]. Glycolysis was found to be associated with grain yield [26]. Fu et al. also confirmed the relationships by analyzing the maize seedling transcriptome [27]. However, oxidizing hexoses to generate ATP, another essential function of glycolysis in plants, reversibly produces hexoses from various low-molecular weight molecules [26]. To control the process of glycolysis, various hormones are involved, and glucosylation of these hormones is highlighted in these modules. In our result, cytokinins-O-glucoside biosynthesis and the flavonol glucosylation pathway were significantly enriched. Glucosylation of cytokinins is a well-recognized modification that plays an important role in hormonal homeostasis [28], and the function of O-glucosylated cytokinins in regulating growth and development was confirmed by genetic manipulation [29]. The glucosylation reactions can accumulate high concentrations of flavonoids, particularly the characteristic flavanone and flavone glycosides [30, 31].

**Table 3** Functional analysis on Module 1 in Trait YLD

|  | Name | P-value | Genes |
|---|---|---|---|
| Pathways | Cytokinins-O-glucoside biosynthesis (PWY-2902) | 0.004 | GRMZM2G007012;GRMZM2G476049; GRMZM2G479038 |
|  | Flavonol glucosylation I | 0.018 | GRMZM2G007012; GRMZM2G479038 |
|  | Glycolysis IV (plant cytosol) | 0.078 | GRMZM2G132069;GRMZM2G458728 |
|  | Glycolysis I (GLYCOLYSIS) | 0.085 | GRMZM2G132069;GRMZM2G458728 |
|  | Glycolysis III | 0.087 | GRMZM2G132069;GRMZM2G458728 |
|  | Superpathway of cytosolic glycolysis (plants), pyruvate dehydrogenase and TCA cycle | 0.150 | GRMZM2G132069;GRMZM2G458728 |
| GO | Response to hormone stimulus (GO:0009725) | 0.012 | GRMZM2G081158;GRMZM2G390641 |
|  | Glycolysis (GO:0006096) | 0.160 | GRMZM2G132069;GRMZM2G458728 |

Trait MST is an interesting trait associated with both grain yield and the quality of maize grain. Functional analysis revealed several inner mechanisms related to the modules detected. Table 4 lists the functional analysis result of Module 13. Sugar biosynthesis and degradation are the most obvious functionalities enrichments in this module, such as UDP-L-rhamnose, GDP-mannose, UDP-galactose biosynthe-

**Table 4** Functional analysis on Module 13 in trait MST

|  | Name | P-value | Genes |
|---|---|---|---|
| Pathways | UDP-L-rhamnose biosynthesis (PWY-3261) | 2.303e-5 | GRMZM2G031311; GRMZM2G166767 |
|  | GDP-mannose biosynthesis (PWY-5659) | 0.0014 | GRMZM2G119300; GRMZM2G456471 |
|  | UDP-galactose biosynthesis (salvage pathway from galactose using UDP-glucose) (GALACTMETAB-PWY) | 0.014 | GRMZM2G119300;GRMZM2G166767 |
|  | Stachyose degradation (PWY-6527) | 0.018 | GRMZM2G119300;GRMZM2G166767 |
|  | Galactose degradation III (PWY-3821) | 0.022 | GRMZM2G119300;GRMZM2G166767 |
|  | Colanic acid building blocks biosynthesis (COLANSYN-PWY) | 0.002 | GRMZM2G119300; GRMZM2G166767;GRMZM2G456471 |
|  | Flavonoid and flavonol biosynthesis pathway leading to anthocyanin biosynthesis and accumulation (PWYBWI-410) | 0.019 | GRMZM2G162755; GRMZM2G175076 |
|  | Bassinosteroid biosynthesis II (PWY-2582) | 0.033 | GRMZM2G031311;GRMZM2G166767 |
| GO | Biosynthetic process(GO:0009058) | 6.005e-6 | GRMZM2G008263;GRMZM2G031311; GRMZM2G119300;GRMZM2G151227; GRMZM2G166767;GRMZM2G422750 |
|  | Oxidation-reduction process (GO:0055114) | 0.016 | GRMZM2G025832;GRMZM2G031311; GRMZM2G134134;GRMZM2G138074; GRMZM2G139874;GRMZM2G166767; GRMZM2G167336;GRMZM5G891656 |
|  | Monooxygenase activity (GO:0004497) | 1.700e-4 | GRMZM2G025832;GRMZM2G138074; GRMZM2G139874;GRMZM2G167336; GRMZM5G891656 |
|  | Structural constituent of ribosome (GO:0003735) | 0.140 | GRMZM2G022686;GRMZM2G131516; GRMZM2G134134 |

sis, and stachyose and galactose degradations. Because the major components are sugar related carbohydrates, grain yield in maize is highly related to carbohydrate biosynthesis and degradation. "Anthocyanin biosynthesis and accumulation" are also highly enriched functions. In terms of drying kinetics and final quality of product, vacuum drying had a higher drying rate with a higher conservation of anthocyanin [32]. Breeding practice also revealed that the anthocyanin content was significantly affected by the drying method, drying temperature, and product thickness [33, 34].

Trait P50 is a pollen shed development related trait. Table 5 lists the functional analysis on Module 2 associated with trait P50. "Phosphate acquisition and utilization" was significantly enriched in the analysis, which was consistent with plant development. Phosphorous is an essential macronutrient in plant growth and development, and it is usually absorbed and utilized by the plants in the form of phosphate. Once absorbed, the phosphate is utilized inside the cells at optimum cellular concentration for various developmental and biochemical processes [35].

Trait PHTR3 is highly related to grain yield. Table 6 lists the functional analysis on Module 10 associated with trait PHTR3. "Tryptophan biosynthesis" was significantly enriched in the module. Consistent with the knowledge about plant height trait, L-tryptophan is a precursor of the growth hormone, indole acetic acid, and is known to stimulate plant growth at extremely low concentrations [36].

Trait TWT is the test weight, which is the measure of bulk density or the weight of a specified volume of corn. Twenty-three modules were identified associated with trait TWT. Table 7 lists the functional analysis on Module 9 associated with

**Table 5** Functional analysis on Module 2 in Trait P50

|          | Name | P-value | Genes |
|----------|------|---------|-------|
| Pathways | Cytokinin-O-glucoside biosynthesis (PWY-2902) | 0.004 | GRMZM2G007012; GRMZM2G476049; GRMZM2G479038 |
|          | Flavonol glucosylation I | 0.018 | GRMZM2G007012; GRMZM2G479038 |
|          | Glycolysis IV (plant cytosol) | 0.078 | GRMZM2G132069;GRMZM2G458728 |
|          | Glycolysis I (GLYCOLYSIS) | 0.085 | GRMZM2G132069;GRMZM2G458728 |
|          | Glycolysis III | 0.087 | GRMZM2G132069;GRMZM2G458728 |
|          | Super pathway of cytosolic glycolysis (plants), pyruvate dehydrogenase and TCA cycle | 0.150 | GRMZM2G132069;GRMZM2G458728 |
| GO       | Response to hormone stimulus (GO:0009725) | 0.012 | GRMZM2G081158;GRMZM2G390641 |
|          | Glycolysis (GO:0006096) | 0.160 | GRMZM2G132069;GRMZM2G458728 |

**Table 6** Functional analysis on Module 10 in Trait PHTR3

|          | Name                                      | *P-value* | Genes                               |
|----------|-------------------------------------------|-----------|-------------------------------------|
| Pathways | Tryptophan biosynthesis                   | 4.1e-4    | GRMZM2G003109;GRMZM2G138382         |
|          | Superpathway of tryptophan biosynthesis   | 3.04e-3   | GRMZM2G003109;GRMZM2G138382         |
| GO       | Biosynthetic process (GO:0009058)         | 1.05e-2   | GRMZM2G003109;GRMZM2G138382         |
|          | Nucleotide binding (GO:0000166)           | 0.130     | GRMZM2G014089;GRMZM2G156565         |

**Table 7** Functional analysis on Module 9 in Trait TWT

|          | Name                                              | *P-value* | Genes                                                       |
|----------|---------------------------------------------------|-----------|------------------------------------------------------------|
| Pathways | Glycogen biosynthesis I (from ADP-D-Glucose)      | 8.9e-4    | GRMZM2G008263;GRMZM2G106213                                |
|          | Starch biosynthesis                               | 2.5e-3    | GRMZM2G008263;GRMZM2G106213                                |
| GO       | Glycogen biosynthetic process (GO:0005978)        | 1.7e-3    | GRMZM2G088361;GRMZM2G106213                                |
|          | Biosynthetic process (GO:0009058)                 | 1.8e-3    | GRMZM2G008263;GRMZM2G106213; GRMZM2G118345;GRMZM2G147256   |

trait TWT. The functional analysis revealed that it was significantly associated with glycogen and starch biosynthesis, which is known as related to the main component of the grain yield [37].

## 3.3   Validation Results Using Data Sets across 2 Years

To explore whether our method can capture the intrinsic genetic effect, we compared the results from data sets across 2 years to validate the repeatability of the method in identifying genes and gene pairs. We first considered the repeatability of high-weight genes associated with specific traits. For each trait-dependent gene interacting network, the top $N$ weighted genes from the 2013 dataset were compared with the same number of top weighted genes from the 2014 dataset. The significance of the overlapping top-weighted genes was estimated by the *p-value* (as described in Sect. 2.2.6). The comparison results are shown in Table 8. $N$ was selected as 100, 500, and the whole gene set, identified as the top 100, top 500, and all the genes in the whole gene interacting network, as shown in Table 8.

## 3.4   Candidate Interacting Gene Pairs

Following the method described in Sect. 2.2.4, subsets of trait-associated gene pairs were extracted and served as candidates for the field test. The main idea behind the extraction was that the candidate gene pairs with large Bayes factors were expected

**Table 8** Overlapping of high-weight genes interaction with specific trait across 2 years of data

| Traits | Genes in 2013 data | Genes in 2014 data | Top100 overlapping genes (*p-value*) | Top 500 overlapping genes (*p-value*) | Whole overlapping genes (*p-value*) |
|---|---|---|---|---|---|
| YLD | 1081 | 1443 | 15 (5.24e-09) | 135 (1.34e-24) | 455 (3.26e-47) |
| P50 | 1285 | 1323 | 8 (0.002) | 107 (1.34e-11) | 543 (1.49e-30) |
| MST | 1058 | 941 | 24 (6.63e-19) | 196 (5.38e-68) | 452 (1.70e-95) |
| PHTR3 | 1113 | 967 | 20 (3.50e-14) | 160 (5.59e-40) | 402 (6.23e-54) |
| TWT | 1734 | 1364 | 4 (0.200) | 95 (1.69e-07) | 591 (8.64e-31) |

**Table 9** Number of gene pairs selected for each trait and prediction accuracy for different methods

| Traits | # of gene pairs | Our method | t-test | ANOVA | mRMR |
|---|---|---|---|---|---|
| P50 | 31 | 98% (77%) | 98% (68%) | 98% (71%) | 98% (63%) |
| MST | 71 | 100% (84%) | 98% (84%) | 98% (78%) | 96% (55%) |
| PHTR3 | 91 | 81% (84%) | 84% (83%) | 86% (82%) | 75% (48%) |
| TWT | 41 | 77% (50%) | 77% (57%) | 77% (55%) | 61% (55%) |
| YLD | 61 | 86% (70%) | 84% (77%) | 86% (71%) | 88% (60%) |

Columns 3–6 show the LOOCV accuracies on the 2013 dataset and the accuracies on the 2014 dataset (in parenthesis) for each method

to be significantly related to a specific trait and have high impact in the full network. In Table 9, the number of gene pairs selected for each trait was summarized in the first and second columns for the 2013 and 2014 datasets, respectively. Only dozens of genes are shown for each trait, making the following experimental investigation feasible.

We compared the trait-dependent gene expression patterns for the candidate interacting genes observed during the two-year study. Figure 5 shows one example of the top four ranked gene pairs for trait PHTR3. The top gene pair (No. 1) was GRMZM2G042253-GRMZM2G075124 presented in the first plot of Fig. 5, which was annotated by a functional gene interaction in protein-protein interaction (PPI) networks [38]. From Fig. 5, we can clearly see different patterns under different trait levels (blue and red) and these patterns prevail across 2 years. This consistency in gene expression patterns across 2 years indicates that some genetic interactions in corn populations may impact the repeatability of the trait performance from year to year and that our method can capture these repeatable patterns between genes.

## 3.5 Prediction Power of the Candidate Interacting Genes

To further demonstrate the association between candidate interacting gene pairs and phenotypes, we trained a classification model based on the expression of the candidate gene pairs and evaluated their prediction power by the prediction accuracy of trait levels. The classification model was modified from a standard

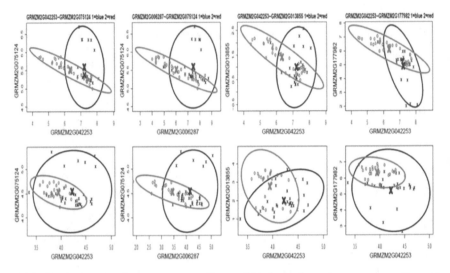

**Fig. 5** Gene-pair expression patterns across 2 years. This figure shows the expression patterns of the top four gene pairs for trait PHTR3 under two different trait levels (blue and red) and across 2 years. The upper plot is generated by the 2013 dataset and the lower plot is generated by the 2014 dataset. The x-axes and y-axes represent gene expression levels for each gene of the pair. Maize hybrids under the two trait levels are differentiated by different dot types and colors. The 95% contours of the bivariate normal density estimated by gene expression levels is shown

Naive Bayes classifier [23] (as described in Sect. 2.2.5). We compared the prediction power using the same classification model on the genes selected by our method and the same number of genes selected by other classical gene selection methods. We compared our method with two single-gene-based methods: the t-test and ANOVA, which considered the changes in mean and the changes in variance, respectively. We also compared with a widely used feature selection method mRMR (minimum redundancy maximum relevance) [39], which also considered gene-gene interactions. For each trait, the leave-one-out cross-validation (LOOCV) accuracy on the 2013 dataset and the prediction accuracy on the 2014 dataset were calculated, as shown in Table 9. According to the accuracy and other comparison results across 2 years, trait TWT showed very poor predictability and repeatability. Because many factors in the field such as moisture, kernel size and shape, slickness of seed coat, and physical characteristics may influence the trait TWT, the poor predictability may be attributed to the complex of environmental or the low heritability of the TWT itself. In general, our method obtained higher accuracies in both 2013 and 2014 datasets compared with other methods. If considering the loss of accuracies from the 2013 dataset to the independent 2014 dataset, the selected gene pairs by our method presented high consistency in terms of prediction power.

# 4 Discussion

Identifying trait-dependent genes is important in trait development through molecular breeding. Correctly identifying trait-dependent genes or gene pairs helps to understand how intrinsic genetic variation impacts traits. In addition, these genes could serve as candidates to modify the traits in the downstream experiments. Beyond the traditional breeding practices, which assume that genes affect the traits independently, in this study, we took gene-gene interactions into consideration and applied a Bayesian method based on data of gene expression traits across a set of maize hybrids to detect complex traits associated gene interactions. The identified gene-gene interactions formed a network and then the trait-dependent gene modules were generated by considering the network topology. These modules demonstrated several biological functions, which associated with a specific trait.

Unlike other machine learning methods applied in detecting trait-dependent genes by seeking high prediction accuracy, our method selects gene pairs by considering both the discrimination power and the influence in the network. From the results across 2 years, the trait-dependent genes and gene-gene interactions selected by our method were demonstrated with some degree of consistency, which suggests that the candidate interacting genes selected by our method are expected to be biologically meaningful for the interested trait. When compared with the traditional single-gene-based methods, the edge-based markers achieved generally higher prediction power for traits with high heritability. Different from other traits, the overall results of trait TWT were relatively poor, which may be due to a combination of its low genetic heritability, low measurement repeatability, and the complexity of its potential biological determinants. TWT is a complex trait that measures the density of the grain and is influenced by many environmental factors such as grain moisture, kernel size and shape as well as other physical characteristics. We may involve the environment factors to improve the prediction power of our method in the future.

From the functional enrichment analyses on the obtained gene modules, most of the modules presented some interesting functions related to the traits. These modules shed some light on the underlying biological mechanisms of the traits. We explored and discussed several biological enrichment results on the presented modules in each trait and found that the genes in these modules may work together to affect the trait development. However, due to the limited knowledge and inadequate annotation of maize species, the biological functional analyses could only explain some mechanisms related to the trait development. It is still a challenge to detail the biological explanation in gene-gene interactions. Some traits have several shared modules. Further exploration on these shared modules may help us to better understand the intricate mechanism associations among these traits.

For each trait, dozens of trait-dependent gene modules and interacting gene pairs were selected, which needed further investigation by downstream experiments. The interacting genes could serve as candidates to modify the traits by expression enhancing or silencing approaches. We plan to do a field test in the future.

**Acknowledgements** The authors would like to acknowledge the support of Monsanto and the National Institutes of Health (R35-GM126985). The high-performance computing infrastructure is supported by the National Science Foundation under grant number CNS-1429294.

# References

1. Alexandratos, N., Bruinsma, J. (2012). World agriculture towards 2030/2050: The 2012 revision. In: ESA Working Paper Rome, FAO.
2. Tokatlidis, I., & Koutroubas, S. (2004). A review of maize hybrids' dependence on high plant populations and its implications for crop yield stability. *Field Crops Research, 88*(2), 103–114.
3. Tollenaar, M., & Wu, J. (1999). Yield improvement in temperate maize is attributable to greater stress tolerance. *Crop Science, 39*(6), 1597–1604.
4. Ray, D. K., Mueller, N. D., West, P. C., & Foley, J. A. (2013). Yield trends are insufficient to double global crop production by 2050. *PLoS One, 8*(6), e66428.
5. Matsuoka, Y., Vigouroux, Y., Goodman, M. M., Sanchez, J., Buckler, E., & Doebley, J. (2002). A single domestication for maize shown by multilocus microsatellite genotyping. *Proceedings of the National Academy of Sciences, 99*(9), 6080–6084.
6. Doust, A. N., Lukens, L., Olsen, K. M., Mauro-Herrera, M., Meyer, A., & Rogers, K. (2014). Beyond the single gene: How epistasis and gene-by-environment effects influence crop domestication. *Proceedings of the National Academy of Sciences, 111*(17), 6178–6183.
7. Bhattacharyya, M., & Bandyopadhyay, S. (2013). Studying the differential co-expression of microRNAs reveals significant role of white matter in early Alzheimer's progression. *Molecular BioSystems, 9*(3), 457–466.
8. de la Fuente, A. (2010). From 'differential expression'to 'differential networking'– identification of dysfunctional regulatory networks in diseases. *Trends in Genetics, 26*(7), 326–333.
9. Brachi, B., Morris, G. P., & Borevitz, J. O. (2011). Genome-wide association studies in plants: The missing heritability is in the field. *Genome Biology, 12*(10), 1.
10. Makowsky, R., Pajewski, N. M., Klimentidis, Y. C., Vazquez, A. I., Duarte, C. W., Allison, D. B., & de Los Campos, G. (2011). Beyond missing heritability: Prediction of complex traits. *PLoS Genetics, 7*(4), e1002051.
11. Purcell, S., Neale, B., Todd-Brown, K., Thomas, L., Ferreira, M. A. R., Bender, D., Maller, J., Sklar, P., de Bakker, P. I. W., & Daly, M. J. (2007). PLINK: A tool set for whole-genome association and population-based linkage analyses. *The American Journal of Human Genetics, 81*(3), 559–575.
12. Zhang, J., Zhang, Q., Lewis, D., & Zhang, M. Q. (2011). A Bayesian method for disentangling dependent structure of epistatic interaction. *American Journal of Biostatistics, 2*(1), 1.
13. Ritchie, M. D., Hahn, L. W., Roodi, N., Bailey, L. R., Dupont, W. D., Parl, F. F., & Moore, J. H. (2001). Multifactor-dimensionality reduction reveals high-order interactions among estrogen-metabolism genes in sporadic breast cancer. *The American Journal of Human Genetics, 69*(1), 138–147.
14. Wang, J., Joshi, T., Valliyodan, B., Shi, H., Liang, Y., Nguyen, H. T., Zhang, J., & Xu, D. (2015). A Bayesian model for detection of high-order interactions among genetic variants in genome-wide association studies. *BMC Genomics, 16*(1), 1.
15. Kayano, M., Shiga, M., & Mamitsuka, H. (2014). Detecting differentially coexpressed genes from labeled expression data: A brief review. *IEEE/ACM Transactions on Computational Biology and Bioinformatics, 11*(1), 154–167.
16. Wang, D., Wang, J., Jiang, Y., Liang, Y., & Xu, D. (2017). BFDCA: A comprehensive tool of using Bayes factor for differential co-expression analysis. *Journal of Molecular Biology, 429*, 446–453.

17. Mortazavi, A. W., Williams, B. A., McCue, K., Schaeffer, L., & Wold, B. (2008). Mapping and quantifying mammalian transcriptomes by RNA-Seq. *Nature Methods, 5*(7), 621–628.
18. Verhaak, R. G., Hoadley, K. A., Purdom, E., Wang, V., Qi, Y., Wilkerson, M. D., Miller, C. R., Ding, L., Golub, T., & Mesirov, J. P. (2010). Integrated genomic analysis identifies clinically relevant subtypes of glioblastoma characterized by abnormalities in PDGFRA, IDH1, EGFR, and NF1. *Cancer Cell, 17*(1), 98–110.
19. Fraley, C., & Raftery, A. E. (2007). Bayesian regularization for normal mixture estimation and model-based clustering. *Journal of Classification, 24*(2), 155–181.
20. Langfelder, P., & Horvath, S. (2008). WGCNA: An R package for weighted correlation network analysis. *BMC Bioinformatics, 9*(1), 1.
21. Rahmatallah, Y., Emmert-Streib, F., & Glazko, G. (2014). Gene sets net correlations analysis (GSNCA): A multivariate differential coexpression test for gene sets. *Bioinformatics, 30*(3), 360–368.
22. Whitney, A. W. (1971). A direct method of nonparametric measurement selection. *IEEE Transactions on Computers, 100*(9), 1100–1103.
23. Leung, K. M. (2007). *Naive bayesian classifier*. Polytechnic University Department of Computer Science/Finance and Risk Engineering.
24. Schaeffer, M. L., Harper, L. C., Gardiner, J. M., Andorf, C. M., Campbell, D. A., Cannon, E. K., Sen, T. Z., & Lawrence, C. J. (2011). MaizeGDB: Curation and outreach go hand-in-hand. *Database, 2011*, bar022.
25. Du, Z., Zhou, X., Ling, Y., Zhang, Z., & Su, Z. (2010). agriGO: A GO analysis toolkit for the agricultural community. *Nucleic Acids Research, 38*, W64–W70.
26. Plaxton, W. C. (1996). The organization and regulation of plant glycolysis. *Annual Review of Plant Biology, 47*(1), 185–214.
27. Fu, J., Thiemann, A., Schrag, T. A., Melchinger, A. E., Scholten, S., & Frisch, M. (2010). Dissecting grain yield pathways and their interactions with grain dry matter content by a two-step correlation approach with maize seedling transcriptome. *BMC Plant Biology, 10*(1), 1.
28. Brzobohaty, B., Moore, I., Kristoffersen, P., Bako, L., Campos, N., Schell, J., & Palme, K. (1993). Release of active Cytokinin by a -glucosidase localized to the maize root meristem. *Science, 262*, 1051–1054.
29. Martin, R. C., Mok, M. C., & Mok, D. W. (1999). Isolation of a cytokinin gene, ZOG1, encoding zeatin O-glucosyltransferase from Phaseolus lunatus. *Proceedings of the National Academy of Sciences, 96*(1), 284–289.
30. Ferreyra, M. L. F., Rius, S. P., & Casati, P. (2012). Flavonoids: Biosynthesis, biological functions, and biotechnological applications. *Frontiers in Plant Science, 3*, 222.
31. Owens, D. K., & McIntosh, C. A. (2009). Identification, recombinant expression, and biochemical characterization of a flavonol 3-O-glucosyltransferase clone from Citrus paradisi. *Phytochemistry, 70*(11), 1382–1391.
32. Ratti, C. (2001). Hot air and freeze-drying of high-value foods: A review. *Journal of Food Engineering, 49*(4), 311–319.
33. Lai, K., Dolan, K., & Ng, P. (2009). Inverse method to estimate kinetic degradation parameters of grape anthocyanins in wheat flour under simultaneously changing temperature and moisture. *Journal of Food Science, 74*(5), E241–E249.
34. Yılmaz, F. M., Yüksekkaya, S., Vardin, H., & Karaaslan, M. (2017). The effects of drying conditions on moisture transfer and quality of pomegranate fruit leather (pestil). *Journal of the Saudi Society of Agricultural Sciences, 16*, 33–40.
35. Yuan, H., & Liu, D. (2008). Signaling components involved in plant responses to phosphate starvation. *Journal of Integrative Plant Biology, 50*(7), 849–859.
36. Ahmad, R., Khalid, A., Arshad, M., Zahir, Z. A., & Mahmood, T. (2008). Effect of compost enriched with N and L-tryptophan on soil and maize. *Agronomy for Sustainable Development, 28*(2), 299–305.
37. Hammer, G. L., Dong, Z., McLean, G., Doherty, A., Messina, C., Schussler, J., Zinselmeier, C., Paszkiewicz, S., & Cooper, M. (2009). Can changes in canopy and/or root system architecture explain historical maize yield trends in the US corn belt? *Crop Science, 49*(1), 299–312.

38. Zhu, G., Wu, A., Xu, X.-J., Xiao, P., Lu, L., Liu, J., Cao, Y., Chen, L., Wu, J., & Zhao, X.-M. (2015). PPIM: A protein-protein interaction database for maize. *Plant Physiology, 02015,* 01821.
39. Ding, C., & Peng, H. (2005). Minimum redundancy feature selection from microarray gene expression data. *Journal of Bioinformatics and Computational Biology, 3*(02), 185–205.

# Molecular Basis of Food Classification in Traditional Chinese Medicine

Xiaosong Han, Haiyan Zhao, Hao Xu, Yun Yang, Yanchun Liang, and Dong Xu

**Abstract** Traditional Chinese Medicine (TCM) started considering the medicinal and health effects of food thousands of years ago. TCM labels are placed on foods based on cold, neutral, and hot properties similar to Chinese herbal medicine. However, it is unclear whether such a classification has any molecular or biochemical basis, and what the relationship is between this TCM classification and the nutrient composition of food. To answer these questions, we collected a large dataset, in which each type of food has both TCM labels and molecular composition records for

**Electronic supplementary material** The online version of this chapter (https://doi.org/10.1007/978-3-030-33416-1_10) contains supplementary material, which is available to authorized users.

X. Han · H. Xu
Key Laboratory of Symbol Computation and Knowledge Engineering of Ministry of Education, College of Computer Science and Technology, Jilin University, Changchun, China
e-mail: hanxiaosong@jlu.edu.cn; xuhao@jlu.edu.cn

H. Zhao
Centre for Artificial Intelligence, FEIT, University of Technology Sydney (UTS), Broadway, NSW, Australia

Y. Yang
Philocafe, San Jose, CA, USA

Y. Liang
College of Computer Science and Technology, Jilin University, Changchun, China

Zhuhai Laboratory of Key Laboratory of Symbol Computation and Knowledge Engineering of Ministry of Education, Department of Computer Science and Technology, Zhuhai College of Jilin University, Zhuhai, China
e-mail: ycliang@jlu.edu.cn

D. Xu (✉)
Department of Electrical Engineering and Computer Science, University of Missouri, Columbia, MO, USA

Christopher S. Bond Life Sciences Center, University of Missouri, Columbia, MO, USA
e-mail: xudong@missouri.edu

© Springer Nature Switzerland AG 2020
Y. Zhao, D.-G. (Din) Chen (eds.), *Statistical Modeling in Biomedical Research*, Emerging Topics in Statistics and Biostatistics, https://doi.org/10.1007/978-3-030-33416-1_10

197

statistical analyses and machine-learning predictions. We applied machine-learning methods by using food molecular composition to predict the hot, neutral or cold label of food, and achieved more than 80% accuracy, which clearly indicated that TCM labels have a significant molecular basis. We also applied ANOVA to analyze the main factors contributing to the TCM labels. The ANOVA analysis shows that some molecular/biochemical compositions and categories, such as Energy, Fat, Protein, Water and Selenium (Se), have the strongest correlations with the TCM labels of food. To the best of our knowledge, this study represents the first effort to quantitatively explore the relationship between TCM labels and the molecular composition of food.

**Keywords** Traditional Chinese medicine · Zheng · Food composition · Health effect of food · Machine learning

## 1 Introduction

Traditional Chinese Medicine (TCM) has been practiced for more than 2500 years in China and in many other Asian countries. It is also gaining more and more popularity in Western countries. TCM includes herbal medicine, acupuncture, massage, exercise, and dietary therapy [1]. In TCM herbal medicine, all kinds of herbs can be categorized based on four properties—hot, warm, cool, and cold. Hot and warm herbs are often used for cold diseases, while cool and cold herbs are often used for hot diseases [2]. One of TCM's typical characteristics is the homology of medicine and food; thus, most common food can be regarded as medicine to treat diseases, which implies there is no strict boundary between food and herbal medicine [3]. In fact, it is stated in a classic TCM Bible "Inner Canon of Huangdi" that food is only food when people are hungry, but turns into medicine when people become sick. Such a homology between medicine and food has been studied extensively [4]. Given such a homology, food also has the four TCM properties, which are used as a guide in dietary therapy and health improvement.

The labels of hot, warm, cool, and cold are hard to define scientifically. They are widely used in TCM. For example, the human body's health status is often based on "ZHENG" when using various body features such as the tongue [5], i.e., hot ZHENG, normal ZHENG, and cold ZHENG [6]. TCM uses "ZHENG" as a key pathological principle to understand the human homeostasis and guide the applications of Chinese herbs [6]. A hot or cold ZHENG or status does not mean high or low in terms of body temperature, but a certain pathological condition or development tendency of an illness [7]. If one has a hot ZHENG/status, it is suggested to take more cold/cool food to achieve balance. If one has a cold ZHENG/status, more hot/warm food is recommended; if one has a normal ZHENG/status, any food is considered okay as long as it is balanced. So far, these food properties are identified empirically with some general guidance. For example, hot food often tastes sweet or spicy, tends to have a red color, is more likely to be present on land, and has more access to sunshine. In contrast, cold food often tastes bitter or sour, tends to have a green color, is more likely to be present in water, and has less access to sunshine.

Although the four properties of food are identified based on people's experience and sense without any scientific theories and methods, some related research has been conducted in China. TCM properties were delineated by Can Hou (a famous TCM expert) in the 1960s [5]. Can Hou studied antibacterial function, antipyretic function, and three other functions of 72 traditional Chinese herbal medicine. According to the comparison of these medicine, he found that the coldest TCM medicine were antibacterial and antipyretic while the hottest TCM medicine were stimulants [5]. In the 1980s, Li et al. [6] indicated that hot medicine and cold medicine have corresponding relations with excitation and inhibition effects on human body based on an analysis of many kinds of medicines such as heat-clearing medicine and diaphoretics, i.e., hot medicine can stimulate the body activities and the cold medicine can inhibit them [5]. In the 1990s, Liang [7] proposed that one of the basic functions of cold medicine was the synthesis and release of the sympathetic medium, based on the sympathetic medium content of 28 patients with hot symptoms and 12 with cold symptoms during pre- and post- treatment. Outside China, some scholars are also interested in the four properties of TCM. For instance, in the1970s, a group in Japan studied different effects on people's health from hot herbs and cold herbs [8]. They found that when rats with inflammation ate cold herbs (such as Sini soup and Huanglian Jiedu soup), the temperature would decrease and the inflammation was inhabited, while hot herbs caused drinking more water and increasing temperature. This result indicated that hot herbs might exacerbate the inflammation while cold herbs could diminish inflammation and inhibit metabolism.

Although hot and cold properties of food are well documented [2], no research has explored the connection between the nutrition composition in food and the TCM properties of food, or whether these properties have any scientific (molecular) basis at all. This paper focuses on the connection between cold/hot properties of food and nutrition composition using data analysis and machine learning methods. If the connection is significant, we can also find out which components of a food affect TCM properties the most. This study also considered ways to predict the hot and cold properties of food based on its molecular composition.

## 2   Data

Many materials about hot and cold properties of food are available online, but their accuracy requires validation. We collected annotations from the '*Encyclopedia of Healthcare Based on Chinese Food*' [9] written by Huanhua Wang, an expert in TCM, especially in Chinese medical recuperation theory. The book collected 556 types of food and each of them is labeled with a unique property—hot, warm, cool, cold or neutral. Table 1 shows some examples. All of these properties are labeled by experts in this field.

**Table 1** Three food properties according to TCM

| Type | Hot/warm food | Neutral food | Cold/cool food |
|---|---|---|---|
| Meat | Lamb, chicken, goose, prawn | Pork, beef | Crab, rabbit, duck |
| Vegetable | Eggplant, onions, chive, garlic, pepper | Potatoes | Seaweed, cabbage, spinach, carrots, celery, cucumbers, tomatoes, green beans |
| Fruit | Longan, litchi, citrus, chestnuts, walnuts | Apricots, peaches, grapes | Melons, watermelons, bananas, pears, persimmons, pineapples |
| Others | Brown sugar, coffee, syrup, wine, curry | Chicken eggs | Sugar, tofu, duck eggs |

**Table 2** Information of U1 and U2 datasets

| | Cold | Neutral | Hot | Total | Features |
|---|---|---|---|---|---|
| U1 | 80 | 102 | 90 | 272 | 25 |
| U2 | 1797 | 2874 | 3036 | 7707 | 99 |

Regarding the food nutrition composition, we collected data mainly from the website *SELFNutritionData* [10] and 'China Food Composition' [11]. The information in the USDA's National Nutrient Database for Standard Information from the USDA Food Composition Databases [12] was used as a supplement. All these resources are authoritative and comprehensive. To coalesce the data, we developed a web crawler based on the WebMagic scalable framework. It includes the whole crawler cycle: downloading, URL management, and content extraction. It provides an application programming interface (API) for html extracting, with multi-thread and distribution support [13]. The input of the crawler is the name of food and a list of nutrition compositions of the corresponding food that can be exported as a file.

With the API, a small dataset (U1) and a large dataset (U2) were obtained (Table 2). The data in the small dataset was manually collected from the 'China Food Composition' Book. It contains 272 entries, and the numbers of hot, neutral and cold food were 80, 102, and 90, respectively. This small dataset contains 25 food compositions are shown in a bold font in column 1 of Table 3. The large dataset has 7707 entries and each of them contained 99 features, which are also shown in Table 3. Some features such as each fatty acid isomer are not considered because the data had too many incomplete entries. There were 1797 entries of cold food, 2874 entries of neutral food, and 3036 entries of hot food in total. Each entry in these two datasets is labeled according to "Encyclopedia of Healthcare Based on Chinese Food" with 0 for cold property, 1 for neutral property and 2 for hot property.

## 3 Methods

Figure 1 is the flowchart of our study, which contains three parts. The first part is data imputing, which allows us to estimate the missing values by a k-nearest neighbor

**Table 3** Features included in U1 and U2 datasets[a]

| Energy | ND rating | Weight loss | Fullness factor |
|---|---|---|---|
| **Ash** | Fluoride | Calories from carbohydrate | Amino acid score |
| **Vitamin B1** | Starch | Galactose | Lactose |
| **Vitamin B3** | Maltose | Total trans-monoenoic fatty acids | Polyunsaturated fat |
| **P** | Total trans fatty acids | Threonine | Methionine |
| **Protein** | Tryptophan | Phenylalanine | Histidine |
| **Fiber** | Cystine | Aspartic acid | Serine |
| **Vitamin B2** | Alanine | Lycopene | Beta carotene |
| **Na** | Weight gain | Gamma tocopherol | Vitamin E (alpha tocopherol) |
| **Cu** | Calories from protein | Vitamin B6 | Dietary folate equivalents |
| **Sugar** | Glucose | Pantothenic acid | Campesterol |
| **Water** | Saturated fat | Calories from alcohol | Caffeine |
| **K** | Total omega-3 fatty acids | Beta-sitosterol | Monounsaturated fat |
| **Ca** | Leucine | Completeness score | Vitamin D |
| **Zn** | Valine | Optimum health | Phytosterols |
| **Fat** | Glycine | Calories from fat | Beta tocopherol |
| **Carotene** | Retinol activity equivalent | Sucrose | Vitamin B12 |
| **Vitamin E** | Vitamin K | Total trans-polyenoic fatty acids | Stigmasterol |
| **Mg** | Food folate | Isoleucine | Theobromine |
| **Mn** | Betaine | Tyrosine | Total Omega-6 fatty acids |
| **Vitamin A** | Cholesterol | Glutamic acid | Proline |
| **Retinol** | Fructose | Lutein+Zeaxanthin | Hydroxyproline |
| **Vitamin C** | Alpha carotene | Delta tocopherol | Beta cryptoxanthin |
| **Fe** | Arginine | Folate | Alcohol |
| **Se** | Folic acid | Choline | |

[a]All the features belong to U2, and features in bold font belong to U1

(k-NN) method. The second part is data analysis. Analysis of variance (ANOVA) was used to assess which features has a strong relation to TCM food labels. The last part is classification. Ensemble learning, deep learning and support vector machine (SVM) were applied to train the prediction models of food labels. The source code of our method is available at https://github.com/squarlhan/foodsvm.

## 3.1 Data Imputing

Dataset U2 contains 99 features for each entry of collected food. These features contain not only common nutrition compositions such as calories, fat, carbohydrates and protein but also have some uncommon compositions like zinc, fluoride and betaine. Features of some entries were unknown. Simply ignoring all these missing

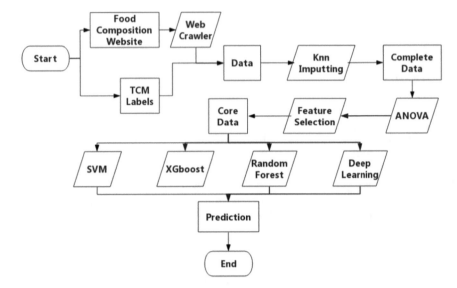

**Fig. 1** Flowchart of the study

values would result in a loss of much information from the data; hence, we estimated some of them.

The missing value rates of all the features are calculated as the ratio of entries with null values:

$$r = n/T \tag{1}$$

where $n$ is the number of null values and $T$ is the total number of all entries for a given feature. Based on Eq. (1), the missing value rates of some features such as calories and fat are less than 1%, while some other features like vitamin D and phytosterols are over 90%. In order to ensure the accuracy of the analyses, high-quality data is needed. We set the threshold from 1% to 25% with a 1% step and exported the features below the threshold as one dataset.

For every null value in the datasets, a value was estimated by the matrix completion algorithm k-NN. $k$ in k-NN was set from 5 to 10, and 54 datasets with different missing value rates were generated from U2 after duplicate removal. The k-NN method identifies the correlation among the variables based on cross-correlation. Assuming the variable $x$ is missing at an entry, and $x$ has a relationship with $y$ and $z$, the test vector will then be formed using the values of $y$ and $z$ in that entry. The training vectors are formed in a similar way. A weighted modification of the Euclidean distance is proposed to measure cross-correlation, which is similar to Mahalanobis distance but can handle missing values in both test and training vectors:

$$d(x, y) = \frac{\sqrt{\sum_{i=1}^{N} (x_i \wedge y_i) \times (x_i - y_i)^2}}{\sum_{i=1}^{N} (x_i \wedge y_i)} \tag{2}$$

where $N$ is the number of variables, and $d(x, y)$ is the distance between $x$ and $y$. Considering an instance $i$ with missing values in position $v$, the value of $v$ is estimated by the weighted cross-correlation with neighbor instances.

$$i^v = \frac{\sum_{j=1}^{k} x_j^v \times d(i, x_j)}{k \bullet \sum_{j=1}^{k} d(i, x_j)} \tag{3}$$

where $k$ is the $k$ value of k-NN, and $x_j^v$ is the value of position $v$ in $j$th neighbor of instance $i$.

## 3.2 Single Factor Analysis

Analysis of variance (ANOVA) [14] was employed to analyze the relationship between molecular compositions and TCM food labels. To assess each molecular composition's effects on the TCM labels of food, ANOVA was first applied to the 25 features in dataset U1, such as energy, sugar, fiber, and so on. After the test, those features with a P-value <0.05 were considered to have significant influence on the final classification results. ANOVA was also applied to 54 datasets generated from dataset U2. The F-test was chosen to compare the factors of the total deviation. In the single-factor ANOVA, statistical significance was tested by comparing the F test statistic:

$$F = \frac{BMSS}{WMSS} = \frac{\sum_i n_i (\overline{Y}_i - \overline{Y}_{total})^2 / (k - 1)}{\sum_i \sum_j (Y_{ij} - \overline{Y}_i)^2 / (N - k)} \tag{4}$$

where $BMSS$ is between the mean sum of squares, $WMSS$ is within the mean sum of squares, $\overline{Y}_i$ is the mean of group $i$, $\overline{Y}_{total}$ is the mean of all cases, $n_i$ is the number of cases in group $i$, $Y_{ij}$ is the $j$-th case in group $i$, $k$ is the total number of groups, and $N$ is the total number of cases. We performed the ANOVA F-test to minimize false negative errors of a fixed rate of false positive errors [15]. ANOVA F-test is recommended as a practical test, because of its robustness against many alternative distributions [16].

## 3.3 Classifier

A variety of machine-learning methods were employed as the classifiers, i.e., ensemble learning, deep learning and SVM. For ensemble learning, random forests and XGboost were used with one deep learning framework, Convolutional neural network (CNN) was also applied. In SVM, the genetic algorithm (GA) was used to select parameters and features.

### 3.3.1 SVM

The SVM algorithm creates nonlinear classifiers by applying the kernel function to maximum-margin hyperplanes [17, 18]. Intuitively, in SVM, a good separation is achieved by the hyperplane that has the largest distance to the nearest training-data point of any class (so-called functional margin); thus, in general, the larger the margin the lower the generalization error of the classifier. In this work, LibSVM [19], a popular open source machine-learning library was used in the experiment. LibSVM implements the SMO algorithm for kernelized SVMs, supporting classification and regression [19]. We selected the Gauss Kernel Function, because it has fewer parameters to optimize. Genetic algorithm (GA) was applied to optimize SVM and select features in the experiment. In particular, the parameter optimization was performed for *gamma* (the width of the kernel function) and *C* (the penalty coefficient). The fitness function of GA is the average accuracy of a tenfold cross-validation. The data was randomly divided into ten portions of equal sizes where nine portions were taken as the training samples and the final one was taken as a test sample. The mean of ten results' accuracies was used as the final fitness value. In addition, feature selection was also conducted to identify significant features. Hybrid encoding was applied in the experiment. Figure 2 is an example chromosome in U1, where 27 genes are encoded in total. The first two genes with decimal coding are parameters of SVM (*gamma*, *C*). The remaining genes with binary coding represent features described as either true or false to indicate whether this feature is selected.

### 3.3.2 Ensemble Learning

In statistics and machine learning, ensemble methods use more multiple learning algorithms to obtain better predictive performance than any of the constituent learning algorithms alone. The random forests algorithm [20] is a method for classification, regression and other tasks. It constructs a multitude of decision trees at training and then outputs the mode of the classes or mean prediction of the individual trees. Random decision forests can help correct the potential problem of decision trees overfitting the training set [21], by averaging the predictions of a set of m trees with individual weight functions [22].

Gradient boosting is another ensemble learning method for regression and classification problems. It produces a prediction model in the form of an ensemble of weak prediction models. It also builds the stage-wise model like other boosting methods and generalizes them by allowing optimization of an arbitrary differen-

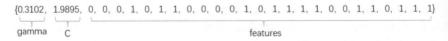

**Fig. 2** GA encoding example

tiable loss function. In this study, we applied Extreme Gradient Boosting (XGboost [23, 24]), an open-source gradient boosting library. XGboost has gained popularity recently as it was the algorithm of choice for many winning teams in a number of machine learning competitions [23].

While both random forests and XGboost belong to ensemble learning, some differences exist between them. The training algorithm for random forests applies the general technique of bootstrap aggregating (bagging) to tree learners while the training algorithm for XGboost applies boosting. Bagging means that users take bootstrap samples (with replacement) of their data set and each subset trains a (potentially) weak learner. Boosting, on the other hand, uses all the data to train each learner, but instances that were misclassified by the previous learners are given more weight so that subsequent learners focus more on them during the training. The classification of XGboost is often more accurate and efficient than random forests. The training sets of random forests are selected randomly and are independent from each other. The training sets of each iteration for XGboost is weighted by the learning results generated by previous iterations.

In this work, we used the classification and regression tree (CART) to create a random forest, and generated ten trees for the forest. The number of features for each CART is set as Eq. (5), where $M$ is the total number of features:

$$Ms = \text{Round}\left(\log_2 M + 1\right) \qquad (5)$$

Regarding XGboost, we set the objective as multiclassification and Softmax. The maximum depth of each tree was set as 6, and the learning step size shrinkage "eta" (used to prevent overfitting) is set to 0.1, which is a very conservative value.

### 3.3.3  Deep Learning

CNN [25, 26] is a powerful and efficient method for discovering local patterns. It is widely used in image-recognition and pattern-recognition problems. In a CNN, the layer of convolutions plays a major role as a feature extractor. Unlike traditional feature extractors, convolution layers extract local features with local windows. Convolution weights are determined in the training process. Figure 3 is the architectural diagram of our CNN model. We used three convolutional layers with a max pooling and then followed by two fully connected layers with each layer including 20 neurons. Each layer in a convolutional layer is a three-dimensional array of size $h \times w \times d$, where $h$ and $w$ are the size of input, and d is the channel dimension. Based on the Bayesian optimization method, the size of $2 \times 1 \times 50$ neurons in each convolutional layer can obtain the best performance. Our model also includes max pooling layers, that reduce the dimension of the features, and the fully connected layers to sum weights of the previous features. In the final layer of CNN, a Softmax function is applied to classify each sample with cross-entropy loss as the objective function for the parameter estimate.

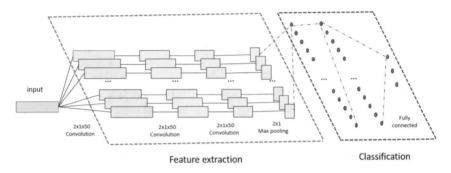

**Fig. 3** Architectural diagram of CNN

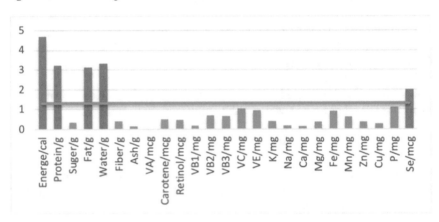

**Fig. 4** Bar diagram of ANOVA analysis for each feature of U1. The x-axis represents the name of each molecular composition, and the y-axis represents the negative base 10 logarithm of the P-value computed by ANOVA

## 4 Experiments

### 4.1 ANOVA Result

ANOVA was performed on the both datasets. It was mainly used to find the features in the dataset with the greatest impact on the hot and cold properties of food. Figure 4 shows the analysis result of ANOVA for U1, where the abscissa line names each nutrition composition, and the vertical ordinate is the negative number of the base 10 logarithm of the P-value computed by ANOVA. The smaller the P-value, the greater impact it has on the property of food, which is the feature. In our experiment, if the P-value of one feature is smaller than 0.05, the feature is considered to be significant. In Fig. 5 we can find that the P-values of five features are smaller than 0.05, including energy, fat, protein, water, and Se. Figure 5 boxplots the three features with the lowest P-values. It shows the distribution of the data for each feature.

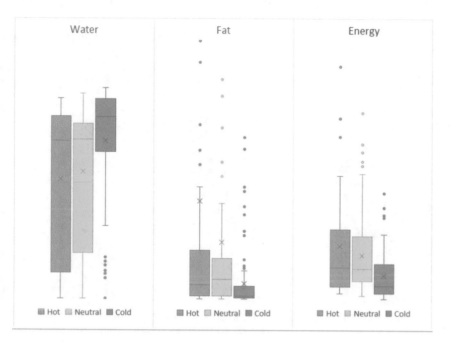

**Fig. 5** Boxplots of 3 top features in U1

The ANOVA analysis of 54 datasets in U2 calculated the P-value of each feature in these datasets. The data are divided into three groups. After the application of Bonferroni's correction, we sorted these P-values and selected those features with smallest P-values, i.e., protein, weight loss, optimum health and calories from protein. The boxplots of the first three features are shown in Fig. 6, which illustrates that TCM labels tend to be hot with high protein abundance. Health indices weight loss and optimum health tend to have high values among food with cold labels.

## 4.2  TCM Label Classification

The above classifiers were all applied on dataset U1, and the results are shown in Table 4. The first dataset, "ALL," is U1 which contains all 25 features. The second dataset "ANOVA5" only includes the five most influential features of which the P-value is smaller than 0.05. The accuracy of optimized SVM using GA is also displayed in the table, and it performed better than the other classifiers.

Table 5 highlights some features including the five most influential features and 12 highlighted features in the second column, selected by GA in the SVM. This table also shows that energy, protein, fat, water and Se are all selected in these two lists.

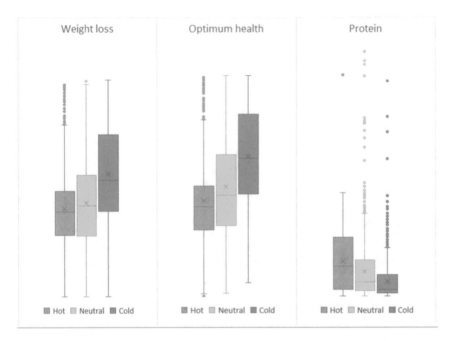

**Fig. 6** Boxplot of 3 top features in U2

**Table 4** The accuracy for each algorithm

| Algorithm framework | Detailed | Accuracy (%) |
|---|---|---|
| SVM | ALL | 64.30 |
| | ANOVA5 | 59.85 |
| | **GA** | **73.20** |
| XGboost (XG) | ALL | 60.50 |
| | ANOVA5 | 64.45 |
| Random Forest (RF) | ALL | 52.60 |
| | ANOVA5 | 51.40 |
| Deep learning | CNN | 60.80 |

These algorithms were also used to train the 54 datasets in U2, and we obtained the accuracy of prediction from these algorithms. Figure 8 is the curve of these algorithms. The abscissa lists 54 datasets, and the ordinate is the prediction accuracy of each dataset resulting from each algorithm. With the increase of missing value rates and $k$, the accuracy predicted by these algorithms increases slowly. In Fig. 7, XGboost is stable and shows a higher accuracy than other algorithms. The orange solid curve is the average value of four algorithms; furthermore, this curve reaches its peak while the missing value rate is 0.25 and $k$ is 6. All four curves are similar. This U3 dataset has a missing value rate of 0.25 and $k$, which is 6, includes the best distributed data.

**Table 5** Most influential features selected by ANOVA and GA in U1

| ANOVA | | GA | |
|---|---|---|---|
| Energy | Vitamin C | Energy | Vitamin C |
| Protein | Vitamin E | Protein | Vitamin E |
| Sugar | K | Sugar | K |
| Fat | Na | Fat | Na |
| Water | Ca | Water | Ca |
| Fiber | Mg | Fiber | Mg |
| Ash | Fe | Ash | Fe |
| Vitamin A | Mn | Vitamin A | Mn |
| Carotene | Zn | Carotene | Zn |
| Retinol | Cu | Retinol | Cu |
| Vitamin B1 | P | Vitamin B1 | P |
| Vitamin B2 | Se | Vitamin B2 | Se |
| Vitamin B3 | | | Vitamin C |

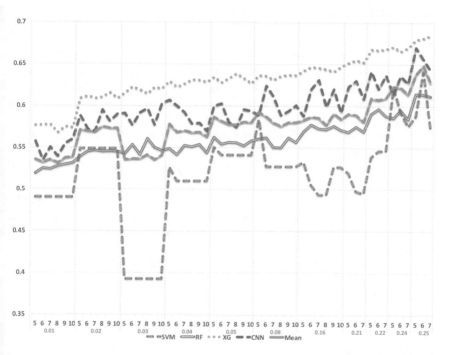

**Fig. 7** The curve plot of the accuracy for each algorithm with different *ks* (first row of x-axis) and missing value rates (second row of x-axis)

Although XGboost and CNN perform better than SVM, the two algorithms have little space to improve by fine tuning. Therefore, in order to get a better prediction accuracy, GA is applied in SVM to adjust the main parameters of SVM. And finally, the GA-SVM with feature selection achieves accuracy at 85.86%, which is higher than any other algorithms. Compared with U1, the classification accuracy in U3 improves a lot. We believe that U3 supplies more samples and features which make

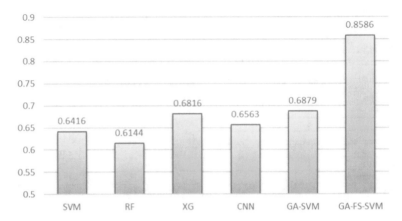

**Fig. 8** The column chart of the accuracy for each algorithm on U3

the classifier performs better. Figure 8 is the column chart of the tenfold cross-validation accuracy for each algorithm in U3. The accuracy of an optimized SVM using GA and feature selection (FS) has the highest accuracy (85.86%). The GA-SVM algorithm without feature selection shows an intermediate value of 68.97%, which is much smaller than the GA-FS-SVM.

The most influential set of features selected by GA in U3 are the following: *Fullness Factor, Fiber, Weight gain, Vitamin C, Glycemic Load, Vitamin B1, Completeness Score, K, Na, Calories, Calories from Fat, Calories from Protein Water, Saturated Fat, Alcohol, Sugar, Ash*

The next set of influential features selected by GA in U3 are the following: *ND Rating, Weight loss, Optimum Health, Calories from Carbohydrate, Protein, Total Fat, Polyunsaturated Fat Monounsaturated Fat, Cholesterol, Vitamin A, Vitamin B2, Vitamin B3, Ca, Fe, Mg, Zn, P.*

In both sets, many features were selected by GA and ANOVA. Fat and protein appear in both the GA and ANOVA datasets. Vitamin A, Ca and P were selected by GA in U1 and U3.

## 5   Discussion

Although these TCM labels are empirical, they have been refined and widely practiced for more than 2000 years. These TCM labels were not established scientifically, but it is worthwhile to study them using a scientific approach. The statistical and machine-learning analyses and predictions clearly show that TCM labels of the hot, neutral, and cold foods have a molecular basis and are predictable based on their food molecular composition. We also identified key molecular compositions that contribute to the TCM labels. The highly-overlapped features selected by ANOVA and GA in U1 and U3 may have the greatest effect on the labels. Fat and Protein are two of the three main macronutrients. In addition, Fig. 5 shows that the food with more energy tends to be hot, while food with less energy tends to be cold. The boxplots in Fig. 6 for U3 illustrate the similar result.

Although this study does not prove the value of TCM food labels in health-care, the key features that drive the TCM labels are highly important in health. Calcium plays an important role in building stronger and denser bones early in life and keeping bones strong and healthy later in life; P is an essential mineral primarily used for growth and repair of body cells and tissues. Lack of P-rich adenosine triphosphate (ATP) can cause hypophosphatemia, including neurological dysfunction and disruption of muscle and blood cells. Too much phosphate can lead to diarrhea and calcification of organs and soft tissue, and can interfere with the body's ability to use Fe, Ca, Mg, and Zn [4]. While a lifelong deficit of Ca can affect bone and tooth formation, over-retention can cause hypercalcemia, impaired kidney function, and decreased absorption of other minerals. Vitamin D is needed to absorb Ca [2]. All these symptoms may be related to the hot or cold status of human body. Food that has more essential nutrients per calorie is considered a better choice for optimum health. We can find that food with the cold label has high scores in optimum health, which shows that cold food is often heathier. Besides, cold food contains less energy, and it helps to control body weight. In the future, we will do more research on this work, with a focus on exploring the health impact of food with different TCM labels.

**Acknowledgements** This work has been partially supported by the National Natural Science Foundation of China (61503150, 61972174), the Jilin Scientific and Technological Development Plan (20160520012JH, 20170204057GX), the Guangdong Key-Project for Applied Fundamental Research (Grant 2018KZDXM076), the Guangdong Premier Key-Discipline Enhancement Scheme (Grant 2016GDYSZDXK036) and the Paul K. and Dianne Shumaker Endowed Fund at University of Missouri.

# References

1. Hobert, O. (2008). Gene regulation by transcription factors and microRNAs. *Science, 319*(5871), 1785–1786.
2. Ergil, M. C., & Ergil, K. (2009). *Pocket atlas of Chinese medicine.* New York: Thieme.
3. Yang, S. (1965). *Grand simplicity of inner canon of Huangdi.* Beijing: People's Medical Publishing House.
4. Zhu, J., Deng, W., et al. (2015). Theoretical origination of medicine and food homology. *Journal of Traditional Chinese Medicine University of Hunan, 35*(12), 27–30.
5. Yu, H., Zhou, H., Xiao, X., Lit, T., Yuan, H., Zhao, Y., & Gao, X. (2001). Advances and prospects of four properties of Chinese traditional medicine. *China Journal of Basic Medicine in Traditional Chinese Medicine, 7*(8), 61–64.
6. Li, S., Zhang, Z. Q., Wu, L. J., Zhang, X. G., Li, Y. D., & Wang, Y. Y. (2007). Understanding ZHENG in traditional Chinese medicine in the context of neuro-endocrine-immune network. *IET Systems Biology, 1*(1), 51–60.
7. Liang, Y. (1998). Study on the therapeutic mechanism of hyperthermia. *Chinese Journal of Integrated Traditional and Western Medicine, 18*(5), 305–306.

8. He, F., Deng, K., et al. (2008). The status and prospect on studies of the four properties for the traditional Chinese Materia medical. *Chinese Journal of Experimental Traditional Medical Formulae, 14*(8), 72–75.

9. Wang, H. (2006). *Encyclopedia of healthcare based on Chinese food.* Guangzhou: Guangdong Travel and Tourism Press.

10. Nutrition Data. (2016). *SELF nutrition data know what you eat.* http://nutritiondata.self.com/

11. Yang, Y. (2009). *China food composition.* Beijing: Peking University Medical Press.

12. USDA, Agriculture Research Service. (2019). *Software developed by the National Agricultural Library v.3.9.5.1_2019-04-03.* Retrieved from https://ndb.nal.usda.gov/ndb/

13. Webmagic (2016). *A scalable web crawler framework for Java.* Retrieved from http://webmagic.io/en/

14. Fisher, R. A. (1921). On the probable error of a coefficient of correlation deduced from a small sample. *Metron, 1,* 3–32.

15. Hinkelmann, K., & Kempthorne, O. (2008). *Design and analysis of experiments. I and II* (2nd ed.). New York: Wiley.

16. Moore, D. S., & McCabe, G. P. (2003). *Introduction to the practice of statistics.* New York: WH Freeman.

17. Boser, B. E., Guyon, I. M., & Vapnik, V. N. (1992). A training algorithm for optimal margin classifiers. In *The workshop on computational learning theory* (Vol. 5, pp. 144–152). New York: ACM.

18. Cortes, C., & Vapnik, V. (1995). Support-vector networks. *Machine Learning, 20*(3), 273–297.

19. Chang, C. C., & Lin, C. J. (2011). *LIBSVM: A library for support vector machines* (Vol. 2, pp. 1–27). New York: ACM.

20. Ho, T. K. (1995). Random decision forests. In *Proceedings of the 3rd international conference on document analysis and recognition*, Montreal, QC, 14–16 (pp. 278–282). Piscataway, NJ: IEEE.

21. Hastie, T., Tibshirani, R., & Friedman, J. (2008). *The elements of statistical learning 2nd end.* Berlin: Springer.

22. Lin Y, Jeon Y (2002). *Random forests and adaptive nearest neighbors* (Technical Report No. 1055). University of Wisconsin .

23. Chen T (2016). *Machine learning challenge winning solutions.* Retrieved from https://github.com/dmlc/xgboost/tree/master/demo#machine-learning-challenge-winning-solutions

24. Chen T (2016). *XGBoost introduction.* Retrieved August 1, 2016, from http://homes.cs.washington.edu/~tqchen/2016/03/10/story-and-lessons-behind-the-evolution-of-xgboost.html

25. LeCun, Y., Bottou, L., Bengio, Y., & Haffner, P. (1998). Gradient-based learning applied to document recognition. *Proceedings of the IEEE, 86*(11), 2278–2324.

26. Krizhevsky, A., Sutskever, I., & Hinton, G. E. (2012). Imagenet classification with deep convolutional neural networks. In *Advances in neural information processing systems* (pp. 1097–1105). Cambridge, MA: MIT.

# Discovery Among Binary Biomarkers in Heterogeneous Populations

**Junxian Geng and Elizabeth H. Slate**

**Abstract** Biomarkers have great potential to improve disease diagnosis and treatment. Disease may arise via multiple pathways, however, each associated with distinct complex interactions among multiple biomarkers, and hence patients exhibit considerable heterogeneity in the biomarker-disease association despite sharing the same clinical diagnosis. Thus identification of clinically useful biomarker combinations requires statistical methods that accommodate population heterogeneity and enable discovery of possibly complex interactions among biomarkers that associate with disease. We address jointly modeling binary and continuous disease outcomes when the association between predictors and these outcomes exhibits heterogeneity. In the context of binary biomarkers, we use ideas from logic regression to find Boolean combinations of these biomarkers that predict the binary disease outcome. The associated continuous outcome is modeled as Gaussian. Heterogeneity is cast as unknown subgroups in the population, with the associations between the joint outcome and biomarkers and other covariates varying by subgroup. We adopt a mixture of finite mixtures (MFM) fully Bayesian formulation to simultaneously estimate the number of subgroups, the subgroup membership structure, and the subgroup-specific relationships between outcomes and predictors. We describe how our model incorporates the Boolean relations as parameters arising from the MFM model and our approach to the associated challenges of specifying the prior distribution and estimation using Markov chain Monte Carlo. We illustrate the performance of the methods using simulation and discuss application.

**Keywords** Bayesian semiparametric model · Clustering · Joint modeling · Markov chain Monte Carlo · Product partition model

J. Geng
Boehringer Ingelheim Pharmaceuticals Inc., Ridgefield, CT, USA
e-mail: junxian.geng@boehringer-ingelheim.com

E. H. Slate (✉)
Department of Statistics, Florida State University, Tallahassee, FL, USA
e-mail: slate@stat.fsu.edu

© Springer Nature Switzerland AG 2020
Y. Zhao, D.-G. (Din) Chen (eds.), *Statistical Modeling in Biomedical Research*, Emerging Topics in Statistics and Biostatistics,
https://doi.org/10.1007/978-3-030-33416-1_11

213

# 1 Introduction

Biomarkers are individual characteristics that have great potential for personalizing and, therefore, improving health care. Biomarkers include demographic, environmental, clinical and biological characteristics such as gender, genotype, protein expression, prognostic status, etc., that can refine risk assessment, aid diagnosis, guide therapeutics and improve our understanding of the disease process. Few diseases, however, are well predicted by any single biomarker. Heterogeneous diseases such as cancer may have different molecular agents (biomarkers) regulating development, growth and ultimate survival of the individual, and may arise from complex interactions among biomarkers. Hence a panel of biomarkers and consideration of interactions among these biomarkers is needed to achieve sensitivity and specificity sufficient for clinical use [18, 31].

This paper is motivated by the problem of predicting a binary disease status using a collection of binary biomarkers. These biomarkers may encode for the occurrence of single nucleotide polymorphisms (SNPs) in the genome or indicate over expression of genes or associated proteins, for instance. Particularly in this case of binary biomarkers as predictors, the interactions may predict disease status far better than only biomarker main effects. We build on the method of logic regression [27], which enables discovery of Boolean combinations of binary predictors to explain a binary response. Briefly, letting $x_1, x_2, \ldots, x_p$ be binary biomarkers, logic regression finds a Boolean combination, $L(x_1, x_2, \ldots, x_p)$, that best predicts the binary response $y$ according to a criterion such as minimizing the misclassification rate. The Boolean relation, $L(\cdot)$, may involve complex interactions among the biomarkers that are discovered through adaptive exploration of all combinations of *and*s, *or*s and *not*s, yet retains an appealing interpretability. We describe logic regression in more detail in Sect. 2.

Complex diseases such as cancer arise via multiple pathways, with different sets of biomarkers integral to the different pathways. Thus, the population (and, correspondingly, the individuals comprising our sample) exhibits latent heterogeneity arising from subpopulations defined by distinct disease pathways and their associated predictive biomarkers. Such subpopulation structure also results from heterogeneity in the stage of disease progression, as different sets of biomarkers may be active at initiation, early and late phases of disease, even when these phases are not clinically apparent. We envision, then, that the population consists of an unknown number of subpopulations, and the disease status in each subpopulation is governed by a different Boolean relation among the binary biomarkers. At first glance, one may think that the disjunction of the collection of Boolean relations is sufficient to capture this structure. But consider the case of two subpopulations with Boolean relations $L_1 = x_1 \vee x_2$ and $L_2 = !x_2 \vee x_3$, respectively. If combined with disjunction, the result is $L_1 \vee L_2 = (x_1 \vee x_2) \vee (!x_2 \vee x_3) = x_1 \vee x_3$, and the role of $x_2$, which is important for both subpopulations and may be a key therapeutic target, is lost!

To accommodate population heterogeneity, a latent class structure can be introduced. The latent class logic regression (LCLR) model [30] postulates the existence of $K$ latent classes that accommodate $K$ subpopulations, each of which has its own Boolean relation between the binary predictors and disease outcome. We let $z_i \in \{1, 2, \ldots, K\}$ be the class membership indicator for observation $i$, $i = 1, 2, \ldots, n$, and note that these are unobservable and hence latent variables. It is straightforward to derive and implement maximum likelihood estimation using the expectation-maximization (EM) [8] algorithm with the $\{z_i\}$ handled as the missing data. However, there are two concerns about this LCLR approach. First, the number of latent classes $K$ must be specified before using the EM algorithm. Thus $K$ may be estimated by means not integrated with the LCLR model, or estimated in a post hoc way, say, by using information criteria. The second concern is that, because our response $y$ is binary, more than one latent class is not strictly identifiable [2]. We propose an approach that handles these two concerns within a Bayesian framework.

A natural solution for simultaneously estimating the number of clusters[1] and the cluster configuration is provided by adopting a Bayesian framework where $K$ is merely another unobservable random variable, i.e., parameter, of the model and hence amenable to inference derived from its posterior distribution. Nonetheless, inference about an unknown number of clusters poses a substantial computational challenge. Historically, the number of clusters was given a prior distribution and Markov chain Monte Carlo (MCMC) used to draw samples from a distribution converging to the posterior distribution. However, implementation typically requires a search algorithm in a variable dimensional parameter space such as reversible jump MCMC [12], which requires complicated Metropolis moves as well as suffers from a lack of scalability and poor mixing.

In this paper, we analytically marginalize over the number of clusters to obtain a more efficient Gibbs sampler and avoid the difficulties brought by the dimension changes in parameter space. One modeling choice is a Bayesian nonparametric approach such as the Dirichlet process mixture model (DPMM), which is also termed the Chinese restaurant process (CRP) [19, 25] for the characteristics of the probability distribution induced on the cluster configuration. While CRPs have long been observed empirically to tend to form tiny extraneous clusters, it has only recently been established that the estimation of the number of clusters from CRPs is inconsistent in a fairly general setting [21]. We use the mixture of finite mixtures (MFM) approach of [21] instead, which prunes the tiny extraneous clusters and, consequently, consistently estimates the number of clusters. Moreover, the MFM model has a Pólya urn scheme similar to the CRP that supports an efficient MCMC algorithm.

---

[1] Henceforth we refer to the classes defining the underlying subpopulation structure as *clusters* for greater consistency with the machine learning and Bayesian literature. The *cluster configuration* is the cluster assignment information encoded by the $\{z_i\}$. Because each individual is assigned to exactly one cluster, the cluster configuration is, equivalently, a *partition* of the $n$ observations into $K$ groups.

To address the strict nonidentifiability of more than one latent cluster, we couple the binary disease status $y$ with a continuous response, $w$, and jointly model the outcome pair $(y, w)$. The continuity of $w$ fills the "information gap" and supports full identifiability of $K \leq n$ clusters under usual conditions on the data. An example scenario is $y$ the indicator for positive diagnosis of prostate cancer, $w$ a serum biomarker such as prostate specific antigen, and the biomarkers $x_1, x_2, \ldots, x_p$ representing SNPs in the genome. The rest of the paper is organized as follows. Section 2 provides an overview of logic regression. The development of our Bayesian model is in Sects. 3 and 4 describes the MCMC algorithm for inference. Section 5 presents a simulation study of the performance of our model and estimation. In Sect. 6, we discuss the model and describe future challenges.

## 2  Logic Regression

In traditional regression problems, a model is developed using prespecified main effects and, perhaps, simple two- or three-way interactions to explain the response. In contrast, logic regression [27] is an adaptive regression methodology that enables discovery of complex interactions among binary predictors associated with a binary response. In this context when all predictors are binary, it is the interactions among many predictors, even more so than the main effects, that may best associate with the response.

Given data on $n$ individuals, $(y_i, \mathbf{x}_i), i = 1, 2, \ldots, n$, where $y_i$ is a binary response and $\mathbf{x}_i = (x_{i1}, x_{i2}, \ldots, x_{ip})^T$ is a vector of $p$ binary markers, logic regression (LR) seeks to recover the underlying Boolean relation, $L(\mathbf{x}_i)$, among the markers that describes $y_i$. In *disjunctive normal form* (DNF) [11], $L$ is a series of conjunctions ($\wedge$) called *prime implicants* (PIs) [29] joined by disjunctions ($\vee$). Thus, for example, a Boolean relation in disjunctive normal form is $L(\mathbf{x}) = (x_1 \wedge x_2) \vee !x_3$, which has two PIs. An advantage of LR is its ability to discern arbitrary, and hence highly flexible, interactions (represented as PIs) among biomarkers predictive of disease. In cancer research [9, 15] and other settings [16, 17], LR has shown modest improvements in sensitivity/specificity compared to traditional statistical methods for binary variables.

The interpretability of Boolean relations, and hence LR, is illustrated by Figure 1 of Mitra et al. [22] (not reproduced here), which depicts three pathways by which bladder cancer may develop. Each of the three pathways requires that a series of events occur; hence each pathway can be expressed as a PI. Taken together, the three pathways can be represented by the following Boolean relation in DNF:

$$I \, (Y = \text{cancer+}) = (\text{HRAS} \wedge \text{FGFR3} \wedge !\text{p53} \wedge !\text{p21}) \vee$$

$$\left(9\text{q}^- \wedge !\text{p53} \wedge !\text{p21}\right) \vee$$

$$(!\text{p53} \wedge \text{Rb}) \, .$$

Here, the variables HRAS and FGFR3 are indicators of activating mutations in the corresponding *HRAS* and *FGFR3* genes; the variables p53 and p21 indicate normal expression of the genes *p53* and *p21*, hence !p53 and !p21 indicate loss of this expression; 9q$^-$ indicates a deletion in chromosome 9; and the variable Rb indicates elevated expression of the protein Rb in hyperphosphorylated form.

Although appealing for its flexibility and interpretability, LR exhibits characteristics of a *weak learner* [28]. In particular, the model fit is unstable when the response is only weakly associated with a PI [32], a likely situation when the biomarker-response association is heterogeneous in the study population.

## 3 Model Description

We develop a Bayesian model to accommodate latent subpopulation structure in the association between biomarkers and response. By incorporating logic regression within a fully Bayesian framework, our approach provides simultaneous estimation of the number of clusters (subpopulations), cluster configuration, and distinct Boolean relations associating biomarkers and response within each cluster. Hence, we retain the ability of logic regression to discover complex, yet interpretable, interactions among binary biomarkers predictive of response, and gain estimation of the underlying subpopulation structure and corresponding disease-response associations.

Recall that we jointly model the binary disease status and a related continuous outcome such as a serum marker or quality of life assessment to ensure identifiability (up to label switching) of the subpopulation structure. Expanding on the notation of Sect. 2, let $Y_i = (y_i, w_i)$ be the joint response, where $y_i$ is binary and $w_i$ is continuous. In addition to the $p$ binary biomarkers $\mathbf{x}_i$, we obtain additional covariates $\mathbf{v}_i$ for modeling $w_i$. Let $F(Y_i \mid \mathbf{x}_i, \mathbf{v}_i, \theta_i)$ denote the joint probability distribution for the bivariate response $Y_i$ depending on individual-specific parameters $\theta_i$ and incorporating the association with the binary biomarkers and additional covariates. The notational dependence on $\mathbf{x}_i$ and $\mathbf{v}_i$ will often be suppressed, and we write $Y_i \mid \theta_i \sim F(\theta_i)$.

The subpopulation structure is handled in our model by clustering among the $\{\theta_i\}$. When $\theta_i = \theta_j$, we view observations $i$ and $j$ as clustered, so that individuals $i$ and $j$ are members of the same subpopulation. This clustering naturally arises from the DPMM, as we describe in Sect. 3.1. Following this, we introduce our preferred MFM formulation in Sect. 3.2. Section 3.3 notes important similarities and differences induced on the distribution of cluster configurations by the DPMM and MFM models. Section 3.4 details our joint model, including all prior distributions.

## 3.1  Dirichlet Process Mixture Model (DPMM)

Given the response $Y_i$, $i = 1, 2, \ldots, n$ for each of $n$ individuals, the DPMM may be written as

$$Y_i \mid \theta_i \sim F(\theta_i), \text{ independently}$$

$$\theta_i \mid G \sim G, \text{ independently}$$

$$G \sim \mathrm{DP}(\alpha, G_0),$$

where $\mathrm{DP}(\alpha, G_0)$ denotes the Dirichlet process with concentration parameter $\alpha$ and base distribution $G_0$. Details of the properties of the Dirichlet process are described in [10], but it may be helpful to note that if $G \sim \mathrm{DP}(\alpha, G_0)$, then the measure of a set $B$ under $G$ has mean $G_0(B)$, and $G(B)$ varies inversely with $\alpha$. In particular, the larger the value of $\alpha$, the more the measure $G$ resembles $G_0$. Because the Dirichlet process yields distributions $G$ that are almost surely discrete [3], the unique values among $\theta_1, \theta_2, \ldots, \theta_n$ induce a natural clustering among the observations. More specifically, observations $i$ and $j$ are clustered when $\theta_i = \theta_j$, in which case we view $Y_i$ and $Y_j$ as having arisen from the same subpopulation. Although this clustering may be viewed as a side effect of the DPMM, it fulfills our goal of accommodating latent subpopulation structure.

There is an equivalent formulation that incorporates the cluster membership indicator $z_i \in \{1, 2, \ldots, K\}$, with $z_i = k$ when observation $i$ arises from subpopulation $k$. With $K \leq n$ distinct subpopulations, let $\boldsymbol{\phi} = (\phi_1, \phi_2, \ldots, \phi_K)$ be the vector of unique values among $\{\theta_1, \theta_2, \ldots, \theta_n\}$. Then $\phi_{z_i}$ are the parameters for the cluster containing observation $i$; that is, $\phi_{z_i} = \theta_i$. Letting $\pi = (\pi_1, \pi_2, \ldots, \pi_K)$ be a vector of probabilities summing to one, the equivalent model is the following:

$$Y_i \mid z_i, \boldsymbol{\phi} \sim F(\phi_{z_i}), \text{ independently}$$

$$z_i \mid \pi \sim \mathrm{Categorical}(\pi_1, \pi_2, \ldots, \pi_K), \text{ independently}$$

$$\phi_k \sim G_0, \text{ independently}$$

$$\pi \sim \mathrm{Dirichlet}_K(\alpha/K, \ldots, \alpha/K),$$

which becomes the DPMM in the limit as $K \to \infty$ [14].

The form of the prior distribution for the cluster configuration in the DPMM leads to conditional distributions that make it straightforward to use the Gibbs sampler to obtain posterior samples [23]. These prior distributions are discussed in Sect. 3.3.

## 3.2 Mixture of Finite Mixtures (MFM)

A mixture of finite mixtures (MFM) model may also be used to represent subpopulation structure. In our context, the MFM model is written as follows:

$$Y_i \mid z_i, \boldsymbol{\phi} \sim F(\phi_{z_i}), \text{ independently}$$

$$z_i \mid \pi, K \sim \text{Categorical}(\pi_1, \pi_2, \ldots, \pi_K), \text{ independently}$$

$$\phi_k \mid K \sim G_0, \text{ independently} \tag{1}$$

$$\pi \mid K \sim \text{Dirichlet}_K(\gamma, \ldots, \gamma),$$

$$K \sim p, \text{ where } p \text{ is a proper distribution on } 1, 2, \ldots.$$

Here, $G_0$ is a base measure on the space of the model parameters $\phi$, and $\gamma > 0$ governs the Dirichlet distribution for the cluster assignment probabilities.

The MFM model shares many attractive properties with the DPMM. As noted in [20], both the MFM model and DPMM may be interpreted as providing a random discrete measure for our model parameters $\{\theta_1, \theta_2, \ldots, \theta_n\}$; both provide for exchangeability; and both induce a simple probability distribution on the cluster configuration that admits a restaurant process. Thus, many DPMM inference algorithms can be applied to the MFM setting directly after minor modifications. Miller [20] notes the following two major advantages of the MFM model over the DPMM:

1. The prior distributions on the number of clusters, $K$, have very different behaviors. In the MFM model prior distribution, the number of clusters converges to a finite value with probability one as the sample size grows. In the DPMM prior distribution, the number of clusters grows to infinity with probability one as the sample size grows.

2. The MFM model prior distribution is such that the sizes of clusters are all the same order of magnitude (asymptotically), a property that Petrone & Raftery [24] termed *balance*. The DPMM prior distribution, on the other hand, exhibits substantial *imbalance* because it favors partitions with some very small clusters relative to the remaining larger clusters.

Miller [21] notes that these properties of the prior distributions for the DPMM and MFM model carry over to the posterior distributions, largely, explaining the extraneous small clusters produced by the DPMM and its overestimation of the number of clusters. We discuss these properties in Sect. 3.3.

However, there are also disadvantages to using a MFM model. A very significant issue is that since the MFM model dislikes small clusters, the mixing time of incremental MCMC samplers, that is, samplers that explore the partition distribution by moving one observation at a time, can be worse than for the DPMM. Another inconvenience is that the coefficients of the partition distribution, $\{V_n(\cdot)\}$ defined in (5) below, need to be precomputed.

## 3.3 The Prior Distribution on the Cluster Assignments

The DPMM and MFM model both accommodate latent subpopulation structure by providing a discrete probability distribution for the individual-specific model parameters $\{\theta_i\}$, which provides a distribution for the cluster assignment variables $\{z_i\}$. This probability distribution on the cluster assignment facilitates simultaneous inference on the number of subpopulations and the assignment of individuals among them. Here we elaborate on key distinctions between the cluster assignment distributions induced by the DPMM and MFM model.

The DPMM induces a distribution on the cluster assignments called the Chinese restaurant process (CRP) [1, 23, 25]. Figure 1 depicts a CRP, so named for the popular Chinese restaurant metaphor: imagine customers arriving to a Chinese restaurant that has infinitely many tables, with the index of each table corresponding to a cluster label. The first customer chooses to sit at the first table, so that $z_1 = 1$. Then $z_i, i = 2, 3, \ldots, n$, have the following conditional distribution (also called a Pólya urn scheme by [4]):

$$\Pr(z_i = k \mid z_1, z_2, \ldots, z_{i-1}) \propto \begin{cases} |k|, & \text{at an existing table labeled } k \\ \alpha, & \text{if } k \text{ is a new table.} \end{cases} \quad (2)$$

Here, $|k|$ refers to the size of table $k$, i.e., the number of customers already seated at table $k$, and $\alpha$ is the concentration parameter of the underlying Dirichlet process. As is evident from Fig. 1, after all $n$ customers have been seated, the tables form a partition of the $n$ customers into a number of clusters corresponding to the number of occupied tables. These clusters capture our subpopulation structure.

The prior distribution on the cluster assignments induces a prior distribution on the sizes of the clusters in the partition. Denote a partition of the observations $\{1, 2, \ldots, n\}$ by $\mathscr{C}$, and let $|\mathscr{C}|$ denote the number of clusters in $\mathscr{C}$. Further, for a partition $\mathscr{C}$ with $|\mathscr{C}| = t$ clusters, let the cluster sizes be $\mathbf{s} = (s_1, s_2, \ldots, s_t)$. The prior distribution on the cluster sizes of the DPMM is given by

$$\Pr_{\mathrm{DP}}(\mathbf{s} = (s_1, s_2, \ldots, s_t) \mid t) \propto (s_1 s_2 \cdots s_t)^{-1}. \quad (3)$$

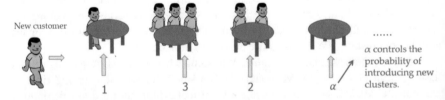

**Fig. 1** An illustration of the Chinese restaurant process. A new customer chooses an existing table with probability proportional to the number of customers already seated at the table, and selects a new table with probability proportional to the Dirichlet process concentration, $\alpha$

From (3), it is clear that the DPMM tends to assign large probabilities to highly imbalanced cluster sizes in which, necessarily, some clusters will be quite small. This provides justification for the tendency of the DPMM to produce small, extraneous clusters. From (2), smaller values of the concentration parameter $\alpha$ have some tendency to curb introduction of new clusters, but the prior distribution on cluster sizes (3) nonetheless pushes toward extraneous clusters. It has recently been established that estimation of the *number of clusters* from DPMMs is inconsistent, even when the sample size grows to infinity [21].

The MFM model described in Sect. 3.2 induces a prior distribution on the cluster assignments that can also be represented as a restaurant process [21, Theorem 4.1]. As illustrated in Fig. 2, the first customer enters the empty restaurant and sits at Table 1. Subsequently, customer $i$ enters and, finding that the previous customers are seated among $t$ tables, chooses a table according to the following conditional distribution:

$$\Pr(z_i = k \mid z_1, z_2, \ldots, z_{i-1}) \propto \begin{cases} |k| + \gamma, & \text{at an existing table labeled } k \\ \dfrac{V_i(t+1)}{V_i(t)}\gamma, & \text{if } k \text{ is a new table.} \end{cases} \tag{4}$$

Recall that $\gamma > 0$ is the parameter of the Dirichlet distribution from which the cluster assignment probabilities arise. The coefficients $V_i(t)$, $i = 2, 3, \ldots, n$ are given by

$$V_i(t) = \sum_{k=1}^{\infty} \frac{k_{(t)}}{(\gamma k)^{(i)}} \, p(k), \tag{5}$$

where $k_{(t)} = k(k-1) \ldots (k-t+1)$, $(\gamma k)^{(i)} = \gamma k(\gamma k+1) \ldots (\gamma k+i-1)$ and $p(\cdot)$, recall, is the prior probability distribution on the number of clusters. (By convention, $x^{(0)} = 1$ and $x_{(0)} = 1$).

While this restaurant process bears close resemblance to the CRP (compare Fig. 2 of the MFM model with Fig. 1 of the DPMM and, similarly, Eqs. (4) and (2)), the introduction of a new $(t + 1)^{\text{st}}$ table at the appearance of customer $i$ is slowed by the factor $V_i(t + 1)/V_i(t)$, which allows a model-based pruning of the tiny extraneous clusters.

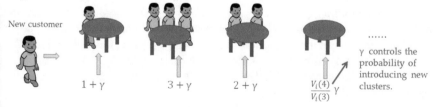

**Fig. 2** The restaurant process associated with the MFM models. New customer $i$ arrives to find the previous $i - 1$ customers seated among $t = 3$ tables. The coefficients $\{V_i(\cdot)\}$ defined in (5) and $\gamma$ determine the probability that this customer starts a new table

Another way to understand the natural pruning of extraneous clusters in the MFM model is through the probability distribution induced on the cluster sizes. Again, let $\mathscr{C}$ be a partition with $t = |\mathscr{C}|$ clusters of sizes $\mathbf{s} = (s_1, s_2, \ldots, s_t)$. In contrast to (3) of the DPMM, the prior probability of the cluster sizes under the MFM model is

$$\text{Pr}_{\text{MFM}}(\mathbf{s} = (s_1, s_2, \ldots, s_t) \mid t) \propto (s_1 s_2 \cdots s_t)^{\gamma-1}. \tag{6}$$

Comparison of (3) and (6) reveals that the MFM model assigns comparatively smaller probability to highly imbalanced cluster sizes than the DPMM. The relative size of the clusters is thus controlled by the parameter $\gamma$; large $\gamma$ gives less variation among the cluster assignment probabilities $\pi = (\pi_1, \pi_2, \ldots, \pi_t)$, and hence more similar cluster sizes, while small $\gamma$ gives more variation among the $\pi$s.

The pruning of small extraneous clusters by the prior distributions of the MFM model induce similar properties in the posterior distributions. Miller [20] proved the consistency of the posterior distribution on the number of clusters in the MFM model, as well as provided careful discussion of the inconsistency of the DPMM in this respect. Because of the desirable feature of consistent estimation of the number of clusters, we use the MFM model (1).

## 3.4   Bayesian Joint Model

We now specify the details of our Bayesian model for the joint response $Y_i = (y_i, w_i)$, where $y_i$ is a binary disease status and $w_i$ is an associated continuous outcome. We use logic regression to allow discovery of interactions among the binary biomarkers, $\mathbf{x}_i$, associated with $y_i$, Gaussian regression to associate the covariates $\mathbf{v}_i$ with $w_i$, and embed this structure within the MFM model (1) to accommodate heterogeneity due to an unknown number of subpopulations. A key assumption is that $y_i$ and $w_i$ are conditionally independent given the cluster assignment $z_i$.

With $K$ subpopulations, let $L_k$ be the Boolean relation governing subpopulation $k$, $k = 1, 2, \ldots, K$, and define the *accuracy* of $L_k$ as $\xi_k = \text{Pr}(y_i = L_k(\mathbf{x}_i) \mid z_i = k, L_k)$. Transforming from the response $y_i$ to the indicators $u_{ik} = I(y_i = L_k(\mathbf{x}_i) \mid z_i = k, L_k)$, we model $u_{ik} \mid z_i = k, L_k, \xi_k \sim \text{Ber}(\xi_k)$, independently. The response $w_i$ is modeled as Gaussian (following transformation, perhaps), again specific to the subpopulation: $w_i \mid z_i = k, \beta_k, \tau_k \sim \text{N}(\mathbf{v}_i^T \beta_k, \tau_k)$, where $\beta_k$ and $\tau_k$ are the regression coefficients and precision, respectively, for subpopulation $k$. Thus, the set of subpopulation-specific parameters is $\phi_k = (L_k, \xi_k, \beta_k, \tau_k)$, and $\phi$ of Sects. 3.1 and 3.2 is the collection of all of these parameters, $\phi = \{(L_k, \xi_k, \beta_k, \tau_k), k = 1, 2, \ldots, K\}$. The conditional independence of $y_i$ and $w_i$ given $z_i$ completes the specification of $F$ in (1), yielding

$$F\left((y_i, w_i) \mid z_i, \boldsymbol{\phi}\right) =$$

$$\xi_{z_i}^{u_{iz_i}} (1 - \xi_{z_i})^{1-u_{iz_i}} \cdot \sqrt{\frac{\tau_{z_i}}{2\pi}} \exp\left(-\frac{\tau_{z_i}}{2} \left[w_i - \mathbf{v}_i^T \beta_{z_i}\right]^2\right), \quad i = 1, 2, \ldots, n. \quad (7)$$

The remainder of our MFM joint model is the choice of prior distribution for the number of subpopulations, $K$, and the conditional prior distribution for the model parameters $\phi_k = (L_k, \xi_k, \beta_k, \tau_k)$ given $K$. As derived by Miller [21], the consistency of the MFM model for the number of subpopulations follows as long as the prior distribution, $K \sim p(\cdot)$, satisfies $p(k) > 0$, $k = 1, 2, \ldots$. Miller also notes, however, that it is desirable to avoid heavy tails in $p$ to make computation of the coefficients $\{V_n(\cdot)\}$ in (5) more efficient. (When $p$ has thin tails, the infinite sum in (5) converges rapidly and fewer terms are needed for accurate approximation of $V_n$.) We use $K - 1 \sim \text{Poisson}(\lambda)$, *a priori*, a choice also studied by Miller [21].

We take the parameters in the conditional submodels for $y_i$ and $w_i$ to be *a priori* independent. Thus, the prior $G_0$ for $\phi_k$ factors into the product of the prior distribution for $(L_k, \xi_k)$ of the logic regression and the prior distribution for $(\beta_k, \tau_k)$ of the Gaussian regression. We further model $L_k$ and $\xi_k$ as *a priori* independent, take $\xi_k$ to follow a beta distribution, and adopt the conjugate normal-gamma prior for $(\beta_k, \tau_k)$. Thus, the prior distribution has the form

$$G_0(\phi_k) = \Pr(L_k) \cdot \text{Beta}(\xi_k; a, b) \cdot \text{N}(\beta_k; \mu_\beta, \tau_k^{-1}\mathbf{V}_\beta) \cdot \text{Gamma}(\tau_k; a', b'), \quad (8)$$

where the parameterizations are such that the beta distribution has mean $a/(a + b)$ and the gamma distribution has mean $a'/b'$. In the simulation of Sect. 5, we take $a = 50$, $b = 10$, $\mu_\beta = \mathbf{0}$, $\mathbf{V}_\beta$ the identity matrix, and $a' = b' = 1.5$. The values of $a$ and $b$ ensure that identified subpopulations have meaningfully accurate Boolean relations.

Building on ideas from Bayesian CART [5] and BART [6], we define the prior distribution on the Boolean relation $L_k$ constructively via the following four steps:

1. Select the number of PIs, denoted $N_{\text{PI}}$, for $L_k$ according to the distribution

$$\Pr(N_{\text{PI}} = q) \propto \delta q^{-\epsilon} - \delta(q + 1)^{-\epsilon}, \quad 0 < \delta < 1, \ \epsilon \geq 0, \ q = 1, 2, \ldots. \quad (9)$$

The probability is a decreasing function of $q$, making larger numbers of PIs less likely. In practice, this distribution is truncated at a maximum size, maxQ, say.
2. Select the number of biomarkers to be included in each PI, denoted $M$, again using probabilities of the form (9), though truncated above at $\text{maxVar} \leq p$.
3. Select the specific biomarkers for each PI uniformly.
4. Negate each selected biomarker with probability 0.5.

These steps yield a Boolean relation in DNF. The corresponding prior probability associated with a Boolean relation $L$ can be computed as

$$\Pr(L) = \sum_{q=1}^{\max Q} \Pr(L \mid N_{\text{PI}} = q) \Pr(N_{\text{PI}} = q)$$

$$= \sum_{q=1}^{\max Q} \left\{ \prod_{j=1}^{q} \sum_{m=1}^{\max \text{Var}} \binom{p}{m}^{-1} 2^{-m} \Pr(M = m \text{ in PI } j) \right\} \Pr(N_{\text{PI}} = q).$$

## 4 Estimation

We perform estimation in the joint MFM model using an MCMC procedure that marginalizes over the number of subpopulations by sampling directly from the induced distribution on the cluster assignments. Because a realization of the cluster assignment corresponds precisely to a partition of the $n$ observations, it provides also a realization of $K$, the number of clusters. Consequently, the MFM model (1) can be written equivalently using the restaurant process for the cluster assignments, the distribution for the distinct parameter values $\{\phi_k\}$ associated with the clusters, and the common distribution of the outcomes for all observations in the same cluster, $\{Y_i : z_i = k\}$. That is, MFM model (1) may be formulated as follows:

$$(z_1, z_2, \ldots, z_n) \sim \text{restaurant process in (4)}$$

$$\phi_k \mid (z_1, z_2, \ldots, z_n) \sim G_0, \text{ independently, for } k \in \{z_1, z_2, \ldots, z_n\} \quad (10)$$

$$(y_i, w_i) \mid \boldsymbol{\phi}, (z_1, z_2, \ldots, z_n) \sim F(\phi_{z_i}), \text{ independently.}$$

Here, the joint distribution of $z_1, z_2, \ldots, z_n$ is obtained from the series of conditional distributions in (4), and the effect of the prior distribution on the number of clusters, $p(\cdot)$, enters through the coefficients $\{V_n\}$ in (5). In the second line of (10), $k$ assumes only the unique values among the cluster assignments.

The model formulation (10) has marginalized over the number of subpopulations, thereby enabling estimation using a Gibbs sampling MCMC procedure with no need to explore model spaces of varying dimension. Let $z_{-i}$ denote the cluster assignments for the $n - 1$ observations excluding observation $i$. Also, let $\mathbb{Y}_k$ be the set of data from the individuals currently in subpopulation $k$, i.e., $\mathbb{Y}_k = \{Y_i = (y_i, w_i) \mid z_i = k\}$, and similarly define $\mathbb{B}_k = \{y_i \mid z_i = k\}$ and $\mathbb{W}_k = \{w_i \mid z_i = k\}$ as the data specific to the binary and continuous outcomes, respectively, among individuals currently in subpopulation $k$. We first sample from the conditional posterior distribution on $\{z_i\}$, that is $\Pr(z_i \mid z_{-i}, Y_i, \boldsymbol{\phi})$, $i = 1, 2, \ldots, n$, in order to have a summary about the number of clusters and cluster assignment. Then we sample from $P(\phi_k \mid \mathbb{Y}_k)$ for each unique value $k$ among $\{z_1, z_2, \ldots, z_n\}$. This sampling of $\phi_k$ involves drawing the Boolean relation and its accuracy for each cluster from $P(L_k, \xi_k \mid \mathbb{B}_k)$, as well as the Gaussian regression parameters from $P(\beta_k, \tau_k \mid \mathbb{W}_k)$.

The algorithm used here is Algorithm 4.4.2 in [20] (similar to Neal's algorithm 8 [23] for the DPMM), which iterates the following updates until convergence:

1. Update the cluster assignments, $\{z_i\}$: For $i = 1, 2, \ldots, n$, if observation $i$ is the sole member of cluster $z_i$, set $\phi^* = \phi_{z_i}$. Otherwise, draw parameters for a potential new cluster as $\phi^* \sim G_0$ given in (8). Then draw a new cluster assignment $z_i$ from the full conditional distribution induced by the MFM model:

$$\Pr(z_i = k \mid z_{-i}, Y_i, \phi) \propto \begin{cases} (|k| + \gamma) \, F(Y_i \mid \phi_k) & \text{for an existing cluster } k \\ \dfrac{V_n(t+1)}{V_n(t)} \, \gamma \, F(Y_i \mid \phi^*) & \text{if } k \text{ is a new cluster,} \end{cases}$$

where $t$ is the number of clusters after removing observation $i$ and $|k|$ is the size of cluster $k$.

2. Update the cluster parameters, $\{\phi_k\}$: For each unique $k \in \{z_1, \ldots, z_n\}$, draw $\phi_k \sim P(\phi \mid \mathbb{Y}_k)$. Because of the structure of our model, we may draw the Boolean relation and associated accuracy $(L_k, \xi_k) \sim P(L_k, \xi_k \mid \mathbb{B}_k)$ based on the information from the binary outcome and separately draw the Gaussian parameters $(\beta_k, \tau_k) \sim P(\beta_k, \tau_k \mid \mathbb{W}_k)$ based on the continuous outcome.

Note that the full conditional distribution for the cluster assignments in Step 1 is a restaurant process of the same form as the prior distribution (4). Because these are full conditional distributions, the coefficients $\{V_i\}$ defined in (5) need be precomputed only for $i = n$. The sampling in Step 2 is straightforward due to the conjugate nature of our model, apart from the sampling of the Boolean relation, $L_k$. We use a Metropolis-Hastings algorithm to obtain the new $L_k^{\text{new}}$ from $P(L_k \mid \mathbb{B}_k)$ with the proposal distribution consisting of a random selection among a set of "tweaks" to the existing relation, $L_k$. Then we draw the corresponding accuracy $\xi_k^{\text{new}} \sim P(\xi_k \mid L_k^{\text{new}}, \mathbb{B}_k)$ using the conjugate beta structure.

We initialize the algorithm by generating values for each parameter from their prior distributions. Convergence can be assessed in the usual ways for parameters apart from the Boolean relations. In practice, we observe that the Boolean relations have the slowest convergence rate, thus we deem the Markov chain as having converged once the Boolean relations are stable.

# 5 Simulation Study

We use a simulation study to illustrate the performance of the estimation procedure described in Sect. 4 for the joint model of Sect. 3.4 based on the MFM formulation, and also provide comparison with the DPMM. Data are generated according to the joint model with $K = 3$ subpopulations, each having a distinct Boolean function relating the binary biomarkers and binary disease outcome. We explore the effects of increasing the number of nonpredictive binary biomarkers and decreasing the informativeness of the continuous outcome about the distinction among subpopulations.

A simulated data set consists of $n = 300$ individuals with 100 in each of the $K = 3$ subpopulations. For a given number of binary biomarkers, $p$, the binary biomarkers $\mathbf{x}_i$ are generated for each individual as $x_{i1}, x_{i2}, \ldots, x_{ip} \sim \text{Ber}(0.5)$, independently. The Boolean relation for the first subpopulation is $L_1(\mathbf{x}) = (x_1 \wedge x_2) \vee (x_3 \wedge x_4)$ and the binary disease outcome in this subpopulation is determined as $y_i = L_1(\mathbf{x}_i)$ with probability $\xi_1 = 0.99$, $i = 1, 2, \ldots, 100$. The binary outcome is generated similarly for the individuals in subpopulations 2 and 3 with $L_2(\mathbf{x}) = x_5 \wedge x_6$, $\xi_2 = 0.95$, $L_3(\mathbf{x}) = x_7 \wedge !x_8$, and $\xi_3 = 0.90$. Thus, there are six informative biomarkers among the $p$ biomarkers in $\mathbf{x}$, with different sets of biomarkers pertinent to each of the subpopulations. The Boolean relation is most complex and has the highest accuracy for the first subpopulation. The continuous outcome, $w_i$, for individual $i$ in subpopulation $k$ is generated as Gaussian with mean $\beta_{k0} + \beta_{k1} v_i$ and variance 1, where $v_i \sim \text{Uniform}(0, 2)$, independently. Three simulation cases are distinguished by three sets of subpopulation-specific coefficients $\{\beta_k, k = 1, 2, 3\}$. These values are given in Table 1, which summarizes the simulation settings. Figure 3 shows density estimates for the generated values of $w_i$ for each of the three subpopulations in each of the three simulation cases. The impact of the predictor $v_i$ and the coefficients $\beta_k$ is apparent in these distributions, apart from subpopulation 2, for which the associated regression coefficient is zero. The subpopulation distributions are progressively less well distinguished across the three cases (in order), and hence the continuous outcome $w$ provides increasingly less information about the underlying cluster structure. For each simulation case, we also vary the number of binary predictors $p \in \{20, 50, 100\}$. The comparison to DPMM is provided for $p = 20$.

For each replicate, the Gibbs sampler described in Sect. 4 is run for 2000 burn-in iterations and an additional 3000 iterations for inference. The hyperparameters are fixed as $\text{maxQ} = 3$, $\text{maxVar} = 3$, $\delta = 1$, $\epsilon = 0.6$, $a = 50$, $b = 10$, $a' = 1.5$, $b' = 1.5$, $\lambda = 1$ and $\gamma = 1$.

**Table 1** Data for the simulation are generated from $K = 3$ subpopulations with the Boolean relations, accuracies and Gaussian regression coefficients shown here

|  | Cluster 1 | Cluster 2 | Cluster 3 |
|---|---|---|---|
| *Binary disease outcome* $y_i$ | | | |
| Boolean relation | $L_1(\mathbf{x}) = (x_1 \wedge x_2) \vee (x_3 \wedge x_4)$ | $L_2(\mathbf{x}) = x_5 \wedge x_6$ | $L_3(\mathbf{x}) = x_7 \wedge !x_8$ |
| Boolean accuracy | $\xi_1 = 0.99$ | $\xi_2 = 0.95$ | $\xi_3 = 0.90$ |
| Membership proportion | $\pi_1 = 1/3$ | $\pi_2 = 1/3$ | $\pi_3 = 1/3$ |
| *Continuous outcome* $w_i$ | | | |
| Case I | $\beta_1^T = (-5.0, 10)$ | $\beta_2^T = (0, 0)$ | $\beta_3^T = (-10, 5.0)$ |
| Case II | $\beta_1^T = (-2.5, 5.0)$ | $\beta_2^T = (0, 0)$ | $\beta_3^T = (-5.0, 2.5)$ |
| Case III | $\beta_1^T = (-2.5, 3.5)$ | $\beta_2^T = (0, 0)$ | $\beta_3^T = (-5.0, 2.5)$ |

The Boolean relations and accuracies are the same for the three simulation cases. The regression coefficients differ for the three cases, with the distribution of $w$ differing the most among subpopulations in Case I, and the least among subpopulations in Case III

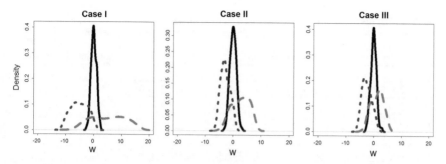

**Fig. 3** The realized distribution of the continuous outcomes $w$ in the simulation. The red dashed line corresponds to cluster 1, the solid black line to cluster 2 and the blue dotted line to cluster 3. The three clusters are most distinguishable in Case I and least distinguishable in Case III

The model fit for a replicate is then summarized by the following quantities: an estimated number of clusters, the estimated Boolean relations for each cluster, the Rand index comparing the estimated and true cluster assignments, and the accuracy of predictions for the binary response. The estimated number of clusters is the posterior mode, determined as the most frequently occurring value among the post burn-in iterations. The estimated Boolean relations, the Rand index and prediction accuracy are determined from the best post burn-in iteration selected using Dahl's method [7]. This best iteration has the cluster configuration best supported by the post burn-in iterations in a least squares sense. It provides a single realization of the cluster assignments and all model parameters. The Rand index evaluates the quality of the estimated cluster assignments as the proportion of pairs of observations that are correctly clustered together or apart. The prediction accuracy is the proportion of individuals for whom the binary response is correctly predicted when using the estimated Boolean relation for the individual's assigned cluster.

For ten replicates, we report the set of cluster-specific Boolean relations appearing most frequently among the selected best iterations and, in parentheses in the table, the proportion of replicates yielding this set; the average of the resulting Rand indices; and the average prediction accuracy.

## 5.1 Simulation Results

Table 2 provides the results of the simulation. The posterior mode of the number of clusters accurately captures the $K = 3$ subpopulations in all three simulation cases and consistently as the number of noise biomarkers gets large, e.g., $p = 100$. The Boolean relations within each subpopulation are also recovered very well when the distributions for the continuous response have separation (Cases I and II) and are robust to increasing $p$. Recovery of the exact Boolean relations used to generate the data ranges from 40 to 60% in Cases I and II as $p$ varies, and in all of these Case

**Table 2** Results of the simulation study of the MFM model

| | # of clusters | Boolean relations | | Rand index | Prediction accuracy |
|---|---|---|---|---|---|
| *Case I* | | | | | |
| $p = 20$ | 3 | $(x_1 \wedge x_2) \vee (x_3 \wedge x_4), x_5 \wedge x_6, x_7 \wedge !x_8$ | (0.6) | 0.74 | 0.93 |
| $p = 50$ | 3 | $(x_1 \wedge x_2) \vee (x_3 \wedge x_4), x_5 \wedge x_6, x_7 \wedge !x_8$ | (0.5) | 0.74 | 0.92 |
| $p = 100$ | 3 | $(x_1 \wedge x_2) \vee (x_3 \wedge x_4), x_5 \wedge x_6, x_7 \wedge !x_8$ | (0.4) | 0.73 | 0.93 |
| *Case II* | | | | | |
| $p = 20$ | 3 | $(x_1 \wedge x_2) \vee (x_3 \wedge x_4), x_5 \wedge x_6, x_7 \wedge !x_8$ | (0.6) | 0.50 | 0.91 |
| $p = 50$ | 3 | $(x_1 \wedge x_2) \vee (x_3 \wedge x_4), x_5 \wedge x_6, x_7 \wedge !x_8$ | (0.5) | 0.52 | 0.91 |
| $p = 100$ | 3 | $(x_1 \wedge x_2) \vee (x_3 \wedge x_4), x_5 \wedge x_6, x_7 \wedge !x_8$ | (0.4) | 0.51 | 0.89 |
| *Case III* | | | | | |
| $p = 20$ | 3 | $x_1 \wedge x_2, x_5 \wedge x_6, x_7 \wedge !x_8$ | (0.3) | 0.39 | 0.89 |
| $p = 50$ | 3 | $x_3 \wedge x_4, x_5 \wedge x_6, x_7 \wedge !x_8$ | (0.4) | 0.35 | 0.88 |
| $p = 100$ | 3 | $x_1, x_5 \wedge x_6, x_7 \wedge !x_8$ | (0.3) | 0.36 | 0.88 |

The estimated number of clusters is the posterior mode. The estimated Boolean relations are the set that occurred most frequently among the summary iterates from the ten replications. The Rand index and prediction accuracy are the average values over the replicates. Details are given in the text

I and Case III replicates, the four most frequently occurring PIs among the 3000 inferential MCMC iterates are correctly identified, namely $x_1 \wedge x_2$, $x_3 \wedge x_4$, $x_5 \wedge x_6$ and $x_7 \wedge !x_8$.

Even in Case III where there is considerable overlap in the distributions of $w$ for the three subpopulations, the recovery of informative biomarkers is very strong. In Case III, examination of the inferential MCMC iterations reveals that the top four most frequently appearing PIs are $x_5 \wedge x_6$, $x_7 \wedge !x_8$, $x_1$ and $x_3 \wedge x_4$ for all values of $p$ and all replicates, implying the algorithm successfully finds important features.

The estimated cluster configuration (Rand index) is stable with increasing $p$, but becomes worse as the separation among the distributions of the continuous response in the subpopulations decreases. This degradation of the estimated cluster assignment is not surprising given that the subpopulation structure is purely latent. Nonetheless, the resulting prediction of the binary response is relatively robust at near 90% accuracy. In contrast, if the underlying heterogeneity is ignored and a single logic regression is used, the average prediction accuracy for the binary response is approximately 70%.

Table 3 provides the results of the comparison of the MFM and DPMM formulations for $p = 20$. While the prediction of the binary response is similar for two models, the DPMM tends to overestimate the number of clusters by identifying tiny extraneous clusters, behavior that is consistent with our discussion in Sect. 3.3. The estimated Boolean relations for these extraneous clusters are highly variable in the posterior distribution, which complicates summarization of the fitted Boolean relations in the DPMM. We report the estimated Boolean relations as the set that occurred most frequently among the summary iterates from the ten replications. As

**Table 3** Comparison of the MFM and DPMM formulations with $p = 20$

| | # of clusters | Boolean relations | | Rand index | Prediction accuracy |
|---|---|---|---|---|---|
| *Case I* | | | | | |
| MFM | 3 | $(x_1 \wedge x_2) \vee (x_3 \wedge x_4), x_5 \wedge x_6, x_7 \wedge !x_8$ | (0.6) | 0.74 | 0.93 |
| DPMM | 3 | $(x_1 \wedge x_2) \vee (x_3 \wedge x_4), x_5 \wedge x_6, x_7 \wedge !x_8$ | (0.4) | 0.73 | 0.93 |
| *Case II* | | | | | |
| MFM | 3 | $(x_1 \wedge x_2) \vee (x_3 \wedge x_4), x_5 \wedge x_6, x_7 \wedge !x_8$ | (0.6) | 0.50 | 0.91 |
| DPMM | 4 | $(x_1 \wedge x_2) \vee (x_3 \wedge x_4), x_5 \wedge x_6, x_7 \wedge !x_8$ | (0.2) | 0.49 | 0.90 |
| *Case III* | | | | | |
| MFM | 3 | $x_1 \wedge x_2, x_5 \wedge x_6, x_7 \wedge !x_8$ | (0.3) | 0.39 | 0.89 |
| DPMM | 4 | $x_3 \wedge x_4, x_5 \wedge x_6, x_7 \wedge !x_8$ | (0.3) | 0.38 | 0.89 |

The estimated number of clusters is the posterior mode. The estimated Boolean relations are the set that occurred most frequently among the summary iterates from the ten replications. The Rand index and prediction accuracy are the average values over the replicates. Details are given in the text

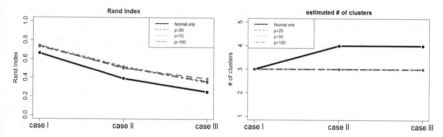

**Fig. 4** Exploration of the added value of the binary response in the joint model. When the MFM model is fit to only the continuous response in the simulated data, the cluster configuration is not recovered as accurately as from the joint model

shown in Table 3, this set contained three Boolean relations in all cases, even if the posterior mode of the number of clusters was higher.

## 5.2 Added Value of the Binary Response

Theoretically, the continuous response alone is sufficient to identify the subpopulation structure. It is natural, then, to ask "What is the contribution of the binary response to recovering the cluster configuration?" To address this question, we fit the MFM model for only the continuous response $w$ to the same simulated datasets. We used the same estimation algorithm to fit model (10) with the response distribution $F$ in (7) modified to only the Gaussian part, $F(w_i \mid z_i, \boldsymbol{\phi})$. The results are shown in Fig. 4. The average (over the ten replicates) of the Rand indices drops to 0.66, 0.39 and 0.25 for the three simulation cases, respectively. Moreover, the posterior mode over estimates the number of clusters in Cases II and III. This illustrates that incorporating the binary response through the joint modeling does improve recovery of the cluster configuration in these settings.

# 6 Discussion

We have proposed a fully Bayesian joint model for discovery of interactions among binary biomarkers predictive of disease while accommodating latent subpopulation heterogeneity. The model enables simultaneous estimation of the number of subpopulations, subpopulation membership and distinct associations between the response and predictors within each subpopulation. The Bayesian hierarchical framework provides borrowing-of-strength across the discovered subgroups that can enhance within-group estimation. Our contributions include incorporating Boolean relations among the binary biomarkers as parameters arising from a MFM model and addressing the associated challenges both in terms of specification of the prior distributions and estimation using an MCMC approach.

Our focus is to capture heterogeneity of the predictor-response association using the postulated subgroup structure. This contrasts with analyses that cluster the responses themselves, or the predictors themselves, perhaps as initial steps toward discovery of predictive interactions. The simulation study shows that estimation of the number of clusters, cluster configuration and cluster-specific relations is robust to a moderately increasing number of noise predictors and improves with greater separation of the underlying clusters.

The identifiability of our model requires sufficient variation in the data such that there is no collinearity among the biomarkers $x$, the covariates $v$, and how these relate to the responses $y$ and $w$, among other conditions. We have not derived details, but techniques such as those used for latent class regression models [13] or latent class joint models [26] could be adapted to study global and local identifiability carefully. We advise ensuring, at minimum, that $x$ and $v$ are full column rank and do not induce singularities in combination with the responses, properties expected for reasonably large sample sizes. We noted that the strict identifiability of more than one latent cluster in the association between the biomarkers and binary disease status requires additional information. We have opted to couple the binary disease status $y$ with a continuous response, $w$, which is often available in our experience. Recall our motivating example is the association between SNPs and presence of prostate cancer, for which the continuous prostate specific antigen level provides a meaningful value for $w$. Even in cases when $w$ is not available, we have found that the modified version of our model utilizing only the binary disease status $y$ and biomarkers $x$ reliably identifies Boolean relations that improve prediction accuracy of $y$.

The model may be extended to handle data with a large number of predictors, but estimation presents some computational challenges. The Bayesian sampler itself may be used as a variable screening tool, as it has demonstrated the ability to identify features useful for response prediction. However, variable pre-screening or additional variable selection methods incorporated in the model may improve efficiency.

**Acknowledgements** The authors were partially supported by grants R01MH104423, R01HD078410 and R01HD093055 from the National Institutes of Health. Portions of this work were revised while E. Slate was the Visiting Scholar in Honor of David C. Jordan at AbbVie, Inc. in North Chicago, IL and also a Research Fellow with the Statistical and Applied Mathematical Sciences Institute in Durham, NC. Additional support from the Graduate School and Department of Statistics at Florida State University is gratefully acknowledged. Figures 1 and 2 were adapted from a figure provided by Dr. Zhengwu Zhang, Univ. of Rochester. The authors thank the reviewers for comments that led to improvement of this manuscript.

# References

1. Aldous, D. J. (1985). *Exchangeability and related topics*. Berlin: Springer.
2. Allman, E. S., Matias, C., & Rhodes, J. A. (2009). Identifiability of parameters in latent structure models with many observed variables. *The Annals of Statistics, 3099–3132.*
3. Antoniak, C. E. (1974). Mixtures of Dirichlet processes with applications to Bayesian nonparametric problems. *The Annals of Statistics, 1152–1174.*
4. Blackwell, D. & MacQueen, J. B. (1973). Ferguson distributions via Pólya urn schemes. *The Annals of Statistics, 353–355.*
5. Chipman, H. A., George, E. I., & Mcculloch, R. E. (1998). Bayesian CART model search. *Journal of the American Statistical Association, 93*(443), 935–960.
6. Chipman, H. A., George, E. I., & McCulloch, R. E. (2010). BART: Bayesian additive regression trees. *The Annals of Applied Statistics, 4*(1), 266–298.
7. Dahl, D. B. (2006). Model-based clustering for expression data via a Dirichlet process mixture model. *Bayesian inference for gene expression and proteomics, 4,* 201–218.
8. Dempster, A. P., Laird, N. M., & Rubin, D. B. (1977). Maximum likelihood from incomplete data via the EM algorithm. *Journal of the Royal Statistical Society. Series B (Methodological), 39*(1), 1–38.
9. Etzioni, R., Falcon, S., Gann, P. H., Kooperberg, C. L., Penson, D. F., & Stampfer, M. J. (2004). Prostate-specific antigen and free prostate-specific antigen in the early detection of prostate cancer: Do combination tests improve detection? *Cancer Epidemiology Biomarkers and Prevention, 13*(10), 1640–1645.
10. Ferguson, T. S. (1973). A Bayesian analysis of some nonparametric problems. *The Annals of Statistics,* 209–230.
11. Fleisher, H., Tavel, M., & Yeager, J. (1983). Exclusive-OR representation of Boolean functions. *IBM Journal of Research and Development, 27*(4), 412–416.
12. Green, P. J. (1995). Reversible jump Markov chain Monte Carlo computation and Bayesian model determination. *Biometrika, 82*(4), 711–732.
13. Huang, G.-H., & Bandeen-Roche, K. (2004). Building an identifiable latent class model with covariate effects on underlying and measured variables. *Psychometrika, 69*(1), 5–32.
14. Ishwaran, H., & Zarepour, M. (2002). Dirichlet prior sieves in finite normal mixtures. *Statistica Sinica, 12,* 941–963.
15. Janes, H., Pepe, M., Kooperberg, C., & Newcomb, P. (2005). Identifying target populations for screening or not screening using logic regression. *Statistics in Medicine, 24*(9), 1321–1338.

16. Kooperberg, C., Bis, J. C., Marciante, K. D., Heckbert, S. R., Lumley, T., & Psaty, B. M. (2007). Logic regression for analysis of the association between genetic variation in the renin-angiotensin system and myocardial infarction or stroke. *American Journal of Epidemiology, 165*(3), 334–343.
17. Kooperberg, C., & Ruczinski, I. (2005). Identifying interacting SNPs using Monte Carlo logic regression. *Genetic Epidemiology, 28*(2), 157–70.
18. Lo, S. H., & Zhang, T. (2002). Backward haplotype transmission association (BHTA) algorithm – A fast multiple-marker screening method. *Human Heredity, 53*(4), 197–215.
19. MacEachern, S. N., & Muller, P. (1998). Estimating mixture of Dirichlet process models. *Journal of Computational and Graphical Statistics, 7*(2), 223–238.
20. Miller, J. W. (2014). *Nonparametric and variable-dimension Bayesian mixture models: Analysis, comparison, and new methods.* Ph.D. Thesis, Brown University.
21. Miller, J. W., & Harrison, M. T. (2018). Mixture models with a prior on the number of components. *Journal of the American Statistical Association, 113*(521), 340–356.
22. Mitra, A. P., Datar, R. H., & Cote, R. J. (2006). Molecular pathways in invasive bladder cancer: New insights into mechanisms, progression, and target identification. *Journal of Clinical Oncolology, 24*(35), 5552–5564.
23. Neal, R. M. (2000). Markov chain sampling methods for Dirichlet process mixture models. *Journal of Computational and Graphical Statistics, 9*(2), 249–265.
24. Petrone, S., & Raftery, A. E. (1997). A note on the Dirichlet process prior in Bayesian nonparametric inference with partial exchangeability. *Statistics & Probability Letters, 36*(1), 69–83.
25. Pitman, J. (1995). Exchangeable and partially exchangeable random partitions. *Probability Theory and Related Fields, 102*(2), 145–158.
26. Proust-Lima, C., Séne, M., Taylor, J. M., & Jacqmin-Gadda, H. (2014). Joint latent class models for longitudinal and time-to-event data: A review. *Statistical Methods in Medical Research, 23*(1), 74–90.
27. Ruczinski, I., Kooperberg, C., & LeBlanc, M. (2003). Logic regression. *Journal of Computational and graphical Statistics, 12*(3), 475–511.
28. Schapire, R. E., & Freund, Y. (2012). *Boosting: Foundations and Algorithms.* Cambridge: The MIT Press.
29. Schwender, H., & Ickstadt, K. (2008). Identification of SNP interactions using logic regression. *Biostatistics, 9*(1), 187–198.
30. Slate, E. H., Geng, J., Wolf, B. J., & Hill, E. G. (2014). Discovery among binary biomarkers. In *JSM Proceedings, WNAR.* Alexandria: American Statistical Association.
31. Srivastava, S. (2005). Cancer biomarkers: an emerging means of detecting, diagnosing and treating cancer. *Cancer Biomarkers, 1*(1), 1–2.
32. Vermeulen, S. H., Den Heijer, M., Sham, P., & Knight, J. (2007). Application of multi-locus analytical methods to identify interacting loci in case-control studies. *Annals of Human Genetics, 71*, 689–700.

# Part IV
# Biomedical Research and the Modelling

# Heat Kernel Smoothing on Manifolds and Its Application to Hyoid Bone Growth Modeling

Moo K. Chung, Nagesh Adluru, and Houri K. Vorperian

**Abstract** We present a unified heat kernel smoothing framework for modeling 3D anatomical surface data extracted from medical images. Due to image acquisition and preprocessing noises, it is expected the medical imaging data is noisy. The surface data of the anatomical structures is regressed using the weighted linear combination of Laplace-Beltrami (LB) eigenfunctions to smooth out noisy data and perform statistical analysis. The method is applied in characterizing the 3D growth pattern of human hyoid bone between ages 0 and 20 obtained from CT images. We detected a significant age effect on localized parts of the hyoid bone.

**Keywords** Heat kernel smoothing · Hyoid bone growth · Random field theory · Laplace Beltrami eigenfunctions · Diffusion on manifolds

## 1 Introduction

For normally developing children, age and sex could be major factors that affect the structure and function of growing hyoid bone. As in other developmental studies [22, 55, 56], we expect highly localized complex growth pattern to emerge between

M. K. Chung (✉)
Department of Biostatistics and Medical Informatics, University of Wisconsin, Madison, WI, USA
e-mail: mkchung@wisc.edu

N. Adluru
Waisman Laboratory for Brain Imaging and Behavior, University of Wisconsin, Madison, WI, USA
e-mail: adluru@wisc.edu

H. K. Vorperian
Vocal Tract Development Laboratory, Waisman Center, University of Wisconsin, Madison, WI, USA
e-mail: vorperian@waisman.wisc.edu

© Springer Nature Switzerland AG 2020
Y. Zhao, D.-G. (Din) Chen (eds.), *Statistical Modeling in Biomedical Research*, Emerging Topics in Statistics and Biostatistics,
https://doi.org/10.1007/978-3-030-33416-1_12

ages 0 and 20 in the hyoid bone. Growth is expected to extend laterally with respect to the surface of the bone. However, it is unclear what specific parts of the hyoid bone are growing. This provides a biological motivation for a need to develop a local surface-based morphometric technique beyond simple volumetric techniques that cannot detect localized subtle anatomical changes along the surface of the hyoid bone composting of three segments—a central hyoid body with two greater cornua (horns) [11, 21].

The end results of existing surface-based morphometric studies in medical imaging are statistical parametric maps (SPM) that show the statistical significance of growth at each surface mesh vertex [22, 48, 64]. In order to obtain stable and robust SPM, various signal smoothing and filtering methods have been proposed. Among them, diffusion equations, kernel smoothing, and wavelet-based approaches are probably the most popular. Diffusion equations have been widely used in image processing as a form of noise reduction starting with Perona and Malik in 1990s [46]. Although numerous techniques have been developed for performing diffusion along surfaces [2, 21, 22, 43, 51–53], many approaches are nonparametric and requires the finite element or finite difference schemes which are known to suffer various numerical instabilities [16, 18].

Recently, few regression models are proposed on manifolds. In [40], Laplace-Beltrami operator based functional principal component analysis was proposed. In [25], Fréchet mean based regression model was proposed on manifolds. Kernel smoothing based models have been also proposed for surface and manifolds data [6, 17, 18]. The kernel methods basically smooth data as the weighted average of neighboring mesh vertices using mostly a Gaussian kernel and its iterative application is supposed to approximate the diffusion process. Recently, wavelets have been popularized for surface and graph data [33, 36, 38]. Spherical wavelets have been used on brain surface data that has been mapped onto a sphere [8, 44]. Since wavelet basis functions have local support in both space and scale, the wavelet coefficients from the scale-space decomposition using the spherical wavelets provide shape features that describe local shape variation at a variety of scales and spatial locations. However, spherical wavelets have an intrinsic problem that they require to establish a smooth mapping from the surface to a unit sphere, which introduces a serious metric distortion. The spherical mapping such as conformal mapping introduces serious metric distortion which usually compounds SPM [28, 34]. Furthermore, such basis functions defined on a sphere seem to be suboptimal than those directly defined on anatomical surfaces in detecting locations or scales of shape variations. To remedy the limitation of the spherical wavelets, the spectral graph wavelet transform defined on a graph has been applied to arbitrary surface meshes by treating surface meshes as graphs [3, 29, 38]. The wavelet transform is a powerful tool decomposing a signal or function into a collection of components localized at both location and scale. Although all three methods (diffusion-, kernel- and wavelet-based) look different from each other, it is possible to develop a unified framework that relates all of them in a coherent mathematical framework [16].

Starting with a symmetric positive definite kernel, we propose a unified kernel smoothing framework within the Hilbert space theory [23]. The proposed kernel smoothing works for any symmetric positive definite kernel, which behaves like weights between two functional data. We show how this facilitates a coherent statistical inference for functional signals defined on an arbitrary manifold. The focus of this paper is on the development of the proposed kernel smoothing on manifolds.

The structure of this paper is as follows. First, we present a unified bivariate kernel smoothing that is related to diffusion-like equations on manifolds. The proposed kernel regression inherits various mathematical and statistical properties of diffusion-like equations. Then, we show the relationship between the kernel smoothing and recently popular spectral graph wavelets for manifolds. The proposed kernel smoothing is shown to be equivalent to the wavelet transform. This mathematical equivalence levitates a need for constructing wavelets using a complicated computational machinery as often done in previous diffusion wavelet constructions [3, 29, 36, 38]. A unified statistical inference framework is then developed for the kernel method via Worsley's random field theory [54, 63]. This levitates the need for using time consuming nonparametric procedures such as false discovery rates (FDR) [7, 27] or permutation tests [9, 15, 20, 31] that do not have explicate control over the scale and smoothness of models. Finally, we illustrate how the kernel smoothing procedure can be used to localize the disconnected hyoid bone growth pattern in human.

## 2 Preliminary

Let us illustrate two statistical problems in the Euclidean space that motivate the development of the proposed kernel smoothing on manifolds. Consider measurements $f_i$ sampled at point $p_i \in \mathbb{R}^d$. The measurements are usually modeled as

$$f_i = h(p_i) + \epsilon_i$$

with mean zero noise $\epsilon_i$ and unknown mean function $h$ that has to be estimated. In the traditional kernel regression framework [6, 24, 45], the mean function $h$ is estimated in the weighted least squares fashion:

$$\widehat{h}(p) = \sum_{j=1}^{k} G(p - p_i) f_i,$$

where $G$ is given by Nadaraya-Waton type of normalized kernels. In the local polynomial regression framework [24], $h$ is estimated as

$$\widehat{h}(p) = \arg\min_{\beta_0, \cdots, \beta_k} \sum_{i=1}^{n} G(p - p_i) \left| f_i - \sum_{j=0}^{k} \beta_j (p - p_i)^j \right|^2. \tag{1}$$

In many related local polynomial or kernel regression frameworks, kernel $G$ and polynomial basis $\{p^j\}$ are translated by the amount of $p_i$ in fitting the data locally. In this fashion, at each data point $p_i$, exactly the same shape of kernel and distance can be used. However, one immediately encounters a difficulty of directly generalizing the Euclidean formulation (1) to an arbitrary surface since it is unclear how to translate the kernel and basis in a coherent fashion. To remedy this problem, many recent kernel regression frameworks on manifolds use bivariate kernel $G(p, q)$ and bypass the problem of translating a univariate kernel [6]. By simply changing the second argument, it has the effect of translating the kernel.

A similar problem is also encountered in wavelets in the Euclidean space. Consider wavelet basis $W_{t,q}(p)$ obtained from a mother wavelet $W$ with scale parameter $t$ and translation parameter $q$:

$$W_{t,q}(p) = \frac{1}{t} W\left(\frac{p-q}{t}\right). \tag{2}$$

Scaling a function on a surface is trivial. But the difficulty arises when one tries to define a mother wavelet and translate it on a surface. It is not straightforward to generalize the Euclidean formulation (2) to an arbitrary manifold. If one tries to modify the existing spherical wavelets to an arbitrary surface [8, 44], one also encounters the lack of regular grids on the surface. The recent work based on the spectral graph wavelet transform bypass this problem by also taking a bivariate kernel as a mother wavelet [3, 29, 38, 42]. To remedy these two different but related problems, we propose to use a bivariate kernel and bypass the problem of translating a univariate kernel. By simply changing the second argument, it has the effect of translating the kernel.

## 3   Methods

In many anatomical surface studies in medical imaging, measurements are sampled densely at each mesh vertex so it is more practical to model the measurements as smooth functions. Consider a functional measurement $f$ defined on a manifold $\mathcal{M} \subset \mathbb{R}^d$. We assume the following additive model:

$$f(p) = h(p) + \epsilon(p), \tag{3}$$

where $h$ is the unknown signal to be estimated and $\epsilon$ is a zero-mean random field, possibly Gaussian. The manifold $\mathcal{M}$ can be a single connected component or multiple disjoint components as our hyoid bone application (Fig. 1). We further assume $f \in L^2(\mathcal{M})$, the space of square integrable functions on $\mathcal{M}$ with the inner product

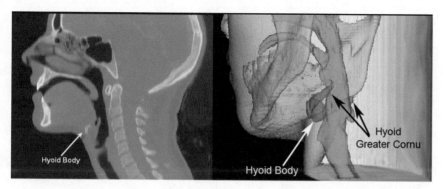

**Fig. 1** CT image showing the location of the hyoid bone (left), and 3D model (right) showing the relative location of the hyoid bone (red) with respect to the mandible (gray) and vocal tract (green)

$$\langle f, g \rangle = \int_{\mathcal{M}} f(p)g(p) \, d\mu(p),$$

where $\mu$ is the Lebesgue measure. $\mu(\mathcal{M})$ will measure the volume of $\mathcal{M}$ in $d$-dimension [11, 16]. Define a self-adjoint operator $\mathscr{L}$ satisfying

$$\langle g_1, \mathscr{L}g_2 \rangle = \langle \mathscr{L}g_1, g_2 \rangle$$

for all $g_1, g_2 \in L^2(\mathcal{M})$. Then $\mathscr{L}$ induces the eigenvalues $\lambda_j$ and eigenfunctions $\psi_j$ on $\mathcal{M}$ (Fig. 2):

$$\mathscr{L}\psi_j = \lambda_j \psi_j. \tag{4}$$

Without loss of generality, we can order the eigenvalues

$$0 = \lambda_0 \leq \lambda_1 \leq \lambda_2 \leq \cdots .$$

We can show that the eigenfunctions $\psi_j$ form an orthonormal basis in $L^2(\mathcal{M})$. We will consider a smooth symmetric positive definite kernel of the form

$$K(p, q) = \sum_{j=0}^{\infty} \tau_j \psi_j(p)\psi_j(q) \tag{5}$$

for some $\tau_j$ in this paper. The constants $\tau_j$ are identified as follows. Apply the kernel convolution on the eigenfunction $\psi_j$:

$$K * \psi_j(p) = \int_{\mathcal{M}} K(p, q)\psi_j(q) \, d\mu(q). \tag{6}$$

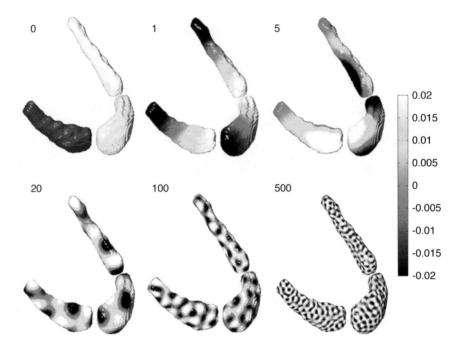

**Fig. 2** Laplace-Beltrami eigenfunctions $\psi_j$ of various degrees ($j = 0, 1, 5, 20, 100, 500$) on the template. The first eigenfunction is constant in each component. As the degree increases, the spatial frequency increases

Substituting (5) into (6), we have

$$K * \psi_j(p) = \tau_j \psi_j(p)$$

indicating $\tau_j$ and $\psi_j$ must be the eigenvalues and eigenfunctions of the convolution (6). Note $\psi_j$ are eigenfunctions of self-adjoint operator $\mathscr{L}$ and kernel convolution at the same time.

*Example 1* For $\tau_j = e^{-\lambda t}$, we have heat kernel

$$K(p, q) = \sum_{j=0}^{\infty} e^{-\lambda t} \psi_j(p) \psi_j(q), \tag{7}$$

where $t$ is the bandwidth of kernel. The heat kernel has been often used in numerous studies but without much theoretical justification [16, 32, 37, 49]. For this study, we will denote the heat kernel as $H_t(p, q)$ to explicitly show that the spread of the kernel is determined by diffusion time $t$ [17, 18].

## 3.1 Kernel Smoothing on Manifolds

Consider subspace $\mathcal{H}_k \subset L^2(\mathcal{M})$ spanned by the orthonormal basis $\{\psi_j\}$, i.e.,

$$\mathcal{H}_k = \{\sum_{j=0}^{k} \beta_j \psi_j(p) : \beta_j \in \mathbb{R}\}.$$

Then the least squares estimation (LSE) of $h$ in $\mathcal{H}_k$ is given by the shortest distance from $f$ to $\mathcal{H}_k$ [14, 16]:

$$\widehat{h}(p) = \arg \min_{h \in \mathcal{H}_k} \int_{\mathcal{M}} |f(p) - h(p)|^2 \, d\mu(p) = \sum_{j=0}^{k} f_j \psi_j(p), \qquad (8)$$

where $f_j = \langle f, \psi_j \rangle$ are the Fourier coefficients. Figure 3 shows an example of LSE with $\mathcal{L}$ as the Laplace-Beltrami operator and $k = 1000$. This is a special case of Fourier series expansion that tends to suffer the Gibbs phenomenon, i.e., ringing artifact [13, 26]. The Gibbs phenomenon can be effectively removed if the Fourier series expansion converges fast enough as the number of basis functions goes to infinity. By weighting the Fourier coefficients exponentially smaller, we can make

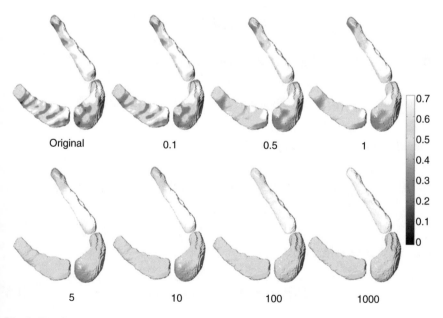

**Fig. 3** Heat kernel smoothing using different bandwidth between 0.1 and 1000. As the bandwidth increases, the kernel regression becomes inversely proportional to the square root of the surface area

the representation converges faster; this can be achieved by additionally weighting the squared residuals in Eq. (8) with some weights. Thus, we propose to estimate $h$ by minimizing the weighted distance to the space $\mathcal{H}_k$:

$$\widehat{h}(p) = \arg \min_{h \in \mathcal{H}_k} \int_{\mathcal{M}} \int_{\mathcal{M}} K(p,q) \Big| f(q) - h(p) \Big|^2 \, d\mu(q) \, d\mu(p). \tag{9}$$

Without loss of generality, we will assume the kernel to be a probability distribution

$$\int_{\mathcal{M}} K(p,q) \, d\mu(q) = 1$$

for all $p \in \mathcal{M}$. The solution of (9) has the following analytic expression.

**Theorem 1**

$$\widehat{h}(p) = \arg \min_{h \in \mathcal{H}_k} \int_{\mathcal{M}} \int_{\mathcal{M}} K(p,q) \Big| f(q) - h(p) \Big|^2 \, d\mu(q) \, d\mu(p) = \sum_{j=0}^{k} \tau_j f_j \psi_j,$$

where $f_j = \langle f, \psi_j \rangle$ are Fourier coefficients.

**Proof** Any function $h \in \mathcal{H}_k$ can be expressed as

$$h(p) = \sum_{j=0}^{k} \beta_j \psi_j(p). \tag{10}$$

Then by plugging (10) into the inner integral $I(p)$, it becomes

$$I(p) = \int_{\mathcal{M}} K(p,q) \Big| f(q) - \sum_{j=0}^{k} \beta_j \psi(p) \Big|^2 \, d\mu(q).$$

Simplifying the expression, we obtain

$$I(p) = \sum_{j=0}^{k} \sum_{j'=0}^{k} \psi_j(p) \psi_{j'}(p) \beta_j \beta_{j'} - 2K * f(p) \sum_{j=0}^{k} \psi_j(p) \beta_j + K * f^2(p). \tag{11}$$

The kernel can be written as

$$K(p,q) = \sum_{j'=0}^{\infty} \tau_{j'} \psi_{j'}(p) \psi_{j'}(q). \tag{12}$$

The convolution is then written as

$$K * f(p) = \sum_{j'=0}^{\infty} \tau_{j'} f_{j'} \psi_{j'}(p).$$

Since $I$ is an unconstrained positive semidefinite quadratic program (QP) in $\beta_j$, there is no unique global minimizer of $I$ without additional linear constraints. Integrating $I$ further with respect to $d\mu(p)$, we collapses (11) to a positive definite QP, which yields a unique global minimizer:

$$\int_{\mathcal{M}} I(p) \, d\mu(p) = \sum_{j=0}^{k} \beta_j^2 - 2 \sum_{j=0}^{k} \tau_j f_j \beta_j + \text{const.}$$

The minimum of the above integral is obtained when all the partial derivatives with respect to $\beta_j$ vanish, i.e.

$$\int_{\mathcal{M}} \frac{\partial I}{\partial \beta_j} \, d\mu(p) = 2\beta_j - 2\tau_j f_j = 0$$

for all $j$. Hence $\sum_{j=0}^{k} \tau_j f_j \psi_j$ must be the unique minimizer. $\qquad\square$

Theorem 1 generalizes the weighted spherical harmonic (SPHARM) representation on a unit sphere to an arbitrary manifold [14]. Theorem 1 implies that the kernel regression can be performed by simply computing the Fourier coefficients $f_j = \langle f, \psi_j \rangle$ without doing any numerical optimization. The numerically difficult optimization problem is then reduced to the problem of computing Fourier coefficients. If the kernel $K$ is the Dirac-delta function, the kernel regression simply collapses to the least squares estimation (LSE) which results in the standard Fourier series, i.e.

$$\widehat{h}(p) = \arg\min_{h \in \mathcal{H}_k} \int_{\mathcal{M}} \left| f(q) - h(q) \right|^2 d\mu(q) = \sum_{j=0}^{k} f_j \psi_j.$$

It can be also shown that as $k \to \infty$, the kernel regression

$$\widehat{h} = \sum_{j=0}^{k} \tau_j f_j \psi_j$$

converges to convolution $K * f$ establishing the connection to the manifold-based kernel smoothing framework [5, 18]. Hence, asymptotically the proposed kernel regression should inherit many statistical properties of the usual kernel smoothing.

## 3.2   Properties of Kernel Smoothing

Kernel smoothing can be shown to be related to the following diffusion-like Cauchy problem [13, 14].

**Theorem 2** *For an arbitrary self-adjoint differential operator $\mathscr{L}$, the unique solution of the following initial value problem*

$$\frac{\partial g(p, t)}{\partial t} + \mathscr{L}g(p, t) = 0, g(p, t = 0) = f(p) \tag{13}$$

*is given by*

$$g(p, t) = \sum_{j=0}^{\infty} e^{-\lambda_j t} f_j \psi_j(p). \tag{14}$$

***Proof*** For each fixed $t$, $g(p, t)$ can be written as

$$g(p, t) = \sum_{j=0}^{\infty} c_j(t) \psi_j(p). \tag{15}$$

Then

$$\mathscr{L}g(p, t) = \sum_{j=0}^{\infty} c_j(t) \lambda_j \psi_j(p). \tag{16}$$

Substituting (15) and (16) into (13), we obtain

$$\frac{\partial c_j(t)}{\partial t} + \lambda_j c_j(t) = 0 \tag{17}$$

for all $j$. The solution of equation (17) is given by $c_j(t) = b_j e^{-\lambda_j t}$. So we have a solution

$$g(p, t) = \sum_{j=0}^{\infty} b_j e^{-\lambda_j t} \psi_j(p).$$

At $t = 0$, we have

$$g(p, 0) = \sum_{j=0}^{\infty} b_j \psi_j(p) = f(p).$$

The coefficients $b_j$ must be the Fourier coefficients, i.e.,

$$b_j = \langle f, \psi_j \rangle = f_j.$$

$\square$

For a particular choice of kernel $K$ with $\tau_j = e^{-\lambda_j t}$, the proposed kernel regression $\widehat{h} = \sum_{j=0}^{k} \tau_j f_j \psi_j$ should converge to the solution of the diffusion-like equation.

*Example 2* If $\mathscr{L}$ is the Laplace-Beltrami operator, (13) becomes an isotropic diffusion equation as a special case and we are then dealing with heat kernel

$$H_t(p, q) = \sum_{j=0}^{\infty} e^{-\lambda_j t} \psi_j(p) \psi_j(q),$$

which is often explored mathematical objects in various areas [5, 18].

In order to construct wavelets on an arbitrary graph and mesh, diffusion wavelet transform has been proposed recently [3, 29, 38]. The diffusion wavelet construction has been fairly involving so far. However, its mathematical structure is related to the proposed kernel smoothing. For scale function $g$ that satisfies the admissibility conditions [3, 29, 36, 38], diffusion wavelet $W_{t,p}(p)$ at position $p$ and scale $t$ is given by

$$W_{t,q}(p) = \sum_{j=0}^{k} g(\lambda_j t) \psi_j(p) \psi_j(q).$$

If we let $\tau_j = g(\lambda_j t)$, the diffusion wavelet transform is given by

$$\langle W_{t,p}, f \rangle = \int_{\mathscr{M}} W_{t,q}(p) f(p) \, d\mu(p) = \sum_{j=0}^{k} \tau_j f_j \psi_j(q),$$

which is the exactly kernel smoothing we introduced. Hence, the diffusion wavelet transform can be simply obtained by doing the kernel smoothing with specific scale function $g$ [38]. If we let $g(\lambda_j t) = e^{-\lambda_j t}$, we have

$$W_{t,p}(q) = H_t(p, q),$$

which is a heat kernel. The bandwidth $t$ of heat kernel controls resolution while the translation is done by shifting one argument in the kernel. Thus, although heat kernel smoothing is not exactly diffusion wavelet, it shares the same algebraic formalism and behaves similarly. Although the kernel smoothing is constructed using global basis functions $\psi_j$, the kernel regression at each point $p$ coincides with the diffusion wavelet transform at that point. Hence, just like wavelets, the kernel smoothing will have the localization property of wavelets.

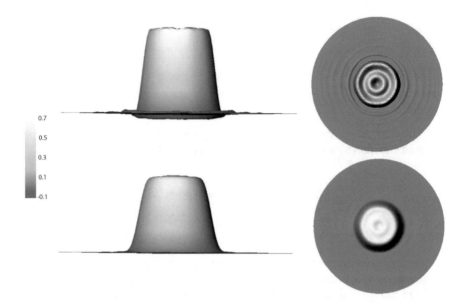

**Fig. 4** The Gibbs phenomenon on a hat shaped simulated surface showing the ringing effect on the SPHARM expansion (top) and the reduced effect on the heat kernel smoothing (bottom) [12, 13]. 7225 basis functions were used for the both cases and the bandwidth $t = 0.001$ is used for heat kernel smoothing

Another important property of heat kernel smoothing is the ability to reduce the Gibbs phenomenon, which often occurs when we tried to represent signals with rapid changes [12–14]. Example 3 illustrates how heat kernel smoothing can be use in reducing ringing artifacts in a 3D step function.

*Example 3* A hat-shaped step function is simulated in 3D as $z = 1$ for $x^2 + y^2 < 1$ and $z = 0$ for $1 \le x^2 + y^2 \le 2$ (Fig. 4). Then the step function is reconstructed using the SPHARM expansion via LSE (top) and kernel regression (bottom). In the both cases, up to 7225 basis functions were used. For the kernel regression, the heat kernel with bandwidth $t = 0.0001$ is used. LSE clearly shows the visible Gibbs phenomenon, i.e., ringing artifact [13, 26] compared to the kernel regression.

## 3.3 Numerical Implementation

In this study, the Laplace-Beltrami operator is chosen as the self-adjoint operators $\mathscr{L}$ of choice. The eigenfunctions of the Laplace-Beltrami operator on an arbitrary curved surface is analytically unknown. So it is necessary to discretize (4) using the Cotan formulation as a generalized eigenvalue problem [19, 47, 66]:

$$\mathbf{C}\psi = \lambda \mathbf{A}\psi, \tag{18}$$

where $\mathbf{C}$ is the stiffness matrix, $\mathbf{A}$ is the mass matrix and $\boldsymbol{\psi} = (\psi(p_1), \cdots, \psi(p_n))'$ is the eigenfunction evaluated at $n$ mesh vertices. Once we obtained the basis functions $\psi_j$, the corresponding LB-eigenfunction expansion coefficients $\beta_j$ are estimated as

$$\beta_j = \mathbf{f}'\mathbf{A}\boldsymbol{\psi}_j,$$

where $\mathbf{f} = (f(p_1), \cdots, f(p_n))'$ and $\boldsymbol{\psi}_j = (\psi_j(p_1), \cdots, \psi_j(p_n))'$ [66]. Figure 2 shows few representative LB-eigenfunctions on the hyoid surface. For heat kernel smoothing, we used the bandwidth $t = 5$ and 500 LB-eigenfunctions on the surface of the hyoid bone. The number of eigenfunctions used is more than sufficient to guarantee relative error less than 0.3% in our data. The MATLAB code for computing the eigenfunctions and performing heat kernel smoothing is available at http://www.stat.wisc.edu/~mchung/mandible.

## 3.4 Statistical Inference

We are interested in determining the significance of functional signals on manifolds. We borrow the statistical parametric mapping (SPM) framework for analyzing and visualizing statistical tests on surfaces that is often used in brain image analysis [2, 17, 39, 57, 62, 65]. Since test statistics are constructed over all mesh vertices on the surfaces, the multiple comparisons correction is needed. For continuous functional data, the random field theory is often used [54, 62, 63]. The random field theory assumes the measurements to be a smooth Gaussian random field. Heat kernel smoothing will make the data more smooth and Gaussian and increase the signal-to-noise ratio [17].

Consider a functional measurements $f_1, \cdots, f_n$ on manifold $\mathcal{M}$. In the simplest statistical setting, the measurements can be modeled as

$$f_i(p) = h(p) + \epsilon_i(p),$$

where $h$ is an unknown group level signal and $\epsilon_i$ is a zero-mean Gaussian random field [63]. At each fixed point $p$, we are assuming $\epsilon_i \sim N(0, \sigma^2)$.

We are interested in determining the significance of $h$, i.e.

$$H_0 : h(p) = 0 \text{ for all } p \in \mathcal{M} \quad \text{vs.} \quad H_1 : h(p) > 0 \text{ for some } p \in \mathcal{M}. \quad (19)$$

Note that any point $p_0$ that gives $h(p_0) > 0$ is considered as signal. The hypothesis (19) is an infinite dimensional multiple comparisons problem for continuously indexed hypotheses over the manifold $\mathcal{M}$. The underlying group level signal $h$ is estimated using the proposed heat kernel smoothing. Subsequently, a test statistic is given by a T-field $T(p)$ or a F-field, which is simply given by the square of the T-field [62, 63].

Under $H_0$, the type-I error of testing hypotheses (19) is given by

$$
\begin{aligned}
\alpha &= P(T(p) > z \text{ for some } p \in \mathcal{M}) \\
&= 1 - P(T(p) \leq z \text{ for all } p \in \mathcal{M}) \\
&= 1 - P\left( \sup_{p \in \mathcal{M}} T(p) \leq z \right) \\
&= P\left( \sup_{p \in \mathcal{M}} T(p) > z \right)
\end{aligned}
$$

for observed threshold $z$, which is the maximum $T(p)$ in the whole region $\mathcal{M}$. Note we are taking the sup operator over all $\mathcal{M}$. For sufficiently high threshold $z$, the multiple comparisons corrected type-I error of testing hypothesis (19) is given by

$$
P\left( \sup_{p \in \mathcal{M}} T(p) > z \right) = \sum_{j=0}^{d} \mu_j(\mathcal{M}) \rho_j(z),
$$

where $\mu_d(\mathcal{M})$ is the $j$-th Minkowski functional or intrinsic volume of $\mathcal{M}$ and $\rho_j$ is the $j$-th Euler characteristic (EC) density of T-field [1, 54, 59, 63]. Since the hyoid bone is compact with no boundary but has three disconnected components, the Minkowski functionals are simply

$$
\begin{aligned}
\mu_2(\mathcal{M}) &= \text{area}(\mathcal{M})/2 \\
\mu_1(\mathcal{M}) &= 0 \\
\mu_0(\mathcal{M}) &= \chi(\mathcal{M}) = 3 \times 2.
\end{aligned}
$$

The term $\mu_1$ is zero since there is no boundary and $\mu_0$ is simply the Euler characteristic of the template surface. Note that the Euler characteristic of a closed surface with no hole or handle is 2 and there are three such surfaces. The EC-densities of the T-field with $\nu$ degrees of freedom is given by

$$
\rho_0(z) = 1 - P(T_\nu \leq z),
$$

$$
\rho_1(z) = \frac{1}{\sqrt{2t^2}} \cdot \frac{1}{2\pi} \left( 1 + \frac{z^2}{\nu} \right)^{-(\nu-1)/2},
$$

$$
\rho_2(z) = \frac{1}{2t^2} \cdot \frac{1}{(2\pi)^{3/2}} \frac{\Gamma(\frac{\nu+1}{2})}{(\frac{\nu}{2})^{1/2}\Gamma(\frac{\nu}{2})} z \left( 1 + \frac{z^2}{\nu} \right)^{-(\nu-1)/2}.
$$

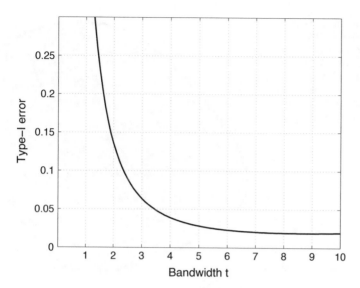

**Fig. 5** The type-I error plot over bandwidth $t$ of kernel smoothing for testing the difference between the groups I and III on the middle hyoid bone. As the bandwidth increases, the multiple comparisons corrected type-I error decreases. The bandwidth 5 is chosen for the study. The choice of the bandwidth around 5 does not change the over-all type-I error much

The EC-density of the F-field is similarly given in [54, 63]. The EC-density has the kernel bandwidth $t$ in the formulation so the inference is done at a particular smoothing scale. Figure 5 shows the type-I error plot over different bandwidth $t$ of the kernel regression in our application. As the bandwidth $t$ goes to zero, the type-I error increases. When $t = 0$, the kernel regression collapse to the usual Fourier series expansion. Note that the LB-eigenfunction expansion with 500 eigenfunctions is close to the original data without any smoothing. Hence, the proposed kernel smoothing can be viewed as having substantially smaller type-I error compared to the LB-eigenfunction expansion and the original data demonstrating a better statistical performance. The type-II error and the statistical power can be similarly computed.

**Theorem 3** *The statistical power $\mathscr{P}$ of testing the hypotheses*

$$H_0 : h(p) = 0 \text{ for all } p \in \mathscr{M} \text{ vs. } H_1 : h(p) = c\sigma > 0 \text{ for some } p \in \mathscr{M}.$$

*using the T random field $T(p)$ is given by*

$$\mathscr{P}(n) \approx 1 - \exp\left[ -\sum_{j=0}^{d} \mu_j(\mathscr{M}_1)\rho_j(t_\alpha^* - c\sqrt{n}) \right],$$

**Fig. 6** Schematic of the
hypothesis testing in
Theorem 3 when $H_1$ is true.
Since the hyoid bone is
composed of three structures
(hyoid body and two greater
horns), we can have multiple
disconnected $\mathcal{M}_1$, where
$c > 0$

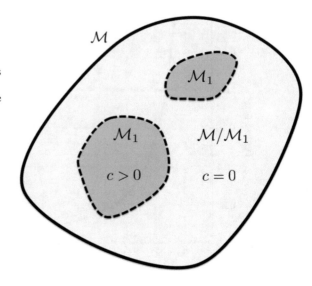

where $t_\alpha^*$ is the $\alpha$-quantile given by

$$\alpha = P\left( \sup_{p \in \mathcal{M}} T(p) > t_\alpha^* \right).$$

**Proof** In the region $\mathcal{M}_0 = \mathcal{M} / \mathcal{M}_1$ corresponding to $H_0$,

$$f^i(p) \sim N(0, \sigma^2).$$

In the region $\mathcal{M}_1$ corresponding to $H_1$,

$$f^i(p) \sim N(c\sigma, \sigma^2).$$

Figure 6 illustrates this setting, where $\mathcal{M}_1$ can be disconnected sets. Consider the test statistic

$$T(p) = \frac{\bar{f}(p)}{S(p)/\sqrt{n}}, \tag{20}$$

where $\bar{f}$ and $S$ are the sample mean and standard deviation of the measurements $f^i, \cdots, f^n$. In $\mathcal{M}_0$, $T(p)$ is a T random field with $n - 1$ degrees of freedom [1]. In $\mathcal{M}_1$, $T(p)$ can be written as

$$T(p) = T'(p) + \frac{c\sigma}{S(p)/\sqrt{n}},$$

where $T'(p)$ a T random field with $n-1$ degrees of freedom. Since $\sigma$ is usually estimated using the standard deviation, approximately, we have $S(p) = \sigma$ and the test statistic becomes $T(p) = T'(p) + c\sqrt{n}$ in $\mathcal{M}_1$. At each fixed $p$, $T(p)$ is no longer a T random field but a non-central T random field [30]. Subsequently the power $\mathscr{P}$ at the $\alpha$-level is given by

$$\mathscr{P}(n) = P\left( \sup_{p \in \mathcal{M}_1} T(p) > t_\alpha^* \right) \tag{21}$$

$$= P\left( \sup_{p \in \mathcal{M}_1} T'(p) > t_\alpha^* - c\sqrt{n} \right), \tag{22}$$

where $t_\alpha^*$ is the $\alpha$-quantile of $\sup_{p \in \mathcal{M}} T(p)$ under $H_0$, i.e.

$$\alpha = P\left( \sup_{p \in \mathcal{M}} T(p) > t_\alpha^* \right).$$

Although (22) is intractable to directly compute, we can approximate (22) using the expected Euler characteristic (EC) [59, 61]. The power (22) can be written as

$$\mathscr{P}(n) = \sum_{j=0}^{d} \mu_j(\mathcal{M}_1) \rho_j(t_\alpha^* - c\sqrt{n}),$$

where $\mu_d(\mathcal{M})$ is the $j$-th Minkowski functional or intrinsic volume of $\mathcal{M}$ and $\rho_j$ is the $j$-th EC-density of T-field [1, 54, 59, 60]. The expansion only works for sufficiently large $t_\alpha^* - c\sqrt{n}$. The rate of the convergence is given in terms of probability as $O((t_\alpha^*)^{-1/2})$ [58]. For small thresholds, the power may not be bounded between 0 and 1. Thus, it is necessary to use the exponential transform to bound the power [30]. For small $\mathscr{P}(n)$, using the Taylor expansion, we can write $\exp\left[-\mathscr{P}(n)\right] \approx 1 - \mathscr{P}(n)$. Equivalently, it is written as $\mathscr{P}(n) \approx 1 - \exp\left[-\mathscr{P}(n)\right]$. This transformation guarantees the power estimation to be bounded between 0 and 1 [30]. Subsequently, the power is given by

$$\mathscr{P}(n) = 1 - \exp\left[ -\sum_{j=0}^{d} \mu_j(\mathcal{M}_1) \rho_j(t_\alpha^* - c\sqrt{n}) \right]. \tag{23}$$

Figure 7 displays the power $\mathscr{P}(n)$ over the sample size $n$ for effect sizes $c = 0.1, 0.2, 0.5$ based on (23). The actual surface of the hyoid bone is taken as $\mathcal{M}$ and 10% of surface area is taken as the signal region $\mathcal{M}_1$.

$\square$

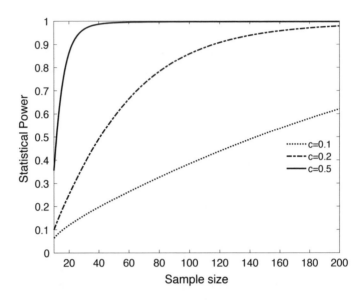

**Fig. 7** Statistical power over the sample size under the multiple comparisons. $c$ is the effect size using formula (23). The surface of the hyoid bone is taken as $\mathcal{M}$ and 10% of surface area is taken as the signal region $\mathcal{M}_1$

## 3.5  Validation

The proposed method is validated against the *iterated kernel smoothing* [17, 18], which smooth data as weighted average of neighboring mesh vertices using a Gaussian kernel and its iterative application is supposed to approximate the diffusion process. The iterated Gaussian kernel smoothing was also used as the baseline method in [40]. We performed two simulations with small and large signal to noise ratio (SNR) settings on a T-junction surface with three different curvatures: convex, concave and almost flat regions (Fig. 8). Surface smoothing methods perform differently under different curvatures. Three signal regions of different sizes (colored red in Fig. 8) were taken as the ground truth at these regions and 60 independent functional measurements on the surface were simulated as $|N(0, \gamma^2)|$, the absolute value of normal distribution with mean 0 and variance $\gamma^2$, at each mesh vertex. Value 1 was then added to the regions in 30 of the measurements, which served as group II, while the other 30 measurements were taken as group I. Group I has distribution $|N(0, \gamma^2)|$ while group II has distribution $|N(1, \gamma^2)|$ in the signal regions. Larger variance $\gamma^2$ corresponds to smaller SNR.

In Study I, $\gamma^2 = 2^2$ was used to simulate smaller SNR. Figure 8 shows the simulation results. For iterated kernel smoothing [17, 18], we used bandwidth $t = 0.5$ and 100 iterations (second column). The expansion with 1000 LB eigenfunction is used to smooth data, which is equivalent to heat kernel smoothing with zero bandwidth (third column). For heat kernel smoothing, bandwidth $t = 0.5$ and 1000

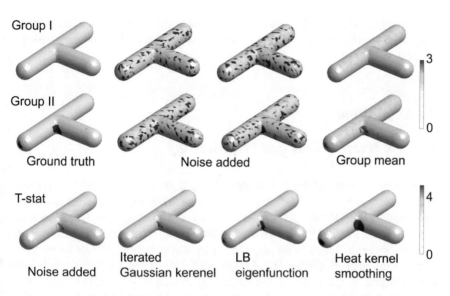

**Fig. 8** Simulation study on a T-junction shaped surface where three regions of different sizes are taken as the ground truth (colored red in group II - ground truth). 60 independent functional measurements on the T-junction were simulated as $|N(0, \gamma^2)|$ at each mesh vertex. Value 1 was added to the ground truth region in 30 measurements, which served as group II while the other 30 measurements were taken as group I. T-statistics are shown for these simulations (original) and three techniques with bandwidth 0.5. Heat kernel smoothing performed the best in detecting the ground truth regions

eigenfunctions were used (fourth column). We then performed a two sample $t$-test with the random field theory corrected threshold of 4.90 to detect the group difference at $\alpha = 0.05$ level. The noise added raw data were able to correctly identify only 3% of signal regions but also detected 3% of non-signal regions as signal. Iterated kernel smoothing also was able to identify only 3% of signal regions as signal but also detected 3% of non-signal regions as signal. The LB eigenfunction expansion were able to correctly identify 25% of signal regions but did not detect any signal in non-signal regions as signal. In comparison, heat kernel correctly identified 94% of the signal regions and incorrectly identified 0.4% of non-signal regions as signal. The proposed heat kernel smoothing performed very well in the small SNR setting.

In Study II, $\gamma^2 = 1$ was used to simulate functional measurements with substantially larger SNR. The same parameters were used as in Study I. The noise added raw data was able to correctly identify 88% of signal regions and did not detect any signal in non-signal regions as signal. Iterated kernel smoothing was able to correctly identify 91% of signal regions and did not detect any signal in non-signal regions as signal. LB eigenfunction expansion was able to correctly identify only 94% of signal regions and did not detect any signal in non-signal regions as signal. In comparison, heat kernel correctly identified 97% of the signal regions and incorrectly identified 1.5% of non-signal regions as signal. Although all the methods performed well in small SNR setting, the proposed heat kernel smoothing performed the best.

## 4 Application

### 4.1 CT Imaging Data and Preprocessing

This study consists of high resolution CT images of 70 typically developing individuals ages between 0 and 20 years (mean age $8.0 \pm 11.3$ years). CT scans were converted to DICOM format and Analyze 8.1 software package (AnalyzeDirect, Inc., Overland Park, KS) was then used in segmenting binary hyoid bone images by a trained individual rater in the native space by simple image intensity thresholding and careful manual editing [10, 16]. A nonlinear image registration using the diffeomorphic shape and intensity averaging technique with cross-correlation as similarity metric was performed through Advanced Normalization Tools (ANTS) [4]. Some individual may have larger hyoid than others so it was necessary to remove the global size differences in local shape modeling. From the affine transformed individual hyoid surfaces, we performed the diffeomorphic nonlinear image registration to the template. A study-specific template was constructed as follows. We chose a 12 year old female identified as F155 as the initial template and aligned the remaining 69 hyoids to this template affinely to remove the overall size variability. F155 was carefully chosen among all other segmentation results by visual inspection to have no segmentation artifacts. Further, it was constantly used as a reference template in previous studies [49, 50]. By averaging the inverse deformation fields from the initial template to individual hyoid, we obtained the yet another final template. Since the final template is the average of all other surfaces, the final localized growth pattern is not much influenced by the choice of the initial template.

Image acquisition error, discretization error, and image preprocessing noises in segmentation and registration often result in noisy deformation fields. The proposed heat kernel smoothing was applied to the displacement vector fields to smooth out high frequency noises. 70 individuals are binned into three age groups: ages between 0 and 6 years (group I), between 7 and 12 years (group II), and between 13 and 19 years (group III). There are 26, 14 and 30 individuals in group I, II and III respectively. The main biological hypothesis of interest is if there is any localized hyoid bone growth spurts between these specific age groups. The age range is chosen based on prior bone growth studies [35], where similar age binning is used in modeling the growth of mandible, which is located in the close proximity to the hyoid bone.

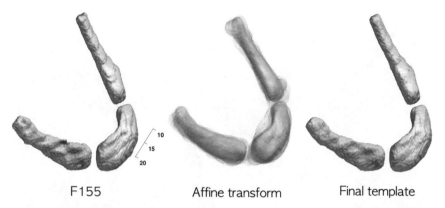

F155        Affine transform        Final template

**Fig. 9** Left: Hyoid F155 which forms an initial template $\mathcal{M}_I$. All other hyoids are affine registered to F155. Middle: The superimposition of affine registered hyoids showing local misalignments. Diffeomorphic registration is then performed to register misaligned affine transformed hyoids. Right: The average of deformation with respect to F155 provides the final population average template $\mathcal{M}_F$ where statistical parametric maps will be constructed

## 4.2 Results

Figure 9 shows the initial and final templates. The isosurface of the final template volume is extracted using the marching cubes algorithm [41]. The displacement from the template to an individual surface is obtained at each mesh vertex. Figure 10 shows the mean displacement differences between the groups I and II (top) and II and III (bottom). Each row shows the group differences of the displacement: group II–group I (first row) and group III–group II (second row). The arrows are the growth direction given by the mean displacement differences and colors indicate their lengths in mm. We are interested in localizing the regions of hyoid bone growth between the age groups.

Since the length measurement provides a much easier biological interpretation, we used the length of displacement vector as a response variable among many other possible features. Since the length on the template surface is expected to be noisy due to image acquisition, segmentation and image registration errors, it is necessary perform the proposed kernel regression and subsequently reduce the type-I error and obtain more stable SPM. Figure 3 shows an example of kernel smoothing on our data. The kernel smoothing increases the signal-to-noise ratio (SNR) and improves the smoothness and Gaussianness of data. Subsequently, the heat kernel smoothing of the displacement length is taken as the response variable. We have chosen $t = 5$ as the bandwidth for the study since the bandwidth 5 is where the type-I error starts to flatten out in Fig. 5. Note that the LB-eigenfunction expansion with 500 eigenfunctions is close to the original data (relative error of less than 0.3%). Hence, performing the proposed kernel regression before the statistical analysis can substantially smaller type-I error demonstrating its effectiveness.

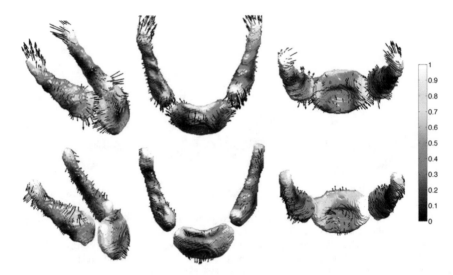

**Fig. 10** Hyoid bones are binned into three age groups: group I (ages 0 and 6), group II (ages 7 and 12) and group III (ages 13 and 19) and the mean displacements between the groups are visualized. Each row shows the mean group differences of the displacement: group II–group I (first row) and group III–group II (second row). The arrows are the mean displacement differences and colors indicate their lengths in mm

After the displacement lengths are smoothed, we constructed the F-field, or equivalently the T-field square, for testing the length difference between the age groups I and II, II and III, and I and III showing the regions of growth spurts between different age range (Fig. 11). Since test statistics are constructed over all mesh vertices on the hyoid bone, multiple comparisons were account for using the random field theory [62, 63].

For testing the differences between the groups I and II, II and III, and I and III, they are based on F-field with 1 and 38, 1 and 42, and 1 and 54 degrees of freedom respectively. The result is displayed in Fig. 11, where the significant results were only found between the groups II and III (middle), and I and III (bottom) at $\alpha = 0.1$ level. Between the groups I and II, we obtained maximum $F$-statistic value of 4.58 (left hyoid), which is not significant enough. Between the groups II and III, we the maximum F-statistic value of 9.36 (right hyoid), which corresponds to the $p$-value of 0.13 (corrected). Between the groups I and III, we obtained the maximum $F$-statistic value of 10.55 (middle hyoid), which corresponds to the $p$-value of 0.074 (corrected). The multiple comparisons were done over the whole hyoid bone. If we perform the multiple comparisons for each of the three components of the hyoid bone, we can boost the signal a bit. For instance, restricted to the middle hyoid bone, the maximum $F$-statistic value of 10.55 will correspond to the $p$-value of 0.028.

# F-stat (Group II - I)

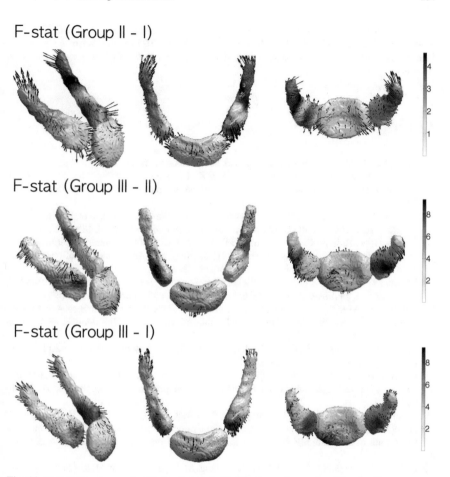

# F-stat (Group III - II)

# F-stat (Group III - I)

**Fig. 11** F-statistic maps on hyoid showing age effect between the groups. The significant growth regions (red) are identified only between groups II and III, and I and III. The growth is highly localized near the regions that connect the disconnected hyoid bones

## 5 Conclusions

We have developed a new kernel regression framework on a manifold that unifies bivariate kernel regression, heat diffusion and wavelets in a single coherent mathematical framework. The kernel regression is robust both globally and locally in that it uses global basis functions to perform regression but locally related to the diffusion wavelet transform. The proposed framework is demonstrated to reduce the type-I error in modeling shape variations compared to the usual LB-eigenfunction expansion. The method is then used in developing a statistical inference procedure for functional signals on manifolds.

**Acknowledgements** This work was supported by NIH Research Grants R01 DC6282, R01 EB022856, UL1TR000427 and P-30 HD03352 and U54 HD090256 to the Waisman Center. We thank Vikas Singh and Won Hwa Kim of University of Wisconsin-Madison for discussion on wavelets.

# References

1. Adler, R. J. (1981). *The geometry of random fields.* London: Wiley.
2. Andrade, A., Kherif, F., Mangin, J., Worsley, K. J., Paradis, A., Simon, O., et al. (2001). Detection of fMRI activation using cortical surface mapping. *Human Brain Mapping, 12,* 79–93.
3. Antoine, J.-P., Roşca, D., & Vandergheynst, P. (2010). Wavelet transform on manifolds: Old and new approaches. *Applied and Computational Harmonic Analysis, 28,* 189–202.
4. Avants, B. B., Epstein, C. L., Grossman, M., & Gee, J. C. (2008). Symmetric diffeomorphic image registration with cross-correlation: Evaluating automated labeling of elderly and neurodegenerative brain. *Medical Image Analysis, 12,* 26–41.
5. Belkin, M., & Niyogi, P. (2002). Laplacian eigenmaps and spectral techniques for embedding and clustering. In *Advances in Neural Information Processing Systems* (pp. 585–592)
6. Belkin, M., Niyogi, P., & Sindhwani, V. (2006). Manifold regularization: A geometric framework for learning from labeled and unlabeled examples. *The Journal of Machine Learning Research, 7,* 2399–2434.
7. Benjamini, Y., & Yekutieli, D. (2001). The control of the false discovery rate in multiple testing under dependency. *Annals of Statistics, 29,* 1165–1188.
8. Bernal-Rusiel, J., Atienza, M., & Cantero, J. (2008). Detection of focal changes in human cortical thickness: Spherical wavelets versus gaussian smoothing. *NeuroImage, 41,* 1278–1292.
9. Bullmore, E. T., Suckling, J., Overmeyer, S., Rabe-Hesketh, S., Taylor, E., & Brammer, M. J. (1999). Global, voxel, and cluster tests, by theory and permutation, for adifference between two groups of structural MR images of the brain. *IEEE Transactions on Medical Imaging, 18,* 32–42.
10. Chuang, Y. J., Doherty, B. M., Adluru, N., Chung, M. K., & Vorperian, H. K. (2018). A novel registration-based semiautomatic mandible segmentation pipeline using computed tomography images to study mandibular development. *Journal of Computer Assisted Tomography, 42,* 306–316.
11. Chung, M.K. (2012). *Computational neuroanatomy: The methods.* Singapore: World Scientific.
12. Chung, M. K., Dalton, K.M., & Davidson, R. J. (2008). Tensor-based cortical surface morphometry via weighted spherical harmonic representation. *IEEE Transactions on Medical Imaging, 27,* 1143–1151.
13. Chung, M. K., Dalton, K. M., Shen, L., Evans, A. C., & Davidson, R. J. (2007). Weighted Fourier representation and its application to quantifying the amount of gray matter. *IEEE Transactions on Medical Imaging, 26,* 566–581.
14. Chung, M. K., Hartley, R., Dalton, K. M., & Davidson, R. J. (2008). Encoding cortical surface by spherical harmonics. *Statistica Sinica, 18,* 1269–1291.
15. Chung, M. K., Lee, H., Solo, V., Davidson, R. J., & Pollak, S. D. (2017). Topological distances between brain networks. *International Workshop on Connectomics in Neuroimaging. Lecture Notes in Computer Science* (pp. 161–170).
16. Chung, M. K., Qiu, A., Seo, S., & Vorperian, H. K. (2015). Unified heat kernel regression for diffusion, kernel smoothing and wavelets on manifolds and its application to mandible growth modeling in CT images. *Medical Image Analysis, 22,* 63–76.

17. Chung, M. K., Robbins, S., Dalton, K. M., Davidson, R. J., Alexander, A. L., & Evans, A. C. (2005). Cortical thickness analysis in autism with heat kernel smoothing. *NeuroImage, 25*, 1256–1265.
18. Chung, M. K., Robbins, S., & Evans, A. C. (2005). Unified statistical approach to cortical thickness analysis. In *Information Processing in Medical Imaging (IPMI). Lecture Notes in Computer Science* (Vol. 3565, pp. 627–638)
19. Chung, M. K., & Taylor, J. (2004). Diffusion smoothing on brain surface via finite element method. In *Proceedings of IEEE International Symposium on Biomedical Imaging (ISBI)* (Vol. 1, pp. 432–435).
20. Chung, M. K., Vilalta-Gil, V., Lee, H., Rathouz, P. J., Lahey, B. B., & Zald, D. H. (2017). Exact topological inference for paired brain networks via persistent homology. In *Information Processing in Medical Imaging (IPMI). Lecture Notes in Computer Science* (Vol. 10265, pp. 299–310).
21. Chung, M. K., Worsley, K. J., Paus, T., Cherif, D. L., Collins, C., Giedd, J., et al. (2001). A unified statistical approach to deformation-based morphometry. *NeuroImage, 14*, 595–606.
22. Chung, M. K., Worsley, K. J., Robbins, S., Paus, T., Taylor, J., Giedd, J. N., et al. (2003). Deformation-based surface morphometry applied to gray matter deformation. *NeuroImage, 18*, 198–213.
23. Courant, R., & Hilbert, D. (1953). *Methods of mathematical physics*. New York: Interscience. English edition.
24. Fan, J., & Gijbels, I. (1996). *Local polynomial modelling and its applications*. Boca Raton: Chapman & Hall/CRC.
25. Fletcher, T. (2011). Geodesic regression on Riemannian manifolds. In *Proceedings of the Third International Workshop on Mathematical Foundations of Computational Anatomy-Geometrical and Statistical Methods for Modelling Biological Shape Variability* (pp. 75–86).
26. Gelb, A. (1997). The resolution of the Gibbs phenomenon for spherical harmonics. *Mathematics of Computation, 66*, 699–717.
27. Genovese, C. R., Lazar, N. A., & Nichols, T. (2002). Thresholding of statistical maps in functional neuroimaging using the false discovery rate. *NeuroImage, 15*, 870–878.
28. Gu, X., Wang, Y. L., Chan, T. F., Thompson, T. M., & Yau, S. T. (2004). Genus zero surface conformal mapping and its application to brain surface mapping. *IEEE Transactions on Medical Imaging, 23*, 1–10.
29. Hammond, D. K., Vandergheynst, P., & Gribonval, R. (2011). Wavelets on graphs via spectral graph theory. *Applied and Computational Harmonic Analysis, 30*, 129–150.
30. Hayasaka, S., Peiffer, A. M., Hugenschmidt, C. E., & Laurienti, P. J. (2007). Power and sample size calculation for neuroimaging studies by non-central random field theory. *NeuroImage, 37*, 721–730.
31. Hayasaka, S., Phan, K. L., Liberzon, I., Worsley, K. J., & Nichols, T. E. (2004). Nonstationary cluster-size inference with random field and permutation methods. *Neuroimage, 22*, 676–687.
32. Hendriks, H. (1990). Nonparametric estimation of a probability density on a Riemannian manifold using Fourier expansions. *The Annals of Statistics, 18*, 832–849.
33. Hosseinbor, A. P., Kim, W. H., Adluru, N., Acharya, A., Vorperian, H. K., & Chung, M. K. (2014). The 4D hyperspherical diffusion wavelet: A new method for the detection of localized anatomical variation. In *International Conference on Medical Image Computing and Computer-Assisted Intervention* (Vol. 8675, pp. 65–72).
34. Hurdal, M. K., & Stephenson, K. (2004). Cortical cartography using the discrete conformal approach of circle packings. *NeuroImage, 23*, S119–S128.
35. Kelly, M. P., Vorperian, H. K., Wang, Y., Tillman, K. K., Werner, H. M., Chung, M. K., et al. (2017). Characterizing mandibular growth using three-dimensional imaging techniques and anatomic landmarks. *Archives of Oral Biology, 77*, 27–38.
36. Kim, H. J., Adluru, N., Collins, M. D., Chung, M. K., Bendlin, B. B., Johnson, S. C., et al. (2014). Multivariate general linear models (MGLM) on Riemannian manifolds with applications to statistical analysis of diffusion weighted images. In *Proceedings of the IEEE Conference on Computer Vision and Pattern Recognition* (pp. 2705–2712).

37. Kim, S.-G., Chung, M. K., Seo, S., Schaefer, S. M., van Reekum, C., & Davidson, R. J. (2011). Heat kernel smoothing via Laplace-Beltrami eigenfunctions and its application to subcortical structure modeling. In *Pacific-Rim Symposium on Image and Video Technology (PSIVT)*. Lecture Notes in Computer Science (Vol. 7087, pp. 36–47).

38. Kim, W. H., Pachauri, D., Hatt, C., Chung, M. K., Johnson, S., & Singh, V. (2012). Wavelet based multi-scale shape features on arbitrary surfaces for cortical thickness discrimination. In *Advances in Neural Information Processing Systems* (pp. 1250–1258).

39. Lerch, J. P., & Evans, A. C. (2005). Cortical thickness analysis examined through power analysis and a population simulation. *NeuroImage, 24*, 163–173.

40. Lila, E., Aston, J. A. D., & Sangalli, L. M. (2016). Smooth principal component analysis over two-dimensional manifolds with an application to neuroimaging. *The Annals of Applied Statistics, 10*, 1854–1879.

41. Lorensen, W. E., & Cline, H. E. (1987). Marching cubes: A high resolution 3D surface construction algorithm. In *Proceedings of the 14th Annual Conference on Computer Graphics and Interactive Techniques* (pp. 163–169).

42. Mahadevan, S., & Maggioni, M. (2006). Value function approximation with diffusion wavelets and laplacian eigenfunctions. *Advances in Neural Information Processing Systems, 18*, 843.

43. Malladi, R., & Ravve, I. (2002). Fast difference schemes for edge enhancing Beltrami flow. In *Proceedings of Computer Vision-ECCV. Lecture Notes in Computer Science* (Vol. 2350, pp. 343–357).

44. Nain, D., Styner, M., Niethammer, M., Levitt, J. J., Shenton, M. E., G. Gerig, et al. (2007). Statistical shape analysis of brain structures using spherical wavelets. In *IEEE Symposium on Biomedical Imaging ISBI* (Vol. 4, pp. 209–212).

45. Öztireli, A. C., Guennebaud, G., & Gross, M. (2009). Feature preserving point set surfaces based on non-linear kernel regression. In *Computer Graphics Forum* (Vol. 28, pp. 493–501).

46. Perona, P., & Malik, J. (1990). Scale-space and edge detection using anisotropic diffusion. *IEEE Trans. Pattern Analysis and Machine Intelligence, 12*, 629–639.

47. Qiu, A., Bitouk, D., & Miller, M.I. (2006). Smooth functional and structural maps on the neocortex via orthonormal bases of the Laplace-Beltrami operator. *IEEE Transactions on Medical Imaging, 25*, 1296–1396.

48. Qiu, A., & Miller, M. I. (2008). Multi-structure network shape analysis via normal surface momentum maps. *NeuroImage, 42*, 1430–1438.

49. Seo, S., Chung, M. K., & Vorperian, H. K. (2010). Heat kernel smoothing using Laplace-Beltrami eigenfunctions. In *Medical Image Computing and Computer-Assisted Intervention — MICCAI 2010. Lecture Notes in Computer Science* (Vol. 6363, pp 505–512).

50. Seo, S., Chung, M. K., & Voperian, H. K. (2011). Mandible shape modeling using the second eigenfunction of the Laplace-Beltrami operator. In *Proceedings of SPIE Medical Imaging* (Vol. 7962, pp. 79620Z).

51. Sochen, N., Kimmel, R., & Malladi, R. (1998). A general framework for low level vision. *IEEE Transactions on Image Processing, 7*, 310–318.

52. Tang, B., Sapiro, G., & Caselles, V. (1999). Direction diffusion. In *The Proceedings of the Seventh IEEE International Conference on Computer Vision* (Vol. 2, pp. 1245–1252).

53. Taubin, G. (2000). Geometric signal processing on polygonal meshes. In *EUROGRAPHICS*. Geneve: Eurographics Association.

54. Taylor, J. E., & Worsley, K. J. (2007). Detecting sparse signals in random fields, with an application to brain mapping. *Journal of the American Statistical Association, 102*, 913–928. .

55. Vorperian, H. K., Wang, S., Schimek, E. M., Durtschi, R. B., Kent, R. D., Gentry, L. R., et al. (2011). Developmental sexual dimorphism of the oral and pharyngeal portions of the vocal tract: an imaging study. *Journal of Speech, Language and Hearing Research, 54*, 995–1010. .

56. Wang, Y., Chung,, M. K., & Vorperian, H. K. (2016). Composite growth model applied to human oral and pharyngeal structures and identifying the contribution of growth types. *Statistical Methods in Medical Research, 25*, 1975–1990.

57. Wang, Y., Zhang, J., Gutman, B., Chan, T. F., Becker, J. T., Aizenstein, H. J., et al. (2010). Multivariate tensor-based morphometry on surfaces: Application to mapping ventricular abnormalities in HIV/AIDS. *NeuroImage, 49*, 2141–2157.
58. Worsley, K. J. (1994). Local maxima and the expected Euler characteristic of excursion sets of $\chi^2$, $f$ and $t$ fields. *Advances in Applied Probability, 26*, 13–42.
59. Worsley, K. J. (2003). Detecting activation in fMRI data. *Statistical Methods in Medical Research, 12*, 401–418.
60. Worsley, K. J., Cao, J., Paus, T., Petrides, M., & Evans, A. C. (1998). Applications of random field theory to functional connectivity. *Human Brain Mapping, 6*, 364–367.
61. Worsley, K. J., Marrett, S., Neelin, P., Vandal, A. C., Friston, K. J., & Evans, A. C. (1996). A unified statistical approach for determining significant signals in images of cerebral activation. *Human Brain Mapping, 4*, 58–73.
62. Worsley, K. J., Poline, J.-B., Vandal, A. C., & Friston, K. J. (1995). Test for distributed, non-focal brain activations. *NeuroImage, 2*, 173–181.
63. Worsley, K. J., Taylor, J. E., Tomaiuolo, F., & Lerch, J. (2004). Unified univariate and multivariate random field theory. *NeuroImage, 23*, S189–195.
64. Xu, Y., Valentino, D. J., Scher, A. I., Dinov, I., White, L. R., Thompson, P. M., Launer, L. J., & Toga, A. W. (2008). Age effects on hippocampal structural changes in old men: The HAAS. *NeuroImage, 40*, 1003–1015.
65. Yushkevich, P. A., Zhang, H., Simon, T. J., & Gee, J. C. (2008). Structure-specific statistical mapping of white matter tracts. *NeuroImage, 41*, 448–461.
66. Zhang, H., Avants, B. B., Yushkevich, P. A., Woo, J. H., Wang, S., McCluskey, L. F., et al. (2007). High-dimensional spatial normalization of diffusion tensor images improves the detection of white matter differences: an example study using amyotrophic lateral sclerosis. *IEEE Transactions on Medical Imaging, 26*(11), 1585–1597.

# Optimal Projections in the Distance-Based Statistical Methods

## Chuanping Yu and Xiaoming Huo

**Abstract** This paper introduces a new way to calculate distance-based statistics, particularly when the data are multivariate. The main idea is to pre-calculate the optimal projection directions given the variable dimension, and to project multidimensional variables onto these pre-specified projection directions; by subsequently utilizing the fast algorithm that is developed in Huo and Székely (Technometrics, 58(4):435–447, 2016) for the univariate variables, the computational complexity can be improved from $O(m^2)$ to $O(nm \cdot \log(m))$, where $n$ is the number of projection directions and $m$ is the sample size. When $n \ll m/\log(m)$, computational savings can be achieved. The key challenge is how to find the optimal pre-specified projection directions. This can be obtained by minimizing the worse-case difference between the true distance and the approximated distance, which can be formulated as a nonconvex optimization problem in a general setting. In this paper, we show that the exact solution of the nonconvex optimization problem can be derived in two special cases: the dimension of the data is equal to either 2 or the number of projection directions. In the generic settings, we propose an algorithm to find approximate solutions. Simulations confirm the advantage of our method, in comparison with the pure Monte Carlo approach, in which the directions are randomly selected rather than pre-calculated.

**Keywords** Distance-based statistical methods · Projection-based methods · Quasi-Monte Carlo · Statistical computing · Random projections

C. Yu · X. Huo (✉)
School of Industrial and Systems Engineering, Georgia Institute of Technology, Atlanta, GA, USA
e-mail: c.yu@gatech.edu; huo@gatech.edu

© Springer Nature Switzerland AG 2020
Y. Zhao, D.-G. (Din) Chen (eds.), *Statistical Modeling in Biomedical Research*, Emerging Topics in Statistics and Biostatistics, https://doi.org/10.1007/978-3-030-33416-1_13

# 1 Introduction

Distances are very important in statistics: a class of hypotheses testing methods are based on distances, such as the energy statistics [16], the distance covariance [10, 17, 18], and many others. This type of testing statistics usually belong to the class of U-statistics or V-statistics [6, 9, 11], which require the calculation of all pairwise distances within the sample. When variables are univariate, assuming the sample size is $m$, both [8] and [4] proposed fast algorithms with computational complexity $O(m\log(m))$ where $m$ is the sample size. Recall that the computational complexity is $O(m^2)$ when the statistics are computed directly based on their definitions. When variables are multivariate, especially when they are high-dimensional, the calculation of the pairwise distances among these multivariate variables can not be implemented directly by the algorithm in [8], and therefore becomes a potential bottleneck. Our paper is aimed at reducing the computation complexity in the multivariate case by projecting the variables along a set of pre-specified optimal directions. When the number of pre-specified optimal directions $n \ll m/\log(m)$, computational savings can be achieved, since the computational complexity is $O(nm \cdot \log(m))$, which would be less than $O(m^2)$.

We use the energy distances [16] as an example to solidify our motivation. The energy statistic is used to test the equality between two distributions. More precisely, suppose $X_1, \ldots, X_{n_1} \in \mathbb{R}^p, p \geq 1$ are independent and identically distributed (i.i.d.), sampled from the distribution $F_X$, and $Y_1, \ldots, Y_{n_2} \in \mathbb{R}^p$ are i.i.d., sampled from the distribution $F_Y$. The two-sample test statistic (also called the energy statistic) for testing the two-sample hypothesis

$$H_0 : F_X = F_Y$$

is defined as [16]:

$$\mathscr{E}_{n_1,n_2} \triangleq \frac{2}{n_1 n_2} \sum_{i=1}^{n_1} \sum_{j=1}^{n_2} \left\| X_i - Y_j \right\| - \frac{1}{n_1^2} \sum_{i=1}^{n_1} \sum_{k=1}^{n_1} \left\| X_i - X_k \right\| - \frac{1}{n_2^2} \sum_{j=1}^{n_2} \sum_{k=1}^{n_2} \left\| Y_j - Y_k \right\|, \tag{1}$$

where $\left\| X_i - Y_j \right\|, \left\| X_i - X_k \right\|, \left\| Y_j - Y_k \right\|$ are the distances from the two samples. Note that the statistic $\mathscr{E}_{n_1,n_2}$ solely depends on three types of inter-point distances: $\left\| X_i - Y_j \right\|, \left\| X_i - X_k \right\|, \left\| Y_j - Y_\ell \right\|, i, k = 1, \ldots, n_1, j, \ell = 1, \ldots, n_2$. Denote $m = n_1 + n_2$. [7] showed that it can be efficiently computed with computational complexity $O(m\log(m))$ in the univariate case (i.e., $p = 1$).

When $X_i$'s and $Y_j$'s are multivariate (i.e., we have $p > 1$), random projections have been proposed to find a fast approximation to the statistic $\mathscr{E}_{n_1,n_2}$. For example, [7] gave a fast algorithm that is based on random projections, which can achieve $O(nm \cdot \log(m))$ computational complexity, where $n$ is the number of random projections. Note that the approach in [7] is a pure Monte Carlo approach. The recent advances in the quasi-Monte Carlo methods [12, 14] have demonstrated that in some settings, utilizing pre-determined projections can lead to better performance than the completely random ones in the pure Monte Carlo approach. Quasi-Monte Carlo methods sometimes enjoy faster rate of convergence, e.g., [1].

Our approach turns a distance calculation in a multivariate situation to the one in a univariate situation. The proposed approach

**P1.** first projects each multivariate variable along some pre-specified optimal directions to corresponding one-dimensional subspaces (the projected values are univariate),

**P2.** then the sum of the $\ell_1$ norm of the projected values is used to approximate the associated distance in the multivariate setting.

More specifically, let's suppose the multivariate variable is $v = (v_1, \ldots, v_p) \in \mathbb{R}^p$. Recall that the norm of $v$ is

$$||v|| = \sqrt{\sum_{i=1}^{p} v_i^2}.$$

For $n \geq 1$, our objective is to identify the projection directions, which can be represented by vectors $u_1, u_2, \ldots, u_n \in \mathbb{R}^p$, and a predetermined constant $C_n \in \mathbb{R}$, such that for any $v \in \mathbb{R}^p$, we have

$$||v|| \approx C_n \sum_{i=1}^{n} \left| u_i^T v \right|. \tag{2}$$

Consequently in step **P2.**, when one needs to compute a distance $\| X_i - Y_j \|$, one can alternatively compute $C_n \sum_{i=1}^{n} \left| u_i^T X_i - u_i^T Y_j \right|$. Note that $u_i^T X_i$ and $u_i^T Y_j$ are univariate. Therefore, the fast algorithm in the one-dimensional case can be utilized.

We continue with the example of the energy distances. Recall that the pre-specified directions are supposed to be $u_1, \ldots, u_n$. The projected values of the corresponding multivariate variables then become

$$X_{wi} = u_w^T X_i \in \mathbb{R}, w = 1, \ldots, n; i = 1, \ldots, n_1; \text{ and}$$

$$Y_{wj} = u_w^T Y_j \in \mathbb{R}, w = 1, \ldots, n; j = 1, \ldots, n_2.$$

The distance between any two multivariate variables can be approximated by the sum of these projections multiplying by a constant:

$$\| X_i - Y_j \| \approx C_n \sum_{w=1}^{n} | X_{wi} - Y_{wj} |.$$

Therefore, the statistic $\mathscr{E}_{n_1, n_2}$ in (1) can be approximated by

$$\mathcal{E}_{n_1,n_2} \approx C_n\Big(\frac{2}{n_1 n_2}\sum_{i=1}^{n_1}\sum_{j=1}^{n_2}\sum_{w=1}^{n}\big\|X_{wi}-Y_{wj}\big\| - \frac{1}{n_1^2}\sum_{i=1}^{n_1}\sum_{k=1}^{n_1}\sum_{w=1}^{n}\big\|X_{wi}-X_{wk}\big\|$$

$$-\frac{1}{n_2^2}\sum_{j=1}^{n_2}\sum_{k=1}^{n_2}\sum_{w=1}^{n}\big\|Y_{wj}-Y_{wk}\big\|\Big)$$

$$= C_n\Big(\frac{2}{n_1 n_2}\sum_{i=1}^{n_1}\sum_{j=1}^{n_2}\sum_{w=1}^{n}\big|X_{wi}-Y_{wj}\big| - \frac{1}{n_1^2}\sum_{i=1}^{n_1}\sum_{k=1}^{n_1}\sum_{w=1}^{n}\big|X_{wi}-X_{wk}\big| \quad (3)$$

$$-\frac{1}{n_2^2}\sum_{j=1}^{n_2}\sum_{k=1}^{n_2}\sum_{w=1}^{n}\big|Y_{wj}-Y_{wk}\big|\Big).$$

The second equation is true because in the one-dimensional case, the $\ell_2$ norm becomes the absolute value. Then one can apply the fast algorithms for univariate variables to calculate the energy statistic in (3).

*Remark* Our method is not restricted to the calculation of the energy statistic, or other distance-based statistics. It can also be applied to the calculation of the distance-based smooth kernel functions.

In this paper, we first give a detailed description of our strategy to find the optimal pre-specified projection directions. We formulate the searching for optimal projection directions problem as a minimax optimization problem. Let $\{u_1, u_2, \cdots, u_n\}$ denote the optimal set of projection directions, they should minimize the worst-case difference between the true distance and the approximate distance. Equation (4) below shows this idea in the mathematical form:

$$\min_{\substack{C_n, u_i: \\ \|u_i\|=1, i=1,\cdots,n}} \quad \max_{v:\|v\|_2 \le 1} \left| C_n \sum_{w=1}^{n}\big|u_w^T v\big| - \|v\| \right|. \qquad (4)$$

Discussion on how to solve the above problem is presented in Sect. 2.

In general, the problem in (4) is a nonconvex optimization problem, which is potentially NP-hard. We found that in two special cases, the optimal directions can be derived analytically: (a) the 2-dimensional case and (b) when the dimension is equal to the number of projections. More details on these two special cases are presented in Sect. 3. In general cases, we propose a greedy algorithm to find the projection directions. Note that the greedy algorithm terminates at a local optimal solution to (4). In this case, we cannot theoretically guarantee that the found directions correspond to the global solution to the problem in (4), which is the case in most nonconvex optimization problems. At the same time, the simulations show that our approach can still outperform the pure Monte Carlo approach in many occasions.

The rest of this paper is organized as follows. Section 2 shows the formulation of our problem. Section 3 provides the analytical solutions to the problem in (4) in two special cases. Section 4 presents the numerical algorithm for the general cases. In Sect. 5, the simulation results of our method are furnished. Section 6 contains the conclusion and a summary of our work. All the technical proofs are relegated to Appendix section.

We adopt the following notations. Throughout this paper, we use $p$ to denote the dimension of the data. The sample size is denoted by $m$. The number of projections is denoted by $n$.

## 2  Problem Formulation

As mentioned above, in order to estimate the distance between two multivariate variables, we project them onto some pre-specified one-dimensional linear subspaces. We present details in the following. Suppose the multivariate variable is $v = (v_1, \ldots, v_p) \in \mathbb{R}^p$. Recall that the norm of vector $v$ is

$$||v|| = \sqrt{\sum_{i=1}^{p} v_i^2}.$$

Our objective is to design $u_1, u_2, \ldots, u_n \in \mathbb{R}^p$, for $n \geq 1$, and $C_n \in \mathbb{R}$, such that for any $v \in \mathbb{R}^p$, we have

$$||v|| \approx C_n \sum_{i=1}^{n} \left| u_i^T v \right|. \tag{5}$$

We would like to turn a distance (i.e., norm) of a multivariate variable $v$ into a weighted sum of the absolute values of some of its one dimensional projections (i.e., $u_i^T v$'s), knowing that the one dimensional projections may facilitate efficient numerical algorithms.

Without loss of generality, we may assume $||v|| = 1$. The approximation problem in (5) can be formulated into the following problem:

$$\min_{C_n, u_1, \ldots, u_n} \max_{v: ||v||_2 = 1} \left| C_n \sum_{i=1}^{n} \left| u_i^T v \right| - 1 \right|. \tag{6}$$

In words, we would like to select $u_1, \ldots, u_n$ and $C_n$ such that the approximation in (5) has the minimal discrepancy in the worst case. One can verify that the problem in (6) and the problem in (4) share the same solution.

To solve the problem in (6), the following two quantities are needed. For fixed $u_1, u_2, \ldots, u_n$, we define

$$V_{\max} = \max_{v:||v||_2=1} \sum_{i=1}^{n} \left| u_i^T v \right|, \tag{7}$$

$$V_{\min} = \min_{v:||v||_2=1} \sum_{i=1}^{n} \left| u_i^T v \right|, \tag{8}$$

where $V_{\max}$ and $V_{\min}$ are the maximum and minimum of $\sum_{i=1}^{n} \left| u_i^T v \right|$ among all possible $v$ under the constraint $||v||_2 = 1$, respectively. With these two quantities (i.e., $V_{\max}$ and $V_{\min}$), we have the following result.

**Theorem 1** *For given* $u_1, u_2, \ldots, u_n \in \mathbb{R}^p$, *the optimal value for* $C_n$ *in the problem* (6) *is*

$$C_n = \frac{2}{V_{\min} + V_{\max}}.$$

*Furthermore, the solutions of* $u_1, u_2, \ldots, u_n$ *in problem* (6) *are identical to the solutions to the following problem:*

$$\max_{\substack{u_1,\ldots,u_n: \\ ||u_i||=1, \forall i, 1 \le i \le n}} \frac{V_{\min}}{V_{\max}}. \tag{9}$$

The above theorem indicates that the minimax problem in (6) is equivalent to the maximization problem in (9). Note that in general, both problems are nonconvex, therefore potentially NP-hard. In our analysis, we found that both formulations (in (6) and (9)) are convenient in various steps of derivation. Both of them are used in later analysis.

## 3  Derivable Analytical Results

We present the two special cases where analytical solutions are derivable. When the dimension is 2 (i.e., $p = 2$), we show in Sect. 3.1 that an analytical solution to the problem in (9) is available. In Sect. 3.2, we present another case (when the dimension of the data is equal to the number of projections, that is we have $n = p$) where an analytic solution to the problem in (9) is derivable.

## 3.1 Special Case When the Dimension is 2

When the multivariate variables are two-dimensional, we can get the exact optimal projections that minimize the worse-case discrepancy. The following theorem describes such a result.

**Theorem 2** When $p = 2$, the 2-dimensional vectors $u_1, u_2, \ldots, u_n$ can be represented by

$$u_i = e^{\sqrt{-1}\theta_i}, i = 1, \ldots, n.$$

The optimal solution in (9) has the form

$$\theta_i = \frac{(i-1)\pi}{n} + k_i \pi, i = 1, \ldots, n \tag{10}$$

where each $k_i \in \mathbb{N}$.

Specially, when $n$ is odd, the optimal solutions can be represented by the equally spaced points on the circle. Furthermore, we can get the error rate in the 2-dimensional case, as in the following theorem.

**Theorem 3** If $u_1, \cdots, u_n$ are chosen according to Theorem 2, we have

$$\mathop{\mathbb{E}}_{v \sim Unif(S^1)} \left\{ \left| C_n \sum_{i=1}^{n} \left| u_i^T v \right| - 1 \right|^2 \right\} = O\left(\frac{1}{n^2}\right).$$

**Remark** Theorem 3 can be used as a guidance of choosing the number of directions. Assume we would like to control the squared error to be $\epsilon$. Then, we can get $\frac{1}{n^2} = \epsilon$, and therefore the number of directions should be larger than $\frac{1}{\sqrt{\epsilon}}$.

In the above theorem, the random vector $v$ is sampled independently from the Uniform distribution on the unit circle $S^1$. Note that the squared error rate is $O(1/n^2)$. The following theorem presents the corresponding rate for the pure random projections.

**Theorem 4** If $u_1, \cdots, u_n$ are selected base on Monte Carlo, we have

$$\mathop{\mathbb{E}}_{u_i, v \sim Unif(S^1)} \left\{ \left| C_n \sum_{i=1}^{n} \left| u_i^T v \right| - 1 \right|^2 \right\} = O\left(\frac{1}{n}\right).$$

In the above theorem, both random vector $v$ and vectors $u_i$'s are independently sampled from the Uniform distribution on the unit circle $(S^1)$. The squared error rate in the pure Monte Carlo case is $O(1/n)$. These two theorems illustrate the theoretical advantage of adopting the pre-calculated projection directions (in relative to the random projections). Such a phenomenon has been discovered in the literature regarding the quasi-Monte Carlo methodology.

## 3.2   Second Special Case with Provable Result

When the dimension is larger than 2, the problem in (6) is challenging. There is some potentially relevant literature in mathematics, such as the searching for algorithms to locate the equally-distributed points on the surfaces of some high-dimensional spheres [3, 5, 15]. We fail to locate the exact solutions to our problem.

Our analysis indicates that when the number of projections is equal to the dimension, an analytical solution to the problem in (6) is derivable. We present details in the following. To derive our analytical solution in a special case, we need to revisit two quantities, $V_{\min}$ and $V_{\max}$, which have been introduced in (7) and (8). The following lemma is about $V_{\max}$.

**Lemma 1**  *For fixed $u_1, u_2, \ldots, u_n \in \mathbb{R}^p$, we have*

$$V_{\max} = \max_{s_i \in \{1, -1\}} \left\| \sum_{i=1}^{n} s_i u_i \right\|. \tag{11}$$

Lemma 1 points out a way to calculate $V_{\max}$, that is, given binary $s_i$'s, finding out the linear combination $\sum_{i=1}^{n} s_i u_i$ with the maximal norm out of the all possible $2^n$ linear combinations. Let $\{s_i^{\max} \in \{1, -1\} : i = 1, \ldots, n\}$ denote the solution for (11) when $u_1, \cdots, u_n$ are given. The Algorithm 1 formally presents the aforementioned approach. Assume we are in the $k$-th loop, where the $u_j$'s are known, which are denoted by $u_1^{(k)}, u_2^{(k)}, \ldots, u_n^{(k)}$. Let $s_i^{(k)}$'s denote the $s_i$'s that can achieve $V_{\max}$ in the $k$-th loop. We have the Algorithm 1.

---

**Algorithm 1** Find $s_i^{\max}$'s in the $k$-loop

---

**Initialization:** Unit vectors $u_1^{(k)}, u_2^{(k)}, \ldots, u_n^{(k)} \in S^{p-1}$ are given.
**Output:** $s_i^{(k)}$'s.
 1: **for all** binary combination of $s_i^{(k)}$'s **do**
 2:     Calculate the value $\left\| \sum_{i=1}^{n} s_i u_i \right\|$.
 3: **end for**
 4: The binary combination that can make the value of $\left\| \sum_{i=1}^{n} s_i u_i \right\|$ be the maximum among all the
       possible values, is the $s_i^{\max}$'s, which is denoted as $s_i^{(k)}$'s.

---

As for $V_{\min}$, suppose $v_{\min}$ is a minimizer of $V_{\min}$. We have the following property for $v_{\min}$.

**Lemma 2** *For fixed $u_1, u_2, \ldots, u_n \in \mathbb{R}^p$, if $\Omega$ is an intersection of $S^{p-1}$ and a linear subspace with at least 2 dimensions, then the solution to the minimization problem*

$$\min_{v \in \Omega} f(v) = \sum_{i=1}^{n} \left| u_i^T v \right|$$

*must have $u_j^T v_{\min} = 0$ for at least one $j$ $(1 \le j \le n)$.*

Geometrically, the above lemma indicates that vector $v_{\min}$ should be orthogonal to at least one of the projection vector $u_j$. For vector $v_{\min}$, we will need the following definition to further our derivation.

**Definition 1 (Maximal Subset)** We call $\Omega(v_{\min})$ a maximal subset of the set $\{u_1, \ldots, u_n\}$ if it satisfies

$$\Omega(v_{\min}) = \left\{ u_j : u_j^T v_{\min} = 0 \right\} \subset \{u_1, \ldots, u_n\},$$

and it cannot be a strict subset for another $\Omega(v'_{\min})$ where $v'_{\min}$ is a minimizer that is different from $v_{\min}$.

Lemma 2 ensures that the set $\Omega(v_{\min})$ cannot be empty. The following lemma shows that the linear subspace that is spanned by the elements of $\Omega(v_{\min})$ must have certain dimensions.

**Lemma 3** *If $\Omega(v_{\min})$ is a maximal subset of $u_1, \ldots, u_n$, we must have*

$$rank(\Omega(v_{\min})) = p - 1,$$

*for any minimizer $v_{\min}$.*

Recall $p$ is the dimension of the data. The above lemma essentially states that the space that is spanned by the elements of $\Omega(v_{\min})$ is the orthogonal complement subspace of the one-dimensional space that is spanned by the vector $v_{\min}$.

One direct corollary of Lemma 3 is that the cardinality of the set $\Omega(v_{\min})$ is at least $p - 1$. Consequently, the total number of possible sets (of $\Omega(v_{\min})$) is no more than $\binom{n}{p-1}$. This inspires us to use Algorithm 2 to find $v_{\min}$ as well as $\Omega(v_{\min})$ if all the $u_j$'s are given. Here suppose we are in the $k$-th loop where the $u_j$'s are known, which are $u_1^{(k)}, u_2^{(k)}, \ldots, u_n^{(k)}$.

From Lemma 3 we can get the exact solution for the special case when the number of projection directions is equal to the dimension of the multivariate variables, which is described in the following theorem.

---

**Algorithm 2** Find $v_{\min}$ and $\Omega(v_{\min})$ in the $k$-loop

**Initialization:** Unit vectors $u_1^{(k)}, u_2^{(k)}, \ldots, u_n^{(k)} \in S^{p-1}$ are given.
**Output:** $v^{(k)}$ and $\Omega(v^{(k)})$.

1: **for all** $(p-1)$ combination of $u_i^{(k)}$'s, denoted as $S_t^u$ **do**
2:    **while** $\text{rank}(S_t^u) < p-1$ **do**
3:       Add another $u_j$ that is not in the set $S_t^u$;
4:    **end while**
5:    Find the orthogonal direction of the set $S_t^u$, which is one of the candidates of $v^{(k)}$, denoted
     as $v_t^{(k)}$, and calculate the value of $f(v_t^{(k)}) = \sum_{i=1}^{n} \left| \left( u_i^{(k)} \right)^T v_t^{(k)} \right|$.
6: **end for**
7: The $v_t^{(k)}$, that can make the value of $f(v_t^{(k)})$ be the minimum among all the possible $f(v_t^{(k)})$
   values, is the $v_{\min}$, which is denoted as $v^{(k)}$, and the corresponding $S_t^u$ set is the set $\Omega(v_{\min})$,
   which is denoted as $\Omega(v^{(k)})$.

---

**Theorem 5** *When the number of projections is equal to the dimension of the data, i.e., we have $n = p$, the optimal solution in (9) satisfies the following condition:*

$$u_i^T u_j = 0, \forall i \neq j. \tag{12}$$

*The above is equivalent to stating that the set $\{u_1, u_2, \cdots, u_n\}$ forms an orthonormal basis in $\mathbb{R}^p$.*

# 4 Numerical Approach in General Cases

When $p > 2$ and $n \neq p$, we propose an algorithm to identify the optimal projections $u_1, u_2, ..., u_n$, such that they solve (9). Per Lemma 1 and the definition of $s_i^{\max}$'s, the $V_{\max}$ can be written as:

$$V_{\max} = \left\| \sum_{i=1}^{n} s_i^{\max} u_i \right\|.$$

According to Lemma 3, we have

$$V_{\min} = \sum_{i=1}^{n} \left| u_i^T v_{\min} \right| = \sum_{u_i \in \Omega(v_{\min})} \left| u_i^T v_{\min} \right| + \sum_{u_i \notin \Omega(v_{\min})} \left| u_i^T v_{\min} \right|$$

$$= \sum_{u_i \notin \Omega(v_{\min})} \left| u_i^T v_{\min} \right|.$$

So when $u_1, \cdots, u_n$ are given, $\frac{V_{\min}}{V_{\max}}$ can be written as

$$\frac{V_{\min}}{V_{\max}} = \frac{\sum\limits_{u_i \notin \Omega(v_{\min})} \left| u_i^T v_{\min} \right|}{\left\| \sum\limits_{i=1}^{n} s_i^{\max} u_i \right\|}, \tag{13}$$

where $v_{\min}$ and $\Omega(v_{\min})$ are defined in Sect. 3.2. We assume that the set $\Omega(v_{\min})$ corresponds to the minimum over all $\binom{n}{p-1}$ possible sets, and $(s_i^{\max})$'s maximize the norm of $\sum\limits_{i=1}^{n} s_i^{\max} u_i$.

We use a method that is similar to the coordinate descent algorithm [13, 19] to search for the optimal solutions of (9). Details of our algorithm can be found in Algorithm 3. The optimal solution can be achieved in circular iterations: maximizing (13) with respect to one $u_i$, while the others are fixed. We then iteratively maximize the objective function in (13) until the value of the objective function (13) cannot be increased.

We derive the iteration strategy in the following. Let $v^{(k)}$ be the minimizer of $\sum\limits_{i=1}^{n} \left| u_i^T v \right|$ at the $k$th iteration. Let $\Omega^{(k)}$ denote the minimum over all $\binom{n}{p-1}$ possible sets at the $k$th iteration. For any $u_j^{(k)} \notin \Omega^{(k)}$, without loss of generality, we assume that $u_1 \notin \Omega^{(k)}$. The objective function in (13) can be written as

$$\frac{V_{\min}}{V_{\max}} = \frac{\left| u_1^T v^{(k)} \right| + \sum\limits_{i>1, u_i \notin \Omega^{(k)}} \left| u_i^T v^{(k)} \right|}{\left\| s_1^{\max} u_1 + \sum\limits_{i=2}^{n} s_i^{\max} u_i \right\|}. \tag{14}$$

Without loss of generality, we can assume $s_1^{\max} = 1$. This is because, recalling that $(s_i^{\max})$'s are binary, we have

$$\left\| s_1^{\max} u_1 + \sum\limits_{i=2}^{n} s_i^{\max} u_i \right\| = \left\| u_1 + \sum\limits_{i=2}^{n} s_1^{\max} s_i^{\max} u_i \right\|.$$

The expression in (14) can then be rewritten as

$$\frac{\left| u_1^T v^{(k)} \right| + A}{\left\| u_1 + B \right\|}, \tag{15}$$

where

$$A = \sum\limits_{i>1, u_i \notin \Omega^{(k)}} \left| u_i^T v^{(k)} \right|, \text{ and } B = \sum\limits_{i=2}^{n} s_i^{\max} u_i.$$

Note that quantities $A$ and $B$ do not depend on $u_1$. Our objective is to derive a strategy to maximize the quantity in (15) as a function of the vector variable $u_1$.

We first solve a constrained version of the above maximization problem. We define $\Sigma(v, \theta) = \{x : \|x\| = 1, \langle x, v \rangle = \theta\}$, for any fixed $\theta \in [0, \pi)$, where $\langle \cdot, \cdot \rangle$ denotes the angle between two vectors. Conditioning on $u_1 \in \Sigma(v, \theta)$, and $v = v^{(k)}$, maximizing the function in (15) is equivalent to maximizing the following function:

$$\frac{|\cos\theta| + A}{\|u_1 + B\|}. \tag{16}$$

Note that the numerator is not a function of $u_1$. Consequently, it is equivalent to minimizing

$$\|x + B\|, \text{ where } x \in \Sigma(v, \theta).$$

The following lemma presents an analytical solution to the above minimization problem.

**Lemma 4** *Given a vector $B$, a constant $\theta \in [0, \pi)$, and a unit-norm vector $v$, the solution to the following problem*

$$\min_{x: \|x\|=1, \langle x, v \rangle = \theta} \|x + B\|^2 \tag{17}$$

*is*

$$x = v \cos\theta + \frac{|\sin\theta|}{\sqrt{B^T B - (v^T B)^2}} \left[ (v^T B)v - B \right]. \tag{18}$$

Using the solution in (18) to substitute the $u_1$ in (16), we have

$$\frac{|\cos\theta| + A}{\|u_1 + B\|} = \frac{|\cos\theta| + A}{\left\| v\cos\theta + B + \frac{|\sin\theta|}{\sqrt{B^T B - (v^T B)^2}} \left[ (v^T B)v - B \right] \right\|}. \tag{19}$$

Maximizing (16) with respect to $\theta$ is equivalent to maximizing (19). For fixed $A$, $B$, and $v$, the right hand side of (19) is a function of $\theta$. The following Theorem 6 gives the solution to the above problem.

**Theorem 6** *The solutions of maximizing (16) with respect to $\theta$ are the zeros of the following function:*

$$g(\theta) = \begin{cases} \sqrt{B^T B} \left[\cos\alpha + A\cos(\alpha - \theta) - \sin\theta\sin(\alpha - \theta)\right] \\ -(1 + B^T B)\sin\theta, & \text{if } \theta \in [0, \frac{\pi}{2}), \\ \sqrt{B^T B} \left[-\cos\alpha + A\cos(\alpha - \theta) + \sin\theta\sin(\alpha - \theta)\right] \\ +(1 + B^T B)\sin\theta & \text{if } \theta \in [\frac{\pi}{2}, \pi), \end{cases} \tag{20}$$

*where $\alpha$ satisfies* $\sin \alpha = \dfrac{v^T B}{\sqrt{B^T B}}$, *and* $\cos \alpha = \dfrac{\sqrt{B^T B - (v^T B)^2}}{\sqrt{B^T B}}$.

The above theorem indicates that one can adopt a line search algorithm to compute for $\theta$.

Based on all the above, the Algorithm 3 (below) furnishes a coordinate ascent scheme to maximize the objective in (9).

---

**Algorithm 3** Optimal projection algorithm

---

**Initialization:** Set a threshold $\Delta > 0$, initial unit vectors $u_1^{(0)}, u_2^{(0)}, \ldots, u_n^{(0)} \in S^{p-1}$. Thus, by Algorithms 1 and 2, we can get the corresponding values $v^{(0)}, \Omega^{(0)}(v^{(0)})$, and $s_i^{(0)}$'s.

1: **repeat**
2:     In the $k$-th loop, suppose the previous $u_1^{(k-1)}, u_2^{(k-1)}, \ldots, u_n^{(k-1)}$ are known.
3:     **for all** $u_j^{(k-1)} \notin \Omega^{(k-1)}(v^{(k-1)})$ **do**
4:         Find the zeros of the function $g(\theta)$ in (20) in Theorem 6, where $v = v^{(k-1)}$, $B = \sum_{i \neq j} s_j^{(k-1)} s_i^{(k-1)} u_i^{(k-1)}$, and denote the zeros as $\theta^*$.
5:         According to Lemma 4, the new $u_j^{(k)}$ would be $v \cos \theta^* + \dfrac{|\sin \theta^*|}{\sqrt{B^T B - (v^T B)^2}} \left[ (v^T B)v - B \right]$.
6:         By Algorithm 1 and 2, we can get the corresponding values $v^{(k)}, \Omega^{(k)}(v^{(k)})$, and $s_i^{(k)}$'s, based on the newly updated $u_j$'s, which also give us the value of $V_{\min}$ and $V_{\max}$.
7:         Compute $V_{\min}/V_{\max}$.
8:     **end for**
9:     Pick the $u_j^{(k)} \notin \Omega^{(k-1)}(v^{(k-1)})$ that gives the maximal value of $V_{\min}/V_{\max}$ in the above loop.
10:     **if** The value of $V_{\min}/V_{\max}$ decreases **then**
11:         Go back to $u_j^{(k-1)}$.
12:     **end if**
13: **until** The increment of $V_{\min}/V_{\max}$ is less than $\Delta$.

---

# 5 Simulations

In the previous section, the optimal projections for both the special cases and the general case are provided. The simulations will follow the same order. The simulations are about the comparison of the Monte Carlo method and our method for the special cases and then for a general case.

According to [7], Monte Carlo method is to select some random directions, denoted as $w_i$, $i = 1, \ldots, n$, on the unit sphere $S^{p-1}$ and project the vector we would like to estimate, that is $v$, along these directions, so the norm of the vector $v$ could be estimated as

$$\|v\| \approx C_p' \frac{1}{n} \sum_{i=1}^n |w_i^T v|,$$

where $C'_p = \frac{\sqrt{\pi}\,\Gamma(\frac{p+1}{2})}{\Gamma(\frac{p}{2})}$.

In all the experiments, we randomly select 100 unit vectors on the sphere as the vectors that we would like to estimate, in order to get the mean squared error for comparison between the Monte Carlo method and the method we propose.

## 5.1   When the Dimension is 2

When the dimension is equal to 2, the exact solution can be found as well as the mean squared error rate. So we randomly select 100 unit vectors on the sphere as the vectors that we would like to estimate. For both the Monte Carlo method and our optimal projection method, we calculate the mean squared error over these 100 vectors. More specifically, the squared error between the true norm of the vector, which is 1, and the estimated norm is calculated for each of the 100 unit vectors when the number of directions is fixed. By taking the mean of the 100 squared errors from the previous step, we get the mean squared error for given number of directions. The number of directions used in our simulation is from 2 to 10,000. Figure 1 shows the comparison between our method and Monte Carlo method regarding the logarithm of the mean squared error and the number of projection directions. From the figure, we can see that our method performs better than the Monte Carlo, and the advantage becomes more obvious when the number of projection directions increases.

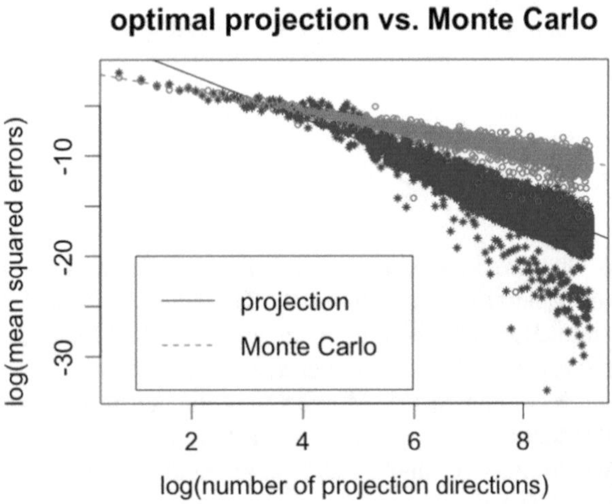

**Fig. 1** Optimal projection vs. Monte Carlo in the 2 dimensional case

## 5.2 When We Have $n = p$

When the dimension $p$ is equal to the number of projection directions $n$, recall that in Theorem 5, we give the exact solution of the pre-specified directions. Similar to what we have done in the 2-dimensional case, we randomly select 100 unit vectors on the sphere $S^{p-1}$, with dimension $p$ varying from 8 to 11. So the number of projection directions is varying from 8 to 11 correspondingly. We calculate the mean squared error of both the Monte Carlo method and our optimal projection method for each $p$ using the same strategy as before. The details are in Fig. 2, where the $x$-axis represents the dimension, and $y$-axis represents the mean squared error.

## 5.3 General Setting: $n > p$

When the dimension $p$ is larger than 2 and $n \neq p$, the exact solution of (9) can not be obtained. Therefore, we adopt the Algorithm 3. Like in previous simulations, we randomly select 100 unit vectors on the sphere $S^{p-1}$, with dimension $p$ varying from 3 to the number of directions minus 1, and the fixed number of directions to be 8, 9, 10, 11, respectively, and calculate the mean squared error of both the Monte Carlo method and our optimal projection method for each $p$ using the same strategy as before. Figures 3, 4, 5 and 6 show the comparison, where the $x$-axis represents the dimension, and $y$-axis represents the mean squared error.

Overall, we can see that our method performs better than the Monte Carlo method.

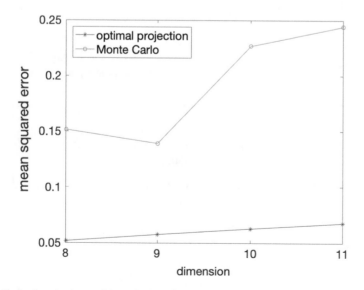

**Fig. 2** Optimal projection vs. Monte Carlo in the $n = p$ case

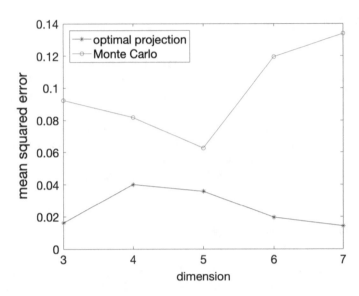

**Fig. 3** Optimal projection vs. Monte Carlo for dimension varying from 3 to 7 in the case $n = 8$

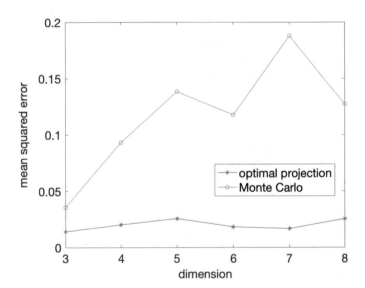

**Fig. 4** Optimal projection vs. Monte Carlo for dimension varying from 3 to 8 in the case $n = 9$

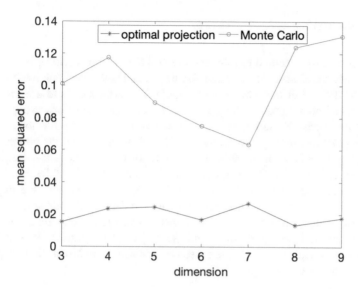

**Fig. 5** Optimal projection vs. Monte Carlo for dimension varying from 3 to 9 in the case $n = 10$

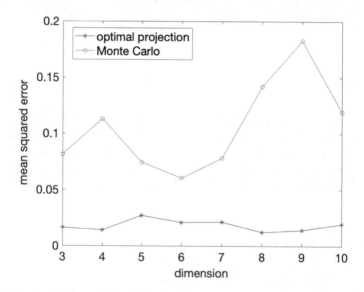

**Fig. 6** Optimal projection vs. Monte Carlo for dimension varying from 3 to 10 in the case $n = 11$

# 6 Conclusion

We propose a new method to calculate the distance, which is critical in computing the distance-based statistics, and can also be utilized in the calculation of the kernel functions that are distance-based and smooth. The main idea is to use the sum of the norms of the projections along a set of pre-calculated directions to approximate the original norm. By doing so, one can utilize the fast algorithm for univariate variables that has been proposed by [8]. The advantage is that the computational complexity is reduced from $O(m^2)$ to $O(m\log(m))$ where $m$ is the sample size. These pre-specified directions can be found by minimizing the difference between the estimated distance and the true value in the worst case. The associated problem is eventually a nonconvex optimization problem. We derive the exact solutions when dimension is equal to either 2 or the number of projection directions. In general cases, we propose an algorithm to find the projection directions. The simulations show the advantage of the proposed method versus the pure Monte Carlo approach, via comparing the mean squared errors.

**Acknowledgements** This project is partially supported by the Transdisciplinary Research Institute for Advancing Data Science (TRIAD), http://triad.gatech.edu, which is a part of the TRIPODS program at NSF and locates at Georgia Tech, enabled by the NSF grant CCF-1740776. Both authors are also partially supported by the NSF grant DMS-1613152.

# Appendix

All the proofs are included in this section, including a proof of Theorem 1, a proof of Theorem 2, a proof of Theorem 3, a proof of Theorem 4, a proof of Lemma 1, a proof of Lemma 2, a proof of Lemma 3, a proof of Theorem 5, a proof of Lemma 4, and a proof of Theorem 6. Some of these proofs involves detailed and potentially tedious derivations. We try to furnish as much details as deemed reasonable.

## *Proof of Theorem 1*

*Proof* By definition of $V_{\min}$ and $V_{\max}$, we have

$$C_n V_{\min} - 1 \le C_n \sum_{i=1}^{n} \left| u_i^T v \right| - 1 \le C_n V_{\max} - 1.$$

The above leads to the following

$$\max_{v:\|v\|_2=1} \left| C_n \sum_{i=1}^{n} |u_i^T v| - 1 \right| = \max \left\{ |C_n V_{\min} - 1|, |C_n V_{\max} - 1| \right\}. \quad (21)$$

Consider the right hand side of the above as a function of $C_n$, it is verifiable that the minimum is achieved when

$$1 - C_n V_{\min} = C_n V_{\max} - 1, \text{ which leads to, } C_n = \frac{2}{V_{\min} + V_{\max}}.$$

Bringing the above to (21), we have

$$\left| \frac{2}{V_{\min} + V_{\max}} V_{\min} - 1 \right| = \frac{V_{\max} - V_{\min}}{V_{\max} + V_{\min}} = \frac{2}{1 + \frac{V_{\min}}{V_{\max}}} - 1. \quad (22)$$

From the above, it is evident that minimizing the right hand of (22) is equivalent to the following

$$\max_{u_1,\dots,u_n:\|u_i\|_2=1} \frac{V_{\min}}{V_{\max}}.$$

From all the above, the lemma is proved. $\square$

## Proof of Theorem 2

**Proof** Without loss of generality, we assume $\theta_i = \alpha_i + k_i \pi$, where $\alpha_1 \leq \alpha_2 \leq \dots \leq \alpha_n \in [0, \pi)$. Then the problem in (9) can be written as

$$\max_{\alpha_i : i=1,\dots,n} \frac{\min_{\theta} f(\theta)}{\max_{\theta} f(\theta)},$$

where $f(\theta) = \sum_{i=1}^{n} |\cos(\alpha_i - \theta)|$.

Let $\delta_i = \alpha_{i+1} - \alpha_i$, $i = 1, \dots, n-1$, and $\delta_n = \alpha_1 - \alpha_n + \pi$. We have

$$\sum_{i=1}^{n} \delta_i = \pi.$$

For given $\alpha_i$, the minimum and the maximum of $f(\theta)$ satisfy

$$\frac{1}{n} \min_{\theta} f(\theta) \leq \frac{1}{n} f(\alpha_i - \frac{\pi}{2}), \text{ for } i = 1, \dots, n, \quad (23)$$

$$\frac{1}{n} \max_{\theta} f(\theta) \geq \frac{1}{n} f\left(\frac{\alpha_i + \alpha_{i+1}}{2} - \frac{\pi}{2}\right), \quad \text{for } i = 1, \ldots, n-1, \tag{24}$$

$$\frac{1}{n} \max_{\theta} f(\theta) \geq \frac{1}{n} f\left(\frac{\alpha_n + \alpha_1}{2}\right). \tag{25}$$

By summing up each side of (23) with $i$ from 1 through $n$, we get

$$\min_{\theta} f(\theta) \leq \frac{1}{n} \sum_{i=1}^{n} f\left(\alpha_i - \frac{\pi}{2}\right). \tag{26}$$

By summing up each side of (24) with $i$ from 1 through $n-1$ and adding it to (25), we have

$$\max_{\theta} f(\theta) \geq \frac{1}{n} \left[\sum_{i=1}^{n-1} f\left(\frac{\alpha_i + \alpha_{i+1}}{2} - \frac{\pi}{2}\right) + f\left(\frac{\alpha_n + \alpha_1}{2}\right)\right]. \tag{27}$$

Based on (26) and (27), for given $\alpha_i$, we have

$$\frac{\min_{\theta} f(\theta)}{\max_{\theta} f(\theta)} \leq \frac{\frac{1}{n} \sum_{i=1}^{n} f\left(\alpha_i - \frac{\pi}{2}\right)}{\frac{1}{n} \left[\sum_{i=1}^{n-1} f\left(\frac{\alpha_i + \alpha_{i+1}}{2} - \frac{\pi}{2}\right) + f\left(\frac{\alpha_n + \alpha_1}{2}\right)\right]}.$$

Therefore, one can verify the following:

$$\max_{\alpha_i : i=1,\ldots,n} \frac{\min_{\theta} f(\theta)}{\max_{\theta} f(\theta)} \leq \max_{\alpha_i : i=1,\ldots,n} \frac{\frac{1}{n} \sum_{i=1}^{n} f\left(\alpha_i - \frac{\pi}{2}\right)}{\frac{1}{n} \left[\sum_{i=1}^{n-1} f\left(\frac{\alpha_i + \alpha_{i+1}}{2} - \frac{\pi}{2}\right) + f\left(\frac{\alpha_n + \alpha_1}{2}\right)\right]}$$

$$= \max_{\alpha_i : i=1,\ldots,n} \frac{\sum_{i=1}^{n} f\left(\alpha_i - \frac{\pi}{2}\right)}{\left[\sum_{i=1}^{n-1} f\left(\frac{\alpha_i + \alpha_{i+1}}{2} - \frac{\pi}{2}\right) + f\left(\frac{\alpha_n + \alpha_1}{2}\right)\right]}. \tag{28}$$

Denote the numerator of the right hand side of (28) as $N_n$, and the denominator as $D_n$. Thus, we have

$$N_n = \begin{cases} 2\sum\limits_{i=1}^{n} |\sin \delta_i| + 2\sum\limits_{i=1}^{n-2} |\sin(\delta_i + \delta_{i+1})| + 2\sum\limits_{i=1}^{n-3} |\sin(\delta_i + \delta_{i+1} + \delta_{i+2})| + \dots \\ +2\sum\limits_{i=1}^{2} |\sin(\delta_i + \delta_{i+1} + \dots + \delta_{i+n-3})|, & \text{if } n \geq 4, \\ 2\sum\limits_{i=1}^{n} |\sin \delta_i| & \text{if } n = 3; \end{cases}$$

and

$$D_n = \sum_{i=1}^{n} 2\left|\sin\frac{\delta_i}{2}\right| + \sum_{i=2}^{n-1}\sum_{j=1}^{i-1}\left|\sin\left(\frac{\delta_i}{2} + \delta_{i-1} + \delta_{i-2} + \dots + \delta_j\right)\right|$$

$$+ \sum_{i=1}^{n-2}\sum_{j=i+1}^{n-1}\left|\sin\left(\frac{\delta_i}{2} + \delta_{i+1} + \dots + \delta_j\right)\right| + \sum_{j=2}^{n-1}\left|\sin\left(\frac{\delta_n}{2} + \delta_1 + \dots + \delta_{j-1}\right)\right|.$$

We would like to show that when all the $\theta_i$'s satisfies (10), $\dfrac{\min\limits_{\theta} f(\theta)}{\max\limits_{\theta} f(\theta)}$ is equal to the right hand side of (28), which means (10) is the optimal solution. In order to do that, we first need to figure out what value the right hand side of (28) is. In the following we use perturbation analysis to show that when $\delta_i = \frac{\pi}{n}$, which is equivalent to (10), the right hand side achieves the maximum value. And then we show that the left side is equal to the right side under the condition of (10). Therefore our proof can be completed.

For $n \geq 4$, $N_n$ and $D_n$ are treated as functions of $\Delta$. Then we have

$$N_n(\delta_1 + \Delta, \delta_2 - \Delta, \delta_3, \dots, \delta_n) = 2|\sin(\delta_1 + \Delta)| + 2|\sin(\delta_2 - \Delta)|$$

$$+2\sum_{j=3}^{n-1}\left|\sin\left(-\Delta + \sum_{i=2}^{j}\delta_i\right)\right| + Const,$$

and

$$\left.\frac{\partial N_n(\delta_1 + \Delta, \delta_2 - \Delta, \delta_3, \dots, \delta_n)}{\partial \Delta}\right|_{\Delta=0} = 2\cos\delta_1\,\mathrm{sign}(\sin\delta_1) - 2\cos\delta_2\,\mathrm{sign}(\sin\delta_2)$$

$$-2\sum_{j=3}^{n-1}\cos\left(\sum_{i=2}^{j}\delta_i\right)\mathrm{sign}\left(\sin\left(\sum_{i=2}^{j}\delta_i\right)\right).$$

When $\delta_i = \frac{\pi}{n}$, $i = 1, \dots, n$, we have

$$\frac{\partial N_n(\delta_1 + \Delta, \delta_2 - \Delta, \delta_3, \ldots, \delta_n)}{\partial \Delta}\bigg|_{\Delta=0}$$

$$= 0 - 2\sum_{j=3}^{n-1}\cos\left(\frac{(j-1)\pi}{n}\right)\text{sign}\left(\sin\left(\frac{(j-1)\pi}{n}\right)\right)$$

$$= 0. \tag{29}$$

Similarly, for $D_n$, we have

$$D_n(\delta_1 + \Delta, \delta_2 - \Delta, \delta_3, \ldots, \delta_n)$$

$$= 2\left|\sin\left(\frac{\delta_1 + \Delta}{2}\right)\right| + 2\left|\sin\left(\frac{\delta_2 - \Delta}{2}\right)\right| + \left|\sin\left(\frac{\Delta}{2} + \delta_1 + \frac{\delta_2}{2}\right)\right|$$

$$+ \sum_{j=3}^{n-1}\left|\sin\left(-\Delta + \sum_{i=2}^{j-1}\delta_i + \frac{\delta_j}{2}\right)\right| + \sum_{j=3}^{n}\left|\sin\left(-\frac{1}{2}\Delta + \frac{\delta_1}{2} + \sum_{i=2}^{j-1}\delta_i\right)\right|$$

$$+ \sum_{j=3}^{n-1}\left|\sin\left(-\frac{1}{2}\Delta + \frac{\delta_2}{2} + \sum_{i=3}^{j}\delta_i\right)\right| + \left|\sin\left(\frac{\delta_n}{2} + \delta_1 + \Delta\right)\right| + Const,$$

and

$$\frac{\partial D_n(\delta_1 + \Delta, \delta_2 - \Delta, \delta_3, \ldots, \delta_n)}{\partial \Delta}\bigg|_{\Delta=0}$$

$$= \cos\frac{\delta_1}{2}\text{sign}(\sin\frac{\delta_1}{2}) - \cos\frac{\delta_2}{2}\text{sign}(\sin\frac{\delta_2}{2}) + \frac{1}{2}\cos\left(\frac{\delta_2}{2} + \delta_1\right)\text{sign}\left(\sin\left(\frac{\delta_2}{2} + \delta_1\right)\right)$$

$$- \sum_{j=3}^{n-1}\cos\left(\sum_{i=2}^{j-1}\delta_i + \frac{\delta_j}{2}\right)\text{sign}\left(\sin\left(\sum_{i=2}^{j-1}\delta_i + \frac{\delta_j}{2}\right)\right)$$

$$- \frac{1}{2}\sum_{j=2}^{n-1}\cos\left(\frac{\delta_1}{2} + \sum_{i=2}^{j}\delta_i\right)\text{sign}\left(\sin\left(\frac{\delta_1}{2} + \sum_{i=2}^{j}\delta_i\right)\right)$$

$$- \frac{1}{2}\sum_{j=3}^{n-1}\cos\left(\frac{\delta_2}{2} + \sum_{i=3}^{j}\delta_i\right)\text{sign}\left(\sin\left(\frac{\delta_2}{2} + \sum_{i=3}^{j}\delta_i\right)\right)$$

$$+ \cos\left(\frac{\delta_n}{2} + \delta_1\right)\text{sign}\left(\sin\left(\frac{\delta_n}{2} + \delta_1\right)\right).$$

When $\delta_i = \frac{\pi}{n}$, $i = 1, \ldots, n$, we have

$$\frac{\partial D_n(\delta_1 + \Delta, \delta_2 - \Delta, \delta_3, \ldots, \delta_n)}{\partial \Delta}\bigg|_{\Delta=0}$$

$$= 0 + \frac{1}{2} \cos\left(\frac{3\pi}{2n}\right) \text{sign}\left(\sin\left(\frac{3\pi}{2n}\right)\right)$$

$$- \sum_{j=3}^{n-1} \cos\left(\frac{(2j-3)\pi}{2n}\right) \text{sign}\left(\sin\left(\frac{(2j-3)\pi}{2n}\right)\right)$$

$$- \frac{1}{2} \sum_{j=2}^{n-1} \cos\left(\frac{(2j-1)\pi}{2n}\right) \text{sign}\left(\sin\left(\frac{(2j-1)\pi}{2n}\right)\right)$$

$$- \frac{1}{2} \sum_{j=3}^{n-1} \cos\left(\frac{(2j-3)\pi}{2n}\right) \text{sign}\left(\sin\left(\frac{(2j-3)\pi}{2n}\right)\right)$$

$$+ \cos\left(\frac{3\pi}{2n}\right) \text{sign}\left(\sin\left(\frac{3\pi}{2n}\right)\right)$$

$$= 0. \tag{30}$$

Define $g(\Delta)$ as the following

$$g(\Delta) = \frac{N_n(\delta_1 + \Delta, \delta_2 - \Delta, \delta_3, \ldots, \delta_n)}{D_n(\delta_1 + \Delta, \delta_2 - \Delta, \delta_3, \ldots, \delta_n)}.$$

Then we have

$$\frac{\partial g(\Delta)}{\partial \Delta}\bigg|_{\Delta=0} = \frac{N_n'\big|_{\Delta=0}}{D_n(0)} - \frac{N_n(0) D_n'\big|_{\Delta=0}}{D_n(0)^2},$$

where

$$N_n'\bigg|_{\Delta=0} = \frac{\partial N_n(\delta_1 + \Delta, \delta_2 - \Delta, \delta_3, \ldots, \delta_n)}{\partial \Delta}\bigg|_{\Delta=0},$$

$$D_n'\bigg|_{\Delta=0} = \frac{\partial D_n(\delta_1 + \Delta, \delta_2 - \Delta, \delta_3, \ldots, \delta_n)}{\partial \Delta}\bigg|_{\Delta=0};$$

$$N_n(0) = N_n(\delta_1, \delta_2, \delta_3, \ldots, \delta_n),$$

$$D_n(0) = D_n(\delta_1, \delta_2, \delta_3, \ldots, \delta_n).$$

According to (29) and (30), we have

$$N_n'\bigg|_{\Delta=0} = D_n'\bigg|_{\Delta=0} = 0.$$

So we can get $\left.\frac{\partial g(\Delta)}{\partial \Delta}\right|_{\Delta=0} = 0 - 0 = 0$.

Similarly, for any two $\delta_i, \delta_j$, simply by giving some perturbation to them, we can get the same result as above. Therefore we can conclude that, for $n \geq 4$, $\{\delta_i = \frac{\pi}{n}, i = 1, \ldots, n\}$ can maximize the function $\frac{N_n}{D_n}$. Furthermore, we can get the maximum of $\frac{N_n}{D_n}$ by letting each $\delta_i$ be $\frac{\pi}{n}$:

$$\left(\frac{N_n}{D_n}\right)_{max} = \frac{2n \sin \frac{\pi}{n} + 2 \sum\limits_{r=2}^{n-2} (n-r) \sin \frac{r\pi}{n}}{2n \sin \frac{\pi}{n} + \sum\limits_{r=1}^{n-2} [2(n-r) - 1] \sin \frac{(2r+1)\pi}{2n}}. \tag{31}$$

Next, we would like to show that when $\delta_i = \frac{\pi}{n}, i = 1, \ldots, n$, we have

$$\frac{\min\limits_{\theta} f(\theta)}{\max\limits_{\theta} f(\theta)} = \left(\frac{N_n}{D_n}\right)_{max}.$$

As $f(\theta) = \sum\limits_{i=1}^{n} \left|\cos\left(\theta - \frac{(i-1)\pi}{n}\right)\right|$, we know $f(\theta) = f\left(\theta - \frac{\pi}{n}\right)$. So we only need to consider $\theta \in [0, \frac{\pi}{n}]$ to get the maximum.

Recall $f(\theta)$ is linear, so the minimum and maximum must be either $\theta = 0$ or $\theta = \frac{\pi}{n}$. By observing the periodicity of the function $f(\theta)$, we can get

$$\min\limits_{\theta} f(\theta) = \begin{cases} f(0) = 2 \sum\limits_{r=1}^{a-1} \sin \frac{r\pi}{2a} + 1 & \text{if } n = 2a, \\ f\left(\frac{\pi}{2(2a+1)}\right) = 2 \sum\limits_{r=1}^{a} \sin \frac{r\pi}{2a+1} & \text{if } n = 2a + 1. \end{cases}$$

$$\max\limits_{\theta} f(\theta) = \begin{cases} f\left(\frac{\pi}{4a}\right) = 2 \sum\limits_{r=1}^{a} \sin \frac{(2r-1)\pi}{4a} & \text{if } n = 2a. \\ f(0) = 2 \sum\limits_{r=1}^{a} \sin \frac{(2r-1)\pi}{2(2a+1)} + 1 & \text{if } n = 2a + 1, \end{cases}$$

From (31) we can get

$$\left(\frac{N_n}{D_n}\right)_{max} = \begin{cases} \dfrac{2 \sum\limits_{r=1}^{a-1} \sin \frac{r\pi}{2a} + 1}{2 \sum\limits_{r=1}^{a} \sin \frac{(2r-1)\pi}{4a}} & \text{if } n = 2a. \\ \dfrac{2 \sum\limits_{r=1}^{a} \sin \frac{r\pi}{2a+1}}{2 \sum\limits_{r=1}^{a} \sin \frac{(2r-1)\pi}{2(2a+1)} + 1} & \text{if } n = 2a + 1, \end{cases} \tag{32}$$

Therefore, we can conclude that when $\delta_i = \frac{\pi}{n}, i = 1, \ldots, n$,

$$\frac{\min\limits_{\theta} f(\theta)}{\max\limits_{\theta} f(\theta)} = \left(\frac{N_n}{D_n}\right)_{\max}.$$

Recall the definition of $\delta_i$'s, we know that (10) is the optimal solution for $n \geq 4$.

For $n = 3$ and 2, by applying the similar strategy, we can get the same result as above. $\qquad\square$

## Propositions We Need in Order to Prove Theorem 3

Before proceeding to the proof of Theorem 3, we need the following Propositions 1 and 2:

**Proposition 1**

$$\sum_{s=1}^{n-1} \sin \frac{s}{n}\pi = cot\frac{\pi}{2n},$$

$$\sum_{s=1}^{n-1} \cos \frac{s}{n}\pi = 0,$$

$$\sum_{s=1}^{n-1} s \sin \frac{s}{n}\pi = \frac{n}{2}cot\frac{\pi}{2n},$$

$$\sum_{s=1}^{n-1} s \cos \frac{s}{n}\pi = -\frac{1}{2}cot^2\frac{\pi}{2n} + \frac{n-1}{2},$$

$$\sum_{s=1}^{n-1} s^2 \cos \frac{s}{n}\pi = -\frac{n}{2}cot^2\frac{\pi}{2n} + \frac{n(n-1)}{2}.$$

**Proof** As the following holds true

$$\sin \frac{s\pi}{N} \sin \frac{\pi}{2n} = \frac{1}{2}\left(\cos \frac{(2s-1)\pi}{2n} - \cos \frac{(2s+1)\pi}{2n}\right),$$

we have

$$\left( \sum_{s=1}^{n-1} \sin \frac{s}{n}\pi \right) \cdot \sin \frac{\pi}{2n}$$

$$= \frac{1}{2} \sum_{s=1}^{n-1} \left( \cos \frac{(2s-1)\pi}{2n} - \cos \frac{(2s+1)\pi}{2n} \right)$$

$$= \frac{1}{2} \left( \cos \frac{\pi}{2n} - \cos \frac{(2n-1)\pi}{2n} \right) = \cos \frac{\pi}{2n}.$$

So by dividing $\sin \frac{\pi}{2n}$ for both sides, we can get

$$\sum_{s=1}^{n-1} \sin \frac{s}{n}\pi = \cot \frac{\pi}{2n}. \tag{33}$$

As we also have

$$\cos \frac{s\pi}{N} \sin \frac{\pi}{2n} = \frac{1}{2} \left( \sin \frac{(2s+1)\pi}{2n} - \sin \frac{(2s-1)\pi}{2n} \right).$$

Therefore, we can get

$$\left( \sum_{s=1}^{n-1} \cos \frac{s}{n}\pi \right) \cdot \sin \frac{\pi}{2n}$$

$$= \frac{1}{2} \sum_{s=1}^{n-1} \left( \sin \frac{(2s+1)\pi}{2n} - \sin \frac{(2s-1)\pi}{2n} \right) = \frac{1}{2} \left( \sin \frac{(2n-1)\pi}{2n} - \sin \frac{\pi}{2n} \right) = 0,$$

which implies

$$\sum_{s=1}^{n-1} \cos \frac{s}{n}\pi = 0. \tag{34}$$

As we also have

$$\sin \frac{s}{n}\pi \cdot \sin \frac{\pi}{2n} = \cos \frac{(2s-1)\pi}{2n} - \cos \frac{(2s+1)\pi}{2n},$$

the following can be derived:

$$\left( \sum_{s=1}^{n-1} s \sin \frac{s}{n}\pi \right) \cdot \sin \frac{\pi}{2n} = \frac{1}{2} \sum_{s=1}^{n-1} s \cdot \left( \cos \frac{(2s-1)\pi}{2n} - \cos \frac{(2s+1)\pi}{2n} \right). \tag{35}$$

Since we have

$$\sum_{s=1}^{n-1} s \cdot \left( \cos \frac{(2s-1)\pi}{2n} - \cos \frac{(2s+1)\pi}{2n} \right)$$

$$= \sum_{s=1}^{n-1} \cos \frac{(2s-1)\pi}{2n} - (n-1) \cos \frac{(2n-1)\pi}{2n}$$

$$= \sum_{s=1}^{n-1} \left( \cos \frac{s}{n}\pi \cos \frac{\pi}{2n} + \sin \frac{s}{n}\pi \sin \frac{\pi}{2n} \right) + (n-1) \cos \frac{\pi}{2n},$$

by plugging the above as well as (33) and (34) into (35), we can get

$$\left( \sum_{s=1}^{n-1} s \sin \frac{s}{n}\pi \right) \cdot \sin \frac{\pi}{2n}$$

$$= \frac{1}{2} \left( \sum_{s=1}^{n-1} \left( \cos \frac{s}{n}\pi \cos \frac{\pi}{2n} + \sin \frac{s}{n}\pi \sin \frac{\pi}{2n} \right) + (n-1) \cos \frac{\pi}{2n} \right)$$

$$= \frac{1}{2} \left( 0 + \cos \frac{\pi}{2n} \right) + \frac{n-1}{2} \cos \frac{\pi}{2n} = \frac{n}{2} \cos \frac{\pi}{2n}. \tag{36}$$

Similarly, since we have

$$\cos \frac{s}{n}\pi \cdot \sin \frac{\pi}{2n} = \sin \frac{(2s+1)\pi}{2n} - \sin \frac{(2s-1)\pi}{2n},$$

by using the similar strategy, we can get

$$\left( \sum_{s=1}^{n-1} s \cos \frac{s}{n}\pi \right) \cdot \sin \frac{\pi}{2n} = -\frac{1}{2} \cos \frac{\pi}{2n} \cot \frac{\pi}{2n} + \frac{n-1}{2} \sin \frac{\pi}{2n}. \tag{37}$$

Therefore, dividing both Eqs. (36) and (37), we can get

$$\sum_{s=1}^{n-1} s \sin \frac{s}{n}\pi = \frac{n}{2} \cot \frac{\pi}{2n}, \tag{38}$$

$$\sum_{s=1}^{n-1} s \cos \frac{s}{n}\pi = -\frac{1}{2} \cot^2 \frac{\pi}{2n} + \frac{n-1}{2}. \tag{39}$$

Since the following holds true,

$$\left(\sum_{s=1}^{n-1} s^2 \cos \frac{s}{n}\pi\right) \cdot \sin \frac{\pi}{2n} = \frac{1}{2}\left\{-\sum_{s=1}^{n-1}(2s-1)\sin \frac{(2s-1)\pi}{2n} + (n-1)^2 \sin \frac{2n-1}{2n}\pi\right\},$$

by simplifying the above equation we can get

$$\left(\sum_{s=1}^{n-1} s^2 \cos \frac{s}{n}\pi\right) \cdot \sin \frac{\pi}{2n}$$

$$= -\sum_{s=1}^{n-1} s\left(\sin \frac{s}{n}\pi \cos \frac{\pi}{2n} - \cos \frac{s}{n}\pi \sin \frac{\pi}{2n}\right) + \frac{1}{2}\sum_{s=1}^{n-1}\left(\sin \frac{s}{n}\pi \cos \frac{\pi}{2n} - \cos \frac{s}{n}\pi \sin \frac{\pi}{2n}\right)$$

$$+ \frac{(n-1)^2}{2}\sin \frac{\pi}{2n}$$

$$= -\left(\sum_{s=1}^{n-1} s \sin \frac{s}{n}\pi\right)\cos \frac{\pi}{2n} + \left(\sum_{s=1}^{n-1} s \cos \frac{s}{n}\pi\right)\sin \frac{\pi}{2n} + \frac{1}{2}\left(\sum_{s=1}^{n-1} \sin \frac{s}{n}\pi\right)\cos \frac{\pi}{2n}$$

$$- \frac{1}{2}\left(\sum_{s=1}^{n-1} \cos \frac{s}{n}\pi\right)\sin \frac{\pi}{2n} + \frac{(n-1)^2}{2}\sin \frac{\pi}{2n}.$$

Plugging (33), (34), (38), and (39) into the above, we can get

$$\left(\sum_{s=1}^{n-1} s^2 \cos \frac{s}{n}\pi\right) \cdot \sin \frac{\pi}{2n} = -\frac{1}{2}\cot^2 \frac{\pi}{2n}\sin \frac{\pi}{2n} + \frac{n(n-1)}{2}\sin \frac{\pi}{2n}.$$

Therefore, dividing $\sin \frac{\pi}{2n}$ on each side, we get

$$\sum_{s=1}^{n-1} s^2 \cos \frac{s}{n}\pi = -\frac{n}{2}\cot^2 \frac{\pi}{2n} + \frac{n(n-1)}{2}.$$

$\square$

**Proposition 2**

$$2\sum_{s=1}^{n-1}(n-s)f(s) = \frac{n}{\pi}\cot \frac{\pi}{2n} + \frac{1}{2}\cot^2 \frac{\pi}{2n} - \frac{n}{2} + \frac{1}{2}.$$

***Proof*** According to the definition of function $f(s)$ in (42), we have

$$2 \sum_{s=1}^{n-1} (n-s) f(s)$$

$$= 2 \sum_{s=1}^{n-1} (n-s) \left( \frac{1}{\pi} \sin \frac{s}{n} \pi + \left( \frac{1}{2} - \frac{s}{n} \right) \cos \frac{s}{n} \pi \right)$$

$$= \frac{2n}{\pi} \sum_{s=1}^{n-1} \sin \frac{s}{n} \pi - \frac{2}{\pi} \sum_{s=1}^{n-1} s \sin \frac{s}{n} \pi + n \sum_{s=1}^{n-1} \cos \frac{s}{n} \pi - 3 \sum_{s=1}^{n-1} s \cos \frac{s}{n} \pi + \frac{2}{n} \sum_{s=1}^{n-1} s^2 \cos \frac{s}{n} \pi.$$

Applying Proposition 1, we have

$$2 \sum_{s=1}^{n-1} (n-s) f(s) = \frac{n}{\pi} \cot \frac{\pi}{2n} + \frac{1}{2} \cot^2 \frac{\pi}{2n} - \frac{n}{2} + \frac{1}{2}.$$

$\square$

## *Proof of Theorem 3*

***Proof*** Recall that $u_i$ can be rewritten as

$$u_i = e^{\sqrt{-1} \frac{i\pi}{n}}, i = 0, 1, \ldots, n-1.$$

And we have

$$\underset{v \sim \text{Unif}(S^1)}{\mathbb{E}} \left\{ \left| C_n \sum_{i=1}^{n} \left| u_i^T v \right| - 1 \right|^2 \right\}$$

$$= C_n^2 \underset{v \sim \text{Unif}(S^1)}{\mathbb{E}} \left\{ \left( \sum_{i=1}^{n} \left| u_i^T v \right| \right)^2 \right\} - 2 C_n \underset{v \sim \text{Unif}(S^1)}{\mathbb{E}} \left\{ \sum_{i=1}^{n} \left| u_i^T v \right| \right\} + 1$$

$$= C_n^2 \sum_{i=1}^{n} \underset{v \sim \text{Unif}(S^1)}{\mathbb{E}} \left( \left| u_i^T v \right|^2 \right) + 2 C_n^2 \sum_{1 \le i < j \le N} \underset{v \sim \text{Unif}(S^1)}{\mathbb{E}} \left( \left| u_i^T v \right| \left| u_j^T v \right| \right)$$

$$- 2 C_n \sum_{i=1}^{n} \underset{v \sim \text{Unif}(S^1)}{\mathbb{E}} \left\{ \left| u_i^T v \right| \right\} + 1. \qquad (40)$$

So we will find out the expected squared error, if for all $i, j = 1, \ldots, n$, we can get the values of

$$\mathop{\mathbb{E}}_{v\sim\mathrm{Unif}(S^1)}\left(\left|u_i^T v\right|^2\right), \qquad \mathop{\mathbb{E}}_{v\sim\mathrm{Unif}(S^1)}\left(\left|u_i^T v\right|\left|u_j^T v\right|\right), \qquad \mathop{\mathbb{E}}_{v\sim\mathrm{Unif}(S^1)}\left\{\left|u_i^T v\right|\right\}.$$

In order to calculate $\mathop{\mathbb{E}}_{v\sim\mathrm{Unif}(S^1)}\left(\left|u_i^T v\right|^2\right)$, we let $u_i = (1,0)'$ and $v = (\cos\theta, \sin\theta)'$ without loss of generality. Then,

$$\mathop{\mathbb{E}}_{v\sim\mathrm{Unif}(S^1)}\left(\left|u_i^T v\right|^2\right) = \mathop{\mathbb{E}}_{\theta\sim\mathrm{Unif}(0,2\pi)}\cos^2\theta = \frac{1}{2} + \frac{1}{2}\mathop{\mathbb{E}}_{\theta\sim\mathrm{Unif}(0,2\pi)}\cos 2\theta = \frac{1}{2}.$$

Without loss of generality, assume $\langle u_i, u_j \rangle = \frac{s}{n}\pi$, for all $1 \le i, j \le n, i \ne j$, which means we can assume

$$u_i = (1,0)', u_j = (\cos\frac{s}{n}\pi, \sin\frac{s}{n}\pi)', s = 1, 2, \ldots, n-1.$$

Therefore, we have

$$\left|u_i^T v\right| \cdot \left|u_j^T v\right| = |\cos\theta|\left|\cos\theta\cos\frac{s}{n}\pi + \sin\theta\sin\frac{s}{n}\pi\right|$$
$$= \left|\cos^2\theta\cos\frac{s}{n}\pi + \cos\theta\sin\theta\sin\frac{s}{n}\pi\right|.$$

As the following equations hold,

$$\cos^2\theta = \frac{1+\cos 2\theta}{2} \text{ and } \cos\theta\sin\theta = \frac{\sin 2\theta}{2},$$

quantity $\left|u_i^T v\right| \cdot \left|u_j^T v\right|$ can be further written as

$$\left|u_i^T v\right| \cdot \left|u_j^T v\right| = \frac{1}{2}\left|\cos 2\theta\cos\frac{s}{n}\pi + \sin 2\theta\sin\frac{s}{n}\pi + \cos\frac{s}{n}\pi\right|$$
$$= \frac{1}{2}\left|\cos\left(2\theta - \frac{s}{n}\pi\right) + \cos\frac{s}{n}\pi\right|.$$

So $\mathop{\mathbb{E}}_{v\sim\mathrm{Unif}(S^1)}\left(\left|u_i^T v\right| \cdot \left|u_j^T v\right|\right)$ can be rewritten as follows:

$$\mathop{\mathbb{E}}_{v\sim\mathrm{Unif}(S^1)}\left(\left|u_i^T v\right| \cdot \left|u_j^T v\right|\right)$$
$$= \frac{1}{2}\mathop{\mathbb{E}}_{\theta\sim\mathrm{Unif}(0,2\pi)}\left\{\left|\cos\left(2\theta - \frac{s}{n}\pi\right) + \cos\frac{s}{n}\pi\right|\right\}$$

$$= \frac{1}{2} \times \frac{1}{2\pi} \left( \int_0^\pi + \int_\pi^{2\pi} \right) \left| \cos\left(2\theta - \frac{s}{n}\pi\right) + \cos\frac{s}{n}\pi \right| d\theta.$$

As we have

$$\int_\pi^{2\pi} \left| \cos\left(2\theta - \frac{s}{n}\pi\right) + \cos\frac{s}{n}\pi \right| d\theta$$

$$= \int_0^\pi \left| \cos\left(2\theta - \frac{s}{n}\pi\right) + \cos\frac{s}{n}\pi \right| d\theta = \int_0^\pi \left| \cos(2\theta) + \cos\frac{s}{n}\pi \right| d\theta$$

$$= \int_{-\frac{\pi}{2}+\frac{s}{2n}\pi}^{\frac{\pi}{2}+\frac{s}{2n}\pi} \left| \cos(2\theta) + \cos\frac{s}{n}\pi \right| d\theta,$$

we can get

$$\mathop{\mathbb{E}}_{v\sim\text{Unif}(S^1)} \left( \left| u_i^T v \right| \cdot \left| u_j^T v \right| \right) = \frac{1}{2\pi} \int_{-\frac{\pi}{2}+\frac{s}{2n}\pi}^{\frac{\pi}{2}-\frac{s}{2n}\pi} \left| \cos(2\theta) + \cos\frac{s}{n}\pi \right| d\theta. \qquad (41)$$

By breaking the integral interval $(-\frac{\pi}{2}+\frac{s}{2n}\pi, \frac{\pi}{2}+\frac{s}{2n}\pi)$ into two subintervals, $(-\frac{\pi}{2}+\frac{s}{2n}\pi, \frac{\pi}{2}-\frac{s}{2n}\pi)$ and $(\frac{\pi}{2}-\frac{s}{2n}\pi, \frac{\pi}{2}+\frac{s}{2n}\pi)$, we have

$$\left| \cos 2\theta + \cos\frac{s}{n}\pi \right| = \begin{cases} \cos 2\theta + \cos\frac{s}{n}\pi, & \theta \in (-\frac{\pi}{2}+\frac{s}{2n}\pi, \frac{\pi}{2}-\frac{s}{2n}\pi), \\ -\left(\cos 2\theta + \cos\frac{s}{n}\pi\right), & \theta \in (\frac{\pi}{2}-\frac{s}{2n}\pi, \frac{\pi}{2}+\frac{s}{2n}\pi). \end{cases}$$

Combining (41), we get

$$\mathop{\mathbb{E}}_{v\sim\text{Unif}(S^1)} \left( \left| u_i^T v \right| \cdot \left| u_j^T v \right| \right)$$

$$= \frac{1}{2\pi} \left( \int_{-\frac{\pi}{2}+\frac{s}{2n}\pi}^{\frac{\pi}{2}-\frac{s}{2n}\pi} + \int_{\frac{\pi}{2}-\frac{s}{2n}\pi}^{\frac{\pi}{2}+\frac{s}{2n}\pi} \right) \left| \cos 2\theta + \cos\frac{s}{n}\pi \right| d\theta$$

$$= \frac{1}{2\pi} \left\{ \int_{-\frac{\pi}{2}+\frac{s}{2n}\pi}^{\frac{\pi}{2}-\frac{s}{2n}\pi} \left(\cos 2\theta + \cos\frac{s}{n}\pi\right) d\theta - \int_{\frac{\pi}{2}-\frac{s}{2n}\pi}^{\frac{\pi}{2}+\frac{s}{2n}\pi} \left(\cos 2\theta + \cos\frac{s}{n}\pi\right) d\theta \right\}$$

$$= \frac{1}{2\pi} \left\{ 2\sin\frac{s}{n}\pi + \left(\pi - \frac{2s}{N}\pi\right) \cos\frac{s}{n}\pi \right\}$$

$$= \frac{1}{\pi} \sin\frac{s}{n}\pi + \left(\frac{1}{2} - \frac{s}{n}\right) \cos\frac{s}{n}\pi.$$

If we define

$$f(s) = \frac{1}{\pi} \sin \frac{s}{n} \pi + \left( \frac{1}{2} - \frac{s}{n} \right) \cos \frac{s}{n} \pi, s = 0, 1, 2, \cdots, n-1. \quad (42)$$

Then we will get

$$\mathop{\mathbb{E}}_{v \sim \text{Unif}(S^1)} \left( \left| u_i^T v \right|^2 \right) = f(0),$$

$$\mathop{\mathbb{E}}_{v \sim \text{Unif}(S^1)} \left( \left| u_i^T v \right| \cdot \left| u_j^T v \right| \right) = f(s), \text{ where } \langle u_i, u_j \rangle = \frac{s}{n} \pi, s = 1, 2, \cdots, n-1.$$

$$(43)$$

Similarly, without loss of generality, if we assume $u_i = (1, 0)'$, $v = (\cos \theta, \sin \theta)'$, the following holds,

$$\mathop{\mathbb{E}}_{v \sim \text{Unif}(S^1)} \left\{ \left| u_i^T v \right| \right\} = \mathop{\mathbb{E}}_{\theta \sim \text{Unif}(-\pi, \pi)} |\cos \theta| = 2 \int_{-\frac{\pi}{2}}^{\frac{\pi}{2}} \frac{1}{2\pi} \cos \theta d\theta = \frac{2}{\pi}. \quad (44)$$

Recall that we have

$$C_n = \frac{2}{V_{\min} + V_{\max}}, \text{ where } V_{\min} = \min_{v: \|v\|=1} \sum_{i=1}^{n} \left| u_i^T v \right|, V_{\max} = \max_{v: \|v\|=1} \sum_{i=1}^{n} \left| u_i^T v \right|.$$

From (32) we can easily verify that

$$V_{\min} + V_{\max} = 2 \sum_{k=1}^{n-1} \sin \frac{k\pi}{2n} + 1.$$

Therefore, $C_n$ can be derived:

$$C_n = \frac{2}{2 \sum_{k=1}^{n-1} \sin \frac{k\pi}{2n} + 1}. \quad (45)$$

As we have

$$\sin \frac{k\pi}{2n} \cdot \sin \frac{\pi}{4n} = \frac{1}{2} \left( \cos \frac{(2k-1)\pi}{4n} - \cos \frac{(2k+1)\pi}{4n} \right),$$

we can get

$$\sin\frac{\pi}{4n}\left(\sum_{k=1}^{n-1}\sin\frac{k\pi}{2n}\right) = \frac{1}{2}\sum_{k=1}^{n-1}\left(\cos\frac{(2k-1)\pi}{4n} - \cos\frac{(2k+1)\pi}{4n}\right)$$

$$= \frac{1}{2}\left(\cos\frac{\pi}{4n} - \sin\frac{\pi}{4n}\right),$$

which leads to

$$\sum_{k=1}^{n-1}\sin\frac{k\pi}{2n} = \frac{\frac{1}{2}\left(\cos\frac{\pi}{4n} - \sin\frac{\pi}{4n}\right)}{\sin\frac{\pi}{4n}} = \frac{1}{2}\cot\frac{\pi}{4n} - \frac{1}{2}. \tag{46}$$

Therefore, by plugging (46) into (45), we have

$$C_n = \frac{2}{\cot\frac{\pi}{4n}} = 2\tan\frac{\pi}{4n}.$$

If we plug in (40) with (43) and (44), we can get

$$\mathop{\mathbb{E}}_{v\sim\text{Unif}(S^1)}\left\{\left|C_n\sum_{i=1}^{n}\left|u_i^T v\right| - 1\right|^2\right\}$$

$$= C_n^2\sum_{i=1}^{n}\mathop{\mathbb{E}}_{v\sim\text{Unif}(S^1)}\left(\left|u_i^T v\right|^2\right) + 2C_n^2\sum_{1\leq i<j\leq N}\mathop{\mathbb{E}}_{v\sim\text{Unif}(S^1)}\left(\left|u_i^T v\right|\left|u_j^T v\right|\right)$$

$$-2C_n\sum_{i=1}^{n}\mathop{\mathbb{E}}_{v\sim\text{Unif}(S^1)}\left\{\left|u_i^T v\right|\right\} + 1$$

$$= 4\tan^2\frac{\pi}{4n}\left(\frac{n}{2} + 2\sum_{s=1}^{n-1}(n-s)f(s)\right) - \frac{8N}{\pi}\tan\frac{\pi}{4n} + 1. \tag{47}$$

In order to calculate the part $\sum_{s=1}^{n-1}(n-s)f(s)$ in (47), we need the Proposition 2.
Applying Proposition 2 on (47), we get

$$\mathop{\mathbb{E}}_{v\sim\text{Unif}(S^1)}\left\{\left|C_n\sum_{i=1}^{n}\left|u_i^T v\right| - 1\right|^2\right\}$$

$$= 4\tan^2\frac{\pi}{4n}\left(\frac{n}{2} + \frac{n}{\pi}\cot\frac{\pi}{2n} + \frac{1}{2}\cot^2\frac{\pi}{2n} - \frac{n}{2} + \frac{1}{2}\right) - \frac{8n}{\pi}\tan\frac{\pi}{4n} + 1$$

$$= 2\tan^2\frac{\pi}{4n}\cot^2\frac{\pi}{2n} + \frac{4n}{\pi}\tan^2\frac{\pi}{4n}\cot\frac{\pi}{2n} + 2\tan^2\frac{\pi}{4n} - \frac{8n}{\pi}\tan\frac{\pi}{4n} + 1. \tag{48}$$

As $\tan x \to x$, as $x \to 0$, we can get

$$\mathop{\mathbb{E}}_{v\sim\text{Unif}(S^1)}\left\{\left|\left|C_n\sum_{i=1}^{n}\left|u_i^T v\right|-1\right|\right|^2\right\} \longrightarrow 2\frac{\pi^2}{16n^2}\frac{4n^2}{\pi^2}+\frac{4n}{\pi}\frac{\pi^2}{16n^2}\frac{2n}{\pi}+2\frac{\pi^2}{16n^2}-\frac{8n}{\pi}\frac{\pi}{4n}+1$$

$$=\frac{\pi^2}{8n^2}.$$

$\square$

## Proof of Theorem 4

**Proof** Monte Carlo method uses random directions to approximate the norm, which means

$$u_i \sim \text{Unif}(S^1),\, i.i.d.$$

We also know that

$$\mathop{\mathbb{E}}_{u_i,v\sim\text{Unif}(S^1)}\left\{\left|\left|C_n\sum_{i=1}^{n}\left|u_i^T v\right|-1\right|\right|^2\right\}$$

$$= C_n^2\mathop{\mathbb{E}}_{u_i,v\sim\text{Unif}(S^1)}\left\{\left(\sum_{i=1}^{n}\left|u_i^T v\right|\right)^2\right\}-2C_n\mathop{\mathbb{E}}_{u_i,v\sim\text{Unif}(S^1)}\left\{\sum_{i=1}^{n}\left|u_i^T v\right|\right\}+1$$

$$= C_n^2\sum_{i=1}^{n}\mathop{\mathbb{E}}_{u_i,v\sim\text{Unif}(S^1)}\left(\left|u_i^T v\right|^2\right)+2C_n^2\sum_{1\leq i<j\leq N}\mathop{\mathbb{E}}_{u_i,u_j,v\sim\text{Unif}(S^1)}\left(\left|u_i^T v\right|\left|u_j^T v\right|\right)$$

$$-2C_n\sum_{i=1}^{n}\mathop{\mathbb{E}}_{u_i,v\sim\text{Unif}(S^1)}\left\{\left|u_i^T v\right|\right\}+1, \tag{49}$$

where $C_n$ satisfies

$$C_n\cdot\int_{u_i\in S^1}\sum_{i=1}^{n}\left|u_i^T v\right|du_i = 1,$$

which implies

$$C_n = \frac{\pi}{2n}.$$

We can find out the expected squared error if we can get the values of

$$
\mathop{\mathbb{E}}_{u_i,v\sim\mathrm{Unif}(S^1)}\left(\left|u_i^T v\right|^2\right),
$$

$$
\mathop{\mathbb{E}}_{u_i,u_j,v\sim\mathrm{Unif}(S^1)}\left(\left|u_i^T v\right|\left|u_j^T v\right|\right),
$$

$$
\mathop{\mathbb{E}}_{u_i,v\sim\mathrm{Unif}(S^1)}\left\{\left|u_i^T v\right|\right\}, \quad \text{for all } i,j=1,\cdots,n.
$$

Let $u_i = (\cos\phi, \sin\phi)'$, $v = (\cos\theta, \sin\theta)'$, where $\phi \sim \mathrm{Unif}(0, 2\pi)$, $\theta \sim \mathrm{Unif}(0, 2\pi)$. Then the above three can be computed as follows:

$$
\mathop{\mathbb{E}}_{u_i,v\sim\mathrm{Unif}(S^1)}\left(\left|u_i^T v\right|^2\right)
$$

$$
= \mathop{\mathbb{E}}_{\phi,\theta\sim\mathrm{Unif}(0,2\pi)} \cos^2(\phi-\theta) = \mathop{\mathbb{E}}_{\phi\sim\mathrm{Unif}(0,2\pi)}\left[\mathop{\mathbb{E}}_{\theta\sim\mathrm{Unif}(0,2\pi)}\left[\cos^2(\phi-\theta)|\phi\right]\right]
$$

$$
= \frac{1}{2},
$$

and

$$
\mathop{\mathbb{E}}_{u_i,u_j,v\sim\mathrm{Unif}(S^1)}\left(\left|u_i^T v\right|\left|u_j^T v\right|\right)
$$

$$
= \mathop{\mathbb{E}}_{\phi_i,\phi_j,\theta\sim\mathrm{Unif}(0,2\pi)}\left\{\left|\cos(\theta-\phi_i)\right|\left|\cos(\theta-\phi_j)\right|\right\}
$$

$$
= \mathop{\mathbb{E}}_{\phi_j,\theta\sim\mathrm{Unif}(0,2\pi)}\left\{\mathop{\mathbb{E}}_{\phi_i\sim\mathrm{Unif}(0,2\pi)}\left[\left|\cos(\theta-\phi_i)\right|\,[\left|\cos(\theta-\phi_j)\right|\,|\phi_j,\theta\right]\right\}
$$

$$
= \mathop{\mathbb{E}}_{\phi_j,\theta\sim\mathrm{Unif}(0,2\pi)}\left\{\left|\cos(\theta-\phi_j)\right|\cdot\frac{2}{\pi}\right\}
$$

$$
= \mathop{\mathbb{E}}_{\theta\sim\mathrm{Unif}(0,2\pi)}\left\{\mathop{\mathbb{E}}_{\phi_j\sim\mathrm{Unif}(0,2\pi)}\left[\left|\cos(\theta-\phi_j)\right|\cdot\frac{2}{\pi}|\theta\right]\right\} = \mathop{\mathbb{E}}_{\theta\sim\mathrm{Unif}(0,2\pi)}\left[\frac{2}{\pi}\cdot\frac{2}{\pi}\right]
$$

$$
= \frac{4}{\pi^2},
$$

and

$$\mathop{\mathbb{E}}_{u_i, v \sim \text{Unif}(S^1)} \left\{ \left| u_i^T v \right| \right\}$$

$$= \mathop{\mathbb{E}}_{\phi, \theta \sim \text{Unif}(0, 2\pi)} |\cos(\phi - \theta)| = \mathop{\mathbb{E}}_{\phi \sim \text{Unif}(0, 2\pi)} \left[ \mathop{\mathbb{E}}_{\theta \sim \text{Unif}(0, 2\pi)} \left[ |\cos(\phi - \theta)| \, |\phi| \right] \right]$$

$$= \mathop{\mathbb{E}}_{\phi \sim \text{Unif}(0, 2\pi)} \frac{2}{\pi} = \frac{2}{\pi}.$$

Therefore by plugging the above results into (49), we eventually get

$$\mathop{\mathbb{E}}_{u_i, v \sim \text{Unif}(S^1)} \left\{ \left| C_n \sum_{i=1}^{n} \left| u_i^T v \right| - 1 \right|^2 \right\}$$

$$= \frac{\pi^2}{4N^2} \left( N \cdot \frac{1}{2} + 2 \frac{N(N-1)}{2} \frac{4}{\pi^2} \right) - 2 \frac{\pi}{2n} \cdot N \cdot \frac{2}{\pi} + 1 = \frac{\pi^2 - 8}{8N}.$$

$\square$

## Proof of Lemma 1

*Proof* Recall that we have

$$V_{\max} = \max_{v: \|v\|_2 = 1} \sum_{i=1}^{n} \left| u_i^T v \right| = \max_{v: \|v\|_2 = 1} \max_{s_i \in \{1, -1\}} \left( \sum_{i=1}^{n} s_i u_i^T \right) v, \qquad (50)$$

where the second equality is based on a standard trick in optimization [2, Chapter 9.2(ii)].

The following is an application of the Cauchy-Schwartz inequality:

$$\left( \sum_{i=1}^{n} s_i u_i^T \right) v \leq \sqrt{ \left\| \sum_{i=1}^{n} s_i u_i \right\|_2^2 \|v\|_2^2 } = \left\| \sum_{i=1}^{n} s_i u_i \right\|,$$

where the equality is due to the condition $\|v\| = 1$.

In the first part, the equality holds if and only if $|v_j| = c \left| \left( \sum_{i=1}^{n} s_i u_i \right)_j \right|, j = 1, \ldots, p.$

Apparently, we must have $c = \left\| \sum_{i=1}^{n} s_i u_i \right\|^{-1}$ (because of $\|v\| = 1$).

So we can have

$$v = \frac{\sum\limits_{i=1}^{n} s_i u_i}{\left\| \sum\limits_{i=1}^{n} s_i u_i \right\|}. \tag{51}$$

Combining (51) and (50), we have (11). $\qquad\qquad\qquad\qquad\qquad\qquad\qquad\square$

## Proof of Lemma 2

**Proof** We start with a special case: the linear subspace is $\mathbb{R}^p$ (the entire space). Obviously the $n$ hyperplanes

$$\left\{ y : u_i^T y = 0 \right\}, \text{ for } i = 1, 2, \ldots, n$$

divide the sphere $S^{p-1}$ into at most $2^n$ sectors. Within each sector, function $f(v)$ is strictly linear, therefore the minima cannot be an interior point. Recall a boundary point $v$ must have $u_j^T v = 0$ for at least one $j$, $1 \leq j \leq n$.

Now we consider a linear subspace with dimension less than $p$, say, $k$. Let $b_1, \ldots, b_k$ be the orthonormal basis of such a linear subspace, we have $\forall x \in \Omega$,

$$x = \sum_{j=1}^{k} c_j b_j,$$

and

$$\sum_{j=1}^{k} c_j^2 = 1, \text{ (Because we have } \|x\| = 1).$$

Therefore, we have

$$f(v) = \sum_{i=1}^{n} \left| u_i^T v \right| = \sum_{i=1}^{n} \left| u_i^T \sum_{j=1}^{k} c_j b_j \right| = \sum_{i=1}^{n} \left| \sum_{j=1}^{k} c_j (u_i^T b_j) \right| = \sum_{i=1}^{n} \left| h_i^T c \right|,$$

where $c = (c_1, \ldots, c_k)^T$ and $h_i^T = \left( u_i^T b_1, \ldots, u_i^T b_k \right)$, $i = 1, \ldots, n$. Note that in the early part of this proof, the $u_i$ can be arbitrary.

The above derivation indicates that the latter case can be converted into the former case, as $c \in \mathbb{R}^k$ is from the entire space. So we can get

$$h_i^T c = 0 \text{ for at least one } i, 1 \leq i \leq n.$$

Since we have $h_i^T c = u_i^T \left( \sum_{j=1}^{k} b_j c_j \right)$, the above is equivalent to

$$u_i^T \left( \sum_{j=1}^{k} b_j c_j \right) = 0 \text{ for at least one } i, \ 1 \le i \le n.$$

Quantity $\sum_{j=1}^{k} b_j c_j$ can also be denoted as $v$, because any vector on the space is a linear combination of the orthonormal basis $b_1, \ldots, b_k$.

From all the above, we proved the lemma.                                                                          $\square$

## Proof of Lemma 3

**Proof** For notational simplicity, let us donate $\Omega = \Omega(v_{\min})$. We can easily verify the following

$$\text{rank}(\Omega) \le p - 1.$$

Otherwise (i.e., $\text{rank}(\Omega) = p$), by the definition of $\Omega$, we will have $v_{\min} = 0$. Now we show that

$$\text{rank}(\Omega) \ge p - 1.$$

We use contradiction. Let us assume that $\text{rank}(\Omega) < p - 1$. Define the following complementary set

$$\Omega^{\perp} = \{x : \|x\| = 1, x \perp \Omega\},$$

where $x \perp \Omega$ stands for that $x$ is perpendicular to the linear space that is spanned by all the $u_j$'s in $\Omega$. Because $v_{\min}$ is a minimizer, we have that

$$f(v_{\min}) = \min_{v \in \Omega^{\perp}} f(v) = \min_{v \in \Omega^{\perp}} \sum_{i=1}^{n} \left| u_i^T v \right| = \min_{v \in \Omega^{\perp}} \sum_{u_i \notin \Omega} \left| u_i^T v \right|$$

Note that if $\text{rank}(\Omega) < p - 1$, we have $\dim(\Omega^{\perp}) \ge 2$.

By Lemma 2, we can declare that there exists $u_j \notin \Omega$, $u_j^T v_{\min} = 0$. However, this contradicts to the definition of $\Omega$, which is supposed to be the maximal subset.
$\square$

## *Proof of Theorem 5*

***Proof*** When $n = p$, we have

$$f(v) = |u_1^T v| + |u_2^T v| + \ldots + |u_p^T v|, \text{ for } u_1, \ldots u_p, v \in \mathbb{S}^{p-1}.$$

According to the Lemma 3, we have

$$\text{rank} \left( \Omega(v_{\min}) \right) = p - 1,$$

where $\Omega(v_{\min}) = \left\{ u_j : u_j^T v_{\min} = 0 \right\}$, and $v_{\min}$ is the minimizer of $f(v)$. So the minimizer of $f(v)$ must satisfy that it is orthogonal to $p - 1$ linearly independent $u_j$'s.

Assume every $p - 1$ $u_j$'s are linearly independent. Then the minimizer is among the vectors that are orthogonal to any $p - 1$ $u_j$'s. We know there are $\binom{p}{p-1} = p$ different combinations of $u_j$'s, and each combination is correspond to 2 unit vectors orthogonal to one of the $p - 1$ $u_j$'s. (These 2 unit vectors are the two directions that are orthogonal to a $p - 1$ spaces in $\mathbb{R}^p$.) Thus there are totally $2p$ unit vectors that might be the minimizer of $f(v)$.

Suppose $p$ of the $2p$ unit vectors are those whose first nonzero entry is positive. Denote them as $v^{-(1)}, v^{-(2)}, \ldots, v^{-(p)}$. Then the other $p$ unit vectors would be $-v^{-(1)}, -v^{-(2)}, \ldots, -v^{-(p)}$. Suppose that for any $i \in \{1, 2, \ldots, p\}$, $v^{-(1)}, v^{-(2)}, \ldots, v^{-(p)}$ satisfy

$$\left( v^{-(i)} \right)^T u_j = 0, \forall j \neq i, j \in \{1, 2, \ldots, p\}.$$

Thus the minimum value of $f(v)$ can be upper bounded by the average of the function values of the $p$ unit vectors:

$$\min_v f(v) \leq \frac{1}{p} \sum_{i=1}^{p} f(v^{-(i)}). \tag{52}$$

We can also bound the maximum value of $f(v)$ by some value:

$$\max_v f(v) \geq \max_{s_i = \pm 1} f \left( \frac{\sum_{i=1}^{p} s_i v^{-(i)}}{\| \sum_{i=1}^{p} s_i v^{-(i)} \|} \right). \tag{53}$$

Because we have

$$f\left(\frac{\sum_{i=1}^{p} s_i v^{-(i)}}{\|\sum_{i=1}^{p} s_i v^{-(i)}\|}\right) = \frac{f\left(\sum_{i=1}^{p} s_i v^{-(i)}\right)}{\|\sum_{i=1}^{p} s_i v^{-(i)}\|},$$

and

$$f\left(\sum_{i=1}^{p} s_i v^{-(i)}\right) = \sum_{j=1}^{p} \left|u_j^T\left(\sum_{i=1}^{p} s_i v^{-(i)}\right)\right| = \sum_{j=1}^{p}\left|\sum_{i=1}^{p} s_i u_j^T v^{-(i)}\right| = \sum_{j=1}^{p}\left|s_j u_j^T v^{-(j)}\right|$$

$$= \sum_{j=1}^{p}\left|u_j^T v^{-(j)}\right| = \sum_{j=1}^{p} f\left(v^{-(j)}\right),$$

we can get

$$f\left(\frac{\sum_{i=1}^{p} s_i v^{-(i)}}{\|\sum_{i=1}^{p} s_i v^{-(i)}\|}\right) = \frac{\sum_{j=1}^{p} f\left(v^{-(j)}\right)}{\|\sum_{i=1}^{p} s_i v^{-(i)}\|}.$$

So (53) becomes

$$\max_v f(v) \geq \max_{s_i=\pm 1} \frac{\sum_{i=1}^{p} f(v^{-(i)})}{\left\|\sum_{i=1}^{p} s_i v^{-(i)}\right\|} = \frac{\sum_{i=1}^{p} f(v^{-(i)})}{\min_{s_i=\pm 1}\left\|\sum_{i=1}^{p} s_i v^{-(i)}\right\|}. \tag{54}$$

Based on (52) and (54), we can get

$$\frac{\min_v f(v)}{\max_v f(v)} \leq \frac{\frac{1}{p}\sum_{i=1}^{p} f(v^{-(i)})}{\frac{\sum_{i=1}^{p} f(v^{-(i)})}{\min_{s_i=\pm 1}\left\|\sum_{i=1}^{p} s_i v^{-(i)}\right\|}} = \frac{1}{p}\min_{s_i=\pm 1}\left\|\sum_{i=1}^{p} s_i v^{-(i)}\right\|.$$

So we have

$$\max_{u_1,\ldots u_p} \frac{\min_v f(v)}{\max_v f(v)} \leq \frac{1}{p}\max_{u_1,\ldots u_p}\min_{s_i=\pm 1}\left\|\sum_{i=1}^{p} s_i v^{-(i)}\right\|. \tag{55}$$

Since solving the problem

$$\max_{u_1,...u_p} \min_{s_i=\pm1} \left\| \sum_{i=1}^{p} s_i v^{-(i)} \right\|$$

is equivalent to solving

$$\max_{u_1,...u_p} \min_{s_i=\pm1} \left\| \sum_{i=1}^{p} s_i v^{-(i)} \right\|^2,$$

we will try to solve the latter one in the following. We have

$$\max_{u_1,...u_p} \min_{s_i=\pm1} \left\| \sum_{i=1}^{p} s_i v^{-(i)} \right\|^2 = \max_{u_1,...u_p} \min_{s_i=\pm1} s^T \Sigma s,$$

where we have $\Sigma \in \mathbb{R}^{p \times p}$ and

$$\Sigma = \begin{pmatrix} 1 & \left(v^{-(1)}\right)^T v^{-(2)} & \left(v^{-(1)}\right)^T v^{-(3)} & \cdots & \left(v^{-(1)}\right)^T v^{-(p)} \\ \left(v^{-(2)}\right)^T v^{-(1)} & 1 & \left(v^{-(2)}\right)^T v^{-(3)} & \cdots & \left(v^{-(2)}\right)^T v^{-(p)} \\ \cdots & \cdots & \cdots & \cdots & \cdots \\ \left(v^{-(p)}\right)^T v^{-(1)} & \left(v^{-(p)}\right)^T v^{-(2)} & \left(v^{-(p)}\right)^T v^{-(3)} & \cdots & 1 \end{pmatrix}.$$

We claim that $\min_{s_i=\pm1} s^T \Sigma s$ is upper bounded by $p$, and $\min_{s_i=\pm1} s^T \Sigma s = p$ when

$$\left(v^{-(i)}\right)^T v^{-(j)} = 0, \forall i \neq j.$$

We can see that if there are some $i, j$ ($i \neq j$), such that $\left(v^{-(i)}\right)^T v^{-(j)} \neq 0$, then there exists some $s$, such that $s^T \Sigma s \leq p$. Suppose there does not exist such $s$, which means for any $s$, the following holds,

$$s^T \Sigma s > p. \tag{56}$$

Since we have

$$\sum_{s_i=\pm1} s^T \Sigma s = \sum_{s \in \{s:s_k=\pm1\}} \sum_{i,j} s_i s_j \Sigma_{ij} = \sum_{s \in \{s:s_k=\pm1\}} \left( p + \sum_{i \neq j} s_i s_j \Sigma_{ij} \right)$$

$$= 2^p p + \sum_{s \in \{s:s_k=\pm1\}} \sum_{i \neq j} s_i s_j \Sigma_{ij} = 2^p p,$$

this will lead to $\sum\limits_{s_i=\pm 1} s^T \Sigma s > 2^p p$, which is a contradiction of (56). So we proved that our claim is true, which says

$$\min_{s_i=\pm 1} s^T \Sigma s \leq p,$$

and when $\left(v^{-(i)}\right)^T v^{-(j)} = 0, \forall i \neq j$, which means $\Sigma = I_p$, we have $\min\limits_{s_i=\pm 1} s^T \Sigma s = p$.

We know that $v^{-(i)}$'s only depends on $u_i$'s, and when $u_i^T u_j = 0, \forall i \neq j$, we have $\left(v^{-(i)}\right)^T v^{-(j)} = 0, \forall i \neq j$. So when the following holds,

$$u_i^T u_j = 0, \forall i \neq j,$$

$\min\limits_{s_i=\pm 1} s^T \Sigma s$ achieves the maximum value, which is $p$. Therefore we get

$$\max_{u_1,\ldots u_p} \min_{s_i=\pm 1} \left\| \sum_{i=1}^{p} s_i v^{-(i)} \right\|^2 = \max_{u_1,\ldots u_p} \min_{s_i=\pm 1} s^T \Sigma s = p,$$

which leads to

$$\max_{u_1,\ldots u_p} \min_{s_i=\pm 1} \left\| \sum_{i=1}^{p} s_i v^{-(i)} \right\| = \sqrt{p}. \tag{57}$$

Based on (55) and (57), we have

$$\max_{u_1,\ldots u_p} \frac{\min\limits_{v} f(v)}{\max\limits_{v} f(v)} \leq \frac{\sqrt{p}}{p}. \tag{58}$$

Next if we can prove that when $u_i^T u_j = 0, \forall i \neq j$, the following holds, $\frac{\min\limits_{v} f(v)}{\max\limits_{v} f(v)} = \frac{\sqrt{p}}{p}$; combined with (58), we can arrive at the conclusion and finish the proof of the Lemma.

Let us assume

$$u_i^T u_j = 0, \forall i \neq j.$$

Without loss of generality, we can assume $u_i = e_i, \forall i \neq j$, where $e_i$'s are the basic vectors of $\mathbb{R}^p$. Then the following holds,

$$f(v) = \sum_{i=1}^{p} |v_i|, v \in \mathbb{S}^{p-1}.$$

We can easily verify the following, $\min_v f(v) = 1$, and $\max_v f(v) = \sqrt{p}$. So when $u_i^T u_j = 0, \forall i \neq j$, we have

$$\frac{\min_v f(v)}{\max_v f(v)} = \frac{\sqrt{p}}{p}.$$

Combined what we get from (58), that is, $\frac{\sqrt{p}}{p}$ is the upper bound of $\max_{u_1,\ldots u_p} \frac{\min_v f(v)}{\max_v f(v)}$, we finished the proof. □

## Proof of Lemma 4

*Proof* As we have

$$\min_{x:\|x\|=1,\langle x,v\rangle=\theta} \|x + B\|^2 = \min_{x:\|x\|=1,\langle x,v\rangle=\theta} 1 + \|B\|^2 + 2\langle x, B\rangle,$$

the problem (17) is equivalent to

$$\min_{x:\|x\|=1,\langle x,v\rangle=\theta} \langle x, B\rangle. \tag{59}$$

Suppose $x^*$ is the solution to the above problem (17). Then $x^*$ is the farthest point to $B$ on the circle that satisfies the constraints $\|x\| = 1$, $\langle x, v\rangle = \theta$. The three points $x^*, v,$ and $B$ must be on a same plane. Therefore, we can assume

$$x^* = av + bB. \tag{60}$$

Bringing (60) into (59), we have

$$\min_{x:\|x\|=1,\langle x,v\rangle=\theta} \langle x, B\rangle = \min_{a,b:\|av+bB\|=1,\langle av+bB,v\rangle=\theta} \langle av + bB, B\rangle,$$

which is equivalent to

$$\min_{a,b} av^T B + bB^T B \tag{61}$$

$$\text{s.t.} \begin{cases} a^2 + b^2\|B\|^2 + 2abv^T B &= 1 \\ a + bv^T B &= \cos\theta. \end{cases} \tag{62}$$

Bringing the second equation in the constraints (62), that is,

$$a = \cos\theta - bv^T B \tag{63}$$

into (61), we have

$$\min_b \ v^T B \cos\theta + b\left(B^T B - (v^T B)^2\right)$$

$$\text{s.t. } b^2\left(B^T B - (v^T B)^2\right) + \cos\theta^2 = 1. \tag{64}$$

Then the solution to (64) is

$$b = \pm\frac{\sin\theta}{\sqrt{B^T B - (v^T B)^2}}.$$

Since $B^T B - (v^T B)^2 \geq 0$, the minimum is achieved when

$$b = -\frac{|\sin\theta|}{\sqrt{B^T B - (v^T B)^2}}. \tag{65}$$

Combining (65) with (63), we can get the solution.                                                                    □


## Proof of Theorem 6

**Proof** If $\theta \in [0, \pi)$, the square of the denominator of (18) becomes

$$1 + 2v^T B \cos\theta + B^T B - 2\sin\theta\sqrt{B^T B - (v^T B)^2} = 1 + B^T B + 2\sqrt{B^T B}\sin(\alpha - \theta),$$

where

$$\sin\alpha = \frac{v^T B}{\sqrt{B^T B}},$$

$$\cos\alpha = \frac{\sqrt{B^T B - (v^T B)^2}}{\sqrt{B^T B}}.$$

Similarly, if $\theta \in [\pi, 2\pi)$, then the square of the denominator of (18) becomes

$$1 + 2v^T B \cos\theta + B^T B + 2\sin\theta\sqrt{B^T B - (v^T B)^2} = 1 + B^T B + 2\sqrt{B^T B}\sin(\alpha + \theta),$$

where $\alpha$ is the same defined as above.

Hence, for $\theta \in [0, \pi)$, we have

$$f(\theta) = \frac{|\cos\theta| + A}{\sqrt{1 + B^T B + 2\sqrt{B^T B}\sin(\alpha - \theta)}};$$

for $\theta \in [\pi, 2\pi)$, we have

$$f(\theta) = \frac{|\cos\theta| + A}{\sqrt{1 + B^T B + 2\sqrt{B^T B}\sin(\alpha + \theta)}},$$

which is equivalent to

$$f(\theta) = \frac{|\cos\theta| + A}{\sqrt{1 + B^T B + 2\sqrt{B^T B}\sin(\alpha + \theta)}},$$

where $\theta \in [-\pi, 0)$, which is also equivalent to

$$f(\theta) = \frac{|\cos\theta| + A}{\sqrt{1 + B^T B + 2\sqrt{B^T B}\sin(\alpha - \theta)}},$$

where $\theta \in [0, \pi)$.

So the problem we want to solve is actually to maximize

$$f(\theta) = \frac{|\cos\theta| + A}{\sqrt{1 + B^T B + 2\sqrt{B^T B}\sin(\alpha - \theta)}}$$

on $\theta \in [0, \pi)$.

Under the first order condition, we have that if $\theta^*$ maximizes $f(\theta)$, then $0 = f'(\theta^*)$.

When $\theta \in [0, \frac{\pi}{2})$, the first order differentiable function of $f(\theta)$ can be written as

$$f'(\theta) = \frac{-(1 + B^T B)\sin\theta + \sqrt{B^T B}\left[\cos\alpha + A\cos(\alpha - \theta) - \sin\theta\sin(\alpha - \theta)\right]}{\left(1 + B^T B + 2\sqrt{B^T B}\sin(\alpha - \theta)\right)^{3/2}};$$

When $\theta \in [\frac{\pi}{2}, \pi)$, the first order differentiable function of $f(\theta)$ can be written as

$$f'(\theta) = \frac{(1 + B^T B)\sin\theta + \sqrt{B^T B}\left[-\cos\alpha + A\cos(\alpha - \theta) + \sin\theta\sin(\alpha - \theta)\right]}{\left(1 + B^T B + 2\sqrt{B^T B}\sin(\alpha - \theta)\right)^{3/2}}.$$

If we define function $g(\theta)$ as the following

$$g(\theta) = \begin{cases} \sqrt{B^T B}\,[\cos\alpha + A\cos(\alpha - \theta) - \sin\theta\sin(\alpha - \theta)] \\ -(1 + B^T B)\sin\theta, & \text{if } \theta \in [0, \frac{\pi}{2}), \\ \sqrt{B^T B}\,[-\cos\alpha + A\cos(\alpha - \theta) + \sin\theta\sin(\alpha - \theta)] \\ +(1 + B^T B)\sin\theta & \text{if } \theta \in [\frac{\pi}{2}, \pi), \end{cases}$$

Then our goal becomes to find the zeros of the function $g(\theta)$. □

# References

1. Asmussen, S., & Glynn, P. W. (2007). *Stochastic simulation: Algorithms and analysis* (Vol. 57). Berlin/Heidelberg: Springer Science & Business Media.
2. Bradley, S., Hax, A., & Magnanti, T. (1977). *Applied mathematical programming*. Boston: Addison-Wesley.
3. Brauchart, J., Saff, E., Sloan, I., & Womersley, R. (2014). QMC designs: Optimal order quasi Monte Carlo integration schemes on the sphere. *Mathematics of Computation, 83*(290), 2821–2851.
4. Chaudhuri, A., & Hu, W. (2018). A fast algorithm for computing distance correlation. Preprint. arXiv:1810.11332.
5. Hesse, K., Sloan, I. H., & Womersley, R. S. (2010). Numerical integration on the sphere. In *Handbook of geomathematics* (pp. 1185–1219). New York: Springer.
6. Hoeffding, W. (1992). A class of statistics with asymptotically normal distribution. In *Breakthroughs in statistics* (pp. 308–334). New York: Springer. .
7. Huang, C., & Huo, X. (2017). An efficient and distribution-free two-sample test based on energy statistics and random projections. Preprint. arXiv:1707.04602.
8. Huo, X., & Székely, G. J. (2016). Fast computing for distance covariance. *Technometrics, 58*(4), 435–447.
9. Korolyuk, V. S., & Borovskich, Y. V. (2013). *Theory of U-statistics* (Vol. 273). Berlin/Heidelberg: Springer Science & Business Media.
10. Lyons, R., et al. (2013). Distance covariance in metric spaces. *The Annals of Probability, 41*(5), 3284–3305.
11. Mises, R. V. (1947). On the asymptotic distribution of differentiable statistical functions. *The Annals of Mathematical Statistics, 18*(3), 309–348 (1947)
12. Morokoff, W. J., & Caflisch, R. E. (1995). Quasi-monte carlo integration. *Journal of Computational Physics, 122*(2), 218–230.
13. Nesterov, Y. (2012). Efficiency of coordinate descent methods on huge-scale optimization problems. *SIAM Journal on Optimization, 22*(2), 341–362 (2012).
14. Niederreiter, H. (1992). *Random number generation and quasi-Monte Carlo methods* (Vol. 63). Philadelphia: SIAM.
15. Sloan, I. H., & Womersley, R. S. (2004). Extremal systems of points and numerical integration on the sphere. *Advances in Computational Mathematics, 21*(1–2), 107–125.
16. Székely, G. J., & Rizzo, M. L. (2004). Testing for equal distributions in high dimension. *InterStat, 5*, 1–6.
17. Székely, G. J., & Rizzo, M. L. (2009). Brownian distance covariance. *The Annals of Applied Statistics, 3*, 1236–1265.
18. Székely, G. J., Rizzo, M. L., Bakirov, N. K., et al. (2007). Measuring and testing dependence by correlation of distances. *The Annals of Statistics, 35*(6), 2769–2794.
19. Wright, S. J. (2015). Coordinate descent algorithms. *Mathematical Programming, 151*(1), 3–34.

# Kernel Tests for One, Two, and $K$-Sample Goodness-of-Fit: State of the Art and Implementation Considerations

Yang Chen and Marianthi Markatou

**Abstract** In this article, we first discuss the fundamental role of statistical distances in the problem of goodness-of-fit and review various existing multivariate two-sample goodness-of-fit tests from both statistics and machine learning literature. The review conducted delivers the fact that there does not exist a satisfactory multivariate two-sample goodness-of-fit test. We introduce a class of one and two-sample tests constructed using the kernel-based quadratic distance, and briefly touch upon their asymptotic properties. We discuss the practical implementation of these tests, with emphasis on the kernel-based two-sample test. Finally, we use simulations and real data to illustrate the application of the kernel-based two-sample test, and compare this test with tests existing in the literature.

**Keywords** Goodness-of-fit · Kernel tests · Quadratic distance · Multivariate · Two-sample methods

## 1 Introduction

An important reason for the popularity of testing is that it is often thought to be a major, if not the main, ingredient of scientific progress [8, 38] and the best way to move from alchemy to science. Further, a frequently expressed goal of testing is decision making. This view of testing and its implementation in statistics, is primarily due to Neyman-Pearson theory of inductive behavior. The decision-theoretic approach to testing has been further elaborated by Wald [50], and from a Bayesian perspective by Savage [42]. However, the modern approach to significance testing starts with Karl Pearson's goodness of fit for large samples.

Y. Chen · M. Markatou (✉)
Department of Biostatistics, University at Buffalo, Buffalo, NY, USA
e-mail: ychen57@buffalo.edu; markatou@buffalo.edu

© Springer Nature Switzerland AG 2020                                    309
Y. Zhao, D.-G. (Din) Chen (eds.), *Statistical Modeling in Biomedical Research*, Emerging Topics in Statistics and Biostatistics,
https://doi.org/10.1007/978-3-030-33416-1_14

The goodness-of-fit problem has a long history in the statistical literature, particularly in the one-dimensional (univariate) case. Examples include Durbin [16], D'Agostino and Stephen [14] and Rayner and Best [39]. Many goodness-of-fit tests for univariate samples have been proposed in the literature. As examples of current literature on the subject, and for the univariate case, we list Cao and Van Keilegom [11] and Cao and Lugosi [10].

In contrast to the voluminous univariate goodness-of-fit testing literature much less is written for the multivariate case. In this paper we first offer a brief review on these multivariate tests. This is actually the first step towards our goal of understanding the performance of existing multivariate goodness-of-fit tests and constructing two and $k$-sample tests based on the concept of statistical distance. In what follows we justify our decision of basing goodness-of-fit procedures on the concept of a statistical distance.

There has been a recent growth of interest in the use of quadratic distance for goodness-of-fit in the scientific literature outside statistics, no doubt because of the modern challenges of very large samples and high dimensions. One area is modern particle physics, where the experimenter is confronted with data in many dimensions and the task of assessing how accurately a model function fits the observed data. Because of the computational and other difficulties encountered with extensions of existing goodness-of-fit tests, Aslan and Zech [2] discuss the construction of energy function-based goodness-of-fit functions $R$. Expressed in our language, $R$ is one-half of the quadratic distance between two distributions $F$, $G$. The proposed kernels are monotonically decreasing functions of the Euclidean distance between points $\mathbf{x}$, $\mathbf{y}$. When $K(\mathbf{x}, \mathbf{y}) = 1/(\| \mathbf{x} - \mathbf{y} \|)$, where $\| \mathbf{x} - \mathbf{y} \|$ is the Euclidean distance, the function $R$ is the electrostatic energy of the two charge distributions of opposite signs; the energy is minimum if the charges neutralize each other.

Another scientific domain where quadratic methods have arisen is biology, where the high dimensional nature of microarray and other "omics" data challenges standard statistical methodology. Szabo et al. [45, 46] use a negative quadratic distance as a test statistic to identify a subset of genes that in some sense differs the most between two subsets of genes. They use Euclidean distance based kernels, and one of the desirable requirements is ease of computation. Szabo et al. [45] discuss how to construct negative definite kernels and how to use the proposed function of the distance to construct two-sample tests.

The field of quasi Monte-Carlo methods requires the use of criteria for measuring whether a set of points is uniformly scattered in the $p$-dimensional unit cube. These criteria, called discrepancies, arise in the error analysis of quasi-Monte Carlo methods for evaluating multiple integrals. In this literature the discrepancy is a measure of the quality of a set of points used to approximate the integral.

A related literature to the aforementioned goodness-of-fit problems comes from machine learning and it is mainly represented by papers such as Gretton et al. [20, 21], Póczos et al. [37], Zaremba et al. [53] and others. Specifically, Gretton et al. [20] introduce a test for the two-sample problem, called Maximum Mean Discrepancy, that is computationally fast and thus, it can be used with large samples and high dimensional data sets.

As rich and interesting as this literature is, there is virtually no discussion of a critical concept for multivariate goodness-of-fit testing. That is, in multivariate goodness-of-fit it is important to construct tunable distances so that one can adjust the operating characteristics of the distances to the dimension of the sample space and sample size. Lindsay et al. [28] are the first to recognize this fundamental issue and propose the concept of a quadratic distance as an extension of Pearson's chi-squared analysis, in continuous distributions. Lindsay et al. [28] show that quadratic distances are functions of nonnegative definite kernels, and they study their application to goodness-of-fit problems. They also show that classical goodness-of-fit tests can be thought of as functions of kernels. Further, Lindsay et al. [27] are the first to actually construct one-sample goodness-of-fit tests in the multivariate case using the concept of a statistical distance and show how to build kernels with targeted power properties. Lindsay et al. [27] discuss the one-sample case, and the choice of kernels $K$ that constitute the backbone of the goodness-of-fit procedures they advocate. They note that the choice of a distance kernel is a matter of design, with important design factors such as the data type, the dimension of the data, the ability to carry out explicit calculations, and the alternatives of interest playing important roles in its construction.

Before we leave this section we would like to mention the work of Székely and Rizzo [49] on energy statistics. Energy statistics are statistical distances between random vectors and they can be expressed as $U$-statistics and $V$-statistics. Székely and Rizzo [49], in an interesting paper, construct one-sample tests for testing multivariate normality, which can be considered as special cases of the quadratic distance based tests presented here, for a specific choice of a kernel. This kernel is the Euclidean distance between two random vectors.

In this paper, we review the existing multivariate two-sample goodness-of-fit tests and introduce the tests constructed using the kernel-based quadratic distance. Section 2 provides a brief review of the multivariate goodness-of-fit tests from statistics literature. In Sect. 3, we elaborate on Maximum Mean Discrepancy, a test from machine learning literature, and discuss the issues pertaining to this test. We introduce the kernel-based quadratic distance in Sect. 4 and present the goodness-of-fit tests constructed using this distance in Sects. 4.1 and 4.2. Section 5 discusses the practical implementation of several tests mentioned in this paper, with emphasis on the kernel-based two-sample tests presented in Sect. 4.2. Sections 6 and 7 use a simulation study and a real-data application to illustrate the performance of the kernel-based test, and to compare it with the existing multivariate two-sample goodness-of-fit tests. Finally, Sect. 8 provides further discussion.

# 2 Relevant Statistical Literature

In this section, we offer a brief review of the multivariate goodness-of-fit tests from statistics literature. We begin with stating some basic notations and the question we are interested in. Let $F(\mathbf{x})$ and $G(\mathbf{y})$ be two unknown continuous distribution functions of two random vectors $\mathbf{X}$ and $\mathbf{Y}$, both defined on $\mathbb{R}^p$ ($p \geq 1$). Let the set of $N = n + m$ points $\mathbf{x}_1, \mathbf{x}_2, \cdots, \mathbf{x}_n$ and $\mathbf{y}_1, \mathbf{y}_2, \cdots, \mathbf{y}_m$ be observations from $\mathbf{X}$ and $\mathbf{Y}$. Let $\mathbf{Z} = \{\mathbf{z}_1, \mathbf{z}_2, \cdots, \mathbf{z}_N\}$ be the pooled sample of $\mathbf{x}_1, \mathbf{x}_2, \cdots, \mathbf{x}_n$ and $\mathbf{y}_1, \mathbf{y}_2, \cdots, \mathbf{y}_m$, with distribution function $H(\mathbf{z})$. Further, $f(\mathbf{x})$, $g(\mathbf{y})$ and $h(\mathbf{z})$ are the corresponding density functions, with $F_n(\mathbf{x})$, $G_m(\mathbf{y})$ and $H_N(\mathbf{z})$ denote the corresponding empirical distribution functions. We would like to test $H_0 : F(\mathbf{x}) = G(\mathbf{y})$ versus a general alternative $H_1 : F(\mathbf{x}) \neq G(\mathbf{y})$.

The first set of tests utilize graph-based multivariate ranking strategies for the extensions of univariate two-sample tests in high dimensional settings. Friedman and Rafsky [19] use the minimal spanning tree (MST) as a multivariate generalization of the univariate ordered list to extend the univariate Wald-Wolfowitz "run" test [51] to multivariate cases. They also point out that the multivariate Kolmogorov-Smirnov (KS) test can be constructed via ranking observations using the rooted MST. It is known that the standard KS test has relatively low power against scale alternatives. Friedman and Rafsky [19] resolve this defect with a modified KS test that can substantially increase the power against scale alternatives at the expense of rendering the test ineffective against location alternatives. Recent work on the graph-based tests also includes Biswas et al. [7] and Chen and Friedman [12]. These two-sample tests concentrate on the limited information captured from ranks of observations within the sorted list of the pooled sample. One possible limitation is that their performance might depend on the distance used. That is, it is possible to obtain different results if different distances are used for these multivariate ranking strategies. However, there is no guideline provided for the selection of the best distance, and only R packages involving Euclidean distance are available.

The second set of tests attempts to extend several famous tests, such as Kolmogorov two-sample test, Anderson-Darling rank test and Cramér-von Mises test. The work includes Maag and Stephens [31], Pettitt [35, 36], Bickel [5], Burke [9]. These five tests use information from permutations of the pooled sample. Only the test proposed by Maag and Stephens [31] provides exact distribution. Although the test proposed by Bickel [5] can handle multivariate cases, it does not have an explicit formula that provides its asymptotic distribution. Only a weighted bootstrap procedure that approximates its limiting distribution is offered by Burke [9].

The third type of tests are based on likelihood methods. Cao and Van Keilegom [11] provide a local empirical likelihood test that reduces testing the multivariate goodness-of-fit to testing the equality of parameters of elliptically contoured distributions. In our opinion, the use of elliptically contoured distributions is actually a limitation, as it does not cover the other types of distributions. For example, the simple mixture of two normal distributions, which is common when studying biomarkers, does not belong to the aforementioned family.

The fourth set of tests concentrate on the application of general "distance" measures, where "distance" in this context means that the measure may not satisfy all the properties in the mathematical definition of a distance. Henze [23, 24] proposes a multivariate two-sample test based on the number of nearest neighbor type coincidences. This test is generalized and extended in various publications, including Schilling [43], Mondal et al. [32], Barakat et al. [3], and Chen et al. [13].

Rosenbaum [41] uses inter-point distances for the construction of optimal bi-partite matchings among the pooled sample and builds a multivariate two-sample test based on the matched pairs. Other inter-point distance-based tests include Hall and Tajvidi [22], Baringhaus and Franz [4], Székely and Rizzo [47], Biswas and Ghosh [6], Liu and Modarres [29]. Other than using inter-point distances to construct tests, Anderson et al. [1] utilize $L_2$ distance between kernel density estimators; Fernández et al. [18] compare the empirical characteristic functions; Aslan and Zech [2], from the field of physics, make use of a positive definite distance function. As a comment, most inter-point distance-based tests use Euclidean distance, and the robustness of the results of these tests to the chosen distances has not been demonstrated in the literature. It is possible that the performance of these tests is affected by the choice of the distance function. For the kernel-based tests, the selection of the bandwidth can be a difficult issue. Anderson et al. [1] are the first to recognize that the performance of kernel-based tests is affected by the selection of the bandwidth. Furthermore, they notice that the bandwidth must be constant for the test to perform well in terms of power and significance level. Lindsay et al. [27], in related work, offer a method for selecting the bandwidth that maximizes the power of the test.

# 3 Relevant Machine Learning Literature: Maximum Mean Discrepancy

Gretton et al. [20] utilize the property of the kernel mean embedding to construct a test statistic, called Maximum Mean Discrepancy (MMD). For a kernel, $K(\mathbf{x}, \mathbf{y}) = < K(\mathbf{x}, .), K(., \mathbf{y}) >$, that is a unit ball in a reproducing kernel Hilbert space (RKHS), the kernel mean embeddings of two random vectors $\mathbf{X}$, $\mathbf{Y}$ with distribution functions $F(\mathbf{x})$, $G(\mathbf{y})$ are $\mu_{\mathbf{X}} = \mathbb{E}_{\mathbf{X}}(K(\mathbf{X}, .))$, $\mu_{\mathbf{Y}} = \mathbb{E}_{\mathbf{Y}}(K(., \mathbf{Y}))$. The kernel mean embedding is injective and can preserve the information on all moments of an embedded distribution for universal kernels [20].

As an example, let us consider a univariate kernel $K(x, y) = e^{xy}$, as well as two univariate random variables $X, Y$ with distribution functions $F(x), G(y)$. Both $F(x)$ and $G(y)$ have moment-generating functions. With the help of Taylor expansion, the kernel mean embeddings of $X, Y$ can be expressed as

$$\mu_X = \mathbb{E}_X\big(K(X, .)\big) = \mathbb{E}_X\Big(1 + yX + \frac{y^2}{2!}X^2 + \frac{y^3}{3!}X^3 + \cdots\Big)$$

$$= 1 + y\mathbb{E}_X(X) + \frac{y^2}{2!}\mathbb{E}_X(X^2) + \frac{y^3}{3!}\mathbb{E}_X(X^3) + \cdots,$$

$$\mu_Y = \mathbb{E}_Y\big(K(Y, .)\big) = \mathbb{E}_Y\Big(1 + xY + \frac{x^2}{2!}Y^2 + \frac{x^3}{3!}Y^3 + \cdots\Big)$$

$$= 1 + x\mathbb{E}_Y(Y) + \frac{x^2}{2!}\mathbb{E}_Y(Y^2) + \frac{x^3}{3!}\mathbb{E}_Y(Y^3) + \cdots.$$

Clearly these are exactly the same as the moment-generating functions of $X$ and $Y$ which contain information on all moments. However, if a polynomial kernel with finite degree is used, the Taylor expansions of the kernel mean embeddings are finite sums and the corresponding kernel mean embeddings cannot preserve the information on all moments. Therefore, the kernel function used in the kernel mean embedding must be carefully selected. To the best of our knowledge, the kernels having exponential form can guarantee the preservation of the information on all moments of an embedded distribution. Furthermore, if either of the moment-generating functions of the two random variables $X$, $Y$ does not exist, the aforementioned way in which the kernel mean embedding preserves the information on all moments breaks down. Under this situation, it is unclear how MMD works. Muandet et al. [33] show that the characteristic function can be also used to explain the mechanism of the kernel mean embedding, but the kernel involved still has limitations.

With the help of the kernel mean embedding, the MMD statistic is defined as

$$MMD^2(\mathbf{X}, \mathbf{Y}) = \| \mu_{\mathbf{X}} - \mu_{\mathbf{Y}} \|_H^2,$$

where $\| . \|_H$ denotes the Hilbert space norm. The corresponding unbiased estimate, in terms of $U$-statistics, is provided as

$$MMD_u^2(\mathbf{X}, \mathbf{Y}) = \frac{1}{n(n-1)} \sum_{j=1}^{n} \sum_{k \neq j}^{n} K(\mathbf{x}_j, \mathbf{x}_k) + \frac{1}{m(m-1)} \sum_{j=1}^{m} \sum_{k \neq j}^{m} K(\mathbf{y}_j, \mathbf{y}_k)$$

$$- \frac{2}{nm} \sum_{j=1}^{n} \sum_{k=1}^{m} K(\mathbf{x}_j, \mathbf{y}_k).$$

The null hypothesis is rejected for large values of $MMD_u^2$. The limiting distribution is showed to be a weighted sum of squared independent Gaussian variables. Bootstrap is recommended to calculate the corresponding critical values in practice.

Gretton et al. [20] use the Gaussian radial basis function kernel $K(\mathbf{x}, \mathbf{y}) = \exp\{-\frac{\|\mathbf{x}-\mathbf{y}\|^2}{2\sigma^2}\}$, where $\sigma$ is a tuning parameter that needs to be selected in order to operationalize the test. They suggest selecting this tuning parameter as the median Euclidean distance between the points in the pooled sample. However there is no guarantee that this selection of tuning parameter is at all optimal. In fact, a fundamental problem here is that the selection of this parameter is not associated with any of the fundamental aspects of the performance of the test. In this sense, it is obvious that there are distributions for which this choice is clearly suboptimal [40]. Furthermore, the issue of the selection of an appropriate kernel for carrying out the MMD test still remains open. The radially symmetric kernel is appropriate for interval scale data, but is not necessarily the case for either categorical or ordinal categorical data.

Recognizing these two drawbacks of MMD, Gretton et al. [21] try to address the issues involved by offering an approach to "optimally" select the kernel. This is done by restricting attention to a family of linear combinations of positive definite kernels, and learning the kernel from the data to be tested by solving an optimization problem. Gretton et al. [21] show that this procedure is equivalent to maximizing the Hodges-Lehmann asymptotic relative efficiency. The procedure is really involved and there is no extensive experience with its use in practice. As a comment, Danafar et al. [15] extend the MMD test by incorporating two penalty terms when sample sizes are small. Eric et al. [17] propose a test, called Maximum Kernel Fisher Discriminant Ratio, which combines both mean element and covariance operator in RKHS.

The review presented in Sects. 2 and 3 clearly suggests that there does not exist a satisfactory multi-dimenional goodness-of-fit testing procedure. MMD is reported to have a better performance than others. But the selection of the kernel and the tuning parameter still remains un-determined, and there is no clear guideline on how this problem could be solved with minimal cost. In the following sections, we introduce goodness-of-fit tests constructed using kernel-based quadratic distances that are capable of handling at least some of these issues.

# 4   Statistical Distance-Based Goodness-of-Fit Tests

In this section, we introduce the kernel-based quadratic distance and the goodness-of-fit tests constructed using this distance. Lindsay et al. [28] define the kernel-based quadratic distance as:

**Definition 1 (Lindsay et al. [28])** Given a nonnegative definite kernel $K(s, t)$, the kernel-based quadratic distance between two probability measures $F$ and $G$ is defined as

$$d_K(F, G) = \iint K(s, t) d(F - G)(s) d(F - G)(t). \tag{1}$$

Kernel based quadratic distances are of interest in statistical work for various reasons, one of which is that the empirical quadratic distance between two distributions $F$ and $G$ has a relatively simple asymptotic distribution theory. Other reasons include the fact that many distances, i.e., Kullback-Leibler distance, are asymptotically quadratic, and many important distances are exactly quadratic, such as Pearson's Chi-squared and Cramér-von Mises statistics. One additional reason justifying the attractiveness of the kernel-based quadratic distance is the fact that when the distance is exactly quadratic, expressed exactly as in relation 1, it is a metric. Furthermore, for a given symmetric kernel $K(s, t)$ there exists a symmetric kernel $K^{\frac{1}{2}}$, called the squared root kernel, satisfying

$$K(s, t) = \int K^{\frac{1}{2}}(s, r)K^{\frac{1}{2}}(r, t)d\sigma(r),$$

where $\sigma(.)$ is a probability measure. We write $d_K(F, G) = \int \left(f^*(r) - g^*(r)\right)^2 d\sigma(r)$, where $f^*(r) = \int K^{\frac{1}{2}}(s, r)dF(s)$ and $g^*(r) = \int K^{\frac{1}{2}}(r, t)dG(t)$. For example, the convolution of the two univariate normal kernels with variances $h_1^2$ and $h_2^2$, produces a normal kernel with variance $h_1^2 + h_2^2$, and we call this property *the convolution property*. This property is also valid for multivariate normal kernels. We work with kernels that exhibit this convolution property. In Sect. 5, we will show that this property can help us with the computation of the corresponding test statistics.

It is also important to note that the distance kernel $K$ that generates a particular distance is not unique. Lindsay et al. [28] discuss this point and introduce the model-centered kernel, defined as follows.

We note here that Sejdinovic et al. [44] introduced a general energy distance using negative definite functions $\rho$. Specifically, Sejdinovic et al. [44] defined this general energy distance as

$$D_{E,\rho}(F, G) = -\int \rho d[(F - G) \times (F - G)],$$

where $\rho$ is a general semimetric of negative definite type. This definition is similar to the definition provided by Lindsay et al. [28], with the difference that Lindsay et al. [28] use general positive definite kernels that are tunable. Székely and Rizzo's energy test [47–49] uses as $\rho$ the Euclidean distance between two multi-dimensional random variables.

**Definition 2** The $G$-centered kernel $K_{cen(G)}$ of a kernel $K$ is defined as

$$K_{cen(G)}(s, t) = K(s, t) - K(s, G) - K(G, t) + K(G, G),$$

where

$$K(s, G) = \int K(s, t)dG(t),$$

$$K(G, t) = \int K(s, t)dG(s),$$

$$K(G, G) = \iint K(s, t)dG(s)dG(t).$$

This $G$-centered kernel plays an important role in obtaining the asymptotic theory of one, two, and $k$-sample goodness-of-fit tests. However, in later sections, we will show that the integration to obtain the $G$-centered kernel could increase the computational cost under certain scenarios.

It is interesting to note that the construction of the function $d\mu$ of Lyons [30] redefines the Lindsay et al. [28] construction on general metric spaces. In the latter case, the kernel is taken to be the distance between two random variables defined on a suitable metric space.

## 4.1 One-Sample Goodness-of-Fit Tests

In the context of one-sample goodness-of-fit, we let $G$ be a null distribution whose distribution function is known and whose fit we wish to assess. After centering the kernel $K$ with respect to the null distribution $G$ to obtain the centered kernel $K_{cen(G)}$, the kernel-based quadratic distance can be written as $d(F, G) = \iint K_{cen(G)}(\mathbf{s}, \mathbf{t}) dF(\mathbf{s}) dF(\mathbf{t})$. Lindsay et al. [27] construct a test statistic based on the $U$-statistic that unbiasedly estimates the true distance $d(F, G)$. The test statistic is provided as

$$U_n = \frac{1}{n(n-1)} \sum_i \sum_{j \neq i} K_{cen(G)}(\mathbf{x}_i, \mathbf{x}_j).$$

Under the simple null hypothesis, the limiting distribution of $U_n$ is

$$nU_n \to \sum_j \lambda_j \left( Z_j^2 - 1 \right) \text{ as } n \to \infty,$$

where $\lambda_j$'s are the nonzero eigenvalues of the centered kernel $K_{cen(G)}$ under the null distribution $G$ and $Z_j$ follows the standard normal distribution. Lindsay et al. [27] also study the limiting distribution of $U_n$ under the composite null hypothesis and provide the exact variance under the alternative.

The selection of the tuning parameter is quite critical to the application of the kernel-based methods. In the context of goodness-of-fit, one cannot expect that a single tuning parameter is capable of obtaining the optimal power for all alternative hypotheses. Lindsay et al. [27] propose a precise strategy to compare the sensitivity of a class of kernels to select the optimal tuning parameter with respect to a specific alternative hypothesis of interest. They provide a very comprehensive simulation study to evaluate the quality of this selection strategy. The simulation study indicates that the proposed strategy indeed provides reasonable guidance without burden of an extensive simulation.

## 4.2 Two and K-Sample Goodness-of-Fit Tests

Compared to the one-sample problem, the luxury of knowing the null distribution $G$ no longer exists in two-sample cases. We let $F_n(\mathbf{x})$ and $G_m(\mathbf{y})$ be the empirical distribution functions of $F(\mathbf{x})$ and $G(\mathbf{y})$. Under $H_0 : F = G = F^*$, the kernel-based quadratic distance can be written as

$$d(F_n, G_m) = \iint K_{cen}(\mathbf{s}, \mathbf{t})d(F_n - F^*)(\mathbf{s})d(F_n - F^*)(\mathbf{t})$$

$$- 2 \iint K_{cen}(\mathbf{s}, \mathbf{t})d(F_n - F^*)(\mathbf{s})d(G_m - F^*)(\mathbf{t})$$

$$+ \iint K_{cen}(\mathbf{s}, \mathbf{t})d(G_m - F^*)(\mathbf{s})d(G_m - F^*)(\mathbf{t}).$$

where $K_{cen}$ is an appropriately centered kernel. The test statistic unbiasedly estimating $d(F_n, G_m)$ is provided as

$$D_{n,m} = \frac{1}{n(n-1)} \sum_{i=1}^{n} \sum_{j \neq i}^{n} K_{cen}(\mathbf{x}_i, \mathbf{x}_j) - \frac{2}{nm} \sum_{i=1}^{n} \sum_{j=1}^{m} K_{cen}(\mathbf{x}_i, \mathbf{y}_j)$$

$$+ \frac{1}{m(m-1)} \sum_{i=1}^{m} \sum_{j \neq i}^{m} K_{cen}(\mathbf{y}_i, \mathbf{y}_j).$$

To obtain the correct limiting theory the kernel must be appropriately centered. Notice that $F^*$, appearing in the expression of the quadratic distance, offers the "appropriate" centering distribution, which needs to be identified. Section 5 of this paper will provide a clear guideline on determining the centering distribution $F^*$ and algorithms to calculate the test statistic as well as critical values.

Under the null hypothesis, the limiting distribution of $D_{n,m}$ is provided as

$$N D_{n,m} \xrightarrow{d} \sum_{k=1}^{\infty} \lambda_k \left[ \left(\frac{1}{\sqrt{\rho_x}} Z_{1k} - \frac{1}{\sqrt{\rho_y}} Z_{2k}\right)^2 - \left(\frac{1}{\rho_x} + \frac{1}{\rho_y}\right) \right] \text{ as } n, m \to \infty, \quad (2)$$

where $Z_{1k}$, $Z_{2k}$ are independent variables that both follow the standard normal distribution; $\lambda_k$'s are the nonzero eigenvalues of $K_{cen}$; $\lim_{n,m\to\infty} \frac{n}{N} = \rho_x$, $\lim_{n,m\to\infty} \frac{m}{N} = \rho_y$ and $0 < \rho_x < 1$. The exact variance of $D_{n,m}$ under the null hypothesis and the limiting distribution under the alternative hypothesis can also be derived. Additionally, optimal tuning parameters used to construct $D_{n,m}$ can be determined by extending the strategy proposed for the one-sample tests by Lindsay et al. [27].

Further, the two-sample tests $D_{n,m}$ can be extended to address the $k$-sample problem by defining a distance matrix with $(i, j)$th element

$$D_{i,j} = \iint K_{cen}(\mathbf{s}, \mathbf{t}) d(F_i - \bar{F})(\mathbf{s}) d(F_j - \bar{F})(\mathbf{t}),$$

where $K_{cen}$ is a centered kernel centered by $\bar{F}$ and $\bar{F} = \frac{\sum_i^k n_i F_i}{\sum_i^k n_i}$ is the grand mean centering distribution. All eigenvectors of this matrix will be contrasts between the densities $F_1, F_2, \cdots, F_k$. Limiting distributional results, understanding the operational characteristics of this formulation, and implementation of the test procedures constitute the contents of our future work on goodness-of-fit testing.

# 5 Practical Implementation

In this section, we discuss the practical implementation of the goodness-of-fit tests mentioned in Sects. 2–4, especially focusing on the issues met in the computation of the kernel-based two-sample tests in Sect. 4.2. Table 1 lists the tests having existing R packages and their associated R packages. It has been demonstrated that the computational cost of Friedman-Rafsky Kolmogorov-Smirnov test, modified Friedman-Rafsky Kolmogorov-Smirnov test, and Friedman-Rafsky Wald-Wolfowitz test increases as the sample size increases because these tests involve ranking the pooled sample, a procedure that is relatively computationally expensive. Rosenbaum's Cross Match test has a sharp rate of increase in the computational cost as dimension increases because its computation involves the calculation of the inverse of a variance covariance matrix, which is time consuming as the dimension grows.

In the content of the kernel-based two-sample test in Sect. 4.2, one important issue involved in the practical implementation is the calculation of $D_{n,m}$ because the integration of the kernel used with respect to the common distribution under the null hypothesis is required to obtain the correct model-centered kernel that is used to construct $D_{n,m}$. Under the assumption that the common null distribution $F^*$ belongs to a family of parametric distribution, the convolution property discussed in Sect. 4 can assist us in this calculation. One example of kernels having the convolution property is the multivariate normal kernel, provided as

**Table 1** Tests and related R packages

| Tests | R packages |
|---|---|
| Friedman-Rafsky Kolmogorov-Smirnov test [19] | "GSAR" |
| Modified Friedman-Rafsky Kolmogorov-Smirnov test [19] | "GSAR" |
| Friedman-Rafsky Wald-Wolfowitztest [19] | "GSAR" |
| Rosenbaum's Cross Match test [41] | "crossmatch" |
| Maximum Mean Discrepancy [20] | "kernlab" |
| Cramer test [4] | "cramer" |
| Energy test [47] | "energy" |

$$\Phi_{\Sigma_h}(\mathbf{s}, \mathbf{t}) = \frac{1}{(2\pi)^{p/2}|\Sigma_h|^{1/2}} exp\left(-\frac{1}{2}(\mathbf{s} - \mathbf{t})^T \Sigma_h^{-1}(\mathbf{s} - \mathbf{t})\right),$$

where $\Sigma_h$ is a matrix of tuning parameters. We now take this kernel as an example to illustrate the algorithm to calculate $D_{n,m}$. Assume the common distribution $F^*$ under the null hypothesis is a multivariate normal distribution with unknown $\mu$, $\Sigma$. The *parametric calculation of* $D_{n,m}$ is described as follows:

- At first, $\mu$, $\Sigma$ are estimated from the pooled sample $\mathbf{z}_1, \cdots, \mathbf{z}_{n+m}$, using Maximum Likelihood Estimation, as $\hat{\mu}$, $\hat{\Sigma}$.
- Then with the help of the convolution property, the integration of the multivariate normal kernel with respect to $F^*$ with $\hat{\mu}$, $\hat{\Sigma}$ produces

$$\int \Phi_{\Sigma_h}(\mathbf{s}, \mathbf{t})dF^*(\mathbf{t}) = \int \Phi_{\Sigma_h}(\mathbf{s}, \mathbf{t})\Phi_{\hat{\Sigma}}(\mathbf{t}, \hat{\mu})d\mathbf{t} = \Phi_{\Sigma_h+\hat{\Sigma}}(\mathbf{s}, \hat{\mu}). \quad (3)$$

And the centered version of $\Phi_{\Sigma_h}(\mathbf{s}, \mathbf{t})$, centered by $F^*$ with $\hat{\mu}$ and $\hat{\Sigma}$, is given as

$$\Phi_{cen(F^*)}(\mathbf{s}, \mathbf{t}) = \Phi_{\Sigma_h}(\mathbf{s}, \mathbf{t}) - \Phi_{\Sigma_h+\hat{\Sigma}}(\mathbf{s}, \hat{\mu}) - \Phi_{\Sigma_h+\hat{\Sigma}}(\hat{\mu}, \mathbf{t}) + \Phi_{\Sigma_h+2\hat{\Sigma}}(\hat{\mu}, \hat{\mu}).$$

- The kernel-based test statistic is now calculated as

$$D_{n,m} = \frac{1}{n(n-1)} \sum_{i=1}^{n} \sum_{j \neq i}^{n} \Phi_{cen(F^*)}(\mathbf{x}_i, \mathbf{x}_j) - \frac{2}{nm} \sum_{i=1}^{n} \sum_{j=1}^{m} \Phi_{cen(F^*)}(\mathbf{x}_i, \mathbf{y}_j)$$

$$+ \frac{1}{m(m-1)} \sum_{i=1}^{m} \sum_{j \neq i}^{m} \Phi_{cen(F^*)}(\mathbf{y}_i, \mathbf{y}_j).$$

Note that the multivariate normal kernel is used because the common distribution under the null hypothesis is assumed as a multivariate normal distribution. In practice, one can assume the common distribution under the null hypothesis as any distribution but appropriate kernels that respect the range and measurement scale of the data must be used.

In the case that the parametric assumption is absent, we can replace Eq. (3) with

$$\int \Phi_{\Sigma_h}(\mathbf{s}, \mathbf{t})dF^*(\mathbf{t}) = \frac{1}{n+m} \sum_{i=1}^{n+m} \Phi_{\Sigma_h}(\mathbf{s}, \mathbf{z}_i).$$

That is, instead of centering the normal kernel with respect to the assumed normal or any other model, we still use the normal kernel and center it with respect to the empirical distribution of the pooled sample. And the centered version of $\Phi_{\Sigma_h}(\mathbf{s}, \mathbf{t})$, centered by $F^*$, is provided as

$$\Phi^*_{cen(F*)}(\mathbf{s},\mathbf{t}) = \Phi_{\Sigma_h}(\mathbf{s},\mathbf{t}) - \frac{1}{n+m}\sum_{i=1}^{n+m}\Phi_{\Sigma_h}(\mathbf{s},\mathbf{z}_i) - \frac{1}{n+m}\sum_{i=1}^{n+m}\Phi_{\Sigma_h}(\mathbf{z}_i,\mathbf{t})$$

$$+ \frac{1}{(n+m)(n+m-1)}\sum_{i=1}^{n+m}\sum_{j\neq i}^{n+m}\Phi_{\Sigma_h}(\mathbf{z}_i,\mathbf{z}_j).$$

The *nonparametric calculation of* $D_{n,m}$ can then be achieved via using $\Phi^*_{cen(F*)}(\mathbf{s},\mathbf{t})$. Generally, in the absence of any distributional assumptions, that is in the case where $F$, $G$ are treated as two unknown distributions, we directly define

$$D_{n,m} = \iint K(\mathbf{s},\mathbf{t})d(F-\bar{F})(\mathbf{s})d(G-\bar{F})(\mathbf{t}),$$

where $K(\mathbf{s},\mathbf{t})$ is the uncentered NND kernel, and $\bar{F}$ is the centering distribution defined as

$$\bar{F} = \frac{n}{n+m}F + \frac{m}{n+m}G.$$

Note that the weights used for $F$, $G$ are functions of the sample sizes. In the case of $n=m$, these weights become $1/2$; and the kernel used is the same with $\Phi^*_{cen(F*)}$. As a comment, involving nonparametric integration indicates an urgent demand of increased computational power and computational algorithms providing high accuracy results.

Another issue closely related to the implementation of the tests proposed in Sect. 4.2 is the calculation of its critical value. Since the eigenvalues of the kernel used are involved in the limiting distribution of the test statistic but they are quite hard to determine in most real cases, it is barely possible to directly obtain the critical value using formula (2). So we adapt the strategy from Lindsay et al. [27] to make use of the normal approximate of the limiting distribution. The exact variance of the test statistic can be derived under the null hypothesis, but we decide to not use it because Lindsay et al. [27] find that the achieved level of the one-sample test using the exact variance shows disturbing results. We concentrate on using the empirical critical value of $D_{n,m}$, which does not require the use of the exact variance and has the ability to achieve higher accuracy. In what follows, we present the parametric and nonparametric calculations of the empirical critical value of $D_{n,m}$.

The *parametric algorithm* to calculate the empirical critical value of $D_{n,m}$ based on the multivariate normal assumption is described as follows:

- Estimate $\mu$, $\Sigma$ from $\mathbf{z}_1, \cdots, \mathbf{z}_{n+m}$, using Maximum Likelihood Estimation, as $\hat{\mu}$, $\hat{\Sigma}$.
- Generate $B$ pairs of independent samples $\mathbf{x}^*_{1,b}, \cdots, \mathbf{x}^*_{n,b}$ and $\mathbf{y}^*_{1,b}, \cdots, \mathbf{y}^*_{m,b}$, $b = 1, \cdots, B$, from the multivariate normal distribution with $\hat{\mu}$, $\hat{\Sigma}$.

- For each pair, compute $D^*_{n,m,b}$, $b = 1, \cdots, B$.
- These $D^*_{n,m,1}, \cdots, D^*_{n,m,B}$ are ordered from smallest to largest. The empirical critical value is determined as the 95th quantile of the above list of values.

Note that one can assume the common distribution under the null hypothesis as any distribution, but appropriate kernels and centering distributions that respect the range and measurement scale of the data must be used.

We next provide two *nonparametric calculations of the empirical critical value of* $D_{n,m}$. The first way is to utilize the help of bootstrap methods. The *bootstrap algorithm* to compute the empirical critical value of $D_{n,m}$ is described as follows:

- Draw $B$ pairs of independent samples (with replacement) $\mathbf{x}^*_{1,b}, \cdots, \mathbf{x}^*_{n,b}$ and $\mathbf{y}^*_{1,b}, \cdots, \mathbf{y}^*_{m,b}$, $b = 1, \cdots, B$, from $\mathbf{z}_1, \cdots, \mathbf{z}_{n+m}$.
- For each pair, compute $D^*_{n,m,b}$, $b = 1, \cdots, B$.
- These $D^*_{n,m,1}, \cdots, D^*_{n,m,B}$ are ordered from smallest to largest. The empirical critical value is determined as the 95th quantile of the above list of values.

The second way is to apply permutation procedures. Let $\sigma(1), \cdots, \sigma(n + m)$ be a permutation of $1, \cdots, n + m$. Then $\mathbf{z}_{\sigma(1)}, \cdots, \mathbf{z}_{\sigma(n+m)}$ is a permutation sample of $\mathbf{z}_1, \cdots, \mathbf{z}_{n+m}$. The *permutation algorithm* to compute the empirical critical value of $D_{n,m}$ is described as follows:

- Generate $B$ permutation samples $\mathbf{z}^*_{\sigma_b(1)}, \cdots, \mathbf{z}^*_{\sigma_b(n+m)}$, $b = 1, \cdots, B$, from $\mathbf{z}_1, \cdots, \mathbf{z}_{n+m}$.
- For each sample, let $\mathbf{x}^*_{i,b} = \mathbf{z}^*_{\sigma_b(i)}$, $i = 1, \cdots, n$, and $\mathbf{y}^*_{j,b} = \mathbf{z}^*_{\sigma_b(n+j)}$, $j = 1, \cdots, m$. Calculate $D^*_{n,m,b}$ using $\mathbf{x}^*_{1,b}, \cdots, \mathbf{x}^*_{n,b}$ and $\mathbf{y}^*_{1,b}, \cdots, \mathbf{y}^*_{m,b}$, $b = 1, \cdots, B$.
- These $D^*_{n,m,1}, \cdots, D^*_{n,m,B}$ are ordered from smallest to largest. The empirical critical value is determined as the 95th quantile of the above list of values.

Note that we are in the process of building an R package to implement the one, two, and $k$-sample tests constructed using kernel-based quadratic distances, as well as the associated procedures.

# 6 Simulation Study

This section presents s a simulation study that is used to evaluate the performance of the kernel-based test, and compare it with the existing multivariate two-sample goodness-of-fit tests that are discussed in Sects. 2 and 3.

## 6.1 Simulation Design

To accomplish these objectives, we design the following simulation study. We simulate data from a $p$-dimensional multivariate normal distribution $MVN_p(\boldsymbol{\mu}_k, \Sigma_k)$,

$k = F, G$, where $\mu_k$ is a $p$-dimensional column vector that presents the mean vector and $\Sigma_k$ is a $p \times p$ non-negative definite matrix that represents the covariance matrix. Note that when carrying out the tests, both of $\mu_k$ and $\Sigma_k$ are treated as unknown.

Samples are obtained by using the R package "distrEllipse". We specify the mean vectors as

$$\mathbb{E}_F(\mathbf{X}) = \mathbf{1} \cdot \mu_F, \ \ \mathbb{E}_G(\mathbf{Y}) = \mathbf{1}_{p*} \cdot \mu_G + (\mathbf{1} - \mathbf{1}_{p*}) \cdot \mu_F,$$

where $\mu_F$, $\mu_G$ correspond to the distributions $F$ and $G$, $p^*$ indicates the number of the coordinates where the means of $F$, $G$ differ, $\mathbf{1}$ is a $p$-dimensional column vector of 1, and $\mathbf{1}_{p*}$ is a $p$-dimensional column vector that has value 1 for the first $p^*$ $(0 \leq p^* \leq p)$ elements and value 0 for the remaining elements. The covariance matrices are specified as

$$\mathrm{Cov}_F(\mathbf{X}) = \mathbf{I} \cdot \sigma_F^2,$$

$$\mathrm{Cov}_G(\mathbf{Y}) = \left( \mathbf{I}_{p*} \cdot \sigma_G + (\mathbf{I} - \mathbf{I}_{p*}) \cdot \sigma_F \right) \mathbf{I} \left( \mathbf{I}_{p*} \cdot \sigma_G + (\mathbf{I} - \mathbf{I}_{p*}) \cdot \sigma_F \right),$$

where $\sigma_F$, $\sigma_G$ correspond to the distributions $F$ and $G$ and $\mathbf{I}_{p*}$ is a $p \times p$ diagonal matrix that has value 1 for the first $p^*$ $(0 \leq p^* \leq p)$ diagonal elements and value 0 for the remaining elements. The sample sizes $(n = m)$ used are 50, 100, 200, 300, 400, 500, and 1000. The dimensions are 5, 10, 20, 30, and 40. And $p^*$ is fixed as 3 for all scenarios.

When applying the kernel-based test, we use the multivariate normal kernel $\Phi_{\Sigma_h}(\mathbf{s}, \mathbf{t})$ where $\Sigma_h$ equals $\mathbf{I} \cdot h$ and $h$ is a tuning parameter that needs to be selected. The parametric calculation of $D_{n,m}$ is used because we know the data are generated from multivariate normal distributions. The common distribution under the null hypothesis is assumed as a multivariate normal distribution with unknown $\mu$ and $\Sigma$, which are estimated using Maximum Likelihood Estimation from the pooled sample. Both the parametric and nonparametric calculations of the empirical critical value of $D_{n,m}$ are implemented, as follows. When applying the distributional assumption (QD-MVN), we assume the common distribution under the null hypothesis is a multivariate normal distribution with unknown $\mu$, $\Sigma$; using maximum likelihood estimators $\hat{\mu}$, $\hat{\Sigma}$ obtained from the pooled sample, we generate $B = 5000$ pairs of independent samples as indicated in the parametric algorithm. When using bootstrap methods (QD-Bootstrap), we generate $B = 5000$ bootstrap samples according to the bootstrap algorithm. When applying the permutation procedure (QD-Permutation), we generate $B = 5000$ permutation samples as discussed in the permutation algorithm. Under the null hypothesis, the kernel-based test is implemented with various tuning parameters to see how the achieved level of the kernel-based test changes for different tuning parameters. Under the alternative hypothesis, the strategy adapted from Lindsay et al. [27] is first implemented to select the most appropriate tuning parameter and the kernel-based test is then applied using the tuning parameter selected. All programs of the kernel-based test are written in R.

We also make comparisons, in terms of achieved level and power, with the existing multivariate two-sample goodness-of-fit tests. These tests are Friedman-Rafsky Kolmogorov-Smirnov test (FR-KS), modified Friedman-Rafsky Kolmo- gorov-Smirnov test (modified FR-KS), Friedman-Rafsky Wald-Wolfowitz test (FR-WW), Rosenbaum's Cross Match test (Cross Match), and Maximum Mean Discrepancy (MMD). The R packages of these tests are listed in Table 1.

All simulations are conducted using R 3.3.0 (64 bit) on the computing cluster located at the State University of New York at Buffalo, and carried out as follows. Each scenario is examined for 1000 simulation runs. In each simulation run, two new data sets are generated from the distributions $F$, $G$ and the kernel-based test with three different ways to determine the empirical critical value, as well as the existing multivariate two-sample goodness-of-fit tests selected, are applied on these data sets to test the null hypothesis. The performance of the tests is summarized as the ratio of rejecting the null hypothesis at the level 0.05 over all 1000 simulation runs. The R package to implement the kernel-based tests is under development, and the R codes used in this manuscript are available from the corresponding author upon reasonable request.

## 6.2   Simulation Results

### 6.2.1   Parametric Case

Here we present results associated with testing the null hypothesis $H_0 : F = G = MVN_p(\mu, \Sigma)$.

We first measure the performance of the kernel-based test in terms of achieved level. Figure 1 presents the achieved level of the test using three different ways to calculate the empirical critical value as a function of the sample size $n = m$ and dimension $p$ for various values of the tuning parameter $h$. Specifically, the $x$-axis plots the dimension used and the $y$-axis plots the achieved level. The horizontal line in the plots indicates the theoretical level $\alpha = 0.05$. In this case, $\mu_F = \mu_G = 0$ and $\sigma_F = \sigma_G = 1$.

Figure 1 indicates that the achieved level of QD-MVN and QD-Permutation is very consistent across different values of $n$, $p$, and $h$. And the achieved level of QD-MVN seems more stable than that of QD-Permutation because data are generated from a multivariate normal distribution which is the same as the assumed distribution under the null hypothesis. Increases of the sample size $n$ can improve the performance of QD-Bootstrap and QD-Permutation for different values of $h$ in the sense that their achieved levels become more stable and closer to the theoretical level $\alpha = 0.05$ as the sample size increases. On the other hand, the achieved level of QD-Bootstrap shows decreasing trends when both $h$ and $n$ are small; and when $h$ and $n$ grow larger, the decreasing trend is mitigated. Especially when $n = m = 1000$ and $h = 16, 20$, the achieved level of QD-Bootstrap is very consistent and close to 0.05. This decreasing trend may be explained by the finding of Karoui and Purdom [26],

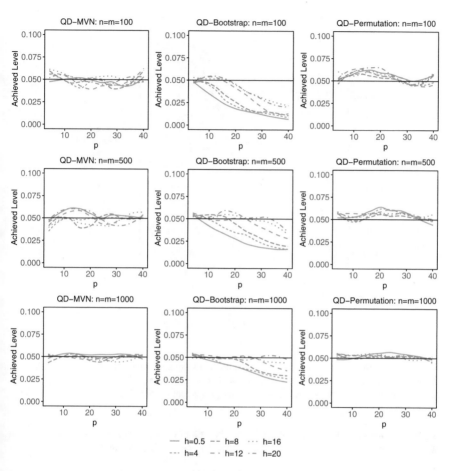

**Fig. 1** Achieved level of the kernel-based test using three different ways to calculate the empirical critical value as a function of the sample size $n = m$ and dimension $p$ for various values of the tuning parameter $h$. The horizontal line indicates the theoretical level $\alpha = 0.05$. The plots are smoothed using LOESS with smoothing parameter 0.6

that is, bootstrap methods have severe loss of power as the ratio $p/n$ grows. Further, the ratio $p/n$ affects the tuning parameter $h$, that is, larger tuning parameters should be used for QD-Bootstrap when the ratio $p/n$ becomes larger. This result is not entirely surprising as the single, most important factor affecting performance (hence selection of $h$) is the dimension of the data.

We next compare the performance of the kernel-based test, in terms of power, with that of the existing multivariate two-sample goodness-of-fit tests. Figure 2 plots the power of the various tests versus the separation between the means of the two distributions $F$, $G$ with $n = m = 100$, $\sigma_F = \sigma_G = 1$, $p = 5$, and $p^* = 3$. The tuning parameter selected for QD-MVN, QD-Bootstrap, QD-Permutation is $h = 14$. It is obvious that the larger the difference between the means of the two distributions

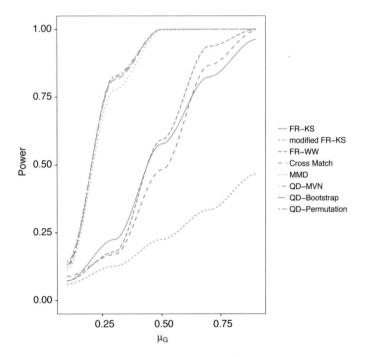

**Fig. 2** Power of the tests studied as a function of the mean difference ($\mu_F = 0$) with $n = m = 100$, $\sigma_F = \sigma_G = 1$, $p = 5$, and $p^* = 3$. The tuning parameter selected for QD-MVN, QD-Bootstrap, QD-Permutation is $h = 14$. The plot is smoothed using LOESS with smoothing parameter 0.6

**Table 2** Tuning parameter selected for QD-MVN, QD-Bootstrap, QD-Permutation as a function of the sample size $n = m$ with $\mu_F = 0$, $\mu_G = 0.2$, $\sigma_F = \sigma_G = 1$, $p = 5$ and $p^* = 3$

| Tests | Sample size ($n = m$) | | |
|---|---|---|---|
| | 100 | 300 | 500 |
| QD-MVN | 14 | 12 | 10 |
| QD-Bootstrap | 14 | 12 | 10 |
| QD-Permutation | 14 | 12 | 10 |

the higher the power is, across all the tests under investigation. The modified FR-KS test has the worst performance because it is designed for scale alternatives. QD-MVN, QD-Bootstrap, QD-Permutation, and MMD present far better performance than the others. Among these top four performers, QD-MVN, QD-Bootstrap, and QD-Permutation have very similar performance, which is generally better than that of MMD. Note that the tuning parameter selected for QD-Bootstrap is not larger than the others because the ratio $p/n$ is fixed and small in this case.

Figure 3 shows the power of the tests investigated as a function of the sample size $n = m$ when the difference occurs in the means ($\mu_F = 0$, $\mu_G = 0.2$). The dimension used is $p = 5$ and $p^*$ is fixed as 3. Correspondingly, Table 2

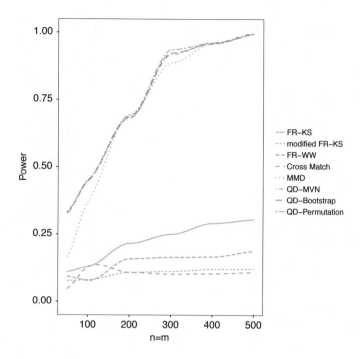

**Fig. 3** Power of the tests studied as a function of the sample size $n = m$ with $\mu_F = 0$, $\mu_G = 0.2$, $\sigma_F = \sigma_G = 1$, $p = 5$ and $p^* = 3$. The tuning parameters selected for QD-MVN, QD-Bootstrap, QD-Permutation are listed in Table 2. The plot is smoothed using LOESS with smoothing parameter 0.6

lists the tuning parameters selected, in the presenting scenario, for QD-MVN, QD-Bootstrap, QD-Permutation. Figure 3 clearly illustrates that all the tests under investigation have better performance as the sample size increases. QD-MVN, QD-Bootstrap, QD-Permutation, and MMD are the top four performers, whose power is much higher than that of the other tests across various sample sizes. Among these four tests, QD-MVN, QD-Bootstrap, QD-Permutation seem to have very similar performance while the power curve of MMD is below its three competitors. Further, from Table 2, we observe that QD-MVN, QD-Bootstrap, QD-Permutation have the same tuning parameter for each sample size studied; the tuning parameters selected decrease as the sample size increases; and QD-Bootstrap does not use larger tuning parameters than the others because the ratio $p/n$ decreases as the sample size increases.

We next illustrate the performance of kernel-based tests in the case of small sample sizes ($n = m = 100$) and relatively high dimensions in relationship to the sample size, with small differences between means.

Figure 4 presents the power of the various tests studied as a function the dimension $p$. The plot shows the case where $n = m = 100$, $\mu_F = 0$, $\mu_G = 0.2$ $\sigma_F = \sigma_G = 1$, and $p^* = 3$. The tuning parameters selected for

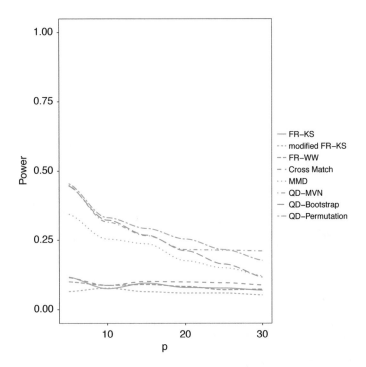

**Fig. 4** Power of the tests studied as a function of the dimension $p$ with $n = m = 100$, $\mu_F = 0$, $\mu_G = 0.2$, $\sigma_F = \sigma_G = 1$, and $p^* = 3$. The tuning parameters selected for QD-MVN, QD-Bootstrap, QD-Permutation are listed in Table 3. The plot is smoothed using LOESS with smoothing parameter 0.6

**Table 3** Tuning parameter selected for QD-MVN, QD-Bootstrap, QD-Permutation as a function of the dimension $p$ with $n = m = 100$, $\mu_F = 0$, $\mu_G = 0.2$, $\sigma_F = \sigma_G = 1$, and $p^* = 3$

| Tests | Dimension ($p$) | | | |
|---|---|---|---|---|
| | 5 | 10 | 20 | 30 |
| QD-MVN | 14 | 15 | 16 | 17 |
| QD-Bootstrap | 14 | 15 | 20 | 24 |
| QD-Permutation | 14 | 15 | 16 | 17 |

QD-MVN, QD-Bootstrap, QD-Permutation are listed in Table 3. Clearly, larger tuning parameters are chosen for higher dimensions. When the dimension is low, the tuning parameters selected for QD-MVN, QD-Bootstrap, QD-Permutation are the same for each dimension $p$. When the dimension becomes higher, QD-MVN and QD-Permutation still have the same tuning parameters; but QD-Bootstrap requires larger tuning parameters. This actually verifies our previous finding, that is, larger tuning parameters should be used for QD-Bootstrap when the ratio $p/n$ grows. Figure 4 illustrates that the power of the tests investigated decreases as the dimension increases. QD-MVN, QD-Bootstrap, QD-Permutation, and MMD are the top four performers, across various dimensions. When the dimension is low (i.e., $p < 20$), QD-MVN, QD-Bootstrap, and QD-Permutation obtain almost the same performance, which is higher than that of MMD. When the dimension grows higher, QD-MVN has the best performance, and although the power for all tests is low, it can keep the power relatively stable; QD-Bootstrap and QD-Permutation present decreasing trends; especially for QD-Bootstrap, its power drops to almost the same value as that of MMD. The severe decreasing trend of QD-Bootstrap may be explained, as we discussed, by the finding that bootstrap methods suffer from severe loss of power as the ratio $p/n$ grows [26].

The aforementioned results illustrate the performance of the kernel-based test as well as the existing multivariate goodness-of-fit tests when the differences between two distributions come from means. We also conduct simulations when the differences come from variances, and here we provide a brief overview of their results. When the differences between two distributions come from variances, QD-MVN, QD-Bootstrap, QD-Permutation, and MMD are still top performers across various scenarios studied. Among these four top performers, the power curves of QD-MVN, QD-Bootstrap, and QD-Permutation are always above that of MMD. Further, QD-Bootstrap tends to have larger tuning parameters selected than QD-MVN and QD-Bootstrap when the ratio $p/n$ grows.

### 6.2.2 Nonparametric Case

We now present results associated with testing $H_0 : F = G$ versus $H_1 : F \neq G$. We have studied the performance of the parametric calculation of the test statistic $D_{n,m}$ using three different ways to compute the empirical critical value. In this paper, we also introduced a completely nonparametric version of the test statistic $D_{n,m}$. In what follows, we provide some results of a simulation study conducted to investigate the performance of this nonparametric calculation.

To measure the performance of the nonparametric calculation of $D_{n,m}$ in terms of achieved level and power, we use the following design. We simulate the data from a $p$-dimensional Laplace distribution ($MVL_p$), whose density function is provided as

$$MVL_p(\mathbf{X}) = \frac{p\Gamma(\frac{p}{2})}{\pi^{\frac{p}{2}}|\Sigma_k|^{\frac{1}{2}}(1+p)2^{1+p}} \exp\left\{ -\frac{1}{2}[(\mathbf{X} - \mu_k)^T \Sigma_k^{-1}(\mathbf{X} - \mu_k)]^{\frac{1}{2}} \right\},$$

where $k = F$ or $G$ corresponds to the densities under testing; $\mu_k$ is a $p$-dimensional column vector that presents the mean vector; and $\Sigma_k$ is a $p \times p$ non-negative definite matrix that does not present the covariance matrix. The covariance matrix is given as

$$\text{Cov}_{MVL_p}(\mathbf{X}) = \frac{4\Gamma(p+2)}{p\Gamma(p)}\Sigma_k.$$

Samples are obtained by using the R package "LaplacesDemon". The mean vectors and covariance matrices of the distributions $F$, $G$ are specified as those used in

Sect. 6.1. The sample size used is $n = m = 100$, and the dimensions are 5, 10, 20, 30, 40. To apply the kernel-based test with the nonparametric calculation of $D_{n,m}$, the multivariate normal kernel $\Phi_{\Sigma_h}(\mathbf{s}, \mathbf{t})$, provided in Sect. 6.1, is implemented. We use the permutation procedure to compute the empirical critical value because it is shown to have better performance, in terms of achieved level and power, than the bootstrap method when the sample size is small. When applying the permutation procedure, we generate $B = 100$ permutation samples as indicated in the permutation algorithm. Each scenario is examined for 100 simulation runs, and the performance of the test is summarized as the ratio of rejecting the null hypothesis at the level of 0.05 over all 100 runs.

Table 4 lists the achieved level of the kernel-based test with the nonparametric calculation of $D_{n,m}$ and the permutation procedure to compute the empirical critical value as a function of the dimension $p$ for various values of the tuning parameter $h$. Clearly, the achieved level of the test is very consistent and close to the theoretical level $\alpha = 0.05$ even if we use only 100 simulation runs.

Table 5 presents the power of the kernel-based test with the nonparametric calculation of $D_{n,m}$ and the permutation procedure to compute the empirical critical value as a function of the dimension $p$. In this case, $n = m = 100$, $\mu_F = 0$, $\mu_G = 0.2$, $\sigma_F = \sigma_G = 1$, and $p^* = 3$. We use the tuning parameter selected for QD-Permutation in Table 3 to illustrate the performance of the nonparametric kernel-based test. It is obvious that the power of this test decreases as the dimension increases.

We also implement the same simulation setting for the nonparametric kernel-based test to investigate the performance of MMD with the exception that 1000 simulation runs are used. The simulation results reveal that the achieved level of MMD is consistent and close to 0.05, but its power curve, across different

**Table 4** Achieved level of the kernel-based test with the nonparametric calculation of $D_{n,m}$ and the permutation procedure to compute the empirical critical value as a function of the dimension $p$ for various values of the tuning parameter $h$

| Dimension ($p$) | Tuning parameter ($h$) | | | | | |
|---|---|---|---|---|---|---|
| | 0.5 | 4 | 8 | 12 | 16 | 20 |
| 5 | 0.07 | 0.06 | 0.05 | 0.05 | 0.07 | 0.07 |
| 10 | 0.04 | 0.05 | 0.07 | 0.05 | 0.07 | 0.04 |
| 20 | 0.05 | 0.04 | 0.04 | 0.06 | 0.05 | 0.05 |
| 30 | 0.05 | 0.05 | 0.06 | 0.05 | 0.04 | 0.06 |
| 40 | 0.06 | 0.05 | 0.05 | 0.07 | 0.06 | 0.05 |

**Table 5** Power of the kernel-based test with the nonparametric calculation of $D_{n,m}$ and the permutation procedure to compute the empirical critical value as a function of the dimension $p$ with $n = m = 100$, $\mu_F = 0$, $\mu_G = 0.2$, $\sigma_F = \sigma_G = 1$, and $p^* = 3$. The tuning parameter used for each dimension is the same as that selected for QD-Permutation in Table 3

| Dimension ($p$) | 5 | 10 | 15 | 20 | 25 | 30 |
|---|---|---|---|---|---|---|
| Power | 0.57 | 0.47 | 0.36 | 0.27 | 0.23 | 0.17 |

dimensions, is clearly below what we can observe in Table 5. In spite of the number of simulation runs used, we believe that the nonparametric kernel-based test already shows a better performance than MMD which takes over the lead among the existing tests even if the tuning parameter used for the nonparametric kernel-based test may not be optimal.

At last, we compare the computational cost of the parametric and nonparametric calculations of $D_{n,m}$. The data are generated from the multivariate normal distribution with the settings described in Sect. 6.1. In this case, $n = m = 50$, $p = 5$, $\mu_F = \mu_G = 0$, and $\sigma_F = \sigma_G = 1$. The multivariate normal kernel $\Phi_{\Sigma_h}(\mathbf{s}, \mathbf{t})$, where $\Sigma_h$ equals $I \cdot 4$, is implemented in both ways of computing $D_{n,m}$. The computational cost is calculated as the average time spent for a single run, in which only one $D_{n,m}$ is computed, over 50 simulation runs. With these settings, the computational cost is 0.288 s for the parametric calculation and 26.177 min for the nonparametric calculation. It is obvious that the computational power required for the nonparametric calculation of $D_{n,m}$ is much higher than that for the parametric calculation. The above simulation was carried out with the sole purpose of measuring the computational time used. To speed up computation, one idea is to adapt the fast computing algorithm proposed by Huo and Székely [25]. This, however, constitutes future work.

Notice that, because of the computational time involved in the nonparametric calculation of the test statistic $D_{n,m}$, we only used a small sample size of 100. When the sample size increases, we believe the power of the test increases as well and the test still outperforms all other tests.

## 7   Real Data Illustration

In this section, we use real data to illustrate the practical application of the kernel-based test introduced in Sect. 4.2, and compare this test with the existing multivariate two-sample goodness-of-fit tests. The data used is Fisher's iris data which has been used by many statisticians to illustrate the application of various statistical procedures. We obtained the data from UCI Machine Learning Repository (https://archive.ics.uci.edu/ml; accessed on April 6, 2019). In this data, there are 150 observations, which belong to three different classes of the flower iris: Setosa, Versicolor, and Virginica; each of these classes contains 50 observations. The data consist of 4 continuous variables: sepal length, sepal width, petal length, and petal width.

We are interested in testing whether Versicolor and Virginica have the same multivariate distribution with respect to all the four variables. Figure 5 presents the density plots of the variables in Versicolor and Virginica. Suppose that we assume the joint distributions of sepal length, sepal width, petal length, and petal width are multivariate normal in Versicolor and Virginica. The null hypothesis is then simplified as

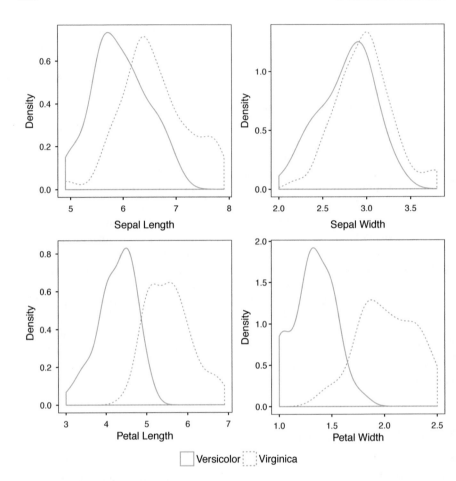

**Fig. 5** Density plot of sepal length, sepal width, petal length, petal width in Versicolor and Virginica. The density estimation uses a Gaussian kernel with the bandwidth automatically selected by the R function "density"

$$H_0 : \mu_{Versicolor} = \mu_{Virginica} \text{ and } \Sigma_{Versicolor} = \Sigma_{Virginica},$$

where $\mu_{Versicolor}$, $\mu_{Virginica}$ are 4 dimensional column vectors that present, from the first to the last row, the means of sepal length, sepal width, petal length, and petal width in Versicolor, Virginica; and $\Sigma_{Versicolor}$, $\Sigma_{Virginica}$ are the corresponding covariance matrices in both classes.

To apply the kernel-based test, we use the multivariate normal kernel $\Phi_{\Sigma_h}(\mathbf{s}, \mathbf{t})$ with $\Sigma_h = \mathbf{I} \cdot h$ where $h$ is the tuning parameter that needs to be selected. Both the parametric and nonparametric calculations of the empirical critical value of $D_{n,m}$ are used. When applying the distributional assumption (QD-MVN), we assume the common distribution under the null hypothesis is a multivariate normal distribution with unknown $\mu$, $\Sigma$ and generate $B = 1000$ pairs of independent samples from a multivariate normal distribution with $\hat{\mu}$, $\hat{\Sigma}$ as discussed in the parametric algorithm. When using bootstrap methods (QD-Bootstrap), we generate $B = 1000$ bootstrap samples from the data according to the bootstrap algorithm. When applying the permutation procedure (QD-Permutation), we generate $B = 1000$ permutation samples as indicated in the permutation algorithm.

Table 6 lists the summary of the variables in Versicolor and Virginica. We can find that the differences between the means of the variables are bigger than those between the variances, skewness and kurtosis; and the mean difference of petal length is almost twice of that of sepal length and petal width while the mean difference of sepal width is close to zero. Therefore, we aim at testing the differences between the means of sepal length, petal length, and petal width in Versicolor and Virginica. The target alternative hypothesis is specified as

$$H_1 : \mu_{Versicolor} = \mu_{Virginica} + \delta \text{ and } \Sigma_{Versicolor} = \Sigma_{Virginica},$$

where $\delta = (\delta, 0, 2\delta, \delta)^T$ and $\delta \neq 0$ is a scalar that indicates the difference between the means. Using the strategy adapted from Lindsay et al. [27], the tuning parameter selected is $h = 4$ for QD-MVN, QD-Bootstrap, and QD-Permutation. We then apply these three versions of the test with the $h$ selected, and find that all of them are in favor of the target alternative hypothesis (test statistic is 0.0006 with critical value 0.000015 for QD-MVN, 0.000028 for QD-Bootstrap, 0.000031 for QD-Permutation).

We also apply Friedman-Rafsky Kolmogorov-Smirnov test (test statistic is 4.4 with p-value $< 0.001$), modified Friedman-Rafsky Kolmogorov-Smirnov test (test statistic is 2.2 with p-value $< 0.001$), Friedman-Rafsky Wald-Wolfowitz test (test statistic is $-8.47$ with p-value $< 0.001$), Rosenbaum's Cross Match test (test statistic is 4 with p-value $< 0.001$), and MMD (test statistic is 28.98 with critical value 2.52) to test the null hypothesis that the variables in Versicolor and Virginica follow the same multivariate distribution. All these tests reject the null hypothesis. Note that Cramer test and Energy test are not implemented as they are very similar to MMD.

**Table 6** Summary of the variables in Versicolor and Virginica

| Summary | Classes | Variable | | | |
|---|---|---|---|---|---|
| | | Sepal length | Sepal width | Petal length | Petal width |
| Mean | Versicolor | 5.936 | 2.770 | 4.260 | 1.326 |
| | Virginica | 6.588 | 2.974 | 5.552 | 2.026 |
| Variance | Versicolor | 0.266 | 0.098 | 0.221 | 0.039 |
| | Virginica | 0.404 | 0.104 | 0.305 | 0.075 |
| Skewness | Versicolor | 0.102 | $-0.352$ | $-0.588$ | $-0.030$ |
| | Virginica | 0.114 | 0.355 | 0.533 | $-0.126$ |
| Kurtosis | Versicolor | 2.401 | 2.552 | 2.926 | 2.512 |
| | Virginica | 2.912 | 3.520 | 2.744 | 2.339 |

To further compare the sensitivities of the kernel-based two-sample test and MMD, we only concentrate on the variable sepal width which has almost the same variance and different means, skewness, kurtosis in Versicolor and Virginica. Regarding the kernel-based two-sample tests, we are interested in testing the null hypothesis that sepal width has the same distribution in both classes versus the alternative that there is a difference between the means. We follow the aforementioned settings to implement QD-MVN, QD-Bootstrap, QD-Permutation, with the exception that we now have a univariate distribution. The tuning parameter selected is $h = 1$ for all the three versions of the kernel-based test; and all the tests are in favor of the alternative hypothesis (test statistic is 0.01 with critical value 0.0006 for QD-MVN, 0.004 for QD-Bootstrap, 0.0035 for QD-Permutation). On the other hand, MMD (test statistic is 2.32 with critical value 2.94) concludes the result of not rejecting the null hypothesis that sepal width follows the same distribution in both classes. The difference between the results of the kernel-based two-sample tests and MMD indicates that the kernel-based tests are more sensitive than MMD.

# 8 Discussion and Conclusions

In this paper, we discuss the fundamental role of statistical distances in the problem of goodness-of-fit and review various existing multivariate two-sample goodness-of-fit tests from both statistics and machine learning literature. The review conducted delivers the fact that there does not exist a satisfactory multivariate two-sample goodness-of-fit test. MMD is reported to have a better performance than other existing tests. But the selection of the kernel used in the MMD test is not discussed often in the literature. The kernel selected is almost by default the Gaussian radial basis function kernel with a specific choice of bandwidth parameter provided by the median heuristic (the median of the inter-point distances between the pooled sample points). As we have previously discussed, this heuristic does not guarantee the optimality of the test performance. And it is unclear how this test can be generalized to the problem of testing equality of more than 2 distribution functions.

We then introduce the kernel-based quadratic distance and the goodness-of-fit tests constructed using this distance. The asymptotic properties of the tests are briefly mentioned, and we point out that there are precise strategies to select the most appropriate kernel tuning parameter that was involved in the construction of the kernel-based tests. We discuss the practical implementation of the kernel-based two-sample test, and introduce various ways to calculate the test statistic and critical value. Our simulation experiments indicate that the kernel-based test is superior to all other existing tests in terms of achieved level and power. The kernel-based test can keep the achieved level stable and close to the theoretical level $\alpha = 0.05$; it also presents better power properties. We also use real data to illustrate that this kernel-based test is more sensitive than MMD.

One issue in the implementation of the kernel-based two-sample tests is the increasing computational cost especially when the distributional assumption is absent. This is because the integration of the kernel used with respect to the common distribution under the null hypothesis is required to obtain the correct model-centered kernel that constructs the test statistic. So it is necessary to have sophisticated computer languages to develop efficient algorithms to speed up the computational procedures. And we are now in the process of building an R package for the implementation of the kernel-based tests. Further, the kernel-based two-sample tests are not applicable to the high dimension low sample size situations. Neuhaus [34] provides a theorem to obtain the limiting distribution of the statistic having the same expression as our test statistic. With the help of this theorem, we may be able to build new tests, using the quadratic distance, that can handle the high dimension low sample size situations, without centering the kernel.

One advantage of the kernel-based tests is the use of the kernel function that has the ability to accommodate different data scales. Data analyzed in real-world applications are rarely comprised of data of exclusively interval scale. Most data are comprised of mixed, continuous and categorical, scale data. This is the case across a diverse range of scientific areas including health care, economics, ecology, biology and other areas. Further, in genetics research, a score test to detect rare genetics variants associated with a disease was developed by Wu et al. [52]. Score tests based on likelihoods are in fact special cases of tests based on general quadratic distances. To apply quadratic distances to genetics research, appropriate kernels need to be constructed.

**Acknowledgement** The work of both authors is supported by The Troup Fund of the Kaleida Health Foundation.

# References

1. Anderson, N. H., Hall, P., & Titterington, D. M. (1994). Two-sample test statistics for measuring discrepancies between two multivariate probability density functions using kernel-based density estimates. *Journal of Multivariate Analysis, 50*(1), 41–54.
2. Aslan, B., & Zech, G. (2005). Statistical energy as a tool for binning-free, multivariate goodness-of-fit tests, two-sample comparison and unfolding. *Nuclear Instruments and Methods in Physics Research Section A: Accelerators, Spectrometers, Detectors and Associated Equipment, 537*(3), 626–636.
3. Barakat, A. S., Quade, D., & Salama, I. A. (1996). Multivariate homogeneity testing using an extended concept of nearest neighbors. *Biometrical Journal, 38*(5), 605–612.
4. Baringhaus, L., & Franz, C. (2004). On a new multivariate two-sample test. *Journal of Multivariate Analysis, 88*(1), 190–206.
5. Bickel, P. J. (1969). A distribution free version of the smirnov two sample test in the p-variate case. *The Annals of Mathematical Statistics, 40*(1), 1–23.
6. Biswas, M., & Ghosh, A. K. (2014). A nonparametric two-sample test applicable to high dimensional data. *Journal of Multivariate Analysis, 123*(1), 160–171.
7. Biswas, M., Mukhopadhyay, M., & Ghosh, A. K. (2014). A distribution-free two-sample run test applicable to high-dimensional data. *Biometrika, 101*(4), 913–926.
8. Blaug, M. (1980). *The methodology of economics: Or, how economists explain.* Cambridge: Cambridge University Press.

9. Burke, M. D. (2000). Multivariate tests-of-fit and uniform confidence bands using a weighted bootstrap. *Statistics and Probability Letters, 46*(1), 13–20.
10. Cao, R., & Lugosi, G. (2005). Goodness-of-fit tests based on the kernel density estimator. *Scandinavian Journal of Statistics, 32*(4), 599–616.
11. Cao, R., & Van Keilegom, I. (2006). Empirical likelihood tests for two-sample problems via nonparametric density estimation. *The Canadian Journal of Statistics, 1*(34), 61–77.
12. Chen, H., & Friedman, J. H. (2017). A new graph-based two-sample test for multivariate and object data. *Journal of the American statistical association, 112*(517), 397–409.
13. Chen, L., Dou, W. W., & Qiao, Z. (2013). Ensemble subsampling for imbalanced multivariate two-sample tests. *Journal of the American Statistical Association, 108*(504), 1308–1323.
14. D'Agostino, R. B., & Stephen, M. A. (1986). *Goodness-of-fit techniques*. New York: Marcel Dekker.
15. Danafar, S., Rancoita, P., Glasmachers, T., Whittingstall, K., & Schmidhuber, J. (2014). Testing hypotheses by regularized maximum mean discrepancy. *International Journal of Computer and Information Technology, 3*(2), 223–232.
16. Durbin, J. (1973). *Distribution theory for tests based on the sample distribution function*. CBMS-NSF, Regional Conference Series in Applied Mathematics. Philadelphia: SIAM.
17. Eric, M., Bach, F. R., & Harchaoui, Z. (2008). Testing for homogeneity with kernel fisher discriminant analysis. In *Advances in neural information processing systems* (Vol. 20, pp. 609–616).
18. Fernández, V. A., Gamero, M. J., & García, J. M. (2008). A test for the two-sample problem based on empirical characteristic functions. *Computational Statistics & Data Analysis, 52*(7), 3730–3748.
19. Friedman, J. H., & Rafsky, L. C. (1979). Multivariate generalizations of the Wald-Wolfowitz and Smirnov two-sample tests. *The Annals of Statistics, 7*(4), 697–717.
20. Gretton, A., Borgwardt, K. M., Rasch, M. J., Schölkopf, B., & Smola, A. (2012a). A kernel two-sample test. *The Journal of Machine Learning Research, 13*(1), 723–773.
21. Gretton, A., Sejdinovic, D., Strathmann, H., Balakrishnan, S., Pontil, M., Fukumizu, K., & Sriperumbudur, B. K. (2012b). Optimal kernel choice for large-scale two-sample tests. *Advances in Neural Information Processing Systems, 25*, 1214–1222.
22. Hall, P., & Tajvidi, N. (2002). Permutation tests for equality of distributions in high dimensional settings. *Biometrika, 89*(2), 359–374.
23. Henze, N. (1984). On the number of random points with nearest neighbors of the same type and a multivariate two-sample test. *Metrika, 31*, 259–273.
24. Henze, N. (1988). A multivariate two-sample test based on the number of nearest neighbor type coincidences. *The Annals of Statistics, 16*(2), 772–783.
25. Huo, X., & Székely, G. J. (2016). Fast computing for distance covariance. *Technometrics, 58*(4), 435–447.
26. Karoui, N. E., & Purdom, E. (2016). Can we trust the bootstrap in high-dimension? arXiv:1608.00696.
27. Lindsay, B. G., Markatou, M., & Ray, S. (2014). Kernels, degrees of freedom, and power properties of quadratic distance goodness-of-fit tests. *Journal of the American Statistical Association, 109*(505), 395–410.
28. Lindsay, B. G., Markatou, M., Ray, S., Yang, K., & Chen, S. C. (2008). Quadratic distances on probabilities: A unified foundation. *The Annals of Statistics, 36*(2), 983–1006.
29. Liu, Z., & Modarres, R. (2011). A triangle test for equality of distribution functions in high dimensions. *Journal of Nonparametric Statistics, 23*(3), 605–615.
30. Lyons, R. (2013). Distance covariance in metrics spaces. *The Annals of Statistics, 41*(5), 3284–3305.
31. Maag, U. R., & Stephens, M. A. (1968). The $v_{nm}$ two-sample test. *The Annals of Mathematical Statistics, 39*(3), 923–935.
32. Mondal, P. K., Biswas, M., & Ghosh, A. K. (2015). On high dimensional two-sample tests based on nearest neighbors. *Journal of Multivariate Analysis, 141*, 168–178.

33. Muandet, K., Fukumizu, K., Sriperumbudur, B., & Schölkopf, B. (2017). Kernel mean embedding of distributions: A review and beyond. *Foundations and Trends in Machine Learning, 10*(1), 1–141.
34. Neuhaus, G. (1977). Functional limit theorems for u-statistics in the degenerate case. *Journal of Multivariate Analysis, 7*(3), 424–439.
35. Pettitt, A. N. (1976a). A two-sample anderson-darling rank statistic. *Biometrika, 63*(1), 161–168.
36. Pettitt, A. N. (1976b). Two-sample cramér-von mises type rank statistics. *Journal of the Royal Statistical Society: Series B, 41*(1), 46–53.
37. Póczos, B., Ghahramani, Z., & Schneider, J. (2012). Copula-based kernel dependency measures. *Proceedings of the 29th International Conference on Machine Learning* (pp. 775–782).
38. Popper, K. R. (1986). *The logic of scientific discovery* (2nd ed.). New York: Harper and Row.
39. Rayner, J. C. W., & Best, D. J. (1986). *Smooth tests of goodness of fit*. Oxford: Oxford University Press.
40. Reddi, S., Ramdas, A., Póczos, B., Singh, A., & Wasserman, L. (2015). On the decreasing power of kernel and distance based nonparametric hypothesis tests in high dimensions. *Proceedings of 29th AAAI Conference on Artificial Intelligence* (pp. 3571–3577).
41. Rosenbaum, P. R. (2005). An exact distribution free test comparing two multivariate distributions based on adjacency. *Journal of the Royal Statistical Society: Series B, 67*(4), 515–530.
42. Savage, L. T. (1972). *The foundations of statistics* (2nd ed.). New York: Dover.
43. Schilling, M. F. (1986). Multivariate two-sample tests based on nearest neighbors. *Journal of the American Statistical Association, 81*(395), 799–806.
44. Sejdinovic, D., Surperumbudur, B., Gretton, A., & Fukumizu, K. (2013). Equivalence of distance-based and RKHS-based statistics in hypothesis testing. *The Annals of Statistics, 41*(3), 2263–2291.
45. Szabo, A., Boucher, K., Carroll, W. L., Klebanov, L. B., Tsodikov, A. D., & Yakovlev, A. Y. (2002). Variable selection and pattern recognition with gene expression data generated by the microarray technology. *Mathematical Biosciences, 176*(1), 71–98.
46. Szabo, A., Boucher, K., Jones, D., Tsodikov, A. D., Klebanov, L. B., & Yakovlev, A. Y. (2003). Multivariate exploratory tools for microarray data analysis. *Biostatistics, 4*(4), 555–567.
47. Székely, G. J., & Rizzo, M. L. (2004). Testing for equal distributions in high dimension. *InterStat, 5*(1), 1–6.
48. Székely, G. J., & Rizzo, M. L. (2005). A new test for multivariate normality. *Journal of Multivariate Analysis, 93*(1), 58–80.
49. Székely, G. J., & Rizzo, M. L. (2013). Energy statistics: A class of statistics based on distances. *Journal of Statistical Planning and Inference, 143*(8), 1249–1272.
50. Wald, A. (1950). *Statistical decision functions*. New York: John Wiley & Sons.
51. Wald, A., & Wolfowitz, J. (1940). On a test whether two samples are from the same population. *The Annals of Mathematical Statistics, 11*(2), 147–162.
52. Wu, M. C., Lee, S., Cai, T., Li, Y., Boehnke, M., & Lin, X. (2011). Rare-variant association testing for sequencing data with the sequence kernel association test. *The American Journal of Human Genetics, 89*(1), 82–93.
53. Zaremba, W., Gretton, A., & Blaschko, M. (2013). B-test: A non-parametric, low variance kernel two-sample test. *Advances in neural information processing systems* (pp. 755–763)

# Hierarchical Modeling of the Effect of Pre-exposure Prophylaxis on HIV in the US

Renee Dale, Yingqing Chen, and Hongyu He

**Abstract**  Pre-exposure chemical prophylaxis has been proposed as a way to slow the growth of the HIV epidemic in the US. This medication reduces the chances of an at-risk, susceptible individual acquiring HIV from an infected partner. The effectiveness of this preventative medication is dependent upon the population that uses it. Individuals susceptible to acquire HIV may engage in risky behaviors such as high partner number. We analyze the effectiveness of chemical prophylaxis on the populations involved in the HIV epidemic in the US using a hierarchical differential equation model. We create a system of nonlinear differential equations representing the system of populations involved in the HIV epidemic, focusing on susceptible and infected individuals. We stratify the susceptible population by behavior risk, and the infected population by behavior risk and HIV status awareness. We further define model parameters for both the national and the urban case, representing low and high sexual network densities. We apply a preventative medication protocol to the susceptible populations to understand the effectiveness. These parameter sets are used to study the predicted population dynamics over the next 5 years. Our results indicate that the undiagnosed high risk infected group is the largest contributor to the epidemic under both national and urban conditions. When medication that prevents contraction of HIV is applied to 35% of the high-risk susceptible population we observe a 40–50% reduction in the growth of the infected population. Little impact is observed when the medication is focused on the low-risk susceptible population.

R. Dale
Department of Biological Sciences, Louisiana State University, Baton Rouge, LA, USA
e-mail: rdale1@lsu.edu

Y. Chen
Biostatistics Program, Fred Hutchinson Cancer Research Center, Seattle, WA, USA
e-mail: yqchen@fhcrc.edu

H. He (✉)
Math Department, Louisiana State University, Baton Rouge, LA, USA

Fred Hutchinson Cancer Research Center, Seattle, WA, USA
e-mail: hhe@lsu.edu

© Springer Nature Switzerland AG 2020
Y. Zhao, D.-G. (Din) Chen (eds.), *Statistical Modeling in Biomedical Research*, Emerging Topics in Statistics and Biostatistics, https://doi.org/10.1007/978-3-030-33416-1_15

The simulations suggest that preventative medication effectiveness extends outside of the group that is taking the drug (herd immunity). Our model suggests that a strategy targeting the high-risk susceptible population would have the largest impact in the next 5 years. We also find that such a protocol has similar effects for the national as the urban case in our model, despite the smaller sexual network and lower transmission chance for rural areas.

**Keywords** Hierarchical differential equations · Nonlinear differential equations · HIV · Pre-exposure prophylaxis · Mathematical modeling

# 1 Introduction

HIV is a disease found across the world that causes autoimmune deficiency syndrome (AIDS). Drugs that treat HIV and prevent AIDS, called anti-retroviral therapies (ART), were first developed in 1985 [1]. It is estimated that 80–95% of HIV infected individuals who are linked to care are prescribed ART [2, 3]. Later it was found that the rate of transmission of HIV was reduced by 44% when HIV-negative at-risk individuals took ART medications as chemoprophylaxis (pre-exposure prophylaxis or PrEP) [4]. It is currently estimated that approximately 135,000 individuals in the US are prescribed chemoprophylaxis, compared to approximately one million infected individuals [5]. However, the HIV infected population shows a steady growth rate [6–8].

To understand what an effective prevalence of PrEP would be, we first need to understand the composition of the susceptible population. Previous research has found that the chance of transmitting HIV is largely dependent on partner number [3, 9]. It is well known that urban and rural populations do not have the same epidemiological dynamics due to differences in population density. In our model we establish two susceptible populations corresponding to an average-density sexual network (national) and high-density sexual network (urban). When considering the effectiveness of P Rep for a given population of susceptibles, we must also consider the many factors involved in those susceptibles contracting HIV. Risky behavior affects transmission events in two ways. High risk susceptibles are more likely to engage in high-risk sexual activities, and they are more likely to do this with a higher partner number. Meanwhile, there is the chance that high risk individuals may not be aware of their status. This can be considered as a generally higher prevalence of risky behavior, and it is reduced by about 50% upon diagnosis [9].

Our model consists of a population of susceptible individuals, stratified by behavior risk, and infected individuals, stratified by both behavior risk and HIV-status awareness. We use our model to look at the effect of a targeted protocol on the rate at which susceptible individuals contract HIV. Our simulations allow us to calculate the optimal target population for PrEP usage based on the projected 5 year population dynamics in high and low risk susceptibles for urban or national (rural and urban) conditions. Our model suggests that targeting the high risk susceptible population is always more effective. While this result is intuitive, we also find that such a protocol is equally effective at the national and urban levels. This demonstrates the unintuitive effect of targeting small sexual networks in the prevention of HIV transmission in the United States.

## 2 Methods

### 2.1 Mathematical Model

To construct our model (Figs. 1 and 2), we first separate the susceptible population into high risk $S_h$ and low risk $S_l$. We use $P(t)$ to describe the growth rate of the susceptibles. We consider new susceptibles to be relatively low risk, and movement into the high risk category is modeled using $g(t)$.

The infected population is stratified by both sexual activity and diagnosis status. High risk undiagnosed individuals are designated as $I_{na}$ (infected not aware active), and diagnosed individuals as $I_{ka}$ (infected knowing active). Movement from undiagnosed to diagnosed is modeled using the diagnosis rate $\delta$. Data suggests that most newly infected individuals are diagnosed within 1 year of contracting the disease [6]. We use $\theta \in [0,1]$ to distribute these individuals between diagnosed and undiagnosed populations proportionally.

We further consider that, regardless of awareness level, some infected individuals may be largely sexually inactive. The transmission of HIV for this group of individuals we consider to be due to rare sexual encounters. We consider low risk individuals' chance of transmitting the disease to be indistinguishable by diagnosis

**Fig. 1** Interactions between populations in the conceptual model of the system of susceptibles $S$, infected $I$, with movement described by the parameters from Table 1

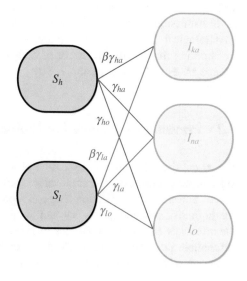

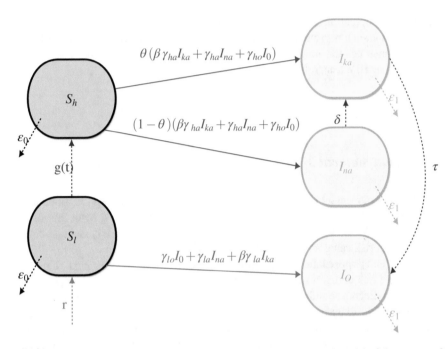

**Fig. 2** Movement of individuals between populations in the conceptual model of the system of susceptibles $S$, infected $I$, with movement described by the parameters from Table 1

status. Both undiagnosed and diagnosed low risk populations are pooled into a single population $I_o$.

Transmission rates are modified according to the relative risk of each group. Infected individuals who are aware are considered to have significant reduction in transmissibility due to reduction in risky behavior, ART usage, and other, psychological factors [3, 9]. Non-active individuals have a very low chance of transmitting the disease, reflective of their low partner number. Death rates of all groups are estimated using data [7, 8].

## 2.2 Preventative Medication Protocol

We model the preventative medication protocol as a control system where the $\pi$'s are control parameters. The removal of individuals from the pool of susceptibles due to preventative medication usage is represented by $\pi$. The rate of PrEP usage for high risk susceptibles is $\pi_h$ and $\pi_l$ for low risk susceptibles. We consider the effects of different magnitudes of preventative effort, from 5% to 30% of the susceptible population yearly. Ideally, one wants to vary $\pi$ to achieve maximal reduction of HIV transmission. We ignore the effect of adherence as preliminary results indicate that even poor adherence (60–70%) provides protection against contraction of the disease [10]. We obtain the following system of equations to describe these dynamics:

$$\frac{dS_h}{dt} = -(1-\pi_h)(\gamma_{ho} \cdot I_o \cdot S_h + \gamma_{ha} \cdot I_{na} \cdot S_h + \beta \cdot \gamma_{ha} \cdot I_{ka} \cdot S_h) - S_h \cdot \epsilon_0 + g(t)$$
(1)

$$\frac{dS_l}{dt} = -(1-\pi_l)(\gamma_{lo} \cdot I_o \cdot S_l + \gamma_{la} \cdot I_{na} \cdot S_l + \beta \cdot \gamma_{la} \cdot I_{ka} \cdot S_l) - S_l \cdot \epsilon_0 + P(t) - g(t)$$
(2)

$$\frac{dI_{ka}}{dt} = \theta(1-\pi_h)(\beta \cdot \gamma_{ha} \cdot S_h \cdot I_{ka} + \gamma_{ho} \cdot I_o \cdot S_h + \gamma_{ha} \cdot S_h \cdot I_{na}) + \delta \cdot I_{na} - \epsilon_1 \cdot I_{ka} - \tau \cdot I_{ka}$$
(3)

$$\frac{dI_{na}}{dt} = (1-\theta)(1-\pi_h)(\beta \cdot \gamma_{ha} \cdot S_h \cdot I_{ka} + \gamma_{ho} \cdot I_o \cdot S_h + \gamma_{ha} \cdot S_h \cdot I_{na}) - \delta \cdot I_{na} - \epsilon_1 \cdot I_{na}$$
(4)

$$\frac{dI_o}{dt} = (1-\pi_l)(\gamma_{lo} \cdot I_o \cdot S_l + \gamma_{la} \cdot I_{na} \cdot S_l + \beta \cdot \gamma_{la} \cdot I_{ka} \cdot S_l) - \epsilon_1 \cdot I_o + \tau \cdot I_{ka}$$
(5)

$$P(t) = r \cdot (S_h + S_l) \tag{6}$$

$$g(t) = \mu \cdot S_l \tag{7}$$

## 2.3 Parameter Estimates

### 2.3.1 National Population Dynamics

We consider the susceptible population to be about ten times larger than the infected population, a conservative estimate since the primary groups affected by the HIV epidemic are MSM and IV drug users [8]. Previous research estimates the size of the high risk population to be about 10% of the susceptible population [3]. Estimates of the undiagnosed population, estimated using the CD4 levels of newly diagnosed individuals, put it at about 20% of the total infected population [6].

The highest transmission rate is between high risk susceptibles and high risk infected who are undiagnosed ($\gamma_{ho}$). Previously it was found that high risk individuals are more likely to get diagnosed in the early stages of the disease, where transmission rate is the highest [11]. We estimate this using the relative differences in transmission rates estimated by fitting epidemiological models to genealogical data [12]. The transmission rate for high risk susceptibles with high risk infected who are aware of their HIV status is reduced in our model by 50% ($\beta$) [9]. Contact between high risk susceptibles and low risk infected is estimated using chronic HIV transmission rates ($\gamma_{ho}$) [12].

Transmission rates for low risk susceptibles engaging with high risk infected who are unaware is estimated using chronic to late stage HIV transmission rates ($\gamma_{la}$) [12]. The transmission rate is reduced by $1 - \beta$ for interaction with diagnosed high risk infected individuals [9]. The transmission rate for low risk susceptibles engaging with low risk infected, $\gamma_{lo}$, is assumed to be the chronic HIV transmission rates [12].

Using data from the CDC, we calculate that approximately 50% of individuals infected between 2006 and 2008 are diagnosed within 1 year [6, 7]. In our model, newly infected susceptibles are immediately moved into the diagnosed category. We set $\theta$ to be $\frac{1}{3}$ since the true number of individuals infected from 2006 to 2008 may not be known until as late as 2018. The diagnosis rate for each year thereafter is estimated as 10% by us, and around 15–16% using other methods [13, 14]. Diagnosis rate is represented as $\delta$ in our model.

The growth rate of the susceptible population is taken to be 1.2%, which is the birth rate of the general U.S. population ($r(S_H + S_L)$) [15]. The mortality of the susceptible population is $\epsilon_0$, the mortality of the general U.S. population. The mortality of the infected population $\epsilon_1$ is obtained from [7]. Movement from low to high risk susceptible ($\mu$) is estimated using the approximate prevalence of high-risk behavior in youth [16]. These rates are not adjusted by the death rate.

We set the proportion of infected individuals as active and aware to be 20% nationally, and 25% in urban areas. CDC data indicates that around 17–30% of HIV-positive MSM engaged in condomless intercourse [3]. Between 3% and 12% of HIV-positive MSM in the same survey reported engaging in condomless intercourse with HIV-negative or unknown HIV status individuals. A survey performed in Los Angeles, CA found that 50–64% of respondents reported engaging in condomless intercourse in the past 3 months [9]. These included both newly diagnosed and known HIV-positive MSM. We use this information to set the proportion of susceptibles that are high risk. We set the national proportion to be 10% and the urban proportion to be 30%. The proportion of unaware and active infected individuals is set at 10% nationally and 15% in high population density areas, as individuals engaging in risky sexual behavior are more likely to seek HIV testing [17].

### 2.3.2 Urban Population Dynamics

Due to the larger infected population and higher diagnosis rates, we consider transmission to be more likely in high population density areas. The data on the HIV infected population in high population density areas indicates a high diagnosis rate, so we increased the number of individuals diagnosed in their first year of infection as well as a higher frequency of diagnosis in the subsequent years. The death rate in Detroit due to HIV infection is approximately six times larger than national [7, 18]. We incorporate this into the model by increasing the death rate of infected individuals.

**Table 1**  Comparison of the parameters for the Urban and General population in the US

| Parameter | Description | Urban | General | Source |
|---|---|---|---|---|
| $\beta$ | Decrease of transmission risk due to diagnosis of infected | 0.5 | 0.5 | [3, 9] |
| $\theta$ | Proportion of individuals diagnosed in first year | **0.4** | $\frac{1}{3}$ | [7, 11] |
| $\tau$ | Proportion of diagnosed high risk individuals becoming low risk | **0.04** | 0.05 | [9, 12] |
| $\gamma_{ha}$ | Transmission rate between high risk $S$ and high risk $I_{na}$ | **0.8** | 0.4 | [12] |
| $\gamma_{ho}$ | Transmission rate between high risk $S$ and low risk $I_0$ | **0.08** | 0.04 | [12] |
| $\gamma_{la}$ | Transmission rate between low risk $S$ and high risk $I_{na}$ | **0.08** | 0.04 | [12] |
| $\gamma_{lo}$ | Transmission rate between low risk $S$ with low risk $I_0$ | **0.02** | 0.01 | [12] |
| $\delta$ | Rate of diagnosis of the general infected population | **0.1** | 0.06 | [7] |
| $\epsilon_0$ | Death rate of susceptibles | 0.017 | 0.017 | |
| $\epsilon_1$ | Death rate of infected | **0.026** | 0.019 | [7] |
| $\mu$ | Susceptible movement from low to high risk | **0.04** | 0.02 | [16] |
| r | Growth rate of susceptible population | 0.015 | 0.012 | |
| | Proportion of $S$ that is active | **0.3** | 0.1 | [3, 11] |
| | Proportion of $I$ that is aware, active | **0.25** | 0.2 | [3, 11] |
| | Proportion of $I$ that is unaware, active | **0.15** | 0.1 | [3, 11] |
| | Proportion of $I$ that is inactive | **0.6** | 0.7 | [3, 11] |

Bolding indicated altered values. Values are taken from the literature when available, or estimated using literature relationships and proportions (primarily [12])

All other parameters are obtained from the literature as stated in Table 1. Simulations were performed in Matlab and code is available as Supplemental. Regional sensitivity analysis of the parameters for the base model and the PrEP model were performed using SAFE toolbox for Matlab [19]. The sensitivity was measured by comparing the proportional changes of the five populations: high risk susceptibles, low risk susceptibles, infected diagnosed active, infected undiagnosed active, and inactive infected. Sensitivities are shown in Figs. 6 and 7.

# 3  Results

In the national case, active undiagnosed infected populations grow up to 50% in 5 years (Fig. 3). The rate of increase for high risk diagnosed infected individuals is 10%, while the rate of increase for high risk undiagnosed infected is 50%. Low risk infected increases by 14% in the fifth year. High risk undiagnosed individuals increase the fastest and remain to be of concern.

We consider the urban situation separately due to the higher population density, which translates into higher density sexual networks. The transmission rates of the

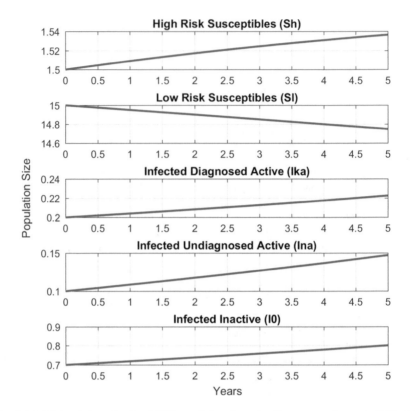

**Fig. 3** Model simulation of national HIV population dynamics. Parameter estimates in Table 1

urban population appear to be much higher than that of the general population. This effect is most likely due to increased ability for larger partner numbers than in rural or small areas. We consider the growth rate of the susceptible population to be equivalent to the national case and reduce the movement of diagnosed active individuals into the inactive pool. We modify the parameters to reflect a larger high risk susceptible population as well as a larger movement from low to high risk of the susceptibles.

In the urban case, the undiagnosed active infected population quadrupled in the same time frame (Fig. 4). The diagnosed active doubled and the inactive population grows at about 25%. Overall, the undiagnosed high risk population is driving the dynamics of HIV infection. Our model suggests that nationally the high risk susceptible population grows, but the high risk susceptible population in high population density areas decreases over time. The high risk susceptible population is clearly a concern (Fig. 5).

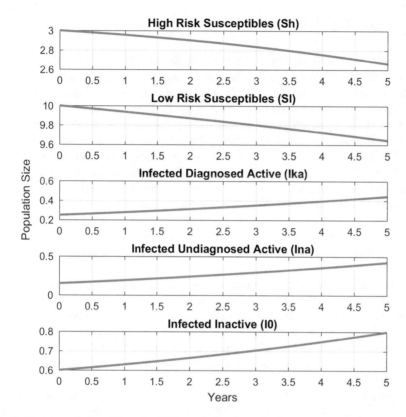

**Fig. 4** Model simulation of the urban HIV population dynamics. Parameters provided in Table 1

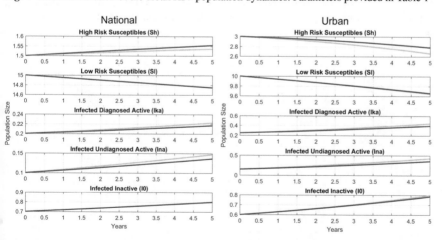

**Fig. 5** No preventative medication (yellow) compared with 20% high risk susceptibles on medication per year (purple) on the national (left) and urban (right) situations. Preventative would appear to be more effective for the population in general than in high density infective populations

## 3.1 Effect of Preventative Medication

We find a linearly increasing reduction on the size of the active infected populations with PrEP usage when applied to high or low risk susceptibles (Table 2). For both national and urban populations PrEP is most effective when applied to high risk susceptibles. In the national case, PrEP usage by high risk susceptibles primarily reduces the infected active aware and unaware populations. In the urban case, a small reduction is also seen in the infected inactive population. If PrEP is primarily used by low risk susceptibles, reduction is primarily observed in the inactive infected population for both national and urban cases. The combination of both low and high risk susceptibles doesn't appear to significantly improve the effects compared to high risk susceptibles alone (Supplemental Figs. 1 and 2).

### 3.1.1 Model Sensitivity Changes with Preventative Medication

The model is most sensitive to parameters that are altered to describe the difference between national and urban dynamics—transmission risk due to diagnosis status ($\beta$), high risk transmission rate ($\gamma_{ha}$), movement from low to high risk susceptible ($\mu$), and proportion of high risk susceptibles and infected non-diagnosed populations (Figs. 6 and 7). Comparing our parameters for the national and urban populations, we double $\gamma_{ha}$ and increase the proportion of high risk susceptibles from 1.2% to 1.5%.

When PrEP is added to the model, the sensitivities change. The proportion of high risk susceptibles on prep and size of high risk susceptibles (phr) determine the dynamics. The dynamics are sensitive to both $\pi_h$ and $\pi_l$, and when comparing the effect of these separately, as well as their combinations, the effect of low-

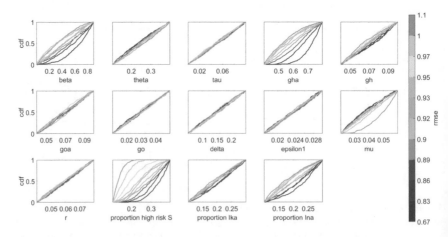

**Fig. 6** Parameter sensitivities for base model ($\pi_h = \pi_l = 0$)

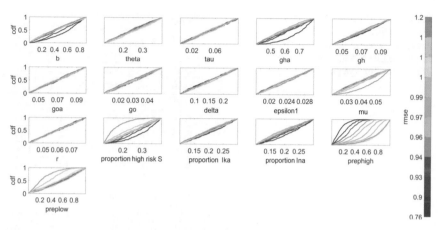

**Fig. 7** Parameter sensitivities when PrEP incorporated

risk susceptible PrEP usage is primarily seen on the low-risk infected group (Supplemental Figs. 2 and 3).

The model suggests that targeting the low risk susceptible population would not be very effective, both in the size of transmission reduction and cost. The low risk susceptible population is estimated to be 10 times larger than the high risk population [3]. A larger effect can be obtained by providing PrEP to high risk susceptibles while reducing the cost by an order of magnitude. The model also suggests that minimal effect would be observed on the inactive infected population. This subpopulation includes both diagnosed and undiagnosed individuals who very rarely interact with susceptibles. We don't expect large changes to occur in this population since they have minimal effect on the HIV epidemic.

# 4 Conclusions

Here we take the control parameters to be constants. We wish to address time variant control parameter in the future. Our results suggest that programmes targeting PrEP to high risk HIV-negative individuals would have similar levels of effectiveness at the national and urban level. The model predicts 40–50% reductions in the size of the diagnosed and undiagnosed active infected populations after 5 years with a medication rate of 35% (Table 2). Previously a 44% reduction in the transmission rate was found in the original study with HIV seronegative men [4]. The increased effectiveness predicted by our model may be due to apparent herd immunity. Not only are individuals taking PrEP protected from HIV transmission, but they confer a degree of immunity to others within the pool of HIV-negative individuals who are at-risk.

**Table 2** Comparison of the effect of a high risk susceptible PreP protocol on the susceptible and infected population after 5 years

| PrEP | $S_h$ | $S_l$ | $I_{ka}$ | $I_{na}$ | $I_o$ |
|------|-------|-------|----------|----------|-------|
| *National* | | | | | |
| 0 | 1.02 | 0.98 | 1.11 | 1.47 | 1.14 |
| 0.05 | 1.03 | 0.98 | 1.11 | 1.44 | 1.14 |
| 0.10 | 1.03 | 0.98 | 1.10 | 1.42 | 1.14 |
| 0.15 | 1.03 | 0.98 | 1.09 | 1.39 | 1.14 |
| 0.20 | 1.04 | 0.98 | 1.09 | 1.36 | 1.14 |
| 0.25 | 1.04 | 0.98 | 1.08 | 1.34 | 1.14 |
| 0.30 | 1.04 | 0.98 | 1.07 | 1.31 | 1.14 |
| 0.35 | 1.05 | 0.98 | 1.07 | 1.27 | 1.14 |
| *Urban* | | | | | |
| 0 | 0.89 | 0.96 | 1.78 | 2.83 | 1.33 |
| 0.05 | 0.90 | 0.96 | 1.73 | 2.71 | 1.33 |
| 0.10 | 0.91 | 0.97 | 1.68 | 2.59 | 1.32 |
| 0.15 | 0.92 | 0.97 | 1.63 | 2.48 | 1.31 |
| 0.20 | 0.93 | 0.97 | 1.59 | 2.37 | 1.31 |
| 0.25 | 0.94 | 0.97 | 1.54 | 2.26 | 1.30 |
| 0.30 | 0.95 | 0.97 | 1.50 | 2.15 | 1.30 |
| 0.35 | 0.96 | 0.97 | 1.45 | 2.05 | 1.29 |

A value $< 1$ indicates a reduction over 5 years, while a value $> 1$ indicates an increase

Targeting PrEP to high risk HIV-negative individuals provides effective protection for the general HIV-negative population according to our model, including those who are lower risk. We also find that targeting rural, smaller sexual networks can effectively curtail the growth of the HIV epidemic. Research suggests that rural individuals have higher risk profiles, as well as more difficulty accessing care [20]. The CDC has reported multiple HIV outbreaks in rural areas involving socioeconomically disadvantaged individuals [21, 22], and the New York Times recently reported on a rural community with a high density of individuals dying due to lacking access to medical attention for their HIV infections [23]. We emphasize that our model makes some assumptions about the sexual network densities of high risk individuals. We expect that, in the real scenario, the benefits provided by herd immunity will increase with increasing PrEP usage over the 35% we consider here.

# Appendix

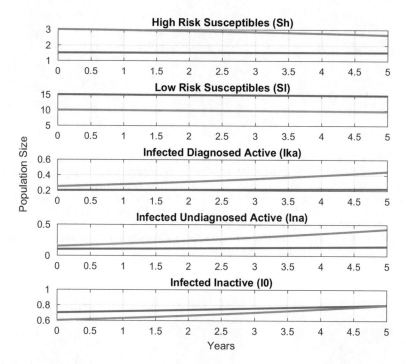

**Supplemental Fig. 1** Comparison between national (blue) and urban (red) dynamics. In the urban case, the infected populations grow much more quickly, while the high risk susceptible population begins to decrease

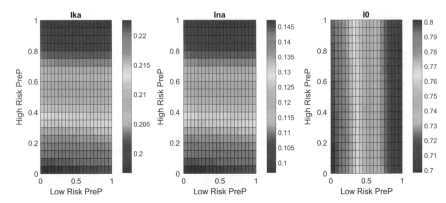

**Supplemental Fig. 2** Effect of PrEP on susceptible populations—national. The effect of PrEP on any combination of low or high risk susceptibles demonstrates that targeting the high risk population is much more effective in the resulting high risk infected populations (Ika, infected diagnosed active; Ina, infected unaware active). As the proportion of low risk susceptibles on PrEP increases, the effect is restricted to reducing the inactive infected population (I0). Hotter (red) values indicate a larger increase in the size of the population. The vertical effect indicates increasing PrEP usage by the high risk susceptible population, while the horizontal effect indicates the effect of low risk susceptible PrEP usage

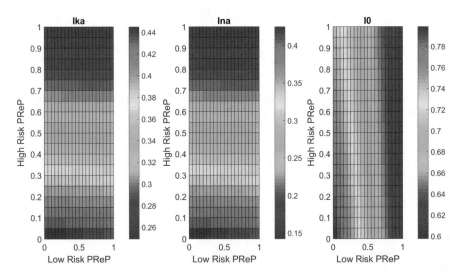

**Supplemental Fig. 3** Effect of PrEP on susceptible populations—urban. The effect of PrEP on any combination of low or high risk susceptibles demonstrates that targeting the high risk population is much more effective in the resulting high risk infected populations (Ika, infected diagnosed active; Ina, infected unaware active). As the proportion of low risk susceptibles on PrEP increases, the effect is restricted to reducing the inactive infected population (I0). Hotter (red) values indicate a larger increase in the size of the population. The vertical effect indicates increasing PrEP usage by the high risk susceptible population, while the horizontal effect indicates the effect of low risk susceptible PrEP usage

# References

1. Broder, S. (2010). The development of antiretroviral therapy and its impact on the HIV-1/AIDS pandemic. *Antiviral Research, 85*, 1–18.
2. Bradley, H., Mattson, C. L., Beer, L., Huang, P., Shouse, R. L., & for the Medical Monitoring Project. (2016). Increased antiretroviral therapy prescription and HIV viral suppression among persons receiving clinical care for HIV infection. *AIDS (London, England), 30*(13), 2117–2124.
3. Centers for Disease Control and Prevention. (2016). *Behavioral and clinical characteristics of persons receiving medical care for HIV infection.* Medical Monitoring Project, United States, 2014 Cycle (June 2014–May 2015). HIV Surveillance Special Report 17.
4. Grant, R. M., Lama, J. R., Anderson, P. L., McMahan, V., Liu, A. Y., Vargas, L., et al. (2010). Preexposure chemoprophylaxis for HIV prevention in men who have sex with men. *New England Journal of Medicine, 363*, 2587–2599.
5. Ryan, B. (2017). *An estimated 136,000 people are on PrEP in the U.S.* Available from https://www.poz.com/article/estimated-136000-people-prep-us
6. Song, R., Hall, H. I., Green, T. A., Szwarcwald, C. L., Pantazis, N. (2017). Using CD4 data to estimate HIV incidence, prevalence, and percent of undiagnosed infections in the United States. *JAIDS Journal of Acquired Immune Deficiency Syndromes, 74*, 3–9.
7. Centers for Disease Control and Prevention. (2016). *HIV Surveillance Report, 2015*, Vol. 27.
8. Centers for Disease Control and Prevention. (2016). *Monitoring selected national HIV prevention and care objectives by using HIV surveillance data: United States and 6 dependent areas, 2014.* HIV Surveillance Supplemental Report 2016 (Vol. 21)(4).
9. Marks, G., Crepaz, N., Senterfitt, J. W., & Janssen, R. S. (2005). Meta-analysis of high-risk sexual behavior in persons aware and unaware they are infected with HIV in the United States: Implications for HIV prevention programs. *JAIDS Journal of Acquired Immune Deficiency Syndromes, 39*, 446–453.
10. Bartlett, J. A. (2002). Addressing the challenges of adherence. *JAIDS, 29*(S1), S2–S10.
11. Davey, D. J., Beymer, M., Roberts, C. P., Bolan, R. K., & Klausner, J. D. (2017). Differences in risk behavior and demographic factors between men who have sex with men with acute and nonacute human immunodeficiency virus infection in a community-based testing program in Los Angeles. *JAIDS Journal of Acquired Immune Deficiency Syndromes, 74*, 97–103.
12. Rasmussen, D. A., Volz, E. M., & Koelle, K. (2014). Phylodynamic inference for structured epidemiological models. *PLoS Computational Biology, 10*, e1003570.
13. Chen, Y., Dale, R., He, H., & Le, Q. A. T. (2017). Posterior estimates of dynamic constants in HIV transmission modeling. *Computational and Mathematical Methods in Medicine, 2017*, 1–8.
14. Pinkerton, S. D. (2012) HIV transmission rate modeling: A primer, review, and extension. *AIDS and Behavior, 16*(4), 791–796.
15. Martin, J. A., Hamilton, B. E., Osterman, M. J. K., Curtin, S. C., & Mathews, T. J. (2017). *Births: Final data for 2015* (National vital statistics report; Vol. 66, No. 1). Hyattsville: National Center for Health Statistics.
16. Levine, D. A., & the Committee on Adolesence. (2013). Office-based care for lesbian, gay, bisexual, transgender, and questioning youth. *Pediatrics, 132*, 297–313.
17. Johnson, B. A., McKenney, J., Ricca, A. V., Rosenberg, E. S., Liu, C., Sharma, A., et al. (2016). Risk factors associated with repeated HIV testing among internet-using men who have sex with men. *AIDS Education and Prevention, 28*, 511–523.
18. Annual HIV Surveillance Report. (2015). Michigan Department of Health and Human Services. City of Detroit.
19. Pianosi, F., Sarrazin, F., & Wagener, T. (2015). *A Matlab toolbox for Global Sensitivity Analysis. Environmental Modelling & Software, 70*, 80–85.
20. Milhausen, R. R., Crosby, R., Yarber, W. L., DiClemente, R. J., Wingood, G. M., Ding, K. (2003). Rural and nonrural African American high school students and STD/HIV sexual-risk behaviors. *American Journal of Health Behavior, 27*(4), 373–379.

21. Conrad, C., Bradley, H. M., Broz, D., Buddha, S., Chapman, E. L., Galang, R. R., et al. (2015). Community outbreak of HIV infection linked to injection drug use of oxymorphone, Indiana, 2015. *Morbidity and Mortality Weekly Report, 64*, 443–444.
22. Yan, A. F., Chiu, Y. W., Stoesen, C. A., & Wang, M. Q. (2007). STD-/HIV-related sexual risk behaviors and substance use among US rural adolescents. *Journal of the National Medical Association, 99*, 1386.
23. Villarosa, L. (2017) America's hidden H.I.V. epidemic. *The New York Times*. Available from https://www.nytimes.com/2017/06/06/magazine/americas-hidden-hiv-epidemic.html?nytmobile=0

# Mathematical Model of Mouse Ventricular Myocytes Overexpressing Adenylyl Cyclase Type 5

Vladimir E. Bondarenko

**Abstract** A compartmentalized mathematical model of transgenic (TG) mouse ventricular myocytes overexpressing adenylyl cyclase type 5 was developed. The model describes well $\beta_1$- and $\beta_2$-adrenergic signaling systems consisting of $\beta_1$- and $\beta_2$-adrenergic receptors ($\beta_1$-ARs and $\beta_2$-ARs), stimulatory and inhibitory G proteins ($G_s$ and $G_i$), adenylyl cyclases types 4–7 (AC4–7), phosphodiesterases type 2–4 (PDE2–4), protein kinase A (PKA), protein phosphatases type 1 and 2A (PP1 and PP2A), G-protein receptor kinase type 2 (GRK2), heat-stable protein kinase inhibitor (PKI), and the inhibitor-1 (I-1). We found that the overexpression of AC5 resulted in an increased basal cAMP production, leading to an increased activation of PKA, prolongation of the action potential, and increased $[Ca^{2+}]_i$ transient. Simulation results suggest blunted response of TG ventricular cells to the stimulation of $\beta$-adrenergic signaling system with isoproterenol comparing to wild type (WT) cells. Simulations of spontaneous $Ca^{2+}$ release showed larger magnitudes of DADs in TG as compared to WT mice. Modeling data were compared to the experimental data obtained from TG mice overexpressing AC5 as well as to the simulations obtained with the mathematical model for WT mice.

**Keywords** Transgenic mice · $\beta_1$- and $\beta_2$-adrenergic receptors · Delayed afterdepolarizations · Phosphodiesterases · Protein kinase A · Isoproterenol

## 1 Introduction

Transgenic mice are important experimental models of the human diseases. Specifically, they have been generated to investigate the heart development and func-

V. E. Bondarenko (✉)
Department of Mathematics and Statistics, Georgia State University, Atlanta, GA, USA

Neuroscience Institute, Georgia State University, Atlanta, GA, USA
e-mail: vbondarenko@gsu.edu

© Springer Nature Switzerland AG 2020
Y. Zhao, D.-G. (Din) Chen (eds.), *Statistical Modeling in Biomedical Research*, Emerging Topics in Statistics and Biostatistics, https://doi.org/10.1007/978-3-030-33416-1_16

tions, as well as the progression and treatment of cardiovascular diseases [1–3]. Of particular interest are the TG mice overexpressing the proteins involved in the $\beta_1$- and $\beta_2$-adrenergic signaling system of cardiac myocytes. It was shown experimentally and in clinical practice that the development of heart failure is accompanied by modifications of the $\beta$-adrenergic signaling system and its components [4]. Because these changes led to the impairment of cardiac function, the idea was to restore it by the specific drugs or by the overexpression of proteins involved in the $\beta$-adrenergic signaling.

Experimental investigations by Engelhardt et al. [5] have shown that the overexpression of $\beta_1$-ARs resulted in a hypertrophy and heart failure. Despite the overexpression level of $\beta_1$-ARs in TG mice was only 15 times the normal expression of wild type (WT) mice, it resulted in the development of cardiac hypertrophy, heart failure, and premature deaths before the age of 14 months. On the other hand, Milano et al. [6] demonstrated an improved cardiac function due to the overexpression of $\beta_2$-ARs. More comprehensive investigation of different levels of overexpression of $\beta_2$-ARs performed by Liggett et al. [7] have shown that cardiac function was dependent on the level of overexpression, and the high levels of overexpression resulted in cardiomyopathy.

The experiments were also carried out with TG mice altering the downstream components of the $\beta$-adrenergic signaling. It was shown that the overexpression or deletion of adenylyl cyclases type 5, 6, or 8 (AC5, AC6, or AC8) can lead to both increased or decreased cardiac function [8]. In particular, TG mice overexpressing AC5 demonstrated an improved baseline cardiac function [9, 10], but the TG mice were more susceptible to arrhythmias upon stimulation of the $\beta$-adrenergic signaling system [11].

To reveal the mechanisms of ventricular myocyte modifications in TG mice overexpressing AC5, we developed and explored a compartmentalized mathematical model of those cells. The model is based on the previously developed mathematical model of the combined $\beta_1$- and $\beta_2$-adrenergic signaling system in mouse ventricular myocytes, which was extensively verified by experimental data [12–15]. In the new model for TG ventricular myocyte, we implemented an overexpression of AC5 by a factor of 26 (according to the experimental finding [9]) and simulated different myocyte behavior found experimentally at baseline and upon stimulation of the $\beta$-adrenergic signaling by 1 $\mu$M isoproterenol.

## 2 Model Development

A mathematical model for TG mouse ventricular myocytes overexpressing AC5 is based on our previously published mathematical models of mouse ventricular myocytes [12–15] (Fig. 1). It contains three major compartments: (1) the caveolar compartment with the cholesterol-rich membrane domain that includes caveolin 3; (2) the extracaveolar compartment with cholesterol-rich lipid rafts that do not include caveolin; (3) the cytosolic compartment associated with the remainder of the cell membrane [12, 15]. The $\beta$-adrenergic receptors ($\beta$1-AR and $\beta$2-AR)

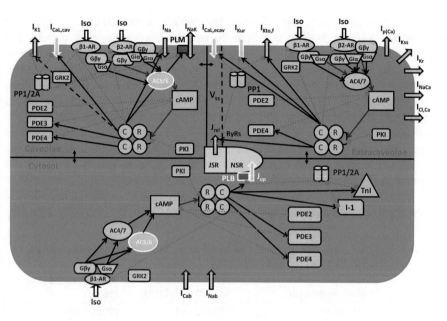

**Fig. 1** A schematic representation of the β-adrenergic signaling system in mouse ventricular myocytes overexpressing type 5 adenylyl cyclase. The cell consists of three compartments (caveolae, extracaveolae, and cytosol). The subspace volume ($V_{ss}$) is localized in the extracaveolae. The signaling system consists of the $\beta_1$-adrenergic receptors (β1-AR), the $\beta_2$-adrenergic receptors (β2-AR), the α-subunit of stimulatory G-protein ($G_{s\alpha}$), the α-subunit of inhibitory G-protein ($G_{i\alpha}$), the βγ-subunit of $G_s$ and $G_i$ ($G_{\beta\gamma}$), the adenylyl cyclases of type 5/6 or 4/7 (AC5/6 or AC4/7, respectively), the phosphodiesterases of type 2, 3, or 4 (PDE2, PDE3, or PDE4, respectively), the cyclic AMP (cAMP), regulatory (R) and catalytic (C) subunits of protein kinase A holoenzyme, the protein kinase A inhibitor (PKI), the G-protein-coupled receptor kinase of type 2 (GRK2), the protein phosphatases of type 1 and 2A (PP1 and PP2A, respectively), the inhibitor-1 (I-1). Targets of the β-adrenergic signaling system are in the caveolae (the fast $Na^+$ current ($I_{Na}$), the L-type $Ca^{2+}$ current ($I_{CaL,cav}$), the $Na^+/K^+$ pump ($I_{NaK}$) which is regulated by phospholemman (PLM), phosphodiesterases PDE2-PDE4, and the time-independent $K^+$ current ($I_{K1}$)), the extracaveolae (the L-type $Ca^{2+}$ current ($I_{CaL,ecav}$), the rapidly recovering transient outward $K^+$ current ($I_{Kto,f}$), the ultra-rapidly activating delayed rectifier $K^+$ current ($I_{Kur}$), ryanodine receptors (RyRs), and phosphodiesterases (PDE2, PDE4)), and cytosol (phospholamban (PLB) and troponin I (TnI)). Stimulatory links are shown by black arrows and inhibitory links are shown by red dashed lines with balls. Other transmembrane currents are the sarcolemmal $Ca^{2+}$ pump ($I_{p(Ca)}$), the $Na^+/Ca^{2+}$ exchanger ($I_{NaCa}$), the rapid delayed rectifier $K^+$ current ($I_{Kr}$), the noninactivating steady-state voltage activated $K^+$ current ($I_{Kss}$), the $Ca^{2+}$ and $Na^+$ background currents ($I_{Cab}$ and $I_{Nab}$), which are not affected by the β-adrenergic signaling systems. The $Ca^{2+}$ fluxes are uptake of $Ca^{2+}$ from the cytosol to the network sarcoplasmic reticulum (NSR) ($J_{up}$) by the SERCA pump and $Ca^{2+}$ release from the junctional sarcoplasmic reticulum (JSR) ($J_{rel}$) through the ryanodine receptors. $[Ca^{2+}]_i$, $[Na^+]_i$, and $[K^+]_i$ are the intracellular $Ca^{2+}$, $Na^+$, and $K^+$ concentrations in the caveolae, extracaveolae, and cytosol; $[Ca^{2+}]_o$, $[Na^+]_o$, and $[K^+]_o$ are the extracellular $Ca^{2+}$, $Na^+$, and $K^+$ concentrations. Proteins which characteristics are modified in transgenic mouse overexpressing AC5 are shown in white. Reproduced with modifications from Bondarenko [12]

were stimulated by isoproterenol (Iso). This leads to activation of the stimulatory G protein ($G_s$) by $\beta_1$-ARs and both $G_s$ and inhibitory G protein ($G_i$) by $\beta_2$-ARs, resulting in activation of adenylyl cyclases AC5/6 in caveolae and cytosol and AC4/7 in extracaveolae and cytosol. AC4–7 generated cyclic AMP (cAMP), which activated protein kinase A (PKA) holoenzyme. Catalytic subunits of PKA phosphorylated multiple targets, such as $\beta_1$- and $\beta_2$-ARs, phosphodiesterases PDE3 and PDE4, the L-type $Ca^{2+}$ current ($I_{CaL}$), the fast $Na^+$ current ($I_{Na}$), the phospholemman (PLM), which regulates the $Na^+$-$K^+$ pump ($I_{NaK}$), the ryanodine receptors (RyRs), the ultra-rapidly activating delayed rectifier $K^+$ current ($I_{Kur}$), the rapidly inactivating transient outward $K^+$ current ($I_{Kto,f}$), the time-independent $K^+$ current ($I_{K1}$), phospholamban (PLB), and troponin I (TnI) (Fig. 1).

Several parameters were changed in the mathematical model of mouse ventricular myocytes overexpressing AC5, found experimentally (Table 1). First, we

**Table 1** Differences between the current model of mouse ventricular myocytes overexpressing AC5 and the model by Rozier and Bondarenko [15]

|  | Parameter definition | WT cell model [15] | TG cell model [this paper] |
|---|---|---|---|
| $[AC]_{tot}$ | Total cellular AC concentration | 0.02622 μM | 0.2295 μM |
| $f_{AC56, AC47}$ | Fraction of AC that is of type 5 or 6 | 0.74 | 0.97029 |
| $G_{CaL}$ | Specific maximum conductivity for L-type $Ca^{2+}$ channel (non-phosphorylated) | 0.3772 mS/μF | 0.32062 mS/μF |
| $G_{CaLp}$ | Specific maximum conductivity for L-type $Ca^{2+}$ channel (phosphorylated) | 0.7875 mS/μF | 0.6694 mS/μF |
| $v_3$ | SR $Ca^{2+}$-ATPase maximum pump rate | 306.0 μM s$^{-1}$ | 918.0 μM s$^{-1}$ |
| $K_{m,up}^{np}$ | Half-saturation constant for SR $Ca^{2+}$-ATPase pump (non-phosphorylated) | 0.41 μM | 0.902 μM |
| $K_{m,up}^{p}$ | Half-saturation constant for SR $Ca^{2+}$-ATPase pump (phosphorylated) | 0.31 μM | 0.682 μM |
| $G_{Kurp}$ | Specific maximum conductance of the ultra-rapidly activating $K^+$ current (phosphorylated)$_*$ | 0.53307 pA/pF | 0.4451 pA/pF |
| $k_{IKur\_PKA}$ | Rate of $I_{Kur}$ phosphorylation by PKA$_*$ | $6.9537 \times 10^{-3}$ μM$^{-1}$ s$^{-1}$ | $1.391 \times 10^{-2}$ μM$^{-1}$ s$^{-1}$ |
| $K_{IKur\_PKA}$ | Relative affinity for $I_{Kur}$ phosphorylation by PKA$_*$ | 0.138115 | 2.0 |
| $k_{IKur\_PP}$ | Rate of $I_{Kur}$ dephosphorylation by PP1$_*$ | $3.170 \times 10^{-2}$ μM$^{-1}$ s$^{-1}$ | $2.536 \times 10^{-2}$ μM$^{-1}$ s$^{-1}$ |
| $K_{IKur\_PP}$ | Relative affinity for $I_{Kur}$ dephosphorylation by PP1$_*$ | 0.23310 | 0.2 |

increased expression of AC5 by a factor of 26 (according to the experimental finding [9]). Then we evaluated an increase in concentration of AC5 in the total concentration of adenylyl cyclases, $[AC]_{tot,TG}$, in TG mice overexpressing AC5 based on the experimental data and our model [15]. Because of experimental difficulties of separation of AC5 and AC6, we used the experimental fact that the ventricular myocytes from transgenic mice with AC5 deletion showed a 35% reduction of basal AC activity [16]. From our simulations [15], we obtained that the fractional contribution of AC activities from different compartments under basal conditions are 11.23%, 9.79%, 72.30%, and 6.68% for AC5/6 in caveolae, AC4/7 in extracaveolae, AC5/6 in cytosol, and AC4/7 in cytosol, respectively. The total contribution of AC5/6 to the total cellular AC activity is, therefore, 83.53%. To obtain a 35% reduction in the total AC activity due to the deletion of AC5, we found that the contributions of AC5 and AC6 should be 41.9% and 58.1% (or 0.419 and 0.581 in fractions), respectively. Out of $[AC]_{tot} = 0.02622$ μM, the fraction of AC5/6 is 0.74 [12], which gives $[AC]_{AC5/6} = 0.01940$ μM, leaving AC4/7 $[AC]_{AC4/7} = 0.00682$ μM. Overexpression of AC5 by 26 times gives the proportional increase of AC5 activity by factor 10.894, with the total AC5/6 concentration increase by factor 10.894 plus 0.581, which is equal to 11.475. Multiplication of 11.475 by $[AC]_{AC5/6} = 0.01940$ μM gives the total concentration of AC5/6 in TG cells, $[AC]_{AC5/6, TG} = 0.2226$ μM.

Assuming that the concentration of $[AC]_{AC4/7} = 0.00682$ μM in TG cell does not change, we obtain the total AC concentration in TG mouse ventricular myocytes is $[AC]_{tot,TG} = 0.00682$ μM $+ 0.2226$ μM $= 0.2295$ μM. In addition, we changed fractional contribution of AC5/6 activity $f_{AC56,AC47}$ from 0.74 in wild type (WT) to 0.97029 in TG cells to reflect the AC5 overexpression.

Further, experimental data by Zhao et al. [11] showed a threefold increase in the expression levels of both SR $Ca^{2+}$ ATPase (SERCA2a) and phospholamban (PLB). In our model, we increased the SR $Ca^{2+}$-ATPase maximum pump rate by threefold as well. We also increased half-saturation constants for SR $Ca^{2+}$-ATPase pump (non-phosphorylated and phosphorylated) by a factor 2.2 to implement a threefold increase in PLB expression. This factor was obtained by the extrapolation data by Luo et al. [17] for PLB knock-out mice and Kadambi et al. [18] for mice with twofold overexpression of PLB.

Moreover, we modified the description of phosphorylation of the ultra-rapidly activating $K^+$ current, $I_{Kur}$ (Table 1). In our mathematical model [12, 13], $I_{Kur}$ includes $K^+$ currents carried by both Kv1.5 and Kv2.1 ion channels, which have different response to β-adrenergic stimulation. Experimental data by Li et al. [19] demonstrated a 35% increase in $I_{Kur}$ in human atrial myocytes upon stimulation with 1 μM isoproterenol. Additional experiments with application of 200 μM of 4-AP, a Kv1.5 inhibitor, with and without 1 μM isoproterenol, have shown that the predominant portion of $I_{Kur}$ in the human atria is Kv1.5 channels. This finding also supported by the experimental data on expression of Kv1.5 and Kv2.1 in the human atria, where the expression level of Kv2.1 is about 1% of that for Kv1.5

[20]. Electrophysiological recording also shows that the magnitude of the remaining component of $I_{Kur}$ in the human atria is about ~15% [21]. In mice, $K^+$ currents encoded by both Kv1.5 and Kv2.1 have approximately equal magnitudes [22, 23]. The effect of PKA on Kv2.1 is quite small, as it was shown experimentally [24, 25]. Therefore, the effect of isoproterenol on $I_{Kur}$ in our mathematical model of mouse ventricular myocytes should be also smaller by a factor 2. Indeed, in our model, presented here, an increase in $I_{Kur}$ upon stimulation with 1 μM isoproterenol is ~15%. We also adjusted $I_{Kur}$ in WT model of mouse ventricular myocytes [15], and the changes are marked by ($_*$) in Table 1.

Finally, we reduced the conductance of the phosphorylated and non-phosphorylated L-type $Ca^{2+}$ channels by a factor 0.85 to obtain experimentally found moderate increase in the basal $I_{CaL}$ (estimated from 16% to 75% [11]) due to increased adenylyl cyclase activity. In our model, $I_{CaL}$ was increased by 27%. This value allowed for matching an experimental increase in the SR $Ca^{2+}$ load in TG mice as compared to WT mice, which was between 23% and 37.5%. Our simulations demonstrated ~40% increase in the SR $Ca^{2+}$ load, which is close to the experimental value.

# 3 Method of Simulation

We used a fourth-order Runge-Kutta method with two different time steps for the solution of the mathematical model consisting of 149 ordinary differential equations. A relatively small time step of 0.000002 ms was used during a 10 ms interval after the initiation of the stimulus current; for all other times we used the time step 0.0001 ms. We used much longer time step, 0.1 ms, for simulation of the cellular behavior without electrical stimulation. The program code was implemented in FORTRAN 90. Computer simulations were performed on a single processor under SUSE Linux 11 on a Dell Precision Workstation T3500 with a six-core Intel Xeon CPU W3670 (3.2 GHz, 12 GB RAM). The model is developed for a room temperature of 25 °C (T = 298°K). Initial conditions were obtained by running the program code without electrical stimulations for 10,000 s to achieve steady-state solution. Action potentials and $[Ca^{2+}]_i$ transients were initiated by a stimulus current ($I_{stim}$ = 80 pA/pF, $\tau_{stim}$ = 1 ms) with the frequency ranged from 0.25 Hz to 5 Hz (electrical stimulation).

# 4 Results

In this paper, we developed a mathematical model of the ventricular myocyte from TG mice overexpressing type 5 adenylyl cyclase. The model includes three major subcellular compartments, caveolae, extracaveolae, and cytosol. It was explored to investigate the effects of stimulation of the β-adrenergic signaling system with isoproterenol under different physiological conditions. Under these physiological conditions, we investigated compartmentalization of cAMP, PKA activation, as well as generation of the action potential and $[Ca^{2+}]_i$ transients. Simulations of spontaneous $Ca^{2+}$ release showed larger magnitudes of pro-arrhythmic events (DADs) in TG as compared to WT mice. Simulation data on TG mice were compared to those obtained for WT mice.

## 4.1 cAMP and PKA Activation in WT and TG Myocytes Overexpressing AC5

Experimental data shows a significant increase in the level of background adenylyl cyclase activity in TG mice overexpressing AC5 as compared to WT mice (26-fold overexpression, Fig. 2b) [9]. In our model, we increased concentration of AC5 by 26 fold as well (Fig. 2a). As result, we were able to match experimental background total adenylyl cyclase activity in ventricular myocytes from TG mice (Fig. 2b). While our simulated WT data shows larger total AC activity (16 pmol/mg/min) than the experimental data by Lai et al. [9] (~8 pmol/mg/min), the former is close to the experimental data obtained by others (18.8 pmol/mg/min [27]) and (22 pmol/mg/min [26], Fig. 2b).

Upon stimulation with isoproterenol, the total AC activity increases in both WT and TG mice, however, to different degrees at maximum stimulation with 10 μM isoproterenol. The simulated maximum AC activity is significantly larger for TG mice overexpressing AC5 than that for WT mice (Fig. 2c). Our simulations show larger AC activity in TG mice without application of isoproterenol, and this relation sustained at high dose of isoproterenol (10 μM). Simulated increase in the total AC activity for WT mice upon application of 5 μM isoproterenol is 4.0 fold as compared to control, which is close to the experimentally found values of 2.7 fold [26] and 3.3 fold [27], but significantly smaller value than ~18 fold increase obtained in [9]. Simulated increase in the total AC activity in TG mice overexpressing AC5 is 2.3 fold upon application of 5 μM isoproterenol, which is close to the experimental value 2.0 [9, 28].

Simulated cAMP concentrations in WT and TG mouse ventricular cells display different dynamics in the three major cellular compartments without and with stimulation by 1 μM isoproterenol. cAMP dynamics is defined by cAMP production by adenylyl cyclases, cAMP degradation by phosphodiesterases, and cAMP diffusion between intracellular compartments. Figure 3 shows the simulated time courses of cAMP concentrations in different subcellular compartments in control (solid black lines for WT and solid gray lines in TG mice) and upon stimulation with 1 μM isoproterenol (dashed black lines for WT and dashed gray lines in TG mice). The modeling data shows different levels of cAMP in different compartments in control both in WT and TG ventricular myocytes. The largest background levels of cAMP are in the caveolar and cytosolic compartments in TG mice, where overexpressed AC5 is localized (23.0 μM and 20.5 μM, respectively). The level of cAMP in

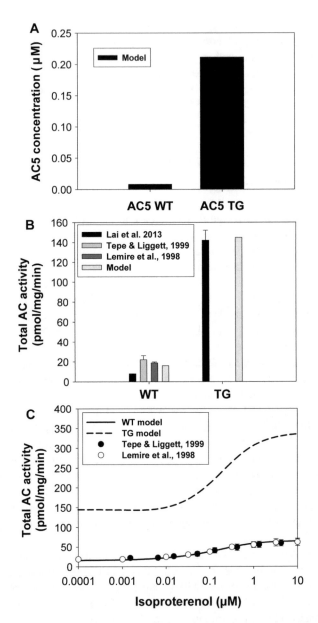

**Fig. 2** Adenylyl cyclase activities in WT and TG mice overexpressing AC5. (**a**) Adenylyl cyclase 5 concentrations in WT and TG mice. (**b**) Experimental and simulated total background adenylyl cyclase activities in WT and TG mice. Experimental data by Lai et al. [9] are shown by black bars; experimental data by Tepe and Liggett [26] for WT mice are shown by a light gray bar; experimental data by Lemire et al. [27] for WT mice are shown by a dark gray bar; simulation data are shown by light gray bars. (**c**) Simulated and experimental total AC activities in WT and TG mice as functions of isoproterenol concentrations. Experimental data by Tepe and Liggett [26] for WT mice are shown by filled circles; experimental data by Lemire et al. [27] are shown by unfilled circles; simulation data are shown by solid (WT mice) and dashed (TG mice) lines. Data in this Figure are shown after 10 min of intervention

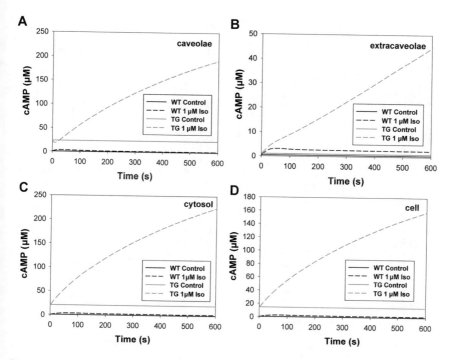

**Fig. 3** Simulated cAMP dynamics in ventricular myocytes from WT and TG mice. (**a–d**) show simulations of cAMP concentration in caveolae, extracaveolae, cytosol, and the whole cell as functions of time. Simulations were performed for four cases: WT control, WT plus 1 μM isoproterenol, TG control, and TG plus 1 μM isoproterenol

the extracaveolar compartment of TG cells is significantly smaller, 1.0 μM; it is determined both by the generation of cAMP by AC4/7 and by the cAMP fluxes from the caveolar and cytosolic compartments. The background cAMP levels in WT mouse cells are significantly smaller in all compartments, caveolae, extracaveolae, and cytosol (0.33 μM, 0.47 μM, and 0.41 μM, respectively).

Myocyte stimulation with 1 μM isoproterenol produces cAMP transients in WT mice with the maxima between 30 s (caveolae) and 70 s (cytosol) and with the values of 3.25 μM, 3.09 μM, and 3.7 μM in the caveolae, extracaveolae, and cytosol, respectively. cAMP behavior in TG mice is remarkably different and demonstrates continuous growth during 10-min simulation interval up to 191.5 μM, 44.7 μM, and 224.5 μM in the caveolar, extracaveolar, and cytosolic compartments, respectively. Comparison of cAMP transients in WT and TG mice in different compartments upon stimulation with 1 μM isoproterenol demonstrates much smaller effects in WT as compared to TG ventricular myocytes (Fig. 3).

Simulated time behavior of the catalytic subunit of PKA reflects that of cAMP (Fig. 4). Considerably higher concentrations of the catalytic subunit of PKA are generated by the TG vs WT mouse model in the three compartments in control due to a significantly higher concentration of cAMP in those compartments (Fig. 4). Upon

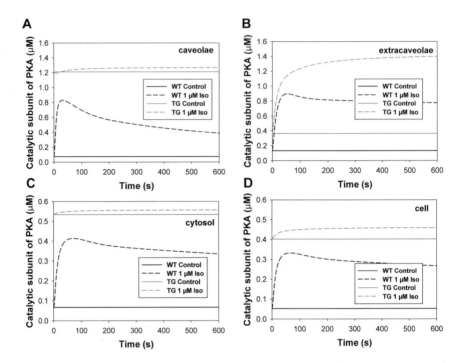

**Fig. 4** Simulated PKA dynamics in ventricular myocytes from WT and TG mice. (**a–d**) show simulations of the catalytic subunit of PKA concentration in caveolae, extracaveolae, cytosol, and the whole cell as functions of time. Simulations were performed for four cases: WT control, WT plus 1 μM isoproterenol, TG control, and TG plus 1 μM isoproterenol

stimulation with 1 μM isoproterenol, simulations demonstrate blunted response of the activation of PKA in the caveolae and cytosol in TG cells while in the extracaveolae activation of PKA shows wider range. In WT myocytes, an increase in concentration of the catalytic subunit of PKA in response to stimulation with isoproterenol is much more significant, from a sixfold increase in the cytosol to an 11-fold increase in the caveolae.

## 4.2 The Effects of Isoproterenol on the Action Potential, $Ca^{2+}$ and $Na^+$ Dynamics in WT and TG Mouse Ventricular Myocytes Overexpressing AC5

Our mathematical model allows for evaluation of the effects of overexpression of AC5 on the action potential, ionic currents, and $Ca^{2+}$ and $Na^+$ dynamics in mouse ventricular myocytes. Experimental data demonstrates an increase in the action potential duration in TG mouse ventricular myocytes as compared to WT cells under basal (control) conditions [11]. Experimentally found increase in $APD_{50}$ was not significant, but an increase in the average value was quite large, about 25% (the interval of variation is from 5% to 50%). Our simulated increase in $APD_{50}$ is moderate, about 13.7%. The larger and significant experimental increase was observed for $APD_{90}$, which was equal on average to 38% (the interval of variation is from 6% to 83%). Our simulated increase in $APD_{90}$ was 29%.

Simulations allow for revealing the mechanism of APD prolongation in TG mice overexpressing AC5, comparing to WT mice. Comparison of Fig. 5c, e shows a quite significant increase in the L-type $Ca^{2+}$ current ($I_{CaL}$) and a reduction in the fast transient outward $K^+$ current ($I_{Kto,f}$) in TG cells as compared to WT cells. Both effects were towards a prolongation of APDs. The effect was partially offset by a moderate increase in the ultra-rapidly activating $K^+$ current ($I_{Kur}$), which promotes a reduction of the action potential duration.

Thus, our model reasonably well reproduced the experimental data on the differences in the action potential durations between WT and TG mouse cells and revealed the mechanism of the action potential prolongation in TG mice overexpressing AC5. Increased APDs in TG mouse ventricular myocytes provide the pro-arrhythmic substrates for their hearts.

Simulations show a significant increase in APDs in WT mice after application of 1 $\mu$M isoproterenol as compared to control. Simulated $APD_{50}$ and $APD_{90}$ increased by 34% and 39%, respectively (Fig. 5). In contrast, the simulated response of TG mouse ventricular myocytes to stimulation with 1 $\mu$M isoproterenol is blunted. Only $APD_{50}$ moderately increased by 11% in TG mice after application of isoproterenol; the changes of other APDs were <10% (Fig. 5). Simulations revealed the major players in the action potential prolongation in WT cells. Figure 5 shows that the application of 1 $\mu$M isoproterenol resulted in a significant increase in the L-type $Ca^{2+}$ current ($I_{CaL}$) and a significant decrease in the fast transient outward $K^+$ current ($I_{Kto,f}$). Both effects were towards the prolongation of APD. The effects of $I_{CaL}$ and $I_{Kto,f}$ were partially reduced by an increase in the ultra-rapidly activating $K^+$ current ($I_{Kur}$), which tends to reduce action potential duration.

The changes in both APDs and underlying ionic currents after application of 1 $\mu$M isoproterenol in TG mice were less apparent. At the initial stage of repolarization, a minor decrease in $I_{Kto,f}$ resulted in a small increase in $APD_{50}$. At the later stage of repolarization, a relatively moderate increase in $I_{CaL}$ and a minor decrease in $I_{Kto,f}$ were compensated by an increase in $I_{Kur}$, producing virtually no change to $APD_{90}$ (Fig. 5a).

Stimulation of the model of WT ventricular myocytes with 1 $\mu$M isoproterenol resulted in a quite large increase in the magnitude of $[Ca^{2+}]_i$ transient (a 3.7-fold increase, Fig. 5b). A smaller increase in $[Ca^{2+}]_i$ transient (a 1.9-fold increase, Fig. 5b) was observed in TG mice overexpressing AC5. Under basal conditions, TG mice have a 1.8-fold larger simulated $[Ca^{2+}]_i$ transient as compared to WT mice, which is comparable to a 1.46-fold experimental increase in $[Ca^{2+}]_i$ [11]. The model was able to reproduce a decrease in the time constant of $[Ca^{2+}]_i$ transient decay. Our simulations show a 71% decrease in the time constant of $[Ca^{2+}]_i$ decay in TG mice as compared to WT mice, which is comparable to the experimental value of

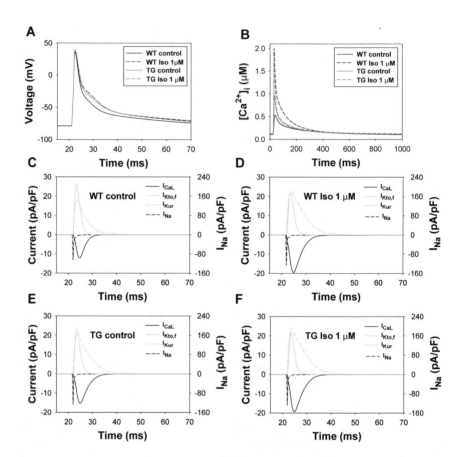

**Fig. 5** The effects of isoproterenol on the action potential, the underlying major ionic currents, and $[Ca^{2+}]_i$ transient in isolated WT and TG mouse ventricular myocyte overexpressing AC5 models. (**a**) Simulated action potentials for control conditions (solid lines) and after application of 1 μM isoproterenol (dashed lines) in WT (black lines) and TG (red lines) ventricular myocytes. (**b**) Simulated $[Ca^{2+}]_i$ transients for control conditions (solid lines) and after application of 1 μM isoproterenol (dashed lines) in WT (black lines) and TG (red lines) ventricular myocytes. (**c**) Major ionic currents underlying WT action potentials for control conditions. (**d**) Major ionic currents underlying WT action potentials after application of 1 μM isoproterenol. (**e**) Major ionic currents underlying TG action potentials for control conditions. (**f**) Major ionic currents underlying TG action potentials after application of 1 μM isoproterenol. Electrical stimulation frequency is 0.5 Hz, $I_{stim} = 80$ pA/pF, $\tau_{stim} = 1.0$ ms. Data is shown after 300 s stimulation. Isoproterenol is applied at the beginning of 300-s stimulation

an 80% decrease. Our model also predicts 40% increase in the SR $Ca^{2+}$ load in TG mice as compared to WT mice, which is comparable to 37.5% increase found experimentally [11].

Thus, our simulations reproduced quite well experimentally observed $Ca^{2+}$ dynamics in WT and TG mouse ventricular myocytes overexpressing AC5.

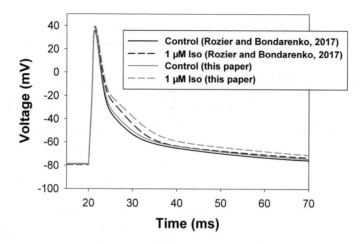

**Fig. 6** Comparison of the effects of isoproterenol on the action potential in isolated WT ventricular myocyte using model presented in this paper and the model published by Rozier and Bondarenko [15]. Simulated action potentials are shown for control conditions (solid lines) and after application of 1 μM isoproterenol (dashed lines) for the model presented in this paper (red lines) and the model published by Rozier and Bondarenko [15] (black lines). Electrical stimulation protocol is the same as in Fig. 5

We should note that the mathematical model of mouse ventricular myocytes presented in this paper differs to some extent from the model published by Rozier and Bondarenko [15]. As we modified the effects of isoproterenol on the ultra-rapidly activating $K^+$ current $I_{Kur}$ (see section "Model development"), it would be interesting to see how this intervention modifies the response of the action potential. Figure 6 shows the action potentials obtained with the current model (red lines) and with the Rozier-Bondarenko model (2017) (black lines). It is seen that the current model demonstrates somewhat larger effects of 1 μM isoproterenol on the action potential durations than the Rozier-Bondarenko model (2017). $APD_{50}$ and $APD_{90}$ obtained with the current model change from 3.20 ms to 4.28 ms (34% increase) and from 27.20 ms to 37.75 ms (39% increase), while $APD_{50}$ and $APD_{90}$ obtained with the Rozier-Bondarenko model (2017) change from 3.3 ms to 3.8 ms (15% increase) and from 26.15 ms to 30.00 ms (15% increase). While both models describe changes in $APD_{50}$ and $APD_{90}$ in response to 1 μM isoproterenol within the experimental variability (see Table 1 from Bondarenko [12]), the current model describes more precisely the response of $I_{Kur}$ to isoproterenol.

We also simulated the time behavior of integral fluxes of the two major intracellular ions, $Ca^{2+}$ and $Na^+$. Their dynamics during the first 1 s of cardiac cycle are shown in Figs. 7 and 8 for WT and TG cells, respectively. Application of 1 μM isoproterenol produced significant increase in integral $Ca^{2+}$ influx through the L-type $Ca^{2+}$ channels in WT mice, from 1.55 μM (Fig. 7a) to 3.36 μM (~117% increase, Fig. 7c), which triggered an increase in the amount of released $Ca^{2+}$, from 37.1 μM to 60.9 μM (~64% increase). In TG mice, the integral $Ca^{2+}$ influx through

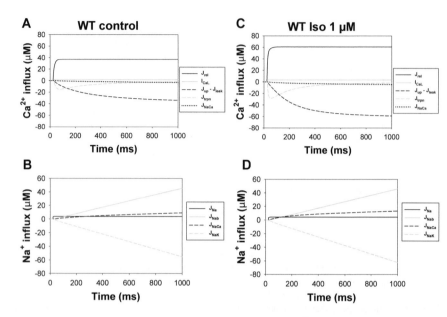

**Fig. 7** Simulated effects of 1 μM isoproterenol on integrated $Ca^{2+}$ and $Na^+$ fluxes (influxes) in WT isolated mouse ventricular myocyte model during first 1 s of cardiac cycle. Simulated $Ca^{2+}$ influxes are shown in (**a, c**). Simulated $Na^+$ influxes are shown in (**b, d**). Simulations for control (basal) conditions are shown in (**a, b**). Simulations for 1 μM isoproterenol are shown in (**c, d**). $Ca^{2+}$ and $Na^+$ fluxes are shown after 300 s of stimulation. In (**c, d**), 1 μM isoproterenol is applied at the beginning of stimulation. Here, $J_{rel}$ is the $Ca^{2+}$ release flux; $J_{CaL}$ is the $Ca^{2+}$ entering the cell through L-type $Ca^{2+}$ channels; $J_{up} - J_{leak}$ is the uptake $Ca^{2+}$ from the cytosol to the network SR with subtracted $Ca^{2+}$ leak from the SR to the cytosol; $J_{trpn}$ is the flux of $Ca^{2+}$ binding by troponin; $J_{Na}$ is the $Na^+$ flux through the fast $Na^+$ channels; $J_{Nab}$ is the $Na^+$ flux through background mechanism; $J_{NaCa}$ is the $Na^+$ flux through the $Na^+/Ca^{2+}$ exchanger; $J_{NaK}$ is the $Na^+$ flux through the $Na^+$-$K^+$ pump. In all *Panels* (**a–d**), electrical stimulation protocol is the same as in Fig. 5

the L-type $Ca^{2+}$ channels increased only from 2.52 μM (Fig. 8a) to 3.40 μM (~35% increase, Fig. 8c). Most of the released $Ca^{2+}$ was pumped back to the SR (34.0 μM and 58.9 μM for control and 1 μM isoproterenol, respectively, in WT mice; 50.2 μM and 54.7 μM for control and 1 μM isoproterenol, respectively, in TG mice). In WT mice, $Ca^{2+}$ extrusion by the $Na^+/Ca^{2+}$ exchanger increased from 3.1 to 4.4 μM at 1 μM isoproterenol (~42% increase), while in TG mice we obtained only ~11% increase (from 3.5 μM to 3.9 μM, Fig. 8). $Ca^{2+}$ balance between the inside and outside of the cell was maintained by the sarcolemmal $Ca^{2+}$ pump and background $Ca^{2+}$ influxes. Thus, our simulations suggest that the major factors that determine the gradual response of $Ca^{2+}$ dynamics to the stimulation of β-ARs in WT mice are the L-type $Ca^{2+}$ current, the $Na^+/Ca^{2+}$ exchanger, and the SERCA pump. In TG mice overexpressing AC5, the effect of stimulation of β-ARs is significantly reduced.

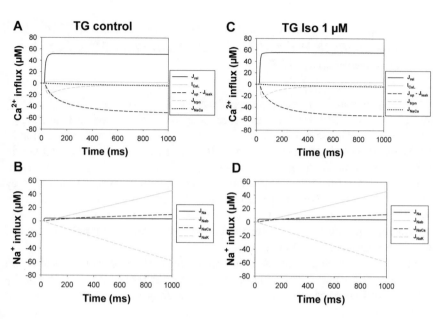

**Fig. 8** Simulated effects of 1 μM isoproterenol on integrated $Ca^{2+}$ and $Na^+$ fluxes (influxes) in the model of isolated TG mouse ventricular myocyte overexpressing AC5 during first 1 s of cardiac cycle. Simulated $Ca^{2+}$ influxes are shown in (**a, c**). Simulated $Na^+$ influxes are shown in (**b, d**). Simulations for control (basal) conditions are shown in (**a, b**). Simulations for 1 μM isoproterenol are shown in (**c, d**). $Ca^{2+}$ and $Na^+$ fluxes are shown after 300 s of stimulation. In (**c, d**), 1 μM isoproterenol is applied at the beginning of stimulation. In all *Panels* (**a–d**), notations are the same as in Fig. 7. Electrical stimulation protocol is the same as in Fig. 5

Simulated integral $Na^+$ influx by the fast $Na^+$ current without isoproterenol in WT mice was 3.9 μM, which was increased to 4.2 μM after application of 1 μM isoproterenol (Fig. 8). Simulated $Na^+$ influx through the $Na^+/Ca^{2+}$ exchanger in mouse cells was 9.2 μM (~16% of total $Na^+$ influx of ~58.6 μM), which increased to 13.2 μM after application of 1 μM isoproterenol. 45.6 μM $Na^+$ entered the cell through background mechanisms in WT cell (~78% of total $Na^+$ influx). In TG mice, the $Na^+$ dynamics was not affected by stimulation of β-ARs. Simulated integral $Na^+$ influx by the fast $Na^+$ current without isoproterenol in TG mice was 4.26 μM, which was basically unchanged (4.23 μM) after application of 1 μM isoproterenol. $Na^+$ influx through the $Na^+/Ca^{2+}$ exchanger in TG mouse cells was only slightly increased from 10.6 μM to 11.8 μM after application of 1 μM isoproterenol. The amount of $Na^+$ entered the cell through background mechanisms was 46.2 μM and was not significantly changed upon stimulation with isoproterenol. $Na^+$ were removed from the cell through the $Na^+$-$K^+$ pump, the activity of which balanced $Na^+$ influx.

## 4.3 Frequency Dependence of the Action Potential and $[Ca^{2+}]_i$ Transients in WT and TG Mouse Ventricular Myocytes Overexpressing AC5

We further explored a frequency dependence of the action potential and $[Ca^{2+}]_i$ transients in WT and TG mice overexpressing AC5. Simulated data on $APD_{25}$, $APD_{50}$, and $APD_{90}$ as functions of the frequency without and with application of 1 μM isoproterenol are shown in Fig. 9. It is seen that the $APD_{25}$ and $APD_{90}$ in WT mice are basically frequency-independent both without and with isoproterenol (Fig. 9a), while $APD_{50}$ demonstrates some increase with the stimulation frequency (increase by 8% without isoproterenol and by 25% with isoproterenol when the stimulation frequency changes from 0.25 to 5 Hz). Application of 1 μM isoproterenol prolongs action potential durations at all levels of repolarization and stimulation frequencies in WT mice.

In TG mice overexpressing AC5 in control, only $APD_{25}$ does not demonstrate frequency dependence (the change is <10%), but $APD_{50}$ and $APD_{90}$ increase by 18% and 16%, respectively, when the stimulation frequency changes from 0.25 to

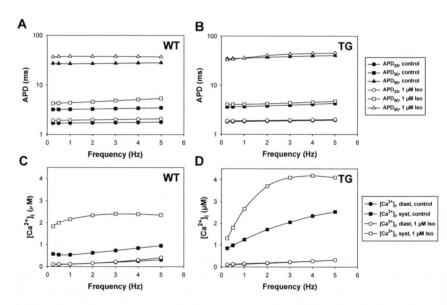

**Fig. 9** Simulated frequency dependences of the action potential durations and $[Ca^{2+}]_i$ transients in WT and TG mouse ventricular myocytes. Simulated $APD_{25}$ (circles), $APD_{50}$ (squares), and $APD_{90}$ (triangles) are shown for WT (**a**) and TG (**b**) mice as functions of stimulation frequency for control conditions (filled symbols) and after application of 1 μM isoproterenol (unfilled symbols). Frequency dependences of diastolic (circles) and systolic (squares) $[Ca^{2+}]_i$ concentrations in WT (**c**) and TG (**d**) mouse ventricular myocytes are shown for control conditions (filled symbols) and after application of 1 μM isoproterenol (unfilled symbols). Electrical stimulation protocol is the same as in Fig. 5, except for $I_{stim}$ was applied at different frequencies

5 Hz (Fig. 9b). $APD_{25}$ does not change with frequency upon application of 1 μM isoproterenol, while $APD_{50}$ and $APD_{90}$ increase by 16% and 37%, respectively.

If we compare the APDs in WT and TG mice at the same frequency and intervention, we observe that the difference in $APD_{25}$ is <10% without and with application of 1 μM isoproterenol. The $APD_{50}$ are greater in TG than in WT mice in control, and the difference increases from 13% to 23% when the frequency increases from 0.25 to 5 Hz. However, when isoproterenol is applied, the difference in $APD_{50}$ between WT and TG cells decreases to <10% for all frequencies. Finally, $APD_{90}$ is more prolong in TG as compared to WT mice in control; the difference changes from 27% at 0.25 Hz to 43% at 5 Hz. Upon application of isoproterenol, the $APD_{90}$ is more prolong in WT mice by ~10% at 0.25 Hz, but it becomes shorter than in TG mice by ~22% at 5 Hz.

More dramatic changes were obtained from the simulations of $[Ca^{2+}]_i$ transients in WT and TG mouse ventricular myocytes (Fig. 9). Both WT and TG mice demonstrated a moderate increase in diastolic $[Ca^{2+}]_i$ concentration when stimulation frequency increased from 0.25 to 5 Hz, from ~0.1 to ~0.3 μM. The change did not depend on the mouse type and intervention.

However, frequency dependences for systolic $[Ca^{2+}]_i$ concentrations are quite different. In the case of control in WT mice, the peak $[Ca^{2+}]_i$ concentration shows a biphasic behavior; it decreases from 0.25 Hz to 1 Hz and increases further up to 5 Hz (Fig. 9c). The peak value varies only between 0.5 and 1.0 μM of $[Ca^{2+}]_i$. Application of 1 μM isoproterenol increased peak $[Ca^{2+}]_i$ values to 1.8–2.5 μM, demonstrating biphasic behavior, starting from an increase between 0.25 and 3 Hz to a decrease from 3 to 5 Hz.

The frequency behavior of the peak $[Ca^{2+}]_i$ in TG mice is quite different. In control, $[Ca^{2+}]_i$ monotonically increased from 0.85 to 2.5 μM when stimulation frequency increased from 0.25 to 5 Hz (Fig. 9d). The absolute values of the peak $[Ca^{2+}]_i$ in control in TG cells are much larger than those in WT cells (compare Fig. 9c, d). Upon stimulation with isoproterenol, we obtained more rapid increase in the peak $[Ca^{2+}]_i$ in TG mice, from 1.3 to 4.2 μM, when frequency increased from 0.25 to 4 Hz, with a subsequent weak decline to 4.1 μM at 5 Hz.

Thus, our simulations demonstrated significant differences in the action potential durations and $[Ca^{2+}]_i$ transients in WT and TG mice overexpressing AC5, when frequency changed in wide range, from 0.25 to 5 Hz. The greater differences are observed in the behavior of $[Ca^{2+}]_i$ transients that suggest their prominent role in the pro-arrhythmic behavior of TG mice.

## 4.4   Simulation of DADs in WT and TG Mouse Ventricular Myocytes Overexpressing AC5

Experimental data shows that TG mouse ventricular myocytes overexpressing AC5 are more susceptible to pro-arrhythmic triggered activities than WT cells [11]. However, we need to note that only fraction of the myocytes demonstrated pro-arrhythmic events both in WT (21%) and TG (46%) mice [11] without application of isoproterenol. To simulate the pro-arrhythmic events in WT and TG cells, we implemented spontaneous release event by an artificial spike of the subspace $Ca^{2+}$ concentration ($[Ca^{2+}]_{ss}$), which was identical to that obtained from electrically stimulated cell with $I_{stim}$ both for WT and TG mice at the stimulation frequency 5 Hz after a 300-s stimulation interval. For both cell types, we first electrically stimulated myocytes by a train of 1500 pulses for 300 s, and then applied 301st $I_{stim}$ pulse at 20 ms after the train, which resulted in a usual action potential and $[Ca^{2+}]_i$ transient. We did not applied $I_{stim}$ further, but we applied $[Ca^{2+}]_{ss}$ transients (which were different for WT and TG cells) from the previous, 301st, pulse at 220 ms after the 1500 pulse train, together with the imitation of the RyR opening by setting $P_{RyR}$ factor to its maximum value, obtained after the 301st stimulation period, for WT ($P_{RyR} = 0.35$) and TG ($P_{RyR} = 0.6$) myocytes for 30 ms. Figure 10 shows the results of simulation of the regular (first) and spontaneous (second) $[Ca^{2+}]_i$ transients for WT (Fig. 10a) and TG (Fig. 10b) mice. As result of this protocol, we observed both normal action potentials and DADs in WT (Fig. 10c) and TG (Fig. 10d) cells. The magnitude of DAD in TG ventricular myocytes (~7.0 mV) was larger by a factor ~3.5 than the DAD in WT myocytes (~2.0 mV) (see insert in Fig. 10c). This result suggests a larger propensity of TG than WT cells to pro-arrhythmic events, as it was observed experimentally [11].

To reveal the mechanism of DAD, we investigated the contribution of depolarization and repolarization currents to the changes in the transmembrane potentials. We found that most of the currents did not changed significantly or were not activated during DADs, except for the time-independent $K^+$ current, $I_{K1}$, and the current produced by the $Na^+/Ca^{2+}$ exchanger, $I_{NaCa}$. The $I_{NaCa}$ current tends to depolarize the membrane potential, while the $I_{K1}$ current tends to repolarize the membrane potential. Figure 10e, f show the $I_{NaCa}$ currents in WT and TG myocytes, respectively, after normal stimulation with $I_{stim}$ (first transient) and after spontaneous $Ca^{2+}$ release (second transient). It is seen that the $I_{NaCa}$ current is much larger in TG cells than in WT cells, and the $I_{K1}$ change does not compensate the difference in the inward $I_{NaCa}$ currents between the two cell types (data not shown). This result supports the conclusion that the DADs in mouse ventricular myocytes are predominantly due to the activation of the $I_{NaCa}$ current and the magnitude of the DADs is larger in TG mice overexpressing AC5 as compared to WT mice due to the larger $I_{NaCa}$ current in TG cells.

# 5   Discussion

In this paper, a new compartmentalized mathematical model for TG mouse ventricular myocytes overexpressing adenylyl cyclase type 5 is developed. The model is based on the previously published model [15] and includes compartmentalization of the $\beta_1$- and $\beta_2$-adrenergic signaling systems and the effects of AC5 overexpression on the action potential, ionic currents, and $Ca^{2+}$ and $Na^+$ dynamics. The new

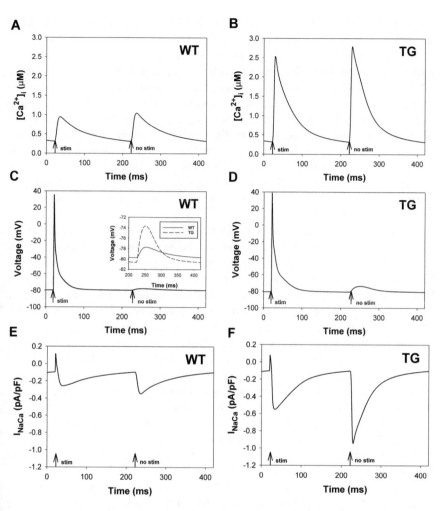

**Fig. 10** Simulated $[Ca^{2+}]_i$ transients (**a**, **b**), transmembrane potentials (**c**, **d**), and $I_{NaCa}$ currents (**e**, **f**) under control conditions after normal electrical stimulation with $I_{stim} = 80$ pA/pF and $\tau_{stim} = 1.0$ ms (stim) at t = 20 ms and during simulated spontaneous $Ca^{2+}$ release (no stim) at t = 220 ms. Data for WT and TG mice are shown in (**a**, **c**, **e**) and (**b**, **d**, **f**), respectively. (**c**, **d**) demonstrate clear delayed afterdepolarizations (DADs) after simulated spontaneous $Ca^{2+}$ release. Insert in (**c**) compares DADs in WT (solid line) and TG (dashed line) mouse cells. Stimulation protocols were applied after a 300-s train of $I_{stim}$ pulses at frequency 5 Hz

model was explored to compare the effects of isoproterenol on WT and TG mice. The model was able to simulate prolongation of action potential duration in TG ventricular myocytes as compared to WT cells under basal conditions and revealed the mechanism of this prolongation. We also explained the larger $[Ca^{2+}]_i$ transients in TG mice due to the enhancement of the L-type $Ca^{2+}$ current and increased SR $Ca^{2+}$ load. Further, we simulated the effects of stimulation of $\beta_1$- and $\beta_2$-ARs on the

$Ca^{2+}$ and $Na^+$ fluxes in WT and TG myocytes. As result, we found blunted effects of isoproterenol in TG as compared to WT cells.

Multiple experimental studies have been performed with transgenic mice with altered expression of the ionic channels as well as the components of the $\beta_1$- and $\beta_2$-adrenergic signaling system to investigate their role in healthy and diseased mouse hearts [1–3, 29]. It was found that cardiac-specific overexpression of $\beta_1$-ARs results in hypertrophy, which lead to heart failure [5]. On the other hand, overexpression of $\beta_2$-ARs improved cardiac function [6]. Further, overexpression of downstream components of the $\beta_1$- and $\beta_2$-adrenergic signaling, such as adenylyl cyclases of type 5, produces pro-arrhythmic activity in the mouse heart [11], while overexpression of adenylyl cyclases of type 6 improved cardiac function [30]. Finally, a moderate overexpression of $G_s$ protein (2.8-fold) in mice did not produce a significant effect on cardiac function [31].

Our mathematical model for WT cells that includes both $\beta_1$- and $\beta_2$-adrenergic signaling systems [15] reproduced most of the experimentally observed effects of the stimulation of the $\beta$-adrenergic signaling in mouse ventricular myocytes. They include an increase in the magnitude of the L-type $Ca^{2+}$ current, $[Ca^{2+}]_i$ transients, increases phosphorylation levels of phospholamban and other proteins, and moderate prolongation of the action potential duration. Simulations revealed mechanism of the changes in response to stimulation with $\beta$-adrenergic receptor agonist isoproterenol in WT type mice. Further, we developed a mathematical model of transgenic mouse ventricular myocytes overexpressing $\beta_2$-ARs [32]. The model simulated the behavior of TG cell at basal conditions and upon stimulation with a specific $\beta_2$-AR agonist zinterol. Simulations demonstrated a significantly increased cAMP production in TG mice overexpressing $\beta_2$-ARs that resulted in almost complete phosphorylation of $\beta_2$-ARs. The model also reproduced $[Ca^{2+}]_i$ transient magnitudes under different physiological conditions in WT and TG cells. It was suggested that the increased $Ca^{2+}$ concentrations can potentially cause deteriorative effects on the activity of the heart during mouse life.

A mathematical model of TG mouse ventricular myocytes overexpressing AC5 presented in this paper predicts similar deterioration effects. The model described an increased cAMP production and increased PKA activity in TG cells under basal conditions and much larger cAMP production upon stimulation with 1 $\mu$M isoproterenol. Even at basal conditions, the prolongation of the action potential duration was quite significant (38% for $APD_{90}$ in the experiment [11] and 29% for simulations), which doubled a number of pro-arrhythmic cells obtained experimentally [11]. Moreover, enormous growth of cAMP concentration in TG cells overexpressing AC5 upon stimulation with 1 $\mu$M isoproterenol can potentially lead to a significant damage of the cellular function as compared, for example, with TG mice overexpressing $\beta_2$-ARs, where stimulated cAMP production was much smaller.

Simulations of frequency dependences of the action potential durations at different levels of repolarization ($APD_{25}$, $APD_{50}$, and $APD_{90}$) and $[Ca^{2+}]_i$ transients in WT and TG mice showed significantly larger $[Ca^{2+}]_i$ transients in TG mice under control conditions and at larger stimulation frequencies upon application of isoproterenol. Simulated spontaneous $Ca^{2+}$ release demonstrated larger amplitudes of DADs in TG mice, suggesting their larger susceptibility to arrhythmias as compared to WT mice. Specifically, we have demonstrated the major role of the sodium-calcium exchanger ($I_{NaCa}$) in generation of pro-arrhythmic DADs in mouse ventricular myocytes.

# 6 Conclusions

We developed a comprehensive experimentally-based compartmentalized mathematical model of the TG mouse ventricular myocyte overexpressing adenylyl cyclase 5. The model simulated major experimental findings on the effects of the overexpression of AC5 in mouse ventricular myocytes. The model describes the dynamics of major signaling molecules in different subcellular compartments; modifications of action potential shape and duration; and $Ca^{2+}$ and $Na^+$ dynamics upon stimulation of β-adrenergic signaling system in control and after application of isoproterenol. The TG myocyte model simulates increased cAMP and PKA transients upon stimulation of β-ARs, as well as larger background $[Ca^{2+}]_i$ transients and a more prolonged $APD_{90}$ compared to the WT cell. We demonstrated that the $[Ca^{2+}]_i$ transients at most stimulation frequencies were larger for TG as compared to WT mice. These differences led to larger magnitudes of DADs in TG mouse myocytes than in WT cells due to larger magnitudes of the sodium-calcium exchanger currents, which suggested larger susceptibility of TG cells to pro-arrhythmic behavior. The simulation results of TG ventricular myocytes overexpressing AC5 are compared to the simulations of WT ventricular myocytes and experimental data obtained from the ventricular myocytes from TG mice.

# References

1. Keys, J. R., & Koch, W. J. (2004). The adrenergic pathway and heart failure. *Recent Progress in Hormone Research, 59*, 13–30.
2. Koch, W. J., Lefkowitz, R. J., & Rockman, H. A. (2000). Functional consequences of altering myocardial adrenergic receptor signaling. *Annual Review of Physiology, 62*, 237–260.
3. Nerbonne, J. M. (2014). Mouse models of arrhythmogenic cardiovascular disease: Challenges and opportunities. *Current Opinion in Pharmacology, 15*, 107–114.
4. Brodde, O. E., & Michel, M. C. (1999). Adrenergic and muscarinic receptors in the human heart. *Pharmacological Reviews, 51*, 651–689.
5. Engelhardt, S., Hein, L., Wiesmann, F., & Lohse, M. J. (1999). Progressive hypertrophy and heart failure in β1-adrenergic receptor transgenic mice. *Proceedings of the National Academy of Sciences of the United States of America, 96*, 7059–7064.
6. Milano, C. A., Allen, L. F., Rockman, H. A., Dolber, P. C., McMinn, T. R., Chien, K. R., Johnson, T. D., Bond, R. A., & Lefkowitz, R. J. (1994). Enhanced myocardial function in transgenic mice overexpressing the β2-adrenergic receptor. *Science, 264*, 582–586.
7. Liggett, S. B., Tepe, N. M., Lorenz, J. N., Canning, A. M., Jantz, T. D., Mitarai, S., Yatani, A., & Dorn, G. W., II. (2000). Early and delayed consequences of β2-adrenergic receptor

overexpression in mouse hearts. Critical role for expression level. *Circulation, 101*, 1707–1714.

8. Ho, D., Yan, L., Iwatsubo, K., Vatner, D. E., & Vatner, S. F. (2010). Modulation of β-adrenergic receptor signaling in heart failure and longevity: Targeting adenylyl cyclase type 5. *Heart Failure Reviews, 15*, 495–512.

9. Lai, L., Yan, L., Gao, S., Hu, C. L., Ge, H., Davidow, A., Park, M., Bravo, C., Iwatsubo, K., Ishikawa, Y., Auwerx, J., Sinclair, D. A., Vatner, S. F., & Vatner, D. E. (2013). Type 5 adenylyl cyclase increases oxidative stress by transcriptional regulation of manganese superoxide dismutase via the SIRT1/FoxO3a pathway. *Circulation, 127*, 1692–1701.

10. Vatner, S. F., Park, M., Yan, L., Lee, G. J., Lai, L., Iwatsubo, K., Ishikawa, Y., Pessin, J., & Vatner, D. E. (2013). Adenylyl cyclase 5 in cardiac disease, metabolism, and aging. *American Journal of Physiology. Heart and Circulatory Physiology, 305*, H1–H8.

11. Zhao, Z., Babu, G. J., Wen, H., Fefelova, N., Gordan, R., Sui, X., Yan, L., Vatner, D. E., Vatner, S. F., & Xie, L. H. (2015). Overexpression of adenylyl cyclase type 5 (AC5) confers a proarrhythmic substrate to the heart. *American Journal of Physiology. Heart and Circulatory Physiology, 308*, H240–H249.

12. Bondarenko, V. E. (2014). A compartmentalized mathematical model of the $\beta_1$-adrenergic signaling system in mouse ventricular myocytes. *PLoS One, 9*, e89113.

13. Bondarenko, V. E., Szigeti, G. P., Bett, G. C. L., Kim, S. J., & Rasmusson, R. L. (2004). Computer model of action potential of mouse ventricular myocytes. *American Journal of Physiology. Heart and Circulatory Physiology, 287*, H1378–H1403.

14. Petkova-Kirova, P. S., London, B., Salama, G., Rasmusson, R. L., & Bondarenko, V. E. (2012). Mathematical modeling mechanisms of arrhythmias in transgenic mouse heart overexpressing TNF-α. *American Journal of Physiology. Heart and Circulatory Physiology, 302*, H934–H952.

15. Rozier, K., & Bondarenko, V. E. (2017). Distinct physiological effects of $\beta_1$- and $\beta_2$-adrenoceptors in mouse ventricular myocytes: Insights from a compartmentalized mathematical model. *American Journal of Physiology. Cell Physiology, 312*, C595–C623.

16. Tang, T., Lai, N. C., Roth, D. M., Drumm, J., Guo, T., Lee, K. W., Han, P. L., Dalton, N., & Gao, M. H. (2006). Adenylyl cyclase type V deletion increases basal left ventricular function and reduces left ventricular contractile responsiveness to β-adrenergic stimulation. *Basic Research in Cardiology, 101*, 117–126.

17. Luo, W., Grupp, I. L., Harrer, J., Ponniah, S., Grupp, G., Duffy, J. J., Doetschman, T., & Kranias, E. G. (1994). Targeted ablation of the phospholamban gene is associated with markedly enhanced myocardial contractility and loss of β-agonist stimulation. *Circulation Research, 75*, 401–409.

18. Kadambi, V. J., Ponniah, S., Harrer, J. M., Hoit, B. D., Dorn, G. W., II, Walsh, R. A., & Kranias, E. G. (1996). Cardiac-specific overexpression of phospholamban alters calcium kinetics and resultant cardiomyocyte mechanics in transgenic mice. *The Journal of Clinical Investigation, 97*, 533–539.

19. Li, G. R., Feng, J., Wang, Z., Fermini, B., & Nattel, S. (1996). Adrenergic modulation of ultrarapid delayed rectifier $K^+$ current in human atrial myocytes. *Circulation Research, 78*, 903–915.

20. Gaborit, N., Le Bouter, S., Szuts, V., Varro, A., Escande, D., Nattel, S., & Demolombe, S. (2007). Regional and tissue specific transcript signatures of ion channel genes in the non-diseased human heart. *The Journal of Physiology, 582*, 675–693.

21. Brandt, M. C., Priebe, L., Böhle, T., Südkamp, M., & Beuckelmann, D. J. (2000). The ultrarapid and the transient outward $K^+$ current in human atrial fibrillation. Their possible role in postoperative atrial fibrillation. *Journal of Molecular and Cellular Cardiology, 32*, 1885–1896.

22. Kodirov, S. A., Brunner, M., Nerbonne, J. M., Buckett, P., Mitchell, G. F., & Koren, G. (2004). Attenuation of $I_{K,slow1}$ and $I_{K,slow2}$ in Kv1/Kv2DN mice prolongs APD and QT intervals but does not suppress spontaneous or inducible arrhythmias. *American Journal of Physiology. Heart and Circulatory Physiology, 286*, H368–H374.

23. London, B., Guo, W., Pan, X. H., Lee, J. S., Shusterman, V., Rocco, C. J., Logothetis, D. A., Nerbonne, J. M., & Hill, J. A. (2001). Targeted replacement of Kv1.5 in the mouse leads to loss of the 4-aminopyridine-sensitive component of $I_{K,slow}$ and resistance to drug-induced QT prolongation. *Circulation Research, 88*, 940–946.
24. Wilson, G. G., O'Neill, C. A., Sivaprasadarao, A., Findlay, J. B. C., & Wray, D. (1994). Modulation by protein kinase A of a cloned rat brain potassium channel expressed in *Xenopus* oocytes. *Pflügers Archiv, 428*, 186–193.
25. Zhou, M. H., Yang, G., Jiao, S., Hu, C. L., & Mei, Y. A. (2012). Cholesterol enhances neuron susceptibility to apoptotic stimuli via cAMP/PKA/CREb-dependent up-regulation of Kv2.1. *Journal of Neurochemistry, 120*, 502–514.
26. Tepe, N. M., & Liggett, S. B. (1999). Transgenic replacement of type V adenylyl cyclase identifies a critical mechanism of β-adrenergic receptor dysfunction in the $G_{\alpha q}$ overexpressing mouse. *FEBS Letters, 458*, 236–240.
27. Lemire, I., Allen, B. G., Rindt, H., & Hebert, T. E. (1998). Cardiac-specific overexpression of $\alpha_{1B}$AR regulates βAR activity via molecular crosstalk. *Journal of Molecular and Cellular Cardiology, 30*, 1827–1839.
28. Iwatsubo, K., Bravo, C., Uechi, M., Baljinnyam, E., Nakamura, T., Umemura, M., Lai, L., Gao, S., Yan, L., Zhao, X., Park, M., Qiu, H., Okumura, S., Iwatsubo, M., Vatner, D. E., Vatner, S. F., & Ishikawa, Y. (2012). Prevention of heart failure in mice by an antiviral agent that inhibits type 5 cardiac adenylyl cyclase. *American Journal of Physiology. Heart and Circulatory Physiology, 302*, H2622–H2628.
29. Nerbonne, J. M., Nichols, C. G., Schwarz, T. L., & Escande, D. (2001). Genetic manipulation of cardiac $K^+$ channel function in mice: What have we learned, and where do we go from here? *Circulation Research, 89*, 944–956.
30. Guellich, A., Gao, S., Hong, C., Yan, L., Wagner, T. E., Dhar, S. K., Ghaleh, B., Hittinger, L., Iwatsubo, K., Ishikawa, Y., Vatner, S. F., & Vatner, D. E. (2010). Effects of cardiac overexpression of type 6 adenylyl cyclase affects on the response to chronic pressure overload. *American Journal of Physiology. Heart and Circulatory Physiology, 299*, H707–H712.
31. Gaudin, C., Ishikawa, Y., Wight, D. C., Mahdavi, V., Nadal-Ginard, B., Wagner, T. E., Vatner, D. E., & Homcy, C. J. (1995). Overexpression of $G_{s\alpha}$ protein in the hearts of transgenic mice. *The Journal of Clinical Investigation, 95*, 1676–1683.
32. Rozier, K., & Bondarenko, V. E. (2018). Mathematical modeling physiological effects of the overexpression of $\beta_2$-adrenoceptors in mouse ventricular myocytes. *American Journal of Physiology. Heart and Circulatory Physiology, 314*, H643–H658.

# Part V
# Survival Analysis with Complex Data Structure and Its Applications

# Non-parametric Maximum Likelihood Estimation for Case-Cohort and Nested Case-Control Designs with Competing Risks Data

Jie-Huei Wang, Chun-Hao Pan, Yi-Hau Chen, and I-Shou Chang

**Abstract** Assuming cause-specific hazards given by Cox's regression model, we provide non-parametric maximum likelihood estimator (NPMLEs) in the nested case-control or case-cohort design with competing risks data. We propose an iterative algorithm based on self-consistency equations derived from score functions to compute NPMLE and compute the predicted cumulative incidence function with their corresponding confidence intervals and bands. Consistency and asymptotic normality are established, together with a consistent estimator of the asymptotic variance based on the observed profile likelihood. Simulation studies show that the numerical performance of NPMLE approach is satisfactory and compares well with that of weighted partial likelihood. Our method is applied to the Taiwan National Health Insurance Research Database (NHIRD) to analyze the occurrences of liver and lung cancers in type 2 diabetic mellitus patients.

**Keywords** Cause-specific hazards · Cohort study · Cox proportional hazards model · Multiple endpoints · Self-consistency

J.-H. Wang
Department of Statistics, Feng Chia University, Taichung, Taiwan
e-mail: jhwang@mail.fcu.edu.tw

Y.-H. Chen (✉)
Institute of Statistical Science, Academia Sinica, Nankang, Taipei, Taiwan
e-mail: yhchen@stat.sinica.edu.tw

C.-H. Pan
Unimicron Technology Corporation, Guishan, Taoyuan, Taiwan

I-S. Chang
Institute of Cancer Research and Division of Biostatistics and Bioinformatics, Institute of Population Health Science, National Health Research Institutes, Zhunan Town, Miaoli County, Taiwan
e-mail: ischang@nhri.org.tw

© Springer Nature Switzerland AG 2020
Y. Zhao, D.-G. (Din) Chen (eds.), *Statistical Modeling in Biomedical Research*, Emerging Topics in Statistics and Biostatistics,
https://doi.org/10.1007/978-3-030-33416-1_17

381

# 1 Introduction

Many epidemiological cohorts are established to learn the effects of some covariates on disease onset, disease recurrence or patient survival. When these covariates are precious, expensive, or labor intensive to collect, for cost consideration, the nested case-control (NCC) or case-cohort (CC) sampling, introduced respectively by Thomas [20] and Prentice [13], are two most popular designs allowing the covariates to be measured only in a subset of the full cohort.

The CC/NCC design uses all incident "cases", i.e., subjects who just develop the targeted disease, and a subsample from the time-matched "controls" or the "risk set", i.e., subjects who have not yet develop the disease by the time a case arises. Compared to the matched case-control study, the CC/NCC design allows reusing controls matched to cases [5, 15, 16]. Furthermore, recent literature indicates that the CC/NCC design also enjoys the ability of reuse of the controls not tied to their matched cases for the study of other endpoints; see, for example, [9, 14, 18, 19]. Reuse or share of controls among different endpoints leads to more effective logistics and efficient statistical analysis.

Saarela et al. [14] and Støer and Samuelsen [19] reported two approaches for the NCC design with multiple competing endpoints, namely the weighted partial likelihood approach (WPL) and the full likelihood approach (FL). However, the WPL approach may be subject to loss of efficiency since it uses only information from the sampled cases and controls, and ignores information from subjects who are not sampled into the NCC sample and hence whose covariate data are not completely measured. On the other hand, the FL approach is based on fully parametric models for hazards functions of the event times and the density for the covariates, which may lead to biased estimation when the assumed models are incorrect. Keogh and White [7] proposed a simple multiple imputation (MI) strategy to impute the missing values for individuals outside the NCC sample based on data available in the full cohort. The MI approach, similar to the FL approach, is subject to biased inference owing to model misspecification. Borgan and Keogh [1] compared the WPL with the MI methods for multiple endpoints via simulation studies.

For a single outcome, Scheike and Juul [16] and Scheike and Martinussen [17] considered the non-parametric maximum likelihood estimation (NPMLE) for the CC/NCC design, and used the EM-algorithm for computation. In this work, we extend the NPMLE method to the CC/NCC design with multiple competing risks.

In Sect. 2, we present the likelihood under the competing risks with the CC/NCC design. Contrary to the parametric likelihood considered in [14], the likelihood in our work is based on the semiparametric Cox's proportional hazards model. We develop the NPMLE in this setting and consider the self-consistency equations derived from score functions. The computation algorithm based on the self-consistency equations is then developed. In Sect. 3, we establish the large sample theorems of NPMLE, together with asymptotic properties of the profile likelihood, and a consistent estimator of the asymptotic variance. In Sect. 4, we provide simulation results for comparing the NPMLE with the WPL approach in terms of estimation bias and efficiency. In Sect. 5 we illustrate the use of the NPMLE method in the analysis of the incidence of liver and lung cancers in type 2 diabetic mellitus (DM) patients with data from Taiwan National Health Insurance Research Database (NHIRD). We conclude this work in Sect. 6 with brief discussion.

# 2 Likelihood Function, Score Function and NPMLE

## 2.1 Likelihood Function

We first define some notations for developing the likelihood function of the CC/NCC sampling with competing risks under the Cox's proportional hazards model. Let the cohort $R = \{1, \cdots, M\}$ consist of $M$ independent subjects. We consider independent CC/NCC studies for each of the $K$ different endpoints in the same cohort. At each event time, $m$ controls are sampled from the individuals still at risk. We collect all cases and sampled controls in the cohort; define the collection $\bar{O}$ as a CC/NCC sample. The covariates of the subjects are measured in the CC/NCC sample.

For the $ith$ individual in the cohort, let $T_i$ be the time-to-event, $C_i$ the censoring time, $X_i = \min(T_i, C_i)$ the observed (censored) time-to-event, $\mathbf{Y}_i$ the always observed covariates which are observed for the full cohort, $\mathbf{Z}_i$ the covariates which are observed only in the CC/NCC sample and are missing for the cohort members not in the CC/NCC sample, and $E_i$ is the failure indicator taking values in $\{0, 1, \cdots, K\}$, with 0 indicating censoring and $k$ the failure from the $kth$ competing event $k = 1, \cdots, K$. We assume $T_i \geq 0$, $C_i \geq 0$, $\mathbf{Y}_i \in \mathfrak{R}^q$ and $\mathbf{Z}_i \in \mathfrak{R}^d$. We assume that the cause-specific proportional hazard of subject $i$ for $E_i = k$ given $\mathbf{Z}_i = \mathbf{z}$ and $\mathbf{Y}_i = \mathbf{y}$ is

$$\lambda_{ik}(t|\mathbf{Z}_i = \mathbf{z}, \mathbf{Y}_i = \mathbf{y}) = \lambda_{0k}(t) \exp\left(\mathbf{y}^T \boldsymbol{\eta}_k\right) \exp\left(\mathbf{z}^T \boldsymbol{\beta}_k\right). \tag{1}$$

Here $\lambda_{0k}(\cdot)$ is an event-specific, non-negative deterministic baseline function, and $\boldsymbol{\eta}_k \in \mathfrak{R}^q$, $\boldsymbol{\beta}_k \in \mathfrak{R}^d$. In this paper, a superscript $T$ denotes transpose of a vector or a matrix. Following conventional survival analysis, we assume that $T$ and $C$ are conditionally independent given covariates, and the censoring time $C$ is non-informative on covariates, that is, the censoring distribution is non-informative on the parameters of interest.

Using a fully parametric approach, Saarela et al. [14] considered the full likelihood under the CC/NCC design with competing risks data given by

$$L(\boldsymbol{\theta}, \mu) \propto \prod_{i \in \bar{O}} p\left(X_i, E_i | \mathbf{Z}_i, \mathbf{y}_i; \boldsymbol{\theta}\right) p\left(\mathbf{Z}_i | \mathbf{y}_i; \mu\right)$$

$$\times \prod_{i \in R \setminus \bar{O}} \int p\left(X_i, E_i | \mathbf{Z}_i, \mathbf{y}_i; \boldsymbol{\theta}\right) p\left(\mathbf{Z}_i | \mathbf{y}_i; \mu\right) dz.$$

Here, $i \in \{1, 2, \cdots, M\}$ indexes the subjects in a cohort. That $O_i = 1$ if $i$ belongs to $\bar{O}$. The observed data in the CC/NCC sample can be defined as $\{(X_i, E_i, Y_i, Z_i \cdot O_i, O_i) \, | i = 1, 2, \cdots, M\}$. The model $p(X, E|z, y; \theta)$ is for the joint density of $(X, E)$ given $(z, y)$, which can be determined by the cause-specific hazard model (1) with $E = 1, \cdots, K$, $\theta = (\theta_1, \cdots, \theta_K)$ with $\theta_k$ the parameters involved in the cause-specific hazard model (1) for the $kth$ competing event. The model $p(Z|y; \mu)$ is for the density of the incompletely observed covariate $Z$ given the completely observed covariate $Y$, and $\mu$ is the associated parameter.

For ease of exposition, we will describe the proposed procedure by omitting the always observed covariates $Y$ tentatively, although in simulation studies and real data analysis we still consider the analysis with such covariates since it can be implemented by simply modifying the following procedure. The more details of how to modify the proposed approach when $Y$ exists and is discrete are given in Appendix 6.

Let $f(z)$ denote the marginal density of $Z$. Then the marginal survival function of $T$ is $G(t) = pr(T \geq t) = \int \exp\left\{-\sum_{k=1}^{K} \Lambda_k(t) \exp\left(z^T \beta_k\right)\right\} f(z) \, dz$, where $\Lambda_k(t) = \int_0^t \lambda_k(s) ds$. The likelihood of the CC/NCC data with competing risks under the Cox's regression model (1) is

$$\tilde{L}_M\left(\beta_1, \cdots, \beta_K, f, \Lambda_1, \cdots, \Lambda_K\right) \tag{2}$$

$$= \prod_{i=1}^{M} \left[\prod_{k=1}^{K} \left(\lambda_k(X_i) \exp\left(Z_i^T \beta_k\right)\right)^{I(E_i=k)} \exp\left(-\sum_{k=1}^{K} \Lambda_k(X_i) \exp\left(Z_i^T \beta_k\right)\right) f(Z_i)\right]^{I(o_i=1)}$$

$$\times [G(X_i)]^{I(o_i=0)},$$

where $O_i = 1$ if $Z_i$ is observed (in the CC/NCC sample) and $O_i = 0$ if not. Because the full likelihood (2) could become arbitrarily large within the class of absolutely continuous $\Lambda_k(\cdot)$ and continuous density $f$, the likelihood function we consider is

$$L_M\left(\beta_1, \cdots, \beta_K, f_e, \Lambda_1, \cdots, \Lambda_K\right) \tag{3}$$

$$= \prod_{i=1}^{M} \left[\prod_{k=1}^{K} \left(\Delta\Lambda_k(X_i) \exp\left(Z_i^T \beta_k\right)\right)^{I(E_i=k)} \exp\left(-\sum_{k=1}^{K} \Lambda_k(X_i) \exp\left(Z_i^T \beta_k\right)\right) f_e(Z_i)\right]^{I(o_i=1)}$$

$$\times [G_e(X_i)]^{I(o_i=0)}.$$

Here, $\Delta\Lambda_k(t) = \Lambda_k(t) - \Lambda_k(t-)$ and $f_e$ and $G_e$ are defined as follows. Assume there are $J$ distinct values for the observed covariates and they are denoted by $(W_1, W_2, \cdots, W_J)$. Let $0 \leq p_j \leq 1$ and $\sum_{j=1}^{J} p_j = 1$. The distribution $f_e$ is defined by

$$f_e(Z) = \sum_{j=1}^{J} p_j I_{Z=W_j}, \tag{4}$$

and the corresponding marginal survival function $G$ of $T$ is

$$
G_e(t) = \sum_{l=1}^{J} \left( \exp\left( -\sum_{k=1}^{K} \Lambda_k(t) \exp\left( W_l^T \beta_k \right) \right) \right) p_l.
$$

This empirical approach to the covariate distribution is similar to that in [4].

The NPMLE we propose is the maximizer of (3) over $\mathscr{B} \times \cdots \times \mathscr{B} \times \mathscr{P} \times \mathscr{L}_* \times \cdots \times \mathscr{L}_*$, where $\mathscr{B}$ is a compact subset of $\Re^d$, $\mathscr{L}_* \subset \mathscr{L}$ comprises step functions, and $\mathscr{P}$ consists of all the empirical distribution of the form in (4), namely $\mathscr{P} = \left[ p = (p_1, \cdots, p_J)^T : p_j \geq 0, \sum_{j=1}^{J} p_j = 1 \right]$. In fact, $\widehat{\Lambda}_k$ has positive jumps precisely at all $X_i$ with $E_i = k$, for $k = 1, \cdots, K$.

## 2.2 Score Functions

In this subsection, we will present the score functions and some integral equations for the NPMLE. From (3), we obtain the log likelihood function

$$
\log L_M \left( \beta_1, \cdots, \beta_K, p, \Lambda_1, \cdots, \Lambda_K \right) = l_M \left( \beta_1, \cdots, \beta_K, p, \Lambda_1, \cdots, \Lambda_K \right)
$$

$$
= \sum_{i=1}^{M} I_{(o_i=1)} \left[ \sum_{k=1}^{K} I_{(E_i=k)} \log \left( \Delta \Lambda_k(X_i) \exp\left( Z_i^T \beta_k \right) \right) \right]
$$

$$
- \sum_{i=1}^{M} I_{(o_i=1)} \left[ \sum_{k=1}^{K} \Lambda_k(X_i) \exp\left( Z_i^T \beta_k \right) + \log\left( \sum_{j=1}^{J} p_j I_{Z_i=W_j} \right) \right]
$$

$$
+ \sum_{i=1}^{M} I_{(o_i=0)} \left[ \log\left( \sum_{j=1}^{J} \exp\left( -\sum_{k=1}^{K} \Lambda_k(X_i) \exp\left( W_j^T \beta_k \right) \right) p_j \right) \right].
$$

Let $BV[0, \tau]$ denote the set of all real-valued functions on $[0, \tau]$ with finite variation. See Sect. 3.1 for the discussions of how to determine $\tau$. For $k = 1, \cdots, K$, $h_{1k} \in \Re^d$, $h_2 \in \Re^J$ and $h_{3k} \in BV[0, \tau]$, let $\Lambda_{k\varepsilon}(t) = \int_0^t (1 + \varepsilon h_{3k}(u)) \, d\Lambda_k(u)$. We define score functions as follows.

$$
l_{1k,\theta}[h_{1k}](X_1, E_1, Z_1 \cdot O_1, O_1)
$$

$$
= \frac{d}{d\varepsilon} \log L_1 \left( \beta_1, \cdots, \beta_k + \varepsilon h_{1k}, \cdots, \beta_K, p, \Lambda_1, \cdots, \Lambda_K \right) \Big|_{\varepsilon=0},
$$

$$
l_{2,\theta}[h_2](X_1, E_1, Z_1 \cdot O_1, O_1)
$$

$$
= \frac{d}{d\varepsilon} \log L_1 \left( \beta_1, \cdots, \beta_K, p + \varepsilon h_2, \Lambda_1, \cdots, \Lambda_K \right) \Big|_{\varepsilon=0},
$$

$$l_{3k,\theta} [h_{3k}] (X_1, E_1, \mathbf{Z}_1 \cdot O_1, O_1)$$

$$= \frac{d}{d\varepsilon} \log L_1 \left( \boldsymbol{\beta}_1, \cdots, \boldsymbol{\beta}_K, \boldsymbol{p}, \Lambda_1, \cdots, \Lambda_{k\varepsilon}, \cdots, \Lambda_K \right) \bigg|_{\varepsilon=0},$$

where $\theta = (\boldsymbol{\beta}_1, \cdots, \boldsymbol{\beta}_K, \boldsymbol{p}, \Lambda_1, \cdots, \Lambda_K)$. Straight-forward calculations, given the following expressions for these score functions.

The score function of $\boldsymbol{\beta}_k, k = 1, \cdots, K$, is

$$l_{1k,\theta} [h_{1k}] (X_1, E_1, \mathbf{Z}_1 \cdot O_1, O_1)$$

$$= I_{(o_1=1)} \left[ \boldsymbol{h}_{1k}^T \left( I_{(E_1=k)} \mathbf{Z}_1 - \Lambda_k (X_1) \mathbf{Z}_1 \exp \left( \mathbf{Z}_1^T \boldsymbol{\beta}_k \right) \right) \right]$$

$$+ I_{(o_1=0)} \left[ -\Lambda_k (X_1) \boldsymbol{h}_{1k}^T \sum_{j=1}^{J} \mathbf{W}_j \exp \left( \mathbf{W}_j^T \boldsymbol{\beta}_k \right) pr \left( \mathbf{Z}_1 = \mathbf{W}_j \middle| T_1 \geq X_1 \right) \right].$$

Here $pr \left( \mathbf{Z}_i = \mathbf{W}_j \middle| T_i \geq X_i \right) = \dfrac{\exp \left( -\sum_{k=1}^{K} \Lambda_k(X_i) \exp \left( \mathbf{W}_j^T \boldsymbol{\beta}_k \right) \right) p_j}{\sum_{l=1}^{J} \exp \left( -\sum_{k=1}^{K} \Lambda_k(X_i) \exp \left( \mathbf{W}_l^T \boldsymbol{\beta}_k \right) \right) p_l}$.

The score function of $\boldsymbol{p}$ is

$$l_{2,\theta} [h_2] (X_1, E_1, \mathbf{Z}_1 \cdot O_1, O_1) = I_{(o_1=1)} \left( \frac{\boldsymbol{\mu}_1^T \boldsymbol{h}_2}{\boldsymbol{\mu}_1^T \boldsymbol{p}} \right) + I_{(o_1=0)} \left( \frac{\boldsymbol{\phi}_1^T \boldsymbol{h}_2}{\boldsymbol{\phi}_1^T \boldsymbol{p}} \right),$$

where $\boldsymbol{p} = (p_1, p_2, \cdots, p_J)^T, \boldsymbol{\mu}_i = \left( I_{\mathbf{Z}_i = \mathbf{W}_1}, I_{\mathbf{Z}_i = \mathbf{W}_2}, \cdots, I_{\mathbf{Z}_i = \mathbf{W}_J} \right)^T$ and $\boldsymbol{\phi}_i = \left( \exp \left( -\sum_{k=1}^{K} \Lambda_k (X_i) \exp \left( \mathbf{W}_1^T \boldsymbol{\beta}_k \right) \right), \cdots, \exp \left( -\sum_{k=1}^{K} \Lambda_k (X_i) \exp \left( \mathbf{W}_J^T \boldsymbol{\beta}_k \right) \right) \right)$

The score function of $\Lambda_k, k = 1, \cdots, K$ is

$$l_{3k,\theta} [h_{3k}] (X_1, E_1, \mathbf{Z}_1 \cdot O_1, O_1)$$

$$= I_{(o_1=1)} \left[ I_{(E_1=k)} h_{3k} (X_1) - \exp \left( \mathbf{Z}_1^T \boldsymbol{\beta}_k \right) \int_0^{X_1} h_{3k} (t) \, d\Lambda_k (t) \right]$$

$$+ I_{(o_1=0)} \left[ \int_0^{X_1} h_{3k} (t) \, d\Lambda_k (t) \sum_{j=1}^{J} \left[ -\exp \left( \mathbf{W}_j^T \boldsymbol{\beta}_k \right) \right] pr \left( \mathbf{Z}_1 = \mathbf{W}_j \middle| T_1 \geq X_1 \right) \right].$$

### 2.3   The NPMLE

It is clear that a necessary condition for $\widehat{\theta}_M = \left( \widehat{\boldsymbol{\beta}}_{1M}, \cdots, \widehat{\boldsymbol{\beta}}_{KM}, \widehat{\boldsymbol{p}}_M, \widehat{\Lambda}_{1M}, \cdots, \widehat{\Lambda}_{KM} \right)$ to be the NPMLE is

$$P_M l_{j,\widehat{\theta}_M} [h_j] = 0,$$

for all large $M$. Here $P_M$ means taking expectation with respect to the empirical measure for the data $\{(X_i, E_i, Z_i \cdot O_i, O_i) | i = 1, 2, \cdots, M\}$. Based on the self-consistency equations derived from the score functions given above, we provide an iterative algorithm to calculate the NPMLE.

The NPMLE $\widehat{\beta}_{kM}$ of $\beta_k, k = 1, \cdots, K$ is given as follows. From $P_M l_{1k, \widehat{\theta}_M}[h_{1k}] = 0$, we get

$$
0 = \sum_{i=1}^{M} I_{(o_i=1)} h_{1k}^T \left[ I_{(E_i=k)} Z_i - \widehat{\Lambda}_{kM}(X_i) Z_i \exp\left(Z_i^T \widehat{\beta}_{kM}\right) \right]
$$

$$
+ \sum_{i=1}^{M} I_{(o_i=0)} \left[ -\widehat{\Lambda}_{kM}(X_i) h_{1k}^T \sum_{j=1}^{J} \left[ W_j \exp\left(W_j^T \widehat{\beta}_{kM}\right) \right] \widehat{\alpha}_{ijM} \right],
$$

where $\widehat{\alpha}_{ijM} = \dfrac{\exp\left(-\sum_{k=1}^{K} \widehat{\Lambda}_{kM}(X_i) \exp\left(W_j^T \widehat{\beta}_{kM}\right)\right) \widehat{p}_{jM}}{\sum_{l=1}^{J} \exp\left(-\sum_{k=1}^{K} \widehat{\Lambda}_{kM}(X_i) \exp(W_l^T \widehat{\beta}_{kM})\right) \widehat{p}_{lM}}$.

Let $h_{1k} = e_l = (0, \cdots, 0, 1_{(l)}, 0, \cdots, 0)_{1 \times d}^T$, we obtain

$$
0 = \sum_{i=1}^{M} I_{(o_i=1)} \left[ I_{(E_i=k)} Z_{i,l} - \widehat{\Lambda}_{kM}(X_i) Z_{i,l} \exp\left(Z_i^T \widehat{\beta}_{kM}\right) \right]
$$

$$
+ \sum_{i=1}^{M} I_{(o_i=0)} \left[ -\widehat{\Lambda}_{kM}(X_i) \sum_{j=1}^{J} \left[ W_{j,l} \exp\left(W_j^T \widehat{\beta}_{kM}\right) \right] \widehat{\alpha}_{ijM} \right].
$$

We can utilize a modified Newton-Raphson method to solve the above equation, namely, the NPMLE of $\beta_k$ is updated by

$$
\beta_k^{(q+1)} = \beta_k^{(q)} - V^{-1}\left(\theta^{(q)}\right) U\left(\theta^{(q)}\right), \tag{5}
$$

where

$$
U\left(\theta^{(q)}\right) = \sum_{i=1}^{M} I_{(o_i=1)} \left[ I_{(E_i=k)} Z_i - \Lambda_k^{(q)}(X_i) Z_i \exp\left(Z_i^T \beta_k^{(q)}\right) \right]
$$

$$
+ \sum_{i=1}^{M} I_{(o_i=0)} \left[ -\Lambda_k^{(q)}(X_i) \sum_{j=1}^{J} \left[ W_j \exp\left(W_j^T \beta_k^{(q)}\right) \right] \alpha_{ij}^{(q)} \right].
$$

$$
V\left(\theta^{(q)}\right) = \sum_{i=1}^{M} I_{(o_i=1)} \left[ -\Lambda_k^{(q)}(X_i) Z_i Z_i^T \exp\left(Z_i^T \beta_k^{(q)}\right) \right]
$$

$$+ \sum_{i=1}^{M} I_{(o_i=0)} \left[ -\Lambda_k^{(q)}(X_i) \sum_{j=1}^{J} \left[ \left( W_j W_j^T \exp\left( W_j^T \beta_k^{(q)} \right) \right) \alpha_{ij}^{(q)} \right] \right]$$

$$+ \sum_{i=1}^{M} I_{(o_i=0)} \left[ -\Lambda_k^{(q)}(X_i) \sum_{j=1}^{J} \left[ \left( W_j \exp\left( W_j^T \beta_k^{(q)} \right) \right) \left[ \frac{\partial}{\partial \beta_k} \alpha_{ij} \right]^{(q)} \right] \right].$$

The NPMLE of $p$ is given as the following updating step. Let $\alpha_{ij}(p) = \frac{\exp\left( -\sum_{k=1}^{K} \Lambda_k^{(q)}(X_i) \exp\left( W_j^T \beta_k^{(q)} \right) \right) p_j}{\sum_{l=1}^{J} \exp\left( -\sum_{k=1}^{K} \Lambda_k^{(q)}(X_i) \exp\left( W_l^T \beta_k^{(q)} \right) \right) p_l}$, and $\alpha(p)$ be the $M \times J$ matrix with $(i, j)$ entry being $\alpha_{ij}(p)$. To facilitate the proposed computation algorithm, we consider results summarized in the following three lemmas.

**Lemma 1** $P_M l_{2, \left( \beta_1^{(q)}, \cdots, \beta_K^{(q)}, p, \Lambda_1^{(q)}, \cdots, \Lambda_K^{(q)} \right)} [h_2] = 0$ for every $h_2 \in \Re^J$ satisfying $\sum_{j=1}^{J} h_{2,j} = 0$ if and only if $p = \left( \frac{1}{M} \mathbf{1}^T \alpha(p) \right)^T$, where $\mathbf{1} = (1, \cdots, 1)_{1 \times M}^T$.

By Lemma 1, we obtain updated value of $p$ at the $(q+1)th$ step as

$$p^{(q+1)} = \left( \frac{1}{M} \mathbf{1}^T \alpha\left( p^{(q)} \right) \right)^T. \tag{6}$$

The NPMLE for $\Lambda_k, k = 1, \cdots, K$, is given by the integral equations given as follows.

**Lemma 2**

$$\widehat{\Lambda}_{kM}(t) = \int_0^t \frac{1}{A_{kM}\left( \widehat{\theta}_M; u \right)} dB_{kM}(u), k = 1, \cdots, K. \tag{7}$$

Here $B_{kM}(u) = \frac{1}{M} \sum_{i=1}^{M} I_{(E_i=k)} I_{(0,u]}(X_i)$ and $A_{kM}(\theta; u) = \frac{1}{M} \sum_{i=1}^{M} \left\{ I_{(o_i=1)} \left[ I_{(0,X_i]}(u) \left( \exp\left( Z_i^T \beta_k \right) \right) \right] + I_{(o_i=0)} \left[ I_{(0,X_i]}(u) \sum_{j=1}^{J} \left[ \exp\left( W_j^T \beta_k \right) \right] \alpha_{ij} \right] \right\}$

**Lemma 3**

$$\Lambda_{k0}(t) = \int_0^t \frac{1}{A_k(\theta_0; u)} dB_k(u), k = 1, \cdots, K.$$

where $A_k(\theta; u) = E A_{k1}(\theta; u)$ and $B_k(u) = E B_{k1}(u)$ with expectation taken under the true parameter $\theta_0$.

Lemma 1 will be proved in Appendix 1, and Lemmas 2 and 3 can be proved using the same methods in proving Lemma 2.1 of Chang et al. [2], we hence omit.

We now present the iterative algorithm for computing the NPMLE. Without loss of generality, we assume there are $K = 2$ types of endpoints. Let $B_1\left( \widehat{\theta}_M \right)$,

$B_2\left(\widehat{\boldsymbol{\theta}}_M\right)$, $P\left(\widehat{\boldsymbol{\theta}}_M\right)$, $L_1\left(\widehat{\boldsymbol{\theta}}_M\right)(t)$, and $L_2\left(\widehat{\boldsymbol{\theta}}_M\right)(t)$ denote respectively the right-hand side of Eqs. (5)–(7). The algorithm consists of the following steps:

(1) Set $q = 0$ and choose a starting value $\left(\boldsymbol{\beta}_1^{(0)}, \boldsymbol{\beta}_2^{(0)}, p^{(0)}, \Lambda_1^{(0)}, \Lambda_2^{(0)}\right)$.

(2) $\boldsymbol{\beta}_1^{(q+1)} = B_1\left(\boldsymbol{\beta}_1^{(q)}, \boldsymbol{\beta}_2^{(q)}, p^{(q)}, \Lambda_1^{(q)}, \Lambda_2^{(q)}\right)$.

(3) $\boldsymbol{\beta}_2^{(q+1)} = B_2\left(\boldsymbol{\beta}_1^{(q+1)}, \boldsymbol{\beta}_2^{(q)}, p^{(q)}, \Lambda_1^{(q)}, \Lambda_2^{(q)}\right)$.

(4) $p^{(q+1)} = P\left(\boldsymbol{\beta}_1^{(q+1)}, \boldsymbol{\beta}_2^{(q+1)}, p^{(q)}, \Lambda_1^{(q)}, \Lambda_2^{(q)}\right)$.

(5) $\Lambda_1^{(q+1)}(t) = L_1\left(\boldsymbol{\beta}_1^{(q+1)}, \boldsymbol{\beta}_2^{(q+1)}, p^{(q+1)}, \Lambda_1^{(q)}, \Lambda_2^{(q)}\right)(t)$.

(6) $\Lambda_2^{(q+1)}(t) = L_2\left(\boldsymbol{\beta}_1^{(q+1)}, \boldsymbol{\beta}_2^{(q+1)}, p^{(q+1)}, \Lambda_1^{(q+1)}, \Lambda_2^{(q)}\right)(t)$.

(7) $q = q + 1$.

(8) Repeat steps (2)–(7) until $q = Q$ when there is evidence of convergence.

## 2.4 The Predicted Cumulative Incidence Function

The model (1) we consider is a regression model based on cause-specific hazards of competing risks under the CC/NCC sampling. In the analysis of competing risks data, it is often of interest to also obtain the cumulative incidence function (CIF) for a particular cause of failure with a given set of covariates $\boldsymbol{Z} = z_0$, which is defined as

$$F_k(t; z_0) = pr\left(T \le t, E = k | \boldsymbol{Z} = z_0\right), k = 1, \cdots, K.$$

Under the Cox's proportional hazards model (1) with the always observed covariates $\boldsymbol{y}$ omitted, the CIF is given by

$$F_k(t; z_0) = \int_0^t \lambda_k(s) \exp\left(z_0^T \boldsymbol{\beta}_k\right) \exp\left(-\sum_{k=1}^{K} \Lambda_k(s) \exp\left(z_0^T \boldsymbol{\beta}_k\right)\right) ds,$$

which can be estimated by

$$\int_0^t \exp\left(-\sum_{k=1}^{K} \widehat{\Lambda}_k(s) \exp\left(z_0^T \widehat{\boldsymbol{\beta}}_k\right)\right) d\widehat{\Lambda}_k(s | z_0),$$

where $d\widehat{\Lambda}_k(s | z_0) = \Delta\widehat{\Lambda}_k(s) \exp\left(z_0^T \widehat{\boldsymbol{\beta}}_k\right)$.

Combining Theorem 3 with the functional delta method, we conclude that for a known, monotone, absolutely continuous transformation $h(\cdot)$,

$$\sqrt{M}\left(h\left(\widehat{F}_k(t; z_0)\right) - h\left(F_k(t; z_0)\right)\right)$$

converges weakly to a Gaussian process.

In order to compute the pointwise confidence interval and simultaneous confidence band for predicted CIF, we need to get the variance estimate of $\sqrt{M}\left(h\left(\widehat{F}_k\left(t;z_0\right)\right)-h\left(F_k\left(t;z_0\right)\right)\right)$. The variance estimate based on the asymptotic theory above mentioned is rather complicated. We thus instead apply the re-sampling method of Lu and Peng [10] to estimate the asymptotic variance for $h\left(\widehat{F}_k\left(t;z_0\right)\right)$. In the re-sampling algorithm, we first generate $M$ i.i.d positive random variable $\boldsymbol{\xi}=\{\xi_i,i=1,\cdots,M\}$ with mean 1 and variance 1. Fixing the data at their observed values, $\boldsymbol{\theta}^*$ is obtained as the solution of

$$P_M\boldsymbol{\xi}l_{j,\boldsymbol{\theta}^*}\left[\boldsymbol{h}_j\right]=0.$$

Generating $\boldsymbol{\xi}=\{\xi_i,i=1,\cdots,M\}$ $J$ times repeatedly, we obtain $J$ realizations of $\boldsymbol{\theta}^*$, and hence the simulated distribution of $\sqrt{M}\left(h\left(F_k^*\left(t;z_0\right)\right)-h\left(\widehat{F}_k\left(t;z_0\right)\right)\right)$, where $F_k^*\left(t;z_0\right)$ is $F_k\left(t;z_0\right)$ evaluated at $\boldsymbol{\theta}^*$. Next, use the simulated distribution of $\sqrt{M}\left(h\left(F_k^*\left(t;z_0\right)\right)-h\left(\widehat{F}_k\left(t;z_0\right)\right)\right)$ to compute an estimate of the variance function, $\sigma^2\left(t;z_0\right)=Var\left\{\sqrt{M}\left(h\left(\widehat{F}_k\left(t;z_0\right)\right)-h\left(F_k\left(t;z_0\right)\right)\right)\right\}$, given as $\widehat{\sigma^2}\left(t;z_0\right)=Var\left\{\sqrt{M}\left(h\left(F_k^*\left(t;z_0\right)\right)-h\left(\widehat{F}_k\left(t;z_0\right)\right)\right)\right\}$.

The $(1-2\alpha)\times 100\%$ pointwise confidence interval for $F_k\left(t;z_0\right)$ can then be constructed using,

$$h^{-1}\left(h\left(\widehat{F}_k\left(t;z_0\right)\right)\pm M^{-1/2}\phi_\alpha\widehat{\sigma}\left(t;z_0\right)\right),$$

where $\phi_\alpha$ is the $\alpha\times 100\%$ quantile of the standard normal distribution. Further, the $(1-2\alpha)\times 100\%$ simultaneous confidence band for $F_k\left(t;z_0\right)$ is obtained by

$$h^{-1}\left(h\left(\widehat{F}_k\left(t;z_0\right)\right)\pm M^{-1/2}c\left(\alpha;z_0\right)\widehat{\sigma}\left(t;z_0\right)\right),$$

where the critical value $c\left(\alpha;z_0\right)$ satisfies

$$\Pr\left[\sup_{t\in[o,\tau]}\frac{\left|\sqrt{M}\left(h\left(F_k^*\left(t;z_0\right)\right)-h\left(\widehat{F}_k\left(t;z_0\right)\right)\right)\right|}{\widehat{\sigma}\left(t;z_0\right)}\leq c\left(\alpha;z_0\right)\right]=1-2\alpha.$$

## 3   Large Sample Theory

This section presents asymptotic theory for the NPMLE. Section 3.1 states the identifiability proposition; Sect. 3.2 gives the consistency of the NPMLE; Sect. 3.3 presents the asymptotic normality of the NPMLE; Sect. 3.4 contains the second order expansion of profile likelihood and a consistent estimator of the asymptotic variance. Without loss of generality, we assume the number of endpoints $K=2$ in developing the following asymptotic properties.

## 3.1 Identifiability

The parameter space is $\Theta = \{(\boldsymbol{\beta}_1, \boldsymbol{\beta}_2, f, \Lambda_1, \Lambda_2) \,|\, \boldsymbol{\beta}_1 \in B, \boldsymbol{\beta}_2 \in B, f \in F, \Lambda_1 \in L, \Lambda_2 \in L\}$. Here $L = \{\Lambda : [0, \tau] \to [0, \infty) | \Lambda(0) = 0\}$, $\Lambda$ is non-decreasing and right continuous, B is a compact subset of $\Re^d$ and $F$ is the set of density functions defined on the non-negative functions. The analysis in this paper is restricted to the interval $[0, \tau]$; in accordance with standard survival analysis, an ideal $\tau$ should be large enough but still satisfy the property that there are subjects whose survival times are larger than $\tau$. Elements of $L$ are the cumulative hazards functions restricted to the interval $[0, \tau]$.

The true parameters $\boldsymbol{\beta}_{10}$ and $\boldsymbol{\beta}_{20}$ are assumed to be interior points of B, and the true cumulative hazard functions $\Lambda_{10}$ and $\Lambda_{20}$ are assumed to have positive and bounded derivatives on $[0, \tau]$. We assume that $pr(T_i \geq \tau, E_i = j | Z_i) > 0$, $j = 1, 2$, and $pr(C_i \leq \tau | Z_i) < 1$ almost surely. We further assume that the support of $Z$ is bounded. Further, we need the following Identifiability proposition.

**Proposition 1 (Identifiability)** *If $\Lambda_1$ is absolutely continuous with respect to $\Lambda_{10}$, and $\Lambda_2$ is absolutely continuous with respect to $\Lambda_{20}$, then $\tilde{L}_{1,\theta} = \tilde{L}_{1,\theta_0}$ a.s. implies $\theta = \theta_0$.*

We omit the proof of Proposition because the detail of the proof can be proved using the same argument in proving "Identifiability" property of Cox-gene model in [2]. Using the arguments in [2], we can show that the identifiability of the likelihood function follow from there exists $0 < t' < \tau$ in the support of the conditional distribution of $C_1$ given $Z_1$ such that if

$$\left(a_1 \frac{\partial}{\partial y_{10}} + a_2 \frac{\partial}{\partial y_{20}} + a_3 \frac{\partial}{\partial y_1} + a_4 \frac{\partial}{\partial y_2}\right)\bigg|_{(y_{10}, y_{20}, y_1, y_2) = \left(\Lambda_{10}(t'), \Lambda_{20}(t'), 1, 1\right)}$$

$$\left[\log \left(\prod_{k=1}^{2} y_k^{I(E_1=k)} \exp\left(-\sum_{k=1}^{2} y_{k0} \exp\left(Z_1^T \boldsymbol{\beta}_{k0}\right)\right)\right)^{I_{(o_1=1)}}\right.$$

$$\left. + \log \left(\int \exp\left(-\sum_{k=1}^{2} y_{k0} \exp\left(Z_1^T \boldsymbol{\beta}_{k0}\right)\right) f_0(Z_1) \, dZ_1\right)^{I_{(o_1=0)}} \right] = 0,$$

for every possible value of $(E_1, Z_1 \cdot O_1, O_1)$, then $a_1 = a_2 = a_3 = a_4 = 0$ in $\Re$.

## 3.2 Consistency of NPMLE

This subsection presents consistency theorem for the NPMLE.

**Theorem 1 (Existence of NPMLE)** *The NPMLE $\left(\widehat{\boldsymbol{\beta}}_{1M}, \widehat{\boldsymbol{\beta}}_{2M}, \widehat{p}_M, \widehat{\Lambda}_{1M}, \widehat{\Lambda}_{2M}\right)$ exists and $\widehat{\Lambda}_{jM}(\tau)$'s are bounded.*

The existence of NPMLE follows from the compactness of $B \times B \times P$ and $\Lambda_1$ and $\Lambda_2$ are of finite dimension. The boundedness of $\widehat{\Lambda}_{jM}(\tau)$'s follows from Lemma 2, and the boundedness of $A_{jM}$'s and $B_{jM}$'s, which is shown in the proof of Theorem 2.

**Theorem 2 (Consistency)** $\left\|\widehat{\beta}_{1M} - \beta_{10}\right\|_d, \left\|\widehat{\beta}_{2M} - \beta_{20}\right\|_d, \left\|\widehat{p}_M - p_0\right\|_J, \sup_{t \in [0,\tau]}$ $\left|\widehat{\Lambda}_{1M}(t) - \Lambda_{10}(t)\right|$, and $\sup_{t \in [0,\tau]} \left|\widehat{\Lambda}_{2M}(t) - \Lambda_{20}(t)\right|$ converge to 0 almost surely, as M tends to infinity.

Here and in the following, $\|\bullet\|_n$ stands for Euclidean norm on $\mathfrak{R}^n$.

We omit the proof of Theorem 2 because the detail of the proof is very long and can be proved using the same argument in proving "Consistency" property of Cox-gene model in [2].

### 3.3  Asymptotic Normality of NPMLE

We will prove the asymptotic normality by verifying the conditions in Theorem 3.3.1 and Lemma 3.3.5 of van der Vaart and Wellner [22], henceforth V&W [22]; details are relegated to Appendix 5.

Let $H = H_1 \times H_2 \times H_3 \times BV[0,\tau] \times BV[0,\tau]$, where $H_1 = \{h_1 \in \mathfrak{R}^d\}$, $H_2 = \{h_2 \in \mathfrak{R}^d\}$ and $H_3 = \left\{h_3 = (h_{3,1}, \cdots, h_{3,J})^T \in \mathfrak{R}^J \mid \sum_{j=1}^{J} h_{3,j} = 0\right\}$. For $h = (h_1, h_2, h_3, h_4, h_5) \in H$. We introduce the norm $\|(h_1, h_2, h_3, h_4, h_5)\|_H = \|h_1\|_d + \|h_2\|_d + \|h_3\|_J + \|h_4\|_V + \|h_5\|_V$, where $\|h\|_V$ is the sum of the absolute value of $h(0)$ and the total variation of $h$ on $[0,\tau]$. Let $H_p$ be the subset of H with $\|(h_1, h_2, h_3, h_4, h_5)\|_H \leq p$ if $p < \infty$. If $p = \infty$, then the previous inequality is strict. Define $\theta(h) = (\beta_1, \beta_2, p, \Lambda_1, \Lambda_2)(h) = h_1^T \beta_1 + h_2^T \beta_2 + h_3^T p + \int_0^\tau h_4 d\Lambda_1 + \int_0^\tau h_5 d\Lambda_2$, and the parameter space $\Theta = \{(\beta_1, \beta_2, p, \Lambda_1, \Lambda_2) \mid \beta_1 \in B, \beta_2 \in B, p \in P, \Lambda_1 \in L, \Lambda_2 \in L\}$ can be considered to be a subset of $l^\infty(H_p)$, which is the space of all bounded real-valued functions on $H_p$ equipped with the norm $\|\theta\|_{l^\infty(H_p)} = \sup_{h \in H_p} |\theta(h)|$. We note that

$$\left(p/\sqrt{d}\right) \left(\|\beta_1 - \beta_{10}\|_d \vee \|\beta_2 - \beta_{20}\|_d \vee \|p - p_0\|_J \vee \|\Lambda_1 - \Lambda_{10}\|_* \vee \|\Lambda_2 - \Lambda_{20}\|_*\right)$$

$$\leq \|\theta - \theta_0\|_{l^\infty(H_p)} = \sup_{h \in H_p} |(\theta - \theta_0)(h)|$$

$$\leq (5p) \left(\|\beta_1 - \beta_{10}\|_d \vee \|\beta_2 - \beta_{20}\|_d \vee \|p - p_0\|_J \vee \|\Lambda_1 - \Lambda_{10}\|_* \vee \|\Lambda_2 - \Lambda_{20}\|_*\right),$$

where $\|\Lambda - \Lambda_0\|_* = \sup_{\|h\|_v \leq 1} \left|\int_0^\tau h d(\Lambda - \Lambda_0)\right|$ is the natural norm for a bounded linear operator on the normed space $BV[0,\tau]$.

Define $\Psi_M : \Theta \to l^\infty(H_p)$ by

$$\Psi_M(\beta_1, \beta_2, p, \Lambda_1, \Lambda_2)(h_1, h_2, h_3, h_4, h_5)$$

$$= P_M \sum_{j=1}^{5} l_{j,(\beta_1,\beta_2,p,\Lambda_1,\Lambda_2)} \left[ h_j \right] (X_i, E_i, Z_i \cdot O_i, O_i)$$

$$= \frac{1}{M} \sum_{i=1}^{M} \sum_{j=1}^{5} l_{j,\theta} \left[ h_j \right] (X_i, E_i, Z_i \cdot O_i, O_i).$$

To simplify the notation, we let

$$\phi_{\theta,h} = \sum_{j=1}^{5} l_{j,\theta} \left[ h_j \right] (X_i, E_i, Z_i \cdot O_i, O_i).$$

Let $\Psi : \Theta \to l^{\infty}(H_p)$ be defined by $\Psi(\theta)(h) = E\Psi_1(\theta)(h)$. Let $lin\Theta$ denote the set of all finite linear combinations of $\theta - \theta_0$, for $\theta \in \Theta$. Then we obtain the following analytic condition on $\Psi$.

**Lemma 4** $\sqrt{M}(\Psi_M(\theta_0) - \Psi(\theta_0))$ *converges weakly to a Gaussian process* $W$ *in* $l^{\infty}(H_p)$ *for every* $0 < p < \infty$.

Lemma 4 can be proved using the same methods in proving Lemma 4.1 of Chang et al. [2], we hence omit.

**Lemma 5** $\left\{ \phi_{\theta,h} - \phi_{\theta_0,h} : \|\theta - \theta_0\|_{l^{\infty}(H_p)} < \delta, h \in H_p \right\}$ *is Donsker.*

We omit the proof of Lemma 5, because it requires only a more complicated version of the proof for Lemma 4.

**Lemma 6** $\lim_{\theta \to \theta_0} \sup_{h \in H_p} E \left( \phi_{\theta,h} - \phi_{\theta_0,h} \right)^2 = 0$.

The proof of Lemma 6 can be seen in Appendix 2.

**Lemma 7 (Fréchet Differentiability)** *Let* $p < \infty$. *There is a continuous linear map* $\dot{\Psi}_{\theta_0} : lin\Theta \to l^{\infty}(H_p)$ *satisfying* $\left\| \Psi(\theta) - \Psi(\theta_0) - \dot{\Psi}_{\theta_0}(\theta - \theta_0) \right\|_{l^{\infty}(H_p)} = o\left( \|\theta - \theta_0\|_{l^{\infty}(H_p)} \right)$. *In addition,* $\dot{\Psi}_{\theta_0}$ *has a continuous inverse on its range, and*

$$\dot{\Psi}_{\theta_0}(\theta - \theta_0)(h)$$

$$= -\sigma_1(h)^T (\beta_1 - \beta_{10}) + \sigma_2(h)^T (\beta_2 - \beta_{20}) + \sigma_3(h)^T (p - p_0)$$

$$+ \int_0^{\tau} \sigma_4(h)(t) d (\Lambda_1(t) - \Lambda_{10}(t)) + \int_0^{\tau} \sigma_5(h)(t) d (\Lambda_2(t) - \Lambda_{20}(t))$$

*for a linear map* $\sigma = (\sigma_1, \sigma_2, \sigma_3, \sigma_4, \sigma_5)$ *from* $H_{\infty}$ *to* $H_{\infty}$.

Lemma 7 can be proved using the same methods in proving Lemma 4.4 of Chang et al. [2], we hence omit.

We note that $\sigma$ is usually called the information operator. Using Lemma 7 and the negative second directional derivative of the log-likelihood of the parametric submodel

$$(\varepsilon_1, \varepsilon_2) \mapsto$$

$$\left( \beta_{10} + \varepsilon_1 h_1 + \varepsilon_2 h_1', \beta_{20} + \varepsilon_1 h_2 + \varepsilon_2 h_2', p_0 + \varepsilon_1 h_3 + \varepsilon_2 h_3', \right.$$

$$\left. \Lambda_{10} + \varepsilon_1 \int_0^{\cdot} h_4 d\Lambda_{10} + \varepsilon_2 \int_0^{\cdot} h_4' d\Lambda_{10}, \Lambda_{20} + \varepsilon_1 \int_0^{\cdot} h_5 d\Lambda_{20} + \varepsilon_2 \int_0^{\cdot} h_5' d\Lambda_{20} \right)$$

for $(\varepsilon_1, \varepsilon_2)$ near 0, we obtain the following equation connecting the information and the score:

$$\sigma_1 (h)^T h_1' + \sigma_2 (h)^T h_2' + \sigma_3 (h)^T h_3' \tag{8}$$

$$+ \int_0^{\tau} \sigma_4 (h) (t) h_4' (t) d\Lambda_{10} (t) + \int_0^{\tau} \sigma_5 (h) (t) h_5' (t) d\Lambda_{20} (t)$$

$$= E \left\{ \left[ \sum_{j=1}^{5} l_{j,\theta_0} [h_j] (X_1, E_1, Z_1 \cdot O_1, O_1) \right] \left[ \sum_{j=1}^{5} l_{j,\theta_0} \left[ h_j' \right] (X_1, E_1, Z_1 \cdot O_1, O_1) \right] \right\},$$

for $(h_1, h_2, h_3, h_4, h_5)$ and $\left( h_1', h_2', h_3', h_4', h_5' \right)$ are in $H_\infty$.

It follows from Lemmas 5 and 6, and the consistency in Theorem 2 that the conditions in Lemma 3.3.5 of V&W [22] are satisfied, and thus the stochastic condition in Theorem 3.3.1 of V&W [22] is satisfied. This together with Lemmas 4 and 7 shows that all the other conditions in Theorem 3.3.1 of V&W [22] are satisfied. Thus

$$\sqrt{M} \left( \hat{\theta}_M - \theta_0 \right) = - \left( \dot{\Psi}_{(\theta_0)} \right)^{-1} \sqrt{M} (\Psi_M - \Psi) (\theta_0) + o_p (1)$$

on $l^\infty (H_p)$.

**Theorem 3 (Asymptotic Normality)** $\sqrt{M} \left( \hat{\theta}_M - \theta_0 \right)$ *converges weakly to a tight Gaussian process* $g \equiv -\dot{\Psi}_{(\theta_0)}^{-1} W$ *on* $l^\infty (H_p)$ *with mean zero and covariance process*

$$cov \left( g (h), g \left( \tilde{h} \right) \right)$$

$$= h_1^T \sigma_1^{-1} \left( \tilde{h} \right) + h_2^T \sigma_2^{-1} \left( \tilde{h} \right) + h_3^T \sigma_3^{-1} \left( \tilde{h} \right) + \int_0^{\tau} h_4 \sigma_4^{-1} \left( \tilde{h} \right) d\Lambda_{10} + \int_0^{\tau} h_5 \sigma_5^{-1} \left( \tilde{h} \right) d\Lambda_2$$

*where* $\left( h, \tilde{h} \right)$ *is in* $H_\infty$, *and* $\left( \sigma_1^{-1}, \sigma_2^{-1}, \sigma_3^{-1}, \sigma_4^{-1}, \sigma_5^{-1} \right) = \sigma^{-1} : H_\infty \to H_\infty$ *is the inverse of* $(\sigma_1, \sigma_2, \sigma_3, \sigma_4, \sigma_5)$.

We omit this proof, because it can be proved using the same arguments in proving the "Asymptotic normality" of Cox-gene model in [2].

## 3.4 A Profile Likelihood Theory for the Estimation of $\beta$

In this subsection, we present a profile likelihood theory for $\beta = (\beta_1, \beta_2)$, focusing our attention on the estimation of $\beta$. One motivation of using profile likelihood theory is to prove the asymptotic normality and efficiency of the NPMLE of $\beta$. Also, we provide variance estimation of the NPMLE of $\beta$ through the profile likelihood and an algorithm to calculate the variance estimator. The corresponding efficient score function, the efficient Fisher information, and the asymptotic normality of $(\widehat{\beta}_{1M}, \widehat{\beta}_{2M})$ are established. We also apply the theory of observed profile information, developed in [11, 12], to obtain a consistent estimator of the asymptotic variance.

For $h \in H_\infty$, let $\left( \sigma_{12}^{-1}(h) \right)^T = \left( \left( \sigma_1^{-1}(h) \right)^T, \left( \sigma_2^{-1}(h) \right)^T \right)$, and $e_i$ be the $D (\equiv 2d)$-dimensional column vector with 1 in the $i$th position and zeros elsewhere. Define the $D \times D$ matrix $\Sigma$ by

$$\Sigma^{-1} = \left( \sigma_{12}^{-1}(e_1, 0, 0, 0), \sigma_{12}^{-1}(e_2, 0, 0, 0), \cdots, \sigma_{12}^{-1}(e_D, 0, 0, 0) \right).$$

We note that $\Sigma$ is positive definite and symmetric (see Appendix 3).

Also, $l_{12,\theta} [h_1, h_2] (X_1, E_1, Z_1 \cdot O_1, O_1) = l_{1,\theta} [h_1] (X_1, E_1, Z_1 \cdot O_1, O_1) + l_{2,\theta} [h_2] (X_1, E_1, Z_1 \cdot O_1, O_1)$ for $h_1, h_2 \in \Re^d$. Viewing $(h_1^T, h_2^T)$ as a D-dimensional row vector, we can consider $l_{12,\theta} [\cdot] (X_1, E_1, Z_1 \cdot O_1, O_1)$ a D-dimensional column vector and abbreviate it as $l_{12,\theta}$.

Define

$$\pi_3 = -\Sigma \begin{pmatrix} \sigma_3^{-1}(e_1, 0, 0, 0)^T \\ \sigma_3^{-1}(e_2, 0, 0, 0)^T \\ \vdots \\ \sigma_3^{-1}(e_D, 0, 0, 0)^T \end{pmatrix}_{D \times J} ;$$

$$\pi_4 = -\Sigma \begin{pmatrix} \sigma_4^{-1}(e_1, 0, 0, 0) \\ \sigma_4^{-1}(e_2, 0, 0, 0) \\ \vdots \\ \sigma_4^{-1}(e_D, 0, 0, 0) \end{pmatrix}_{D \times 1} ; \pi_5 = -\Sigma \begin{pmatrix} \sigma_5^{-1}(e_1, 0, 0, 0) \\ \sigma_5^{-1}(e_2, 0, 0, 0) \\ \vdots \\ \sigma_5^{-1}(e_D, 0, 0, 0) \end{pmatrix}_{D \times 1} .$$

Then we have the following lemmas concerning the efficient score function and the efficient Fisher information; see also [21].

**Lemma 8** *The efficient score function for the estimation of* $\beta = (\beta_1, \beta_2)$ *is*

$$\tilde{l}_0 = l_{12,\theta_0} - \left( l_{3,\theta_0} [\pi_3] + l_{4,\theta_0} [\pi_4] + l_{5,\theta_0} [\pi_5] \right).$$

**Lemma 9** $\Sigma = E\tilde{l}_0\tilde{l}_0^T$.

Lemmas 8 and 9 can be proved using the same ways in proving Lemmas 5.1 and 5.2 of Chang et al. [2], we hence omit.

Then, setting $h = \sigma^{-1}(e_k, 0, 0, 0)$ in Lemma 7, we obtain

$$e_k\sqrt{M}\left(\widehat{\boldsymbol{\beta}}_M - \boldsymbol{\beta}_0\right)$$

$$= \sqrt{M}\,(P_M - P_0)\left(\sum_{j=1}^{5} l_{j,\boldsymbol{\theta}_0}\left[\sigma_j^{-1}(e_k, 0, 0, 0)\right](X_i, E_i, \boldsymbol{Z}_i \cdot O_i, O_i)\right) + o_p\,(1)$$

$$= \sqrt{M}\,(P_M - P_0)\left(e_k^T\Sigma^{-1}\tilde{l}_0\right) + o_p\,(1)\,,$$

which means that

$$\sqrt{M}\left(\widehat{\boldsymbol{\beta}}_M - \boldsymbol{\beta}_0\right) = \Sigma^{-1}\sqrt{M}\,(P_M - P_0)\,\tilde{l}_0 + o_p\,(1)\,. \tag{9}$$

It follows from (9) that $\sqrt{M}\left(\widehat{\boldsymbol{\beta}}_M - \boldsymbol{\beta}_0\right)$ has asymptotic variance $\Sigma^{-1}$, which is proved in Appendix 4. Therefore, $\Sigma$ is called the efficient Fisher information matrix. Because the exact from of $\Sigma^{-1}$ is very complex, we apply the theory of observed profile information to obtain a consistent estimate of the asymptotic variance. First we introduce the least favourable submodel. For $\boldsymbol{\zeta} \in \Re^D$, we define

$$p\,(\boldsymbol{\zeta}, \boldsymbol{\theta}) = p + \left(\left((\boldsymbol{\beta} - \boldsymbol{\zeta})^T\pi_3\right)^T\right.,$$

$$\Lambda_1\,(\boldsymbol{\zeta}, \boldsymbol{\theta}; t) = \int_0^t\left(1 + (\boldsymbol{\beta} - \boldsymbol{\zeta})^T\pi_4\right)(u)\,d\Lambda_1\,(u)\,,$$

$$\Lambda_2\,(\boldsymbol{\zeta}, \boldsymbol{\theta}; t) = \int_0^t\left(1 + (\boldsymbol{\beta} - \boldsymbol{\zeta})^T\pi_5\right)(u)\,d\Lambda_2\,(u)\,.$$

Given $\boldsymbol{\theta}$, the path $\boldsymbol{\zeta} \mapsto (\boldsymbol{\zeta}, p\,(\boldsymbol{\zeta}, \boldsymbol{\theta}), \Lambda_1\,(\boldsymbol{\zeta}, \boldsymbol{\theta}; \cdot), \Lambda_2\,(\boldsymbol{\zeta}, \boldsymbol{\theta}; \cdot))$ defines a parametric submodel, referred to as the submodel indexed by $\boldsymbol{\theta}$. Its log likelihood for the data $(X_1, E_1, \boldsymbol{Z}_1 \cdot O_1, O_1)$ is denoted by $l\,(\boldsymbol{\zeta}, \boldsymbol{\theta}; X_1, E_1, \boldsymbol{Z}_1 \cdot O_1, O_1) \equiv \log L_1\,(\boldsymbol{\zeta}, p\,(\boldsymbol{\zeta}, \boldsymbol{\theta}), \Lambda_1\,(\boldsymbol{\zeta}, \boldsymbol{\theta}; \cdot), \Lambda_2\,(\boldsymbol{\zeta}, \boldsymbol{\theta}; \cdot); X_1, E_1, \boldsymbol{Z}_1 \cdot O_1, O_1)$. Denote by $\dot{l}$ and $\ddot{l}$ the first and second derivatives of $l$ in $\boldsymbol{\zeta}$, respectively.

Thus, the score function at $\boldsymbol{\zeta}$ of the submodel indexed by $\boldsymbol{\theta}$, denoted by $\dot{l}\,(\boldsymbol{\zeta}, \boldsymbol{\theta})$, is equal to

$$l_{12,(\boldsymbol{\zeta},p(\boldsymbol{\zeta},\boldsymbol{\theta}),\Lambda_1(\boldsymbol{\zeta},\boldsymbol{\theta};\cdot),\Lambda_2(\boldsymbol{\zeta},\boldsymbol{\theta};\cdot))} - l_{3,(\boldsymbol{\zeta},p(\boldsymbol{\zeta},\boldsymbol{\theta}),\Lambda_1(\boldsymbol{\zeta},\boldsymbol{\theta};\cdot),\Lambda_2(\boldsymbol{\zeta},\boldsymbol{\theta};\cdot))}\,[\pi_3]$$

$$- \left(l_{4,(\boldsymbol{\zeta},p(\boldsymbol{\zeta},\boldsymbol{\theta}),\Lambda_1(\boldsymbol{\zeta},\boldsymbol{\theta};\cdot),\Lambda_2(\boldsymbol{\zeta},\boldsymbol{\theta};\cdot))}\,[\pi_4] + l_{5,(\boldsymbol{\zeta},p(\boldsymbol{\zeta},\boldsymbol{\theta}),\Lambda_1(\boldsymbol{\zeta},\boldsymbol{\theta};\cdot),\Lambda_2(\boldsymbol{\zeta},\boldsymbol{\theta};\cdot))}\,[\pi_5]\right)\,.$$

Hence,

$$\dot{l}\,(\boldsymbol{\beta}_0, \boldsymbol{\theta}_0) = \tilde{l}_0,$$

which implies that the score function at $\zeta = \beta_0$ of the submodel indexed by $\theta_0 = (\beta_{10}, \beta_{20}, p_0, \Lambda_{10}, \Lambda_{20})$ is equal to the efficient score function $\tilde{l}_0$. Denote by $I_\theta (\zeta, \theta)$ the Fisher information matrix at $\zeta$ of the submodel indexed by $\theta$. Then

$$I_\theta (\beta_0, \theta_0) = -E\ddot{i} (\beta_0, \theta_0) = E\dot{i} (\beta_0, \theta_0) \dot{i} (\beta_0, \theta_0)^T = E\left(\tilde{l}_0 \tilde{l}_0^T\right) = \Sigma.$$

Denote the profile likelihood function for $\beta$ by $pL_M (\beta)$, which is equal to

$$pL_M (\beta) = \sup_{p \in P, \Lambda_1 \in L_*, \Lambda_2 \in L_*} L_M (\beta, p, \Lambda_1, \Lambda_2).$$

**Theorem 4 (Expansion of Profile Likelihood)** *For every random sequence* $\beta_M$ *that converges to* $\beta_0$ *in probability,*

$$\log pL_M (\beta_M) - \log pL_M (\beta_0) \tag{10}$$

$$= (\beta_M - \beta_0)^T \sum_{i=1}^{M} \tilde{l}_0 (X_i, E_i, Z_i \cdot O_i, O_i) - \frac{1}{2} M (\beta_M - \beta_0)^T \Sigma (\beta_M - \beta_0)$$

$$+ o_p \left(\sqrt{M} \left\| (\beta_M - \beta_0)^T \right\| + 1\right)^2$$

We omit the proof of Theorem 4 because the detail of the proof is long and can be proved using the same argument in proving "Observed profile information" property of Cox-gene model of Chang et al. [2, 3].

Utilizing the consistency of $\hat{\beta}_M$ given in Theorem 2, the invertibility of the efficient Fisher information matrix $\Sigma$, and the second order expansion of the profile likelihood (10), we obtain the following theorems following immediately from the profile likelihood theory of Murphy and van der Vaart [12].

**Theorem 5** *The NPMLE* $\hat{\beta}_M = \begin{pmatrix} \hat{\beta}_{1M} \\ \hat{\beta}_{2M} \end{pmatrix}$ *is asymptotically normal and asymptotically efficient at* $\theta_0$; *that is*

$$\sqrt{M} (\hat{\beta}_M - \beta_0) = \Sigma^{-1} \sqrt{M} P_M \tilde{l}_0 + o_p (1) \xrightarrow{d} N\left(0, \Sigma^{-1}\right).$$

### 3.4.1 A Consistent Estimator of the Asymptotic Variance for $\beta$

**Theorem 6** *For all sequences* $v_M \xrightarrow{p} v \in \mathfrak{R}^D$ *and* $\omega_M \xrightarrow{p} 0$ *such that* $\left(\sqrt{M}\omega_M\right)^{-1} = O_p (1)$,

$$-2\frac{\log pL_M (\hat{\beta}_M + \omega_M v_M) - \log pL_M (\hat{\beta}_M)}{M\omega_M^2} \xrightarrow{p} v^T \Sigma v. \tag{11}$$

Using (11), we can obtain that

$$\frac{-1}{M\omega_M^2}\left[\log pL_M\left(\widehat{\boldsymbol{\beta}}_M + \omega_M\boldsymbol{e}_i + \omega_M\boldsymbol{e}_j\right) + \log pL_M\left(\widehat{\boldsymbol{\beta}}_M\right)\right]$$

$$+\frac{1}{M\omega_M^2}\left[\log pL_M\left(\widehat{\boldsymbol{\beta}}_M + \omega_M\boldsymbol{e}_i\right) + \log pL_M\left(\widehat{\boldsymbol{\beta}}_M + \omega_M\boldsymbol{e}_j\right)\right].$$

converges in probability to the $(i, j)_{th}$ entry of $\Sigma$.

To compute the profile log-likelihood, we perform the following iterative algorithm [3]. Let $P(\boldsymbol{\theta})$, $L_1(\boldsymbol{\theta})(t)$, and $L_2(\boldsymbol{\theta})(t)$ denote respectively the right-hand side of Eqs. (6) and (7), and

$$\log pL_M(\boldsymbol{\beta}) = \sup_{\boldsymbol{p}\in P, \Lambda_1\in L_*, \Lambda_2\in L_*} l_M(\boldsymbol{\beta}, \boldsymbol{p}, \Lambda_1, \Lambda_2),$$

the algorithm consists of the following steps:

(1) Set $q = 0$ and choose a starting value $\left(\boldsymbol{p}^{(0)}, \Lambda_1^{(0)}, \Lambda_2^{(0)}\right)$ and set $log\_profile\_likelihood^{(0)} = l_M\left(\boldsymbol{\beta}_1, \boldsymbol{\beta}_2, \boldsymbol{p}^{(0)}, \Lambda_1^{(0)}, \Lambda_2^{(0)}\right).$

(2) $\boldsymbol{p}^{(q+1)} = P\left(\boldsymbol{\beta}_1, \boldsymbol{\beta}_2, \boldsymbol{p}^{(q)}, \Lambda_1^{(q)}, \Lambda_2^{(q)}\right).$

(3) $\Lambda_1^{(q+1)}(t) = L_1\left(\boldsymbol{\beta}_1, \boldsymbol{\beta}_2, \boldsymbol{p}^{(q+1)}, \Lambda_1^{(q)}, \Lambda_2^{(q)}\right)(t).$

(4) $\Lambda_2^{(q+1)}(t) = L_2\left(\boldsymbol{\beta}_1, \boldsymbol{\beta}_2, \boldsymbol{p}^{(q+1)}, \Lambda_1^{(q+1)}, \Lambda_2^{(q)}\right)(t).$

(5) Set $q = q+1.$ and $log\_profile\_likelihood^{(q+1)} = l_M\left(\boldsymbol{\beta}_1, \boldsymbol{\beta}_2, \boldsymbol{p}^{(q+1)}, \Lambda_1^{(q+1)},\right.$ $\left.\Lambda_2^{(q+1)}\right)$

(6) Repeat steps (2)–(5) until $q = Q$ when there is evidence of convergence. Then we set $\log pL_M(\boldsymbol{\beta})$ to be $l_M\left(\boldsymbol{\beta}_1, \boldsymbol{\beta}_2, \boldsymbol{p}^{(Q)}, \Lambda_1^{(Q)}, \Lambda_2^{(Q)}\right).$

Furthermore, we compute the variance estimator of $\boldsymbol{\beta}$,

(1) Given the NPNLE $\widehat{\boldsymbol{\beta}}_M$.

(2) Denote $\boldsymbol{e}_1 = (1, 0, \cdots, 0)^T, \boldsymbol{e}_2 = (0, 1, 0, \cdots, 0)^T, \cdots, \boldsymbol{e}_D = (0, \cdots, 0, 1)^T$, and set $\omega_M = \frac{1}{\sqrt{M}}.$

(3) The $(i, j)_{th}$-entry of $\widehat{\Sigma}$ is

$$\frac{-1}{M\omega_M^2}\left[\log pL_M\left(\widehat{\boldsymbol{\beta}}_M + \omega_M\boldsymbol{e}_i + \omega_M\boldsymbol{e}_j\right) + \log pL_M\left(\widehat{\boldsymbol{\beta}}_M\right)\right]$$

$$+\frac{1}{M\omega_M^2}\left[\log pL_M\left(\widehat{\boldsymbol{\beta}}_M + \omega_M\boldsymbol{e}_i\right) + \log pL_M\left(\widehat{\boldsymbol{\beta}}_M + \omega_M\boldsymbol{e}_j\right)\right].$$

# 4 Simulation Study

In the simulation study, we would like to investigate the performances of the proposed NPMLE analysis, and compared them with those from the WPL analysis and the "Full cohort" analysis assuming that all data are observed for the full cohort and then the Cox regression is performed with the full data.

## 4.1 Multiple Outcomes with Time Matching

In this subsection, we consider the simulation study under the NCC sampling with two competing events and with a cohort of size 2000. The cause-specific hazards functions for the two event times follow the Cox's proportional hazards models

$$\lambda_1 (t \mid z, y) = \lambda_{01} \exp \left( z^T \beta_1 \right) ;$$

$$\lambda_2 (t \mid z, y) = \lambda_{02} \exp \left( z^T \beta_2 \right) .$$

Here $(\lambda_{01}, \lambda_{02}) = (0.15, 0.3)$, the log-relative risk $\beta_1 = (0.5, -0.5)^T$, $\beta_2 = (-1, 1)^T$, and the two covariates $(Z_1, Z_2)$ jointly follow a standard bivariate normal with correlation $corr (Z_1, Z_2) = 0.5$. The censoring time distribution follows a uniform $U(0, 1)$ distribution. We randomly sample one subject from the risk set as a control when a case arises. Simulations are based on 200 simulated cohorts. The mean numbers of the two endpoints are 145 and 349, respectively, and the mean number of sampled subjects is 836 over 200 simulations.

## 4.2 Multiple Outcomes with Stratified Matching

The setup in this simulation is similar to that in the previous one, except that here data on an additional covariate $Y$ are observed for all subjects in the cohort. The cause-specific hazards functions of the two events follow the Cox's proportional hazards models

$$\lambda_1 (t \mid z, y) = \lambda_{01} \exp \left( y^T \eta_1 + z^T \beta_1 \right) ;$$

$$\lambda_2 (t \mid z, y) = \lambda_{02} \exp \left( y^T \eta_2 + z^T \beta_2 \right) .$$

Here $(\lambda_{01}, \lambda_{02}) = (0.1, 0.35)$, $\beta_1 = (0.5, -0.5)^T$, $\beta_2 = (-0.8, 0.8)^T$, and the always observed covariate $Y$ follows a Bernoulli(0.5) distribution and its effects $(\eta_1, \eta_2) = (1, -1)$. Given $Y = y$, the covariates $(Z_1, Z_2)$ follow independent normal distributions with means of $0.5(y+1)$ and variances of 1. When a case occurs, we randomly sample one control from the risk set with the same value of $Y$ as the case has, i.e., the case and control are matched on their $Y$ value. The mean numbers of the two endpoints are 197 and 303, respectively, and the mean number of sampled subjects is 844 over 200 simulations.

## 4.3  Results

The simulation results are summarized as *Mean est.*, which is mean of the estimates over simulations, *Mean est. se*, which is mean of estimated standard errors over simulations, *sd est. se*, which is standard deviation of estimated standard errors over simulations, *Emp. Se*, which is empirical standard deviation of the estimates over simulations, and *CP*, which is the converge probability of the 95% confidence intervals over simulations based on the normal approximation.

From Tables 1 and 2, we can see that most of the differences between *Mean est. se* and *Emp. se* are less than twice of *sd est. se* for the NPMLE approach, and the *CP* values for the NPMLE approach are close to 0.95, implying that the proposed standard error formula (11) and the normal approximation perform well. Also, the values of *Mean est. se* and *Emp. se* for the NPMLE approach are smaller than those of the WPL approach, implying that the NPMLE approach is more efficient than WPL approach. In addition, our further simulation reveals that the MI approach is sensitive to the assumed covariate distribution. When the covariate distribution is misspecified in the MI procedure, the bias for the regression parameter may be unacceptably large (results not shown).

## 5  Example: Application to Liver Cancer in Type 2 DM Patients

Both diabetes mellitus and cancer are common diseases for humans; and both occur more frequently in the same individual. DM has been found to be associated with an increased risk of cancers of liver, pancreas and endometrium [23]. Thiazolidine-diones (TZDs), including pioglitazone and rosiglitazone, are often used to treat type 2 DM patients. We would like to investigate the relative risks of liver and lung cancers in type 2 DM patients who received the TZDs treatment (pioglitazone or rosiglitazone) compared with those type 2 DM patients who did not receive the TZDs treatment.

By analyzing the 2000 Longitudinal Health Insurance Database (LHID) based on the Taiwan National Health Insurance Research Database (NHIRD), we first selected 7851 newly diagnosed diabetic patients without cancer between January

**Table 1** Simulation results for the full cohort, WPL, and NPMLE methods in the first simulation study (Sect. 4.1)

| Method | Mean est. | Mean est. se (sd est. se) | Emp. se | CP (%) |
|--------|-----------|---------------------------|---------|--------|
| **Event1** | | | | |
| *Full cohort* | | | | |
| $\beta_{11}$ | 0.4922 | 0.0996(0.0050) | 0.1014 | 94.5 |
| $\beta_{12}$ | −0.4889 | 0.0995(0.0046) | 0.0997 | 93.0 |
| *WPL* | | | | |
| $\beta_{11}$ | 0.4914 | 0.1134(0.0081) | 0.1115 | 95.5 |
| $\beta_{12}$ | −0.4920 | 0.1141(0.0098) | 0.1129 | 95.0 |
| *NPMLE* | | | | |
| $\beta_{11}$ | 0.4907 | 0.1118(0.0058) | 0.1085 | 95.0 |
| $\beta_{12}$ | −0.4906 | 0.1113(0.0057) | 0.1092 | 94.5 |
| **Event2** | | | | |
| *Full cohort* | | | | |
| $\beta_{21}$ | −1.0074 | 0.0671(0.0023) | 0.0639 | 97.5 |
| $\beta_{22}$ | 1.0085 | 0.0670(0.0023) | 0.0701 | 93.0 |
| *WPL* | | | | |
| $\beta_{21}$ | −1.0176 | 0.0872(0.0079) | 0.0889 | 94.5 |
| $\beta_{22}$ | 1.0172 | 0.0872(0.0079) | 0.0912 | 92.0 |
| *NPMLE* | | | | |
| $\beta_{21}$ | −1.0093 | 0.0815(0.0036) | 0.0782 | 95.5 |
| $\beta_{22}$ | 1.0108 | 0.0815(0.0038) | 0.0817 | 94.5 |

1, 2000 and December 31, 2000. These patients then were followed from the DM diagnosed dates to the earliest of lung or liver cancer diagnosis, dropout, or the date of December 31, 2010.

During the follow-up period, 251 and 206 of the 7851 subjects were identified as liver and lung cancer patients, respectively. In addition to the covariates corresponding to TZDs treatment groups (none, pioglitazone, and rosiglitazone, with the none-TZDs treatment used as the baseline group), we also consider the covariate corresponding to the presence or absence of the chronic liver disease, and that of the chronic lung disease.

Our analysis is based on competing risks consisting of two competing events of liver cancer and lung cancer, with the cause specific hazards for the two events given by Cox's proportional hazards models. At each time where a liver cancer or lung cancer case arose, we randomly sampled 2 subjects from the risk set, i.e., the subjects had not experienced either liver cancer or lung cancer by the time where the case arose, so that the controls were matched on time for the case. A total of 1277 subjects, including the cases and controls, were selected as the NCC sample. The covariate values were observed in the NCC sample, but were missing outside the NCC sample. The hazard ratio parameters of the proportional cause-specific hazards models based respectively on the partial likelihood using only the NCC data, the

**Table 2** Simulation results for the full cohort, WPL, and NPMLE methods in the second simulation study (Sect. 4.2)

| Method | Mean est. | Mean est. se (sd est. se) | Emp. se | CP (%) |
|---|---|---|---|---|
| **Event1** | | | | |
| *Full cohort* | | | | |
| $\eta_1$ | 0.9939 | 0.1676(0.0081) | 0.1622 | 97.0 |
| $\beta_{11}$ | 0.5074 | 0.0738(0.0030) | 0.0787 | 94.0 |
| $\beta_{12}$ | −0.5037 | 0.0738(0.0033) | 0.0665 | 97.0 |
| *WPL* | | | | |
| $\eta_1$ | 1.0040 | 0.1959(0.0098) | 0.1713 | 97.5 |
| $\beta_{11}$ | 0.5150 | 0.0915(0.0066) | 0.0960 | 94.0 |
| $\beta_{12}$ | −0.5177 | 0.0913(0.0066) | 0.0922 | 95.5 |
| *NPMLE* | | | | |
| $\eta_1$ | 1.0010 | 0.1744(0.0126) | 0.1630 | 93.5 |
| $\beta_{11}$ | 0.5086 | 0.0874(0.0051) | 0.0899 | 96.0 |
| $\beta_{12}$ | −0.5048 | 0.0871(0.0050) | 0.0970 | 94.0 |
| **Event2** | | | | |
| *Full cohort* | | | | |
| $\eta_2$ | −1.0073 | 0.1320(0.0048) | 0.1286 | 95.5 |
| $\beta_{21}$ | −0.8088 | 0.0619(0.0027) | 0.0712 | 89.5 |
| $\beta_{22}$ | 0.8064 | 0.0615(0.0026) | 0.0628 | 94.0 |
| *WPL* | | | | |
| $\eta_2$ | −1.0154 | 0.1686(0.0081) | 0.1604 | 95.0 |
| $\beta_{21}$ | −0.8167 | 0.0792(0.0068) | 0.0889 | 91.5 |
| $\beta_{22}$ | 0.8086 | 0.0784(0.0060) | 0.0815 | 93.5 |
| *NPMLE* | | | | |
| $\eta_2$ | −1.0160 | 0.1454(0.0083) | 0.1460 | 96.5 |
| $\beta_{21}$ | −0.8138 | 0.0744(0.0041) | 0.0835 | 88.5 |
| $\beta_{22}$ | 0.8023 | 0.0737(0.0039) | 0.0773 | 94.0 |

conditional logistic regression (CLR, 20), the WPL, and the NPMLE, adjusted for chronic liver and lung diseases, were assessed. We note that the CLR approach is a traditional method used to analyze NCC data.

According to the results of Table 3, we see that all the methods considered identify pioglitazone as a significant protecting factor, and the presence of chronic liver disease as a significant risk factor, for the incidence of liver cancer among type 2 DM patients. The effect of rosiglitazone on the incidence of liver cancer is insignificant, while the effect of the presence of chronic lung disease on the incidence of liver cancer is marginal. Also, we see that pioglitazone is a significant protecting factor for the incidence of lung cancer, while the presence of chronic lung disease is a significant risk factor. The effects of rosiglitazone and the chronic liver disease on the incidence of lung cancer are not statistically significant.

**Table 3** Liver and lung cancers in type 2 DM patients: coefficient estimates (p-value)

| Parameters | CLR.$\beta$(p-value) | WPL.$\beta$(p-value) | NPMLE.$\beta$(p-value) |
|---|---|---|---|
| **Liver cancer** | | | |
| Chronic liver diseases | 0.681(1.0e−04) | 0.704(2.1e−06) | 0.706(1.7e−06) |
| Chronic lung diseases | 0.417(3.5e−02) | 0.301(7.2e−02) | 0.310(6.1e−02) |
| Pioglitazone | −1.530(2.6e−06) | −1.380(4.2e−06) | −1.387(3.9e−06) |
| Rosiglitazone | −0.402(0.1080) | −0.301(0.1630) | −0.296(0.1680) |
| **Lung cancer** | | | |
| Chronic liver diseases | −0.223(0.2806) | −0.238(0.1790) | −0.234(0.1840) |
| Chronic lung diseases | 0.715(4.0e−04) | 0.763(4.4e−06) | 0.762(4.5e−06) |
| Pioglitazone | −1.226(8.0e−04) | −1.351(3.0e−05) | −1.356(3.0e−05) |
| Rosiglitazone | −0.259(0.3606) | −0.475(0.0490) | −0.466(0.0536) |

The conditional logistic regression (CLR) approach to the NCC data

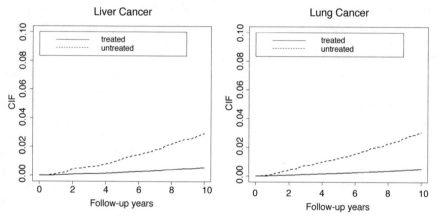

**Fig. 1** Predicted cumulative incidence functions for liver and lung cancers with and without TZDs

Figure 1 shows the predicted CIFs of liver and lung cancers based on the NPMLE for type 2 DM patients with TZDs treatment versus those without any TZDs treatments, in the absence of both chronic liver and lung diseases. From Fig. 1, we clearly observe the pattern of a significant rise in the CIFs of liver and lung cancers for patients without taking TZDs.

# 6  Discussion

We develop the full likelihood approach for the case-cohort and nested case-control designs with multiple competing events under the Cox's regression model. We present a self-consistency iterative algorithm for the computation of NPMLE and its variance estimator. Large sample theory for the NPMLE under the competing risks case-cohort/nested case-control designs is derived. We show by simulation studies that the proposed NPMLE performs better than the WPL estimator, which is as expected since the former method utilizes all the available data in the cohort while the latter method does not. In addition, we derive the predicted cumulative incidence functions for the multiple competing risks under the case-cohort/nested case-control designs, together with the corresponding pointwise confidence intervals and simultaneous confidence bands.

Although we only consider right-censored competing risks data in this paper, our method can be extended naturally to left-truncated data, in a manner similar to Saarela et al. [14]. One limitation of our NPMLE method is that it cannot handle time-dependent covariates. The extension of the NPMLE method to general time-dependent covariate data deserves further studies. In general, such an extension requires full histories for the time-dependent covariates of the cases and controls.

In this work we focus on the cause-specific models for competing risks. The alternative modeling strategies, such as the subdistribution hazard regression [6] and the mixture regression [3] are available for analyzing competing risks data. It is worthwhile to develop the NPMLE for these alternative models for competing risks data under the case-cohort/nested case-control designs.

Finally, the case-cohort and nested case-control designs have been popular strategies for reducing the costs of exposure assessment in cohort studies. Although the likelihood approach in such designs for the estimation of exposure effect is statistically efficient, it is in fact not widely used in practice, partly due to the computational burden [8]. We have developed computer software (R package) for implementing the NPMLE in the case-cohort and nested case-control designs that can accommodate multiple competing risks events. We hope that such a development will be useful for efficient inference in cost-effective epidemiologic studies conducted by case-cohort and nested case-control designs.

**Acknowledgements** We are very grateful to the Editors and referees for their very valuable comments that helped to improve the manuscript.

## Appendix 1: Proof of Lemma 1

$$P_M l_{2, \left( \boldsymbol{\beta}_1^{(q)}, \cdots, \boldsymbol{\beta}_K^{(q)}, p, \Lambda_1^{(q)}, \cdots, \Lambda_K^{(q)} \right)}[\boldsymbol{h}_2] = 0 \text{ means } \sum_{i=1}^{M} \left\{ I_{(o_i=1)} \left( \frac{\boldsymbol{\mu}_i^T \boldsymbol{h}_2}{\boldsymbol{\mu}_i^T \boldsymbol{p}} \right) + I_{(o_i=0)} \right.$$

$$\left. \left( \frac{\boldsymbol{\phi}_i^T \boldsymbol{h}_2}{\boldsymbol{\phi}_i^T \boldsymbol{p}} \right) \right\} = 0. \text{ Here } \boldsymbol{\mu}_i = \left( I_{Z_i=\mathbf{w}_1}, I_{Z_i=\mathbf{w}_2}, \cdots, I_{Z_i=\mathbf{w}_J} \right)^T \text{ and}$$

$$\boldsymbol{\phi}_i = \left( \exp \left( -\sum_{k=1}^{K} \Lambda_k^{(q)} (X_i) \exp \left( \mathbf{W}_1^T \boldsymbol{\beta}_k^{(q)} \right) \right), \right.$$

$$\left. \cdots, \exp \left( -\sum_{k=1}^{K} \Lambda_k^{(q)} (X_i) \exp \left( \mathbf{W}_J^T \boldsymbol{\beta}_k^{(q)} \right) \right) \right)^T.$$

Setting $h_2 = (0, \cdots, 0, 1, 0, \cdots, -1)^T$, having the *l*th and *J*th coordinate equal to 1 and $-1$ respecting and all the other coordinates being 0, we know

$$\sum_{i=1}^{M} \left\{ I_{(o_i=1)} \left( \frac{\mu_{i,l}}{\mu_i^T p} \right) + I_{(o_i=0)} \left( \frac{\phi_{i,l}}{\phi_i^T p} \right) \right\} = \sum_{i=1}^{M} \left\{ I_{(o_i=1)} \left( \frac{\mu_{i,J}}{\mu_i^T p} \right) + I_{(o_i=0)} \left( \frac{\phi_{i,J}}{\phi_i^T p} \right) \right\}.$$

Then

$$\sum_{i=1}^{M} \left[ I_{(o_i=1)} I_{Z_i=W_l} + I_{(o_i=0)} \alpha_{il} \right] = p_l \sum_{i=1}^{M} \left\{ I_{(o_i=1)} \left( \frac{I_{Z_i=W_J}}{p_J} \right) + I_{(o_i=0)} \left( \frac{\alpha_{iJ}}{p_J} \right) \right\}.$$

Straight-forward simplification shows that

$$M = \sum_{l=1}^{J} \sum_{i=1}^{M} \left[ I_{(o_i=1)} I_{Z_i=W_l} + I_{(o_i=0)} \alpha_{il} \right] = \sum_{i=1}^{M} \left\{ I_{(o_i=1)} \left( \frac{I_{Z_i=W_J}}{p_J} \right) + I_{(o_i=0)} \left( \frac{\alpha_{iJ}}{p_J} \right) \right\},$$

then we get that

$$p_l = \frac{1}{M} \sum_{i=1}^{M} \left[ I_{(o_i=1)} I_{Z_i=W_l} + I_{(o_i=0)} \alpha_{il} \right].$$

This shows that

$$p = \left( \frac{1}{M} \mathbf{1}^T \alpha(p) \right)^T,$$

and the proof is complete.

Making use of Lemma 1, we define

$$p^{(q+1)} = \left( \frac{1}{M} \mathbf{1}^T \alpha \left( p^{(q)} \right) \right)^T.$$

# Appendix 2: Proof of Lemma 6

For any $h \in H_p$. If we can show that $\phi_{\theta,h}$ is continuous at $\theta_0$, then we have, for arbitrary $\varepsilon > 0$, there is some $\delta = \delta(\varepsilon, \theta_0) > 0$ such that $\|\phi_{\theta,h} - \phi_{\theta_0,h}\| < \varepsilon$ whenever $\|\theta - \theta_0\| < \delta$. Hence, whenever $\|\theta - \theta_0\| < \delta$,

$$\left| E \left( \phi_{\theta,h} - \phi_{\theta_0,h} \right)^2 \right| \le E \left\| \phi_{\theta,h} - \phi_{\theta_0,h} \right\|^2 \le \varepsilon^2,$$

which means that $E\left(\phi_{\theta,h} - \phi_{\theta_0,h}\right)^2 \to 0$ as $\theta \to \theta_0$ for any $h \in H_p$. Thus,

$$\sup_{h \in H_p} E\left(\phi_{\theta,h} - \phi_{\theta_0,h}\right)^2 \to 0$$

as $\theta \to \theta_0$.

Now, we want to show that $\phi_{\theta,h}$ is continuous at $\theta_0$, for any $h \in H_p$. It is clearly that the following functions $\exp\left(Z_1^T \beta_k\right)$, $\exp\left(W_j^T \beta_k\right)$, $\exp\left(-\sum_{k=1}^2 \Lambda_k(X_1) \exp\left(W_j^T \beta_k\right)\right)$ and $pr\left(Z_1 = W_j | T_1 \geq X_1\right)$ are continuous and we know $\sum_{j=1}^J \exp\left(-\sum_{k=1}^2 \Lambda_k(X_1) \exp\left(W_j^T \beta_k\right)\right) p_j$ is bounded and bounded away from zero. Finally, we may see that $\int_0^{X_1} h(t) d\Lambda_k(t)$ is continuous at $\Lambda_{k0}$, since

$$\sup_{h \in BV[0,\tau]} \int_0^\tau |h(t)| d |\Lambda_k(t) - \Lambda_{k0}(t)| \leq c \int_0^\tau d |\Lambda_k(t) - \Lambda_{k0}(t)|,$$

we know $\|\Lambda_k - \Lambda_{k0}\|_V \to 0$, which means

$$\int_0^\tau d |\Lambda_k(t) - \Lambda_{k0}(t)| = \int_0^\tau \left|(\Lambda_k(t) - \Lambda_{k0}(t))'\right| dt \to 0.$$

This completes the proof.

## Appendix 3: $\Sigma$ is Positive Definite and Symmetric

(i) $\Sigma$ is positive definite.
(ii) $\Sigma$ is symmetric.

**Proof of (i)** Note that $\Sigma^{-1} = \left(\sigma_{12}^{-1}(e_1, 0, 0, 0), \sigma_{12}^{-1}(e_2, 0, 0, 0), \cdots, \sigma_{12}^{-1}\right.$ $(e_D, 0, 0, 0))$. Here we want to show $\Sigma^{-1}$ is positive definite. Let $h_{12} = (y_1, y_2, \cdots, y_D)^T$ be given. Consider

$$h_{12}^T \Sigma^{-1} h_{12}$$

$$= y_1 \sigma_{12}^{-1}(e_1, 0, 0, 0)_1 y_1 + y_2 \sigma_{12}^{-1}(e_1, 0, 0, 0)_2 y_1 + \cdots + y_D \sigma_{12}^{-1}(e_1, 0, 0, 0)_D y_1$$

$$+ y_1 \sigma_{12}^{-1}(e_2, 0, 0, 0)_1 y_2 + y_2 \sigma_{12}^{-1}(e_2, 0, 0, 0)_2 y_2 + \cdots + y_D \sigma_{12}^{-1}(e_2, 0, 0, 0)_D y_2$$

$$+ \cdots$$

$$+ y_1 \sigma_{12}^{-1}(e_D, 0, 0, 0)_1 y_D + y_2 \sigma_{12}^{-1}(e_D, 0, 0, 0)_2 y_D + \cdots + y_D \sigma_{12}^{-1}(e_D, 0, 0, 0)_D y_D$$

$$= y_1 \sigma_{12}^{-1} ((y_1, y_2, \cdots, y_D), 0, 0, 0)_1 + y_2 \sigma_{12}^{-1} ((y_1, y_2, \cdots, y_D), 0, 0, 0)_2$$

$$+ \cdots$$

$$+ y_D \sigma_{12}^{-1} ((y_1, y_2, \cdots, y_D), 0, 0, 0)_D$$

$$= h_{12}^T \sigma_{12}^{-1} (h_{12}, 0, 0, 0) > 0,$$

for $h_{12}$ nonzero. This completes the proof.

**Proof of (ii)** We want to show that $\Sigma^{-1}$ is symmetric. Fix $i$. Choose $h'$ such that Let $h'_1 = \sigma_1^{-1} (e_i, 0, 0, 0)$, $h'_2 = \sigma_2^{-1} (e_i, 0, 0, 0)$, $h'_3 = \sigma_3^{-1} (e_i, 0, 0, 0)$, $h'_4 = \sigma_4^{-1} (e_i, 0, 0, 0)$ and $h'_5 = \sigma_5^{-1} (e_i, 0, 0, 0)$. Choose $h$ such that $h_1 = \sigma_1^{-1} (e_k, 0, 0, 0)$, $h_2 = \sigma_2^{-1} (e_k, 0, 0, 0)$, $h_3 = \sigma_3^{-1} (e_k, 0, 0, 0)$, $h_4 = \sigma_4^{-1} (e_k, 0, 0, 0)$ and $h_5 = \sigma_5^{-1} (e_k, 0, 0, 0)$. It remains to check the following case from (8), we can obtain

$$\sigma_1 (h)^T h'_1 + \sigma_2 (h)^T h'_2 + \sigma_3 (h)^T h'_3$$

$$+ \int_0^\tau \sigma_4 (h) (t) h'_4 (t) \, d\Lambda_{10} (t) + \int_0^\tau \sigma_5 (h) (t) h'_5 (t) \, d\Lambda_{20} (t)$$

$$= e_k^T \sigma_{12}^{-1} (e_i, 0, 0, 0) .$$

$$\sigma_1 \left( h' \right)^T h_1 + \sigma_2 \left( h' \right)^T h_2 + \sigma_3 \left( h' \right)^T h_3$$

$$+ \int_0^\tau \sigma_4 \left( h' \right) (t) h_4 (t) \, d\Lambda_{10} (t) + \int_0^\tau \sigma_5 \left( h' \right) (t) h_5 (t) \, d\Lambda_{20} (t)$$

$$= e_i^T \sigma_{12}^{-1} (e_k, 0, 0, 0) .$$

Hence $e_k^T \sigma_{12}^{-1} (e_i, 0, 0, 0) = e_i^T \sigma_{12}^{-1} (e_k, 0, 0, 0)$. This completes the proof.

# Appendix 4: $\sqrt{M} \left( \widehat{\beta}_M - \beta_0 \right)$ Has Asymptotic Variance $\Sigma^{-1}$

$$var \left( \sqrt{M} \left( \widehat{\beta}_M - \beta_0 \right) \right)$$

$$= var \left( \Sigma^{-1} \sqrt{M} \left( P_M - P_0 \right) \tilde{l}_0 \right)$$

$$= \Sigma^{-1} var \left( \left( \sum_{i=1}^M \tilde{l}_0 (X_i, E_i, Z_i \cdot O_i, O_i) / \sqrt{M} \right) \right) \Sigma^{-1}$$

$$= \Sigma^{-1} var \left( \tilde{l}_0 \right) \Sigma^{-1}$$

$$= \Sigma^{-1} E \left( \tilde{l}_0 \tilde{l}_0^T \right) \Sigma^{-1} - \Sigma^{-1} \left\{ E \left( \tilde{l}_0 \right) E \left( \tilde{l}_0 \right)^T \right\} \Sigma^{-1}$$

$$= \Sigma^{-1}.$$

Because $E \left( \tilde{l}_0 \tilde{l}_0^T \right) = \Sigma$ and

$$e_i^T \Sigma^{-1} \left\{ E \left( \tilde{l}_0 \right) E \left( \tilde{l}_0 \right)^T \right\} \Sigma^{-1} e_k$$

$$= \left\{ e_i^T \Sigma^{-1} E \left( \tilde{l}_0 \right) \left( l_{3,\theta_0} [h_3] + l_{4,\theta_0} [h_4] + l_{5,\theta_0} [h_5] \right) \right\}$$

$$\times \left\{ \left( l_{3,\theta_0} [h_3] + l_{4,\theta_0} [h_4] + l_{5,\theta_0} [h_5] \right)^{-1} E \left( \tilde{l}_0 \right)^T \Sigma^{-1} e_k \right\}$$

$$= 0.$$

This completes the proof.


## Appendix 5: Two Results Due to V&W [22]

We quote two important results used in this paper.

**Theorem 3.3.1 of V&W [22]** Let $\Psi_n$ and $\Psi$ be random maps and a fixed map, respectively, from $\Theta$ into a Banach space such that

$$\sqrt{n} \left( \Psi_n - \Psi \right) \left( \widehat{\theta}_n \right) - \sqrt{n} \left( \Psi_n - \Psi \right) (\theta_0) = o_{p*} \left( 1 + \sqrt{n} \left\| \widehat{\theta}_n - \theta_0 \right\| \right),$$

and such that the sequence $\sqrt{n} \left( \Psi_n - \Psi \right) (\theta_0)$ converges in distribution to a tight random element $Z$. Let $\theta \rightarrow \Psi (\theta)$ be Fréchet differentiable at $\theta_0$ with a continuously invertible derivative $\dot{\Psi}_0$. If $\Psi (\theta_0) = 0$, $\widehat{\theta}_n$ satisfies $\Psi_n \left( \widehat{\theta}_n \right) = o_{p*} \left( n^{-1/2} \right)$, and converges in outer probability to $\theta_0$, then

$$\sqrt{n} \dot{\Psi}_{\theta_0} \left( \widehat{\theta}_n - \theta_0 \right) = -\sqrt{n} \left( \Psi_n - \Psi \right) (\theta_0) + o_{p*} (1).$$

Consequently, $\sqrt{n} \left( \widehat{\theta}_n - \theta_0 \right) \rightarrow -\dot{\Psi}_{\theta_0}^{-1} Z$.

In the case of independent and identically distributed observations, the theorem may be applied with $\Psi_n (\theta) h = P_n \phi_{\theta,h}$ and $\Psi (\theta) h = P \phi_{\theta,h}$ for given measurable functions $\phi_{\theta,h}$, indexed by $\Theta$ and arbitrary index set $H$. In this case, $\sqrt{n} \left( \Psi_n - \Psi \right) (\theta) = \left\{ G_n \phi_{\theta,h} : h \in H \right\}$ is the empirical process indexed by the classes of functions $\left\{ \phi_{\theta,h} : h \in H \right\}$.

**Lemma 3.3.5 of V&W [22]** Suppose that the class of functions

$$\left\{ \phi_{\theta,h} - \phi_{\theta_0,h} : \|\theta - \theta_0\| < \delta, h \in H \right\}$$

is P-Donsker for some $\delta > 0$ and

$$\sup_{h \in H} P \left( \phi_{\theta,h} - \phi_{\theta_0,h} \right)^2 \to 0$$

as $\theta \to \theta_0$.

If $\widehat{\theta}_n$ converges in outer probability to $\theta_0$, then

$$\left\| G_n \left( \phi_{\widehat{\theta}_n,h} - \phi_{\theta_0,h} \right) \right\|_H = o_{p*} \left( 1 + \sqrt{n} \left\| \widehat{\theta}_n - \theta_0 \right\| \right).$$

# Appendix 6: The Conditional Distribution of $Z$ Given $Y$

In modeling the conditional distribution of $Z$ given $Y$ when $Y$ is of discrete type, denote the stratified levels of $Y$ as $SY = (1, \cdots, S)$ and describe $Y$ by using dummy variable according to stratified levels.

Assume that there are $J_s$ distinct values among the observed covariates under $Y$-stratum $s$ and they are denoted by $\left( W_{s1}, W_{s2}, \cdots, W_{sJ_s} \right)$. Let $0 \le p_{sj} \le 1$ and $\sum_{j=1}^{J_s} p_{sj} = 1$ be given. Then the conditional distribution $f_e \left( Z | SY \right)$ is given by

$$f_e \left( Z | SY \right) = \prod_{s=1}^{S} \left[ \sum_{j=1}^{J_s} p_{sj} I_{Z=W_{sj}} \right]^{I_{(SY=s)}},$$

and the corresponding marginal survival function $G$ of $T$ is given by

$$G_e \left( t | SY \right) = \prod_{s=1}^{S} \left[ \sum_{j=1}^{J_s} \left( \exp \left( -\sum_{k=1}^{K} \Lambda_k \left( t \right) \exp \left( Y^T \eta_k + W_{sj}^T \beta_k \right) \right) \right) p_{sj} \right]^{I_{(SY=s)}}.$$

This approach to modeling the covariate distribution is also taken by Scheike and Juul [16]. The proposed NPMLE then applies with the conditional covariate distribution and the marginal survival function of $T$.

When $Y$ is of continuous type, we can apply kernel smoothing techniques to obtain the estimate for the conditional density of $Z$ given $Y$. But this is beyond the scope of this paper and deserves further research.

# References

1. Borgan, ø., & Keogh, R. H. (2015). Nested case-control: Should one break the matching? *Lifetime Data Analysis, 21*, 517–541.
2. Chang, I. S., Hsiung, C. A., Wang, M. C., & Wen, C. C. (2005). An asymptotic theory for the nonparametric maximum likelihood estimator in the Cox-gene model. *Bernoulli, 11*, 863–892.
3. Chang, I. S., Hsiung, C. A., Wen, C. C., Wu, Y. J., & Yang, C. C. (2007). Non-parametric maximum-likelihood estimation in a semiparametric mixture model for competing-risks data. *Scandinavian Journal of Statistics, 34*, 870–895.
4. Chen, H. Y. (2002). Double-semiparametric method for missing covariates in Cox regression models. *Journal of the American Statistical Association, 97*, 565–576.
5. Chen, K. N. (2001). Generalized case-cohort sampling. *Journal of the Royal Statistical Society: Series B, 63*, 791–809.
6. Fine, J. P., & Gray, R. J. (1999). A proportional hazards model for the subdistribution of a competing risk. *Journal of the American Statistical Association, 94*, 496–509.
7. Keogh, R. H., & White, I. R. (2013). Using full-cohort data in nested case–control and case–cohort studies by multiple imputation. *Statistics in Medicine, 32*, 4021–4043.
8. Kim, R. S. (2013). Lesser known facts about nested case-control designs. *Journal of Translational Medicine and Epidemiology, 1*, 1007.
9. Kulathinal, S., & Arjas, E. (2006). Bayesian inference from case-cohort data with multiple end-points. *Scandinavian Journal of Statistics, 33*, 25–36.
10. Lu, W., & Peng, L. (2008). Semiparametric analysis of mixture regression models with competing risks data. *Lifetime Data Analysis, 14*, 231–252.
11. Murphy, S. A., & van der Vaart, A. W. (1999). Observed information in semi-parametric models. *Bernoulli, 5*, 381–412.
12. Murphy, S. A., & van der Vaart, A. W. (2000). On profile likelihood. *Journal of the American Statistical Association, 95*, 449–465.
13. Prentice, R. L. (1986). A case-cohort design for epidemiologic cohort studies and disease prevention trials. *Biometrika, 73*, 1–11.
14. Saarela, O., Kulathinal, S., Arjas, E., & Läärä, E. (2008). Nested case-control data utilized for multiple outcomes: A likelihood approach and alternatives. *Statistics in Medicine, 27*, 5991–6008.
15. Samuelsen, S. O. (1997). A pseudolikelihood approach to analysis of nested case-control studies. *Biometrika, 84*, 379–394.
16. Scheike, T. H., & Juul, A. (2004). Maximum likelihood estimation for Cox's regression model under nested case-control sampling. *Biostatistics, 5*, 193–206.
17. Scheike, T. H., & Martinussen, T. (2004). Maximum likelihood estimation for Cox's regression model under case-cohorts sampling. *Scandinavian Journal of Statistics, 31*, 283–293.
18. Sørensen, P., & Andersen, P. K. (2000). Competing risks analysis of the case-cohort design. *Biometrika, 87*, 49–59.
19. Støer, N. C., & Samuelsen, S. O. (2012). Comparison of estimators in nested case-control studies with multiple outcomes. *Lifetime Data Analysis, 18*, 261–283.
20. Thomas, D. C. (1977). Addendum to "methods of cohort analysis: appraisal by application to asbestos mining," by F. D. K. Liddell, J. C. McDonald and D. C. Thomas. *Journal of the Royal Statistical Society. Series A, 140*, 483–485.
21. van der Vaart, A. W. (1998). *Asymptotic statistics*. Cambridge: Cambridge University Press.
22. van der Vaart, A. W., & Wellner, J. A. (1996). *Weak convergence and empirical processes with application to statistics*. New York: Springer.
23. Vigneri, P., Frasca, L., Sciacca, L., Pandini, G., & Vigneri, R. (2009). Diabetes and cancer. *Endocrine-Related Cancer, 16*, 1103–1123.

# Variable Selection in Partially Linear Proportional Hazards Model with Grouped Covariates and a Diverging Number of Parameters

**Arfan Raheen Afzal and Xuewen Lu**

**Abstract** In regression models with a grouping structure among the explanatory variables, variable selection at the group and within group individual variable level is desired to improve model accuracy and interpretability. In this article, we propose a hierarchical bi-level variable selection approach for censored survival data in the linear part of a partially linear proportional hazards model where the covariates are naturally grouped. The proposed method is capable of conducting simultaneous group selection and individual variable selection within selected groups. Computational algorithms are developed. Rate of convergence, selection consistency and asymptotic normality of the proposed estimators are established. Simulation studies indicate that the hierarchical regularized method outperforms several existing variable selection including LASSO, adaptive LASSO, and SCAD. Application of the proposed method is illustrated with the primary biliary cirrhosis (PBC) data.

**Keywords** Bi-level selection · B-spline · Group variable selection · Partially linear proportional hazards model · Selection consistency

## 1 Introduction

The proportional hazards model [7] has been widely used to study the relationship between multiple covariates and censored event times. The model assumes that the hazard function of a subject related to the covariates $X$ is given by

A. R. Afzal
Department of Mathematics and Statistics, University of Calgary, Calgary, AB, Canada

Tom Baker Cancer Centre, Alberta Health Services, Calgary, AB, Canada

X. Lu (✉)
Department of Mathematics and Statistics, University of Calgary, Calgary, AB, Canada
e-mail: lux@math.ucalgary.ca; xlu@ucalgary.ca

© Springer Nature Switzerland AG 2020    411
Y. Zhao, D.-G. (Din) Chen (eds.), *Statistical Modeling in Biomedical Research*, Emerging Topics in Statistics and Biostatistics,
https://doi.org/10.1007/978-3-030-33416-1_18

$$h(t|X) = h_0(t) \exp\left(\beta^\top X\right), \tag{1}$$

where $h_0(t)$ is an unspecified baseline hazard function, $\beta = (\beta_1, \ldots, \beta_p)^\top$ is the vector of regression coefficients, and $X = (X_1, \ldots, X_p)^\top$ is a $p$-dimensional covariate vector.

In practice, it is possible that not all covariates are linearly related to the hazard, i.e., some of them have a nonlinear effect on the hazard. Considering a purely parametric model is too stringent in this case, while a purely nonparametric model suffers from the so called "curse of dimensionality". Partially linear models (PLMs) in such cases combine the flexibility of nonparametric modeling with the parsimony and easy interpretability of parametric modeling, and avoid the curse of dimensionality of a purely nonparametric model [12, 36]. To incorporate the nonlinear effect of a covariate in a linear model, we consider a partially linear proportional hazards model (PL-PHM) in the same vein as that of Huang [20]. More specifically, we assume that the conditional hazard function is given by

$$h(t|W, X) = h_0(t) \exp\left\{\phi(W) + \beta^\top X\right\}, \tag{2}$$

where $\phi(W) = \sum_{m=1}^{q} \phi_m(W_m)$, $W = (W_1, \ldots, W_q)^\top$ is a $q$ dimensional covariate vector, $\phi_m(\cdot)$ $(m = 1, \ldots, q)$ are unknown possibly nonlinear smooth functions. This model contains both a nonparametric component $\phi(W)$ and a parametric component $\beta^\top X$. In reality, rarely all covariates are important in predicting the response, i.e., some components of $\beta$ are in fact zero. Efficient variable selection in such cases leads to parsimonious models with better prediction accuracy and easier interpretation.

In this paper, we investigate the variable selection problem in the linear part of the PL-PHM given in (2) when covariates in $X$ can be naturally grouped and the dimension of $W$ is fixed and low. The data and model settings are partly motivated by cancer prognosis studies reported in [33] and the variable selection method introduced by Ma and Du [32] in the partly linear accelerated failure time (AFT) model with diverging dimensions in $X$ for right censored data. In their studies, two distinct sets of covariates are measured. The first set $X$ represents high-dimensional genomic measurements such as microarray gene expression or SNPs. The second set $W$ represents low-dimensional clinical and environmental risk factors. For better interpretability and easier computation, the effect of $X$ is usually modeled in a parametric way and the effect of $W$ is modeled with more flexible additive nonparametric functions, since many biological processes are nonlinear. However, variable selection based on such model settings mainly focuses on individual variables such as that in [33]. In some applications, groups of measurements may be taken in the hopes of capturing unobservable latent variables or of measuring different aspects of complex entities [4]. Examples include measurements of gene expression, which can be grouped by gene pathways, and genetic markers, which can be grouped by the gene or haplotype (a set of genetic determinants located on a single chromosome) that they belong to. For example, as Wang et al. [44] explained, when analyzing microarray gene expression data, one can group genes into functionally similar sets as in The Gene Ontology Consortium (2000), or into known biological pathways such as the Kyoto encyclopedia of genes and genomes pathways [25]. In these settings, methods for individual variable selection may perform inefficiently by ignoring the information present in the grouping structure, while making use of the group information, as shown in Wang et al. [44] and [22], can help to identify both pathways and genes within the pathways related to the phenotypes, and hence improves understanding of biological processes.

Many variable selection methods originally proposed for uncensored data later have been extended to the survival models such as the PH model. Examples include LASSO [42], SCAD [14], adaptive LASSO [50], Elastic Net penalty [39], among others, where the focus is on individual variable selection. Since grouping structures are natural in many important practical problems, several authors recently tackled the problem of variable selection with grouped covariates in the PHM. Ma et al. [34] proposed supervised group LASSO in an attempt to select important genes and build predictive model in microarray gene expression data. Kim et al. [26] used group LASSO in gene data to combine clinical and genomic covariates effectively. In these group selection methods, covariates belonging to the same group are either selected or deleted from the model together. However, in gene expression data, a biological pathway can be related to a certain biological outcome although some genes in that pathway may not be related to the same biological outcome. A variable selection method, that can identify important pathways and important genes within important pathways simultaneously, is much more attractive in this case than selecting the entire group. Such a method is popularly known as a bi-level selection method and well studied with uncensored data [3, 4, 15, 23, 40]. Zhou and Zhu [53] proposed a hierarchically penalized method, which is a special case of the group bridge method [23] in the linear regression model. Later, Wang et al. [44] extended the hierarchical penalty to the PHM and established the oracle property of the estimators.

When linear models are extended to partially linear models (PLMs), variable selection in the linear part of a partially linear model has been extensively studied for uncensored data. Examples include [24, 29, 31, 35, 45–47, 51], among others. Relatively fewer works are seen on variable selection in the PL-PHM. Du et al. [11] performed variable selection in the linear part of a PL-PHM using SCAD and adaptive LASSO penalty where they approximated the nonparametric function using smoothing spline ANOVA. Hu and Lian [19] and Lian et al. [28] also performed variable selection applying SCAD penalty in diverging and ultra-high dimensional linear covariates in the PL-PHM, respectively. The latter two papers approximated the nonparametric functions using B-splines. However, all of these above researchers only considered individual variable selection in the linear part.

To the best of our knowledge, in the literature, group selection has not been considered for the partially linear survival models, particularly, for the PL-PHM. To bridge this gap, in this paper, we propose a bi-level variable selection method in the PL-PHM with a diverging number of covariates $X$, assuming a group structure in the linear part and a fixed and low dimensional $W$ for clinical and/or environmental covariates in the nonparametric part. We consider the number of zero coefficients in $X$ is diverging with the sample size. Typically, although the number of covariates collected is large, only a subset of covariates are important in predicting the event times. Therefore, we assume the numbers of non-zero coefficients and non-zero groups are fixed. Such an assumption is often reasonable with high dimensional data.

The remainder of the paper is organized as follows. In Sect. 2, we describe the group variable selection procedure for the PL-PHM. Asymptotic theories and further improvements are discussed in Sect. 3. Section 4 presents the numerical results. Concluding remarks are made in Sect. 5. All the technical proofs are contained in the Appendix.

## 2 Group Variable Selection in the PL-PHM

Suppose a random sample of $n$ subjects is observed. For the $i$-th subject, let $T_i^e$ and $T_i^c$ be the event time and the censoring time respectively, where the hazard function of $T_i^e$ is given by (2). Assume that $T_i^e$ and $T_i^c$ are independent given the covariates, and the censoring mechanism is noninformative. The true nonparametric functions and parameters will be denoted using a superscript 0. The i.i.d. observable random variables are $(T_i, \Delta_i, W_i, X_i)$ where $T_i = \min(T_i^e, T_i^c)$ and $\Delta_i = I[T_i^e \leq T_i^c]$, $I[A]$ is the indicator function of a set $A$, $W_i = \left(W_{i1}, \ldots, W_{iq}\right)^\top \in \mathbb{R}^q$, and $X_i = \left(X_{i1}, \ldots, X_{ip}\right)^\top \in \mathbb{R}^p$ are the covariates in the nonparametric and the parametric part, respectively. Define the at-risk processes $Y_i(t) = I[T_i \geq t]$ and the counting processes $N_i(t) = \Delta_i I[T_i \leq t]$. Note that, $\phi_m$ is identifiable only up to a constant and thus we assume $E\{\phi_m(W_m)\} = 0, m = 1, \ldots, q$.

Following similar strategy of Wang et al. [44], we assume that the $p$ variables in the linear part $X$ can be divided into $G$ groups. Let the $g$-th group have $p_g$ variables. We use $X_{i,(g)} = \left(X_{i,g1}, \ldots, X_{i,gp_g}\right)^\top$ to denote the $p_g$ variables in the $g$-th group for the $i$-th observation, $X_i = \left(X_{i,(1)}^\top, \ldots, X_{i,(G)}^\top\right)^\top$ to denote the total $p$ variables, and $\beta_{(g)} = \left(\beta_{g1}, \ldots, \beta_{gp_g}\right)^\top$ to represent the regression coefficients for the $g$-th group. We assume that the $G$ groups do not overlap, i.e., each variable belongs to only one group. Thus, the partially linear proportional hazards model (2) can be written as

$$
h(t|W, X) = h_0(t) \exp\left\{ \phi(W) + \sum_{g=1}^{G} \sum_{j=1}^{p_g} \beta_{gj} X_{gj} \right\}
$$

$$
= h_0(t) \exp\left\{ \phi(W) + \beta_{(1)}^\top X_{(1)} + \cdots + \beta_{(G)}^\top X_{(G)} \right\}. \tag{3}
$$

Consequently, the partial likelihood is written as

$$L_n(\phi, \beta) = \prod_{i \in D} \frac{\exp\left(\phi(W_i) + \sum_{g=1}^{G} \beta_{(g)}^\top X_{i,(g)}\right)}{\sum_{l \in R_i} \exp\left(\phi(W_l) + \sum_{g=1}^{G} \beta_{(g)}^\top X_{l,(g)}\right)}, \tag{4}$$

where $D$ is the set of indices of observed failures, $R_i$ is the set of indices of the subjects who are at risk at time $T_i$, and $\phi(W_i) = \phi_1(W_{i1}) + \cdots + \phi_q(W_{iq})$. The logarithm of model (4) in counting process notation can be written as

$$l_n(\phi, \beta) = \sum_{i=1}^{n} \Delta_i \left\{ \phi(W_i) + \sum_{g=1}^{G} \beta_{(g)}^\top X_{i,(g)} \right.$$

$$\left. - \log \sum_{l=1}^{n} Y_l(T_i) \exp\left(\phi(W_l) + \sum_{g=1}^{G} \beta_{(g)}^\top X_{l,(g)}\right) \right\}. \tag{5}$$

To estimate parameter $(\phi, \beta)$ in the model (3), since $\phi$ is an infinitely dimensional nonparametric function, we use the sieve method in maximizing the log-likelihood $l_n(\phi, \beta)$ with respect to $(\phi, \beta)$, and construct sieve space for $\phi$. To do that, we use polynomial splines to approximate the nonparametric components. Without loss of generality, we assume $W_m$ ($m = 1, \ldots, q$) have a common support $[0, 1]$. For each non-parametric component $\phi_m(W_m)$, assume $\tau_0 = 0 < \tau_1 < \cdots < \tau_{k'} < 1 = \tau_{k'+1}$ partition $[0, 1]$ into subintervals $[\tau_k, \tau_{k+1})$, $k = 0, \ldots, k'$, with $k'$ internal knots. A polynomial spline of order $r$ is a function whose restriction to each subinterval is a polynomial of degree $r - 1$ and globally $r - 2$ times continuously differentiable on $[0, 1]$. The collection of splines with a fixed sequence of knots has a normalized B-spline basis $\left\{ \tilde{B}_{m1}(x), \ldots, \tilde{B}_{m\tilde{k}}(x) \right\}$ with $\tilde{k} = k' + r$. As $\phi_m$ is identifiable only up to a constant, we put a centering constraint $E\{\phi_m(W_m)\} = 0$, and use the subspace of spline functions: $S_m^0 := \{S : S = \sum_{k=1}^{\tilde{k}-1} \alpha_{mk} B_{mk}(x), \sum_{i=1}^{n} S(W_{im}) = 0\}$ with basis $\left\{ B_{mk}(x) = \sqrt{K}(\tilde{B}_{mk}(x) - \sum_{i=1}^{n} \tilde{B}_{mk}(W_{im})/n), k = 1, \ldots, K = \tilde{k} - 1 \right\}$ (the subspace has a degree $= \tilde{k} - 1$ due to the normalization constraint $\sum_{k=1}^{\tilde{k}} \tilde{B}_{mk}(x) \equiv 1$). The multiplicative constant $\sqrt{K}$ is incorporated in the basis definition to simplify some expression later in the proofs, as done in [43]. Using spline expansions, we can model the nonparametric components by $\phi_m(x) = \sum_{k=1}^{K} \alpha_{mk} B_{mk}(x), 1 \leq m \leq q$. Therefore, the problem of estimating $\phi_m$ is now transformed to the problem of estimating the coefficients $\alpha_{(m)} = (\alpha_{m1}, \ldots, \alpha_{mK})^\top$.

Let $Z = \left(B_{11}(W_1), \ldots, B_{1K}(W_1), \ldots, B_{q1}(W_q), \ldots, B_{qK}(W_q)\right)^\top$ denote the $q \times K$ basis functions and $\alpha = (\alpha_{11}, \ldots, \alpha_{1K}, \ldots, \alpha_{q1}, \ldots, \alpha_{qK})^\top$ denote the corresponding coefficients. Since the $m$-th nonparametric component can be approximated by $\sum_{k=1}^{K} \alpha_{mk} B_{mk}(x)$ ($m = 1, \ldots, q$), it is reasonable to assume that

$B_{m1}(x), \ldots, B_{mK}(x)$ are $K$ variables belonging to one group. Therefore, the $q \times K$ variables in $Z$ can be divided into $q$ groups, where each of the $m$-th group has $K$ variables. We use $Z_{i,(m)} = \left(B_{i,m1}, \ldots, B_{i,mK}\right)^\top$ $(m = 1, \ldots, q; \ k = 1, \ldots, K)$ to denote the $K$ basis functions in the $m$-th group for the $i$-th observation. Similarly, we use $Z_i = \left(Z_{i,(1)}^\top, \ldots, Z_{i,(q)}^\top\right)^\top$ to denote the total $q \times K$ variables for the $i$-th observation, and $\alpha_{(m)} = (\alpha_{m1}, \ldots, \alpha_{mK})^\top$ to represent the regression coefficients for the $m$-th group. We assume that the number of variables in each group is $K$, i.e., we consider the same number of basis functions to approximate each nonparametric function. To simplify computation, since we have assumed $W_m$ $(m = 1, \ldots, q)$ have the same support $[0,1]$, we can assume $B_{mk}(x) = B_{m'k}(x)$ for $m \neq m'$, $1 \leq m, m' \leq q$, $1 \leq k \leq K$.

The partial likelihood in (5) is then equivalent to

$$
l_n(\alpha, \beta) = \sum_{i=1}^n \Delta_i \left[ \sum_{m=1}^q \alpha_{(m)}^\top Z_{i,(m)} + \sum_{g=1}^G \beta_{(g)}^\top X_{i,(g)} \right.
$$

$$
\left. - \log \sum_{l=1}^n \left\{ Y_l(T_i) \exp\left( \sum_{m=1}^q \alpha_{(m)}^\top Z_{l,(m)} + \sum_{g=1}^G \beta_{(g)}^\top X_{l,(g)} \right) \right\} \right]. \quad (6)
$$

To conduct variable selection in the PL-PHM, Hu and Lian [19] and Lian et al. [28] considered individual variable selection in the linear part by maximizing the penalized log partial likelihood objective function for estimating both $\alpha$ and $\beta$ defined in the following:

$$
pl_n(\alpha, \beta) = \frac{1}{n} l_n(\alpha, \beta) - \sum_{g=1}^G \sum_{j=1}^{p_g} p_{\lambda_n}(\beta_{gj}),
$$

where $p_{\lambda_n}(\beta_{gj})$ is a penalty function. Let $(\hat{\alpha}, \hat{\beta})$ be the maximizer of the above penalized partial likelihood, then, the penalized estimators of $\phi_m$ $(m = 1, \ldots, q)$ and $\beta$ are $\hat{\phi}_m = \sum_{k=1}^K \hat{\alpha}_{mk} B_{mk}$ and $\hat{\beta}$, respectively. In this paper, our focus is on group selection, and the above individual variable selection is a special case of the following group selection problem.

To conduct group selection, we introduce notations similar to those in Wang et al.'s [44] procedure. We reparameterize $\beta_{gj}$ as

$$
\beta_{gj} = \gamma_g \theta_{gj} \ (g = 1, \ldots, G; \ j = 1, \ldots, p_g),
$$

where $\gamma_g \geq 0$ for identifiability. This decomposition indicates that all $\beta_{gj}$ $(j = 1, \ldots, p_g)$ belong to the $g$-th group as it treats $\beta_{gj}$ hierarchically. For each $g$, parameter $\gamma_g$ explains $\beta_{gj}$ $(j = 1, \ldots, p_g)$ at the group level and $\theta_{gj}$'s explain differences among individuals within the $g$-th group. Let $\theta_{(g)} = (\theta_{g1}, \ldots, \theta_{gp_g})^\top$, then $\beta_{(g)} = \gamma_g \theta_{(g)}$. The partial likelihood function thus can be written as

$$L_n(\alpha, \gamma, \theta) = \prod_{i \in D} \frac{\exp(\sum_{m=1}^q \alpha_{(m)}^\top Z_{i,(m)} + \sum_{g=1}^G \gamma_g \theta_{(g)}^\top X_{i,(g)})}{\sum_{l \in R_i} \exp(\sum_{m=1}^q \alpha_{(m)}^\top Z_{l,(m)} + \sum_{g=1}^G \gamma_g \theta_{(g)}^\top X_{l,(g)})}.$$

where $\gamma = (\gamma_1, \ldots, \gamma_G)^\top$ and $\theta = (\theta_{11}, \ldots, \theta_{1p_1}, \ldots, \theta_{G1}, \ldots, \theta_{Gp_G})^\top$. Let $l_n(\alpha, \gamma, \theta)$ denote $\log\{L_n(\alpha, \gamma, \theta)\}$. For group selection in the linear part, we consider maximizing the penalized log partial likelihood given by

$$\max_{\alpha_{(m)}, \gamma_g, \theta_{gj}} \left\{ \frac{1}{n} l_n(\alpha, \gamma, \theta) - \lambda_\gamma \sum_{g=1}^G \gamma_g - \lambda_\theta \sum_{g=1}^G \sum_{j=1}^{p_g} |\theta_{gj}| \right\}, \tag{7}$$

subject to $\gamma_g \geq 0$ ($g = 1, \ldots, G$), where $\lambda_\gamma \geq 0$ and $\lambda_\theta \geq 0$ are two tuning parameters, which control the sparsity of the estimation at the group level and within group level, respectively. Similar to the result in [44] for the linear PHM, for fixed $(\alpha, \beta)$ and given values of $\lambda_\gamma$ and $\lambda_\theta$, we obtain that the maximizer of (7) with respect to $(\gamma, \theta)$, where $l_n(\alpha, \gamma, \theta)$ is constant, is unique. To simply computation and theoretical developments, we combine $\lambda_\gamma$ and $\lambda_\theta$ into one tuning parameter $\lambda = \lambda_\gamma \lambda_\theta$ such that (7) is equivalent to

$$\max_{\alpha_{(m)}, \gamma_g, \theta_{gj}} \left\{ \frac{1}{n} l_n(\alpha, \gamma, \theta) - \sum_{g=1}^G \gamma_g - \lambda \sum_{g=1}^G \sum_{j=1}^{p_g} |\theta_{gj}| \right\}, \tag{8}$$

subject to $\gamma_g \geq 0$ ($g = 1, \ldots, G$). Lemma 1 illustrates the meaning of the equivalence.

**Lemma 1** *Let $(\hat{\alpha}^*, \hat{\gamma}^*, \hat{\theta}^*)$ be a local maximizer of (7). Then there exists a local maximizer $(\hat{\alpha}^\dagger, \hat{\gamma}^\dagger, \hat{\theta}^\dagger)$ of (8) such that $\hat{\alpha}^* = \hat{\alpha}^\dagger$ and $\hat{\gamma}_g^* \hat{\theta}_{gj}^* = \hat{\gamma}_g^\dagger \hat{\theta}_{gj}^\dagger$. Similarly, if $(\hat{\alpha}^\dagger, \hat{\gamma}^\dagger, \hat{\theta}^\dagger)$ is a local maximizer of (8), then there exists a local maximizer $(\hat{\alpha}^*, \hat{\gamma}^*, \hat{\theta}^*)$ of (7) such that $\hat{\alpha}^* = \hat{\alpha}^\dagger$ and $\hat{\gamma}_g^* \hat{\theta}_{gj}^* = \hat{\gamma}_g^\dagger \hat{\theta}_{gj}^\dagger$.*

This lemma indicates that the final fitted models from (7) and (8) are the same, although they may provide different $\gamma_g$ and $\theta_{gj}$. This also implies that in practice, we only need to tune one parameter $\lambda = \lambda_\gamma \lambda_\theta$ as in (8), instead of tuning two parameters $\lambda_\gamma$ and $\lambda_\theta$ in (7) separately. Actually, as we can see in the proof, $\lambda_\gamma$ is absorbed into $\hat{\gamma}^\dagger$ and $\hat{\theta}^\dagger$, only $\lambda$ appears in (8). Both Wang et al. [44] and Zhou and Zhu [53] proved similar results. Furthermore, criterion (8) can be written into an equivalent form using the regression coefficients $\alpha$ and $\beta$.

**Lemma 2** *If* $(\hat{\alpha}, \hat{\gamma}, \hat{\theta})$ *is a local maximizer of (8), then* $(\hat{\alpha}, \hat{\beta})$, *where* $\hat{\beta}_{gj} = \hat{\gamma}_g \hat{\theta}_{gj}$, *is a local maximizer of*

$$
\max_{\alpha_{(m)}, \beta_{gj}} \left\{ \frac{1}{n} l_n(\alpha, \beta) - 2\lambda^{1/2} \sum_{g=1}^{G} \left( \sum_{j=1}^{p_g} |\beta_{gj}| \right)^{1/2} \right\}. \tag{9}
$$

*On the other hand, if* $(\hat{\alpha}, \hat{\beta})$ *is a local maximizer of (9), then* $(\hat{\alpha}, \hat{\gamma}, \hat{\theta})$ *is a local maximizer of (8), where* $\hat{\gamma}_g = (\lambda \sum_{j=1}^{p_g} |\hat{\beta}_{gj}|)^{1/2}$ *and* $\hat{\theta}_{gj} = \hat{\beta}_{gj} / \hat{\gamma}_g$ *if* $\hat{\gamma}_g \neq 0$ *and zero otherwise.*

The numerical computation is based on (8) while the proof of asymptotic properties is based on (9). Instead of using $L_2$-norm which performs group LASSO [48], we used $L_1$-norm to the within group coefficients in (9). In addition, the group coefficients are penalized by a bridge-type penalty [16], i.e., $L_{1/2}$-norm. So, the hierarchical penalty can remove unimportant groups and some unimportant variables in the important groups.

To estimate $\alpha$, $\gamma$ and $\theta$ in (8), we use an iterative algorithm. First, we fix $\gamma$ and estimate $(\alpha, \theta)$; then fixing $\theta$, we estimate $(\alpha, \gamma)$. We iterate between these steps until convergence is achieved. Precisely, the algorithm is written as

**Step 0** Center and normalize $X_{gj}$, and obtain an initial value $\gamma_g^{(0)}$ for each $\gamma_g$; for example, $\gamma_g^{(0)} = 1$. Let $s = 1$.

**Step 1** At the $s$-th iteration, let $\tilde{X}_{i,gj} = \gamma_g^{(s-1)} X_{i,gj}$ $(g = 1, \ldots, G; \ j = 1, \ldots, p_g)$ and obtain estimate $(\alpha^{(s)}, \theta^{(s)})$ by

$$
(\alpha^{(s)}, \theta^{(s)}) = \arg\max_{\alpha_{sk}, \theta_{gj}} \frac{1}{n} \log \left\{ \prod_{i \in D} \frac{\exp(\sum_{m=1}^{q} \sum_{k=1}^{K} \alpha_{mk} Z_{i,mk} + \sum_{g=1}^{G} \sum_{j=1}^{p_g} \theta_{gj} \tilde{X}_{i,gj})}{\sum_{l \in R_i} \exp(\sum_{m=1}^{q} \sum_{k=1}^{K} \alpha_{mk} Z_{l,mk} + \sum_{g=1}^{G} \sum_{j=1}^{p_g} \theta_{gj} \tilde{X}_{l,gj})} \right\}
$$
$$
- \lambda \sum_{g=1}^{G} \sum_{j=1}^{p_g} |\theta_{gj}|.
$$

**Step 2** Let $\tilde{X}_{i,g} = \sum_{j=1}^{p_g} \theta_{gj}^{(s)} X_{i,gj}$ $(g = 1, \ldots, G)$ and obtain estimate $(\alpha^{(s)}, \gamma^{(s)})$ by

$$
(\alpha^{(s)}, \gamma^{(s)}) = \arg\max_{\alpha_{sk}, \gamma_g \geq 0} \frac{1}{n} \log \left\{ \prod_{i \in D} \frac{\exp(\sum_{m=1}^{q} \sum_{k=1}^{K} \alpha_{mk} Z_{i,mk} + \sum_{g=1}^{G} \gamma_g \tilde{X}_{i,gj})}{\sum_{l \in R_i} \exp(\sum_{m=1}^{q} \sum_{k=1}^{K} \alpha_{mk} Z_{l,mk} + \sum_{g=1}^{G} \gamma_g \tilde{X}_{l,gj})} \right\} - \sum_{g=1}^{G} \gamma_g
$$

In this step, $\alpha^{(s)}$ is updated from $\alpha^{(s)}$ in step 1.

**Step 3** Repeat Steps 1 and 2 until $\alpha^{(s)}$, $\gamma^{(s)}$, and $\theta^{(s)}$ converge at the $m^*$-th iteration. Let $\hat{\alpha} = \alpha^{(m^*)}$ and $\hat{\beta}_{(g)} = \gamma_g^{(m^*)} \theta_{(g)}^{(m^*)}$ be the final solutions.

Since at each step, the value of objective function (8) is non-decreasing, this algorithm always converges. Step 1 is a LASSO-type problem without penalizing $\alpha$, and the algorithms proposed in [14, 18, 50] or [37] can be used to solve for $\theta$. Step 2 is a nonnegative garrote algorithm without penalizing $\alpha$, and we can use Fan and Li [14] or Yuan and Lin's [49] algorithm to solve for $\gamma$.

# 3 Asymptotic Theory

## 3.1 A General Theorem

For theoretical analysis, we will consider the counting process representation of the partial likelihood. We denote the true risk score by $m^0(W, X) = \phi^0(W) + \beta^{0\top} X$ where $\phi^0(W) = \phi_1^0(W_1) + \cdots + \phi_q^0(W_q)$. Let $R^\top = (W^\top, X^\top)$ be all the covariates and $g, h$ be any functions of $R$ ($h$ can be vector valued). We define

$$S_n^{(0)}(g, t) = n^{-1} \sum_{i=1}^n Y_i(t) \exp[g(R_i)],$$

$$S_n^{(1)}(g, t)[h] = n^{-1} \sum_{i=1}^n Y_i(t) h(R_i) \exp[g(R_i)],$$

$$S_n^{(2)}(g, t)[h] = n^{-1} \sum_{i=1}^n Y_i(t) h(R_i)^{\otimes 2} \exp[g(R_i)],$$

$$G_n(g, t)[h] = S_n^{(1)}(g, t)[h] / S_n^{(0)}(g, t),$$

$$V_n(g, t)[h] = S_n^{(2)}(g, t)[h] / S_n^{(0)}(g, t) - G_n(g, t)[h] G_n^\top(g, t)[h],$$

where for any vector $\xi$, $\xi^{\otimes 2}$ simply means $\xi \xi^\top$. Let $s^{(0)}(g, t) = E(S_n^{(0)}(g, t))$, $s^{(j)}(g, t)[h] = E(S_n^{(j)}(g, t)[h])$, $j = 1, 2$, $G(g, t)[h] = s^{(1)}(g, t)[h] / s^{(0)}(g, t)$, $V(g, t)[h] = s^{(2)}(g, t)[h] / s^{(0)}(g, t) - G(g, t)[h] G^\top(g, t)[h]$. Also, let $P_n$ be the empirical measure of $(T_i, \Delta_i, R_i)$, $1 \leq i \leq n$ and let $P$ be the probability measure of $(T, \Delta, R)$. Let $P_{\Delta n}$ be the empirical subprobability measure of $(T_i, \Delta_i = 1, R_i)$, $1 \leq i \leq n$ and let $P_\Delta$ be one subprobability measure of $(T, \Delta = 1, R)$. It is convenient to use linear functional notation, for example, $P_{\Delta n} f = \int f d P_{\Delta n} = \int \Delta f d P_n = n^{-1} \sum_i \Delta_i f(T_i, \Delta_i, R_i)$ for any $f$ such that this integral is well defined. Let $\|a\|$ denotes the $L_2$ norm of a column vector $a$. The log partial likelihood can be rewritten as

$$l_n(\alpha, \beta) = \sum_{i=1}^n \int_0^\tau \left\{ \omega^\top L_i - \log(S_n^{(0)}(g, t)) \right\} dN_i(t),$$

where $\omega = (\alpha^{\top}, \beta^{\top})^{\top}$, $L_i = L(R_i) = (Z_i^{\top}, X_i^{\top})^{\top}$ is a vector-valued function of $R_i^{\top} = (W_i^{\top}, X_i^{\top})$ and $g$ is a function of $R$ defined by $g(R) = \sum_{m=1}^{q} \alpha_m^{\top} B_m(W_m) + \beta^{\top} X$, which contains $(\alpha, \beta)$, and $Z_m(W_m) = B_m(W_m) = (B_{m1}(W_m), \ldots, B_{mK}(W_m))^{\top}$. We only consider events over a finite interval $[0, \tau]$. The score function and the observed information are given by

$$U_n(\alpha, \beta) = \sum_{i=1}^{n} \int_0^{\tau} \{L_i - G_n(g, t)[L]\} \, dN_i(t),$$

and

$$\Sigma_n(\alpha, \beta) = \sum_{i=1}^{n} \int_0^{\tau} V_n(g, t)[L] dN_i(t),$$

respectively. We first consider the penalized log partial likelihood function with a general penalty function. Let the objective function be

$$Q_n(\alpha, \beta) = \frac{1}{n} l_n(\alpha, \beta) - \sum_{g=1}^{G} p_{\lambda_n}^{(g)}(|\beta_{(g)}|), \tag{10}$$

where $p_{\lambda_n}^{(g)}(|\beta_{(g)}|) = p_{\lambda_n}^{(g)}(|\beta_{g1}|, \ldots, |\beta_{gp_g}|)$ is a general $p_g$-variate penalty function for the linear parameters in the $g$-th group. The penalty functions $p_{\lambda_n}^{(g)}(\cdot)$ ($g = 1, \ldots, G$) in (10) vary between groups and depend on the tuning parameter $\lambda_n$ that varies with $n$. We write the true parameter vector in the sparse linear part as $\beta^0 = (\beta_{\mathcal{A}}^{0\top}, \beta_{\mathcal{B}}^{0\top}, \beta_{\mathcal{C}}^{0\top})^{\top}$, where $\mathcal{A} = \left\{(g, j) : \beta_{gj}^0 \neq 0\right\}$, $\mathcal{B} = \left\{(g, j) : \beta_{gj}^0 = 0, \beta_{(g)}^0 \neq 0\right\}$, and $\mathcal{C} = \left\{(g, j) : \beta_{(g)}^0 = 0\right\}$. Here $\mathcal{A}$, $\mathcal{B}$, $\mathcal{C}$ contain the indices of nonzero coefficients, indices of zero coefficients that belong to nonzero groups, and indices of zero coefficients that belong to zero groups, respectively. Thus, $\mathcal{A}$, $\mathcal{B}$ and $\mathcal{C}$ are disjoint and partition the set of all indices of coefficients. We write $\mathcal{D} = \mathcal{B} \cup \mathcal{C}$, which contains the indices of all zero coefficients. Let

$$a_n = \max_{(g,j)} \left\{ \frac{\partial p_{\lambda_n}^{(g)}(|\beta_{g1}^0|, \ldots, |\beta_{gp_g}^0|)}{\partial |\beta_{gj}|} : \beta_{gj}^0 \neq 0 \right\},$$

$$b_n = \max_{(g,j)} \left\{ \frac{\partial^2 p_{\lambda_n}^{(g)}(|\beta_{g1}^0|, \ldots, |\beta_{gp_g}^0|)}{\partial |\beta_{gj}|^2} : \beta_{gj}^0 \neq 0 \right\}.$$

Lastly, let $s$ be the number of nonzero groups. Without loss of generality, we assume that $\beta^0_{(g)} \neq 0$ $(g = 1, \ldots, s)$ and $\beta^0_{(g)} = 0$ $(g = s+1, \ldots, G)$. Let $s_g$ be the number of nonzero coefficients in group $g$ $(g = 1, \ldots, s)$. Again, without loss of generality, we assume that $\beta^0_{gj} \neq 0$ $(g = 1, \ldots, s; \ j = 1, \ldots, s_g)$ and $\beta^0_{gj} = 0$ $(g = 1, \ldots, s; \ j = s_g + 1, \ldots, p_g)$.

The following technical conditions are used in the study of asymptotic properties:

(B1) The covariate vector $R^\top = (W^\top, X^\top)$ has a bounded support: without loss of generality, the support of $W$ is assumed to be $[0, 1]^q$, with the marginal density of each covariate in $W$ being continuous and bounded away from zero and infinity, and the covariate vector $X$ is also bounded.

(B2) (i) Only observations with event or censored event times in a finite interval $[0, \tau]$ are used in the partial likelihood. At this point $\tau$, the baseline cumulative hazard function $\Lambda_0(\tau) \equiv \int_0^\tau \lambda_0(s)ds < \infty$. (ii) $\Pr(\Delta = 1|R)$ and $\Pr(T^c > \tau|R)$ are both bounded away from zero with probability one.

(B3) Let $\mathcal{H}_d$ be the collection of all functions on support $[0, 1]$ whose $a$-th order derivative satisfying the Hölder condition of order $r$ with $d \equiv a + r$. That is, for each $h \in \mathcal{H}_d$, there exists a constant $M_0 \in (0, \infty)$ such that $\left| h^{(a)}(s) - h^{(a)}(t) \right| \leq M_0|s-t|^r$, for any $s, t \in [0, 1]$. Assume $\varphi^0_m \in \mathcal{H}_d$ $(m = 1, \ldots, q)$, for some $d > 1/2$. The order of the spline satisfies $r > d + 1/2$.

(B4) For $L = L(R) = (Z^\top, X^\top)^\top$, $E \left\{ \sup_{t \in [0, \tau]} Y(t) \|L\|^2 \exp \left( \omega^\top L \right) \right\} = O(K + p)$.

(B5) Let $\Sigma = \int_0^\tau V(m^0, t)[L]s^{(0)}(m^0, t)\lambda_0(t)dt$, where $m^0 = m^0(W, X)$. The eigenvalues of $\Sigma$ are positive and bounded below $O(K^{-1})$.

(B6) The $p_g$-variate penalty function for parameters in the $g$-th group satisfies the following two conditions:

$$p^{(g)}_{\lambda_n}(|\beta_{(g)}|) \geq 0 \quad (\beta_{(g)} \in \mathbb{R}^{p_g}), \quad p^{(g)}_{\lambda_n}(0) = 0; \tag{11}$$

$$p^{(g)}_{\lambda_n}(|\beta_{(g)}|) \geq p^{(g)}_{\lambda_n}(|\beta^*_{(g)}|) \quad (|\beta_{gj}| \geq |\beta^*_{gj}|; \ j = 1, \ldots, p_g). \tag{12}$$

Similar conditions to those listed above have been considered in the literature [19, 44] and are quite reasonable. Condition (B1) places the boundedness condition on the covariates. It is unpleasant, but not too restrictive because in many practical situations continuous covariates may be typically rescaled to fall between 0 and 1. (B2)(i) avoids the unboundedness of the loss function and pseudo-score functions at the end point of the support of the observed event time. (B2)(ii) ensures that the probability of being right censored at $\tau$ and the probability of being observed events are positive and bounded away from zero regardless of the covariate values. (B3) ensures the uniform continuity of the functions. A condition similar to (B4) was considered by Bradic et al. [2] for diverging number of parameters. The positive-definiteness of $\Sigma$ and boundedness of its eigenvalues in (B5) is a reasonable assumption by the following discussion. The term $LL^\top$ appears in the definition of $D$. We see that

$$LL^\top = \begin{pmatrix} Z \\ X \end{pmatrix} (Z^\top, X^\top) = \begin{pmatrix} ZZ^\top & ZX^\top \\ XZ^\top & XX^\top \end{pmatrix}.$$

Under mild assumptions, Huang et al.'s [21] Lemma 3 showed that the eigenvalues of $E(ZZ^\top)$ are bounded below and upper from a positive value proportional to $K^{-1}$, we can expect that the eigenvalues of $E(LL^\top)$ are bounded below from a positive value proportional to $K^{-1}$ as well if the eigenvalues of $E(XX^\top)$ are bounded below away from zero, and $Z$ and $X$ are linearly independent. Wang et al. [44] used the condition (B6) for hierarchical group variable selection in the PHM. Under these conditions, to emphasize the dependence on $n$, in the sequel, we denote $K_n \equiv K$ and $p_n \equiv p$, we have the following theoretical results.

**Theorem 1** *Let* $\gamma_n = \sqrt{(K_n + p_n)/n} + K_n^{-d}$. *Under the regularity conditions (B1)–(B6), assume that* $q, s$ *and* $s_g$ *is fixed,* $K_n \to \infty$, $p_n \to \infty$, $(K_n + p_n)/n \to 0$, $\gamma_n (K_n + p_n)^{3/2} = O(1)$, $a_n = O_p(\gamma_n)$ *and* $b_n \to 0$, *as* $n \to \infty$, *then there exists a local maximizer* $(\hat{\alpha}^\top, \hat{\beta}^\top)^\top$ *in (10) and* $\hat{\phi}_m = \sum_{k=1}^{K_n} \hat{\alpha}_{mk} B_{mk}$, $\hat{\phi}(w) = \sum_{m=1}^{q} \hat{\phi}_m(w_m)$ *such that* $\left\| \hat{\phi} - \phi^0 \right\| + \left\| \hat{\beta} - \beta^0 \right\| = O_p \left( \sqrt{(K_n + p_n)/n} + K_n^{-d} \right)$.

**Theorem 2** *Let* $\gamma_n = \sqrt{(K_n + p_n)/n} + K_n^{-d}$ *and* $(\hat{\alpha}^\top, \hat{\beta}_A^\top, \hat{\beta}_B^\top, \hat{\beta}_C^\top)^\top$ *be the local maximizer of* $Q_n(\alpha, \beta)$ *in (10). For* $(g, j) \in \mathcal{D}$, *i.e.,* $\beta_{gj}^0 = 0$, *under the same conditions as in Theorem 1, if* $\gamma_n^{-1} \partial p_{\lambda_n}^{(g)}(|\hat{\beta}_{g1}|, \ldots, |\hat{\beta}_{gp_g}|)/\partial |\beta_{gj}| \to \infty$ *as* $n \to \infty$, *then we have* $\hat{\beta}_{gj} = 0$ *with probability approaching 1.*

In the following section, we show how to construct penalty functions $p_{\lambda_n}^{(g)}$ such that the conditions in Theorem 2 are satisfied.

## 3.2 Adaptive Hierarchical Penalty

The results in Theorems 1 and 2 are obtained for a general penalty. Following [44], here we will show the asymptotic results hold for the hierarchically penalized PL-PHM based on criterion (9). If we write $\lambda_n = 2\lambda^{1/2}$ in (9), then based on Theorems 1 and 2 we have

**Corollary 1** *Let* $\gamma_n = \sqrt{(K_n + p_n)/n} + K_n^{-d}$. *If* $\lambda_n = O_p(\gamma_n)$, *then there exists a local maximizer* $(\hat{\alpha}^\top, \hat{\beta}^\top)^\top = (\hat{\alpha}^\top, \hat{\beta}_A^\top, \hat{\beta}_B^\top, \hat{\beta}_C^\top)^\top$ *for the hierarchically penalized PL-PHM in (9) such that* $\left\| \hat{\phi} - \phi^0 \right\| + \left\| \hat{\beta} - \beta^0 \right\| = O_p(\gamma_n)$; *if further* $p_n^{-1/2} \gamma_n^{-3/2} \lambda_n \to \infty$ *as* $n \to \infty$, *then* $\hat{\beta}_C = 0$ *with probability tending to 1.*

Comparing Corollary 1 with Theorem 2, we see that although the hierarchical penalty can effectively remove unimportant groups because $\hat{\beta}_{\mathcal{C}} = 0$ with probability approaching to 1, it cannot effectively remove unimportant variables within the important groups as $\hat{\beta}_{\mathcal{D}} = 0$ with probability tending to 1 may not hold. To understand this intuitively, as Zou [54] showed, the Lasso procedure does not in general have the oracle properties (selection consistency), while adaptive Lasso is an oracle procedure. In the hierarchical penalty method, we applied the bridge penalty to $L_1$ norm, it inherits the property of Lasso, which in general does not have selection consistency at the individual level. To tackle this limitation, we apply the adaptive idea used in [5, 30, 38, 44, 50, 52, 54, 55], and others, which is to penalize different coefficients differently. To do so, we maximize the following objective function

$$Q_n^w(\alpha, \beta) = \frac{1}{n} l_n(\alpha, \beta) - \lambda_n \sum_{g=1}^{G} \left\{ \sum_{j=1}^{p_g} w_{n,gj} |\beta_{gj}| \right\}^{1/2}, \tag{13}$$

where $w_{n,gj}$'s are pre-specified non-negative weights. The next theorem shows that, by controlling weights properly, the adaptive hierarchically penalized PL-PHM has the selection consistency as stated in Theorem 2.

**Theorem 3** *Let us define*

$$w_{n,\max}^{\mathcal{A}} = \max\left\{ w_{n,gj} : (g, j) \in \mathcal{A} \right\}, \quad w_{n,\min}^{\mathcal{A}} = \min\left\{ w_{n,gj} : (g, j) \in \mathcal{A} \right\};$$

$$w_{n,\max}^{\mathcal{D}} = \max\left\{ w_{n,gj} : (g, j) \in \mathcal{D} \right\}, \quad w_{n,\min}^{\mathcal{D}} = \min\left\{ w_{n,gj} : (g, j) \in \mathcal{D} \right\}.$$

*Let $\gamma_n = \sqrt{(K_n + p_n)/n} + K_n^{-d}$. Under the same conditions as assumed in Theorem 1, if $\gamma_n^{-1} \lambda_n w_{n,\max}^{\mathcal{A}} \left( w_{n,\min}^{\mathcal{A}} \right)^{-1/2} \to 0$, $\lambda_n \left( w_{n,\max}^{\mathcal{A}} \right)^2 \left( w_{n,\min}^{\mathcal{A}} \right)^{-3/2} \to 0$, and $\gamma_n^{-1} \lambda_n w_{n,\min}^{\mathcal{D}} / (w_{n,\max}^{\mathcal{A}} + w_{n,\max}^{\mathcal{D}})^{1/2} \to \infty$ as $n \to \infty$, there exists a local maximizer $(\hat{\alpha}^\top, (\hat{\beta}_{\mathcal{A}}^\top, \hat{\beta}_{\mathcal{D}}^\top))^\top$ in (13) such that $\left\| \hat{\phi} - \phi^0 \right\| + \left\| \hat{\beta} - \beta^0 \right\| = O_p(\gamma_n)$ and $\hat{\beta}_{\mathcal{D}} = 0$ with probability tending to 1.*

Finally, we specify the tuning parameter $\lambda_n$ and the weights $w_{n,gj}$ that satisfy conditions in Theorem 3, which are given by the following corollary.

**Corollary 2** *Let $\gamma_n = \sqrt{(K_n + p_n)/n} + K_n^{-d}$ and $\tilde{\beta}_n$ be an estimator such that, $\left\| \tilde{\beta}_n - \beta^0 \right\| = O_p(\gamma_n)$. If $\lambda_n = \gamma_n / \log(n)$ and $w_{n,gj} = 1/|\tilde{\beta}_{n,gj}|^r$, where $r > 0$, then there exists a local maximizer $(\hat{\alpha}^\top, (\hat{\beta}_{\mathcal{A}}^\top, \hat{\beta}_{\mathcal{D}}^\top))^\top$ in (13) such that $\left\| \hat{\phi} - \phi^0 \right\| + \left\| \hat{\beta} - \beta^0 \right\| = O_p(\gamma_n)$ and $\hat{\beta}_{\mathcal{D}} = 0$ with probability tending to 1.*

In practice, we choose $(\tilde{\alpha}_n, \tilde{\beta}_n) = \arg\max_{\alpha, \beta} l_n(\alpha, \beta)$, the estimator from the unpenalized score function when $p$ is diverging with $n$ and $p < n$. From

Corollaries 1 and 2, we notice that the rates of convergence of the estimators are the same but the selection performance of the adaptive hierarchically penalized method is superior to that of the hierarchically penalized method, because the adaptive method possesses the individual variable selection consistency, while the non-adaptive method holds only group selection consistency.

In the following theorem, we provide the asymptotic normality of the estimator for the linear coefficients. Further notation and assumptions are required to obtain the theorem. To do that, we follow the lines in [19]. Let $a^*$ and $h^*$ be $\mathbb{R}$-valued $L_2$ functions that minimize $E\{\Delta \parallel X - a(T) - h(W) \parallel^2\}$. Define $\Sigma^* = E\{\Delta \parallel X - a^*(T) - h^*(W) \parallel^{\otimes 2}\}$. Then $\Sigma^*$ can be written as $\int_0^\tau V(m_0, t)[X - h^*(W)]S^{(0)}(m_0, t)\lambda_0(t)dt$, which is thus the information matrix for the linear part derived by Huang [20]. The $p = p_n$ components of $h^*$ are denoted by $h_j^*$, $1 \le j \le p_n$. We make the following additional assumption:

(B7)   All $h^*$, $1 \le j \le p_n$, are in $\mathcal{H}_d$. The eigenvalues of $\Sigma^*$ are bounded away from zero below and bounded by a positive constant upper.

**Theorem 4** *Under the same conditions as in Theorem 2, further, (B7) holds and $p_n^3/n \to 0$, let $s^* = \sum_{g=1}^s s_g =$ the cardinality of the set $\mathcal{A}$, then*

$$\sqrt{n} v_n^\top \Sigma_{11}^{*1/2}(\hat{\beta}_{\mathcal{A}} - \beta_{\mathcal{A}}^0) \longrightarrow N(0, 1),$$

*where $\Sigma_{11}^*$ is the $s^* \times s^*$ principal submatrix of $\Sigma^*$ and $v_n$ is a unit $s^*$-vector.*

Theorem 4 indicates that the estimator $\hat{\beta}_{\mathcal{A}}$ for the nonzero coefficients has the same asymptotic distribution as it would have if the zero coefficients were known in advance, therefore, it possesses the oracle property of Fan and Li [13].

# 4   Numerical Results

## 4.1   Simulation Studies

To evaluate the finite-sample performance of the hierarchically penalized (HP) method and its adaptive version (AHP) in the PL-PHM, we conducted two simulation studies. In Example 1, the number of groups is moderately large, the group sizes are equal and relatively large, and within each group the coefficients are either all nonzero or all zero. In Example 2, the group sizes vary and there are zero coefficients in a nonzero group. In each example, we set sample size $n = 200$ and baseline hazard functions $h_0(t) = 1.0$. The censoring variable is generated from a uniform distribution over $[0, C_0]$, where $C_0$ is chosen to yield censoring rate $= 30\%$. For each of these settings, we replicate 500 simulations.

We compared the results with those based on some existing individual (LASSO, Adaptive LASSO, SCAD, MCP) and group (Group SCAD or G-SCAD, Group MCP or G-MCP) variable selection methods developed for linear models. LASSO, Adaptive LASSO (A-LASSO) and SCAD have been used for variable selection in the PLMs [19, 32]. The asymptotic theory for G-SCAD and G-MCP under PLMs has not studied in the literature, we used them only for comparison purpose and leave the asymptotic theory for future research. We expect that similar results to those for AHP method will also hold for G-SCAD and G-MCP penalties. In our simulation studies we used R packages ncvreg and Coxnet for individual variable selection penalties and grpreg for computing G-SCAD and G-MCP estimates. We used these penalties for variable selection in the linear part after linearizing the nonparametric functions $\phi(\cdot)$ using B-splines where the tuning parameter $\lambda_n$ is chosen by the built-in fivefold cross validation method. For computation of our AHP group selection method in the PL-PHM, we used the R package penalized and R program written by Wang et al. [44] for the linear PHM, where the tuning parameter $\lambda_n$ is chosen to be 10 for HP and 20 for AHP methods based on a trial and error method. Five performance measures are used to compare different group selection methods: number of true groups selected (TG), number of zero group selected (FG), number of true nonzero variables selected as nonzero (TP), number of true zero variables selected as nonzero (FP), and $L_2$-prediction error (PE) in the excess risk defined as

$$\left\| \left\{ \hat{\beta}^{\top} Z + \hat{\phi}_1(W_1) + \hat{\phi}_2(W_2) \right\} - \left\{ \beta^{\top} Z + \phi_1(W_1) + \phi_2(W_2) \right\} \right\|.$$

As a benchmark, we compute the oracle estimates, which are obtained by maximizing (6) for model (3) which includes only important variables and groups. To estimate nonparametric functions, we use B-splines, see details in Sect. 2 for centering the B-splines in general. Specifically, we centered $\phi_1(W_1)$ and $\phi_2(W_2)$ such that $E\{\phi_1(W_1)\} = E\{\phi_2(W_2)\} = 0$. We approximated the nonlinear functions using cubic B-spline functions. Lian et al. [28] used 5–8 basis functions in their simulations and found similar results. They reported the results only for 6 basis functions. To ease the computational burden, we also choose $K = 6$ as the number of basis functions in B-splines. This choice of $K$ is small enough to avoid overfitting and big enough to flexibly approximate the smooth functions [6, 17].

*Example 1* In this example, there are 7 groups in the linear part, each with 5 covariates, and two nonparametric functions. For the linear covariates, the covariate vector is $X^{\top} = (X_1^{\top}, \ldots, X_7^{\top})$. The subvector of covariates that belong to the same group is $X_j^{\top} = (X_{5(j-1)+1}, \ldots, X_{5(j-1)+5})$; $j = 1, \ldots, 7$. To generate the covariates $X_1, \ldots, X_{35}$, we first simulate 35 random variables $R_1, \ldots, R_{35}$ independently from the standard normal distribution. Then $Z_j$ $(j = 1, \ldots, 7)$ are simulated from a multivariate normal distribution with mean zero and an AR(1) covariance structure such that $\text{cov}(Z_{j1}, Z_{j2}) = 0.4^{|j_1 - j_2|}$ for $j_1, j_2 = 1, \ldots, 7$. The covariates $X_1, \ldots, X_{35}$ are generated as $X_j = (Z_{g_j} + R_j)/6$ $(j = 1, \ldots, 35)$, where $g_j$ is the smallest integer greater than $(j - 1)/5$ and the $X_j$'s with the same value of $g_j$ belong to the same group. Similar correlation structure was considered in [23]. The nonparametric functions are $\phi_1(W_1) = W_1^2 - (25/12)$ and $\phi_2(W_2) = \exp(-W_2) - 2\sinh(5/2)/5$, where the covariates $W$'s are sampled from $U(-2.5, 2.5)$. Such nonparametric functions were considered in [8] in a nonparametric additive regression model. The event times in Example 1 are generated from an exponential distribution with a hazard rate given as follows:

$$h(t|X, W) = h_0(t) \exp\left\{\beta^\top X + \phi_1(W_1) + \phi_2(W_2)\right\},$$

where $\beta = (\underbrace{1.2, \ldots, 1.2}_{5}, \underbrace{3.6, \ldots, 3.6}_{5}, \underbrace{2.4, \ldots, 2.4}_{5}, \underbrace{0, \ldots, 0}_{5}, \underbrace{0, 0, \ldots, 0}_{5}, \underbrace{0, 0, \ldots, 0}_{5},$
$\underbrace{0, \ldots, 0}_{5})^\top.$

In this example, there exist three important groups and all variables within each group are important. This example illustrates that the proposed group selection methods have the ability to identify important groups.

*Example 2* In this example, the group size differs across groups and some groups have a mixture of important and unimportant variables. There are seven groups: three groups each of size 8 and four groups each of size 4. The covariate vector is $X^\top = (X_1^\top, \ldots, X_7^\top)$, where the seven subvectors of covariates are $X_j^\top = (X_{8(j-1)+1}, \ldots, X_{8(j-1)+8})$, for $j = 1, 2, 3$, and $X_j^\top = (X_{4(j-1)+13}, \ldots, X_{4(j-1)+16})$, for $j = 4, 5, 6, 7$. To generate the covariates $X_1, \ldots, X_{40}$, we first simulate $Z_i$ $(i = 1, \ldots, 7)$ and $R_1, \ldots, R_{40}$ independently from the standard normal distribution. For $j = 1, \ldots, 24$, let $g_j$ be the largest integer less than $j/8 + 1$ and, for $j = 25, \ldots, 40$, let $g_j$ be the largest integer less than $(j - 24)/4 + 1$. The covariates $X_1, \ldots, X_{40}$ are obtained as $X_j = (Z_{g_j} + R_j)/6$ $(j = 1, \ldots, 40)$. The nonparametric functions are generated in the same way as of Example 1. Therefore, the corresponding coefficients in Example 2 are

$$\beta = (\underbrace{1.2, \ldots, 1.2}_{8}, \underbrace{3.6, 3.4, 3.2, 3.0, 2.8, 0, 0, 0}_{8}, \underbrace{0, \ldots, 0}_{8}, \underbrace{2.4, 0, 0, 0}_{4}, \underbrace{0, \ldots, 0}_{4},$$
$$\underbrace{0, \ldots, 0}_{4}, \underbrace{0, \ldots, 0}_{4})^\top.$$

This example considers three important groups in a more complex structure than that in Example 1. These three groups represent three different settings: all variables within the group are important, many variables within the group are important and very few variables within the group are important, respectively.

Tables 1 and 2 summarize variable selection results for Examples 1 and 2 by using the LASSO, A-LASSO, SCAD, MCP, G-SCAD, G-MCP, HP and AHP, respectively. The first four penalties perform individual variable selection, the

**Table 1** Example 1: Simulation results with median and standard deviations (in parentheses) of $L_2$-PE, TG, FG, TP and FP over 500 simulations

|         | $L_2$-PE     | TG        | FG        | TP         | FP        |
|---------|--------------|-----------|-----------|------------|-----------|
| LASSO   | 18.79 (5.76) | 3 (0.00)  | 4 (0.73)  | 15 (0.09)  | 6 (2.49)  |
| A-LASSO | 10.45 (3.95) | 3 (0.00)  | 2 (1.16)  | 15 (0.37)  | 3 (2.18)  |
| SCAD    | 11.18 (4.77) | 3 (0.00)  | 2 (1.17)  | 15 (0.50)  | 3 (2.50)  |
| MCP     | 11.24 (4.75) | 3 (0.00)  | 1 (1.14)  | 15 (0.71)  | 1 (1.82)  |
| HP      | 9.39(3.89)   | 3 (0.00)  | 2 (0.99)  | 15 (0.06)  | 5 (3.27)  |
| G-SCAD  | 9.45 (4.53)  | 3 (0.00)  | 0 (0.75)  | 15 (0.00)  | 0 (3.73)  |
| G-MCP   | 9.42 (4.45)  | 3 (0.00)  | 0 (0.39)  | 15 (0.00)  | 0 (1.93)  |
| AHP     | 8.63 (3.67)  | 3 (0.60)  | 0 (0.60)  | 15 (0.22)  | 0 (1.00)  |
| Oracle  | 8.87 (4.26)  | 3 (0.00)  | NA        | 15 (0.00)  | NA        |

**Table 2** Example 2: Simulation results with median and standard deviations (in parentheses) of $L_2$-PE, TG, FG, TP and FP over 500 simulations

|         | $L_2$-PE     | TG        | FG        | TP         | FP        |
|---------|--------------|-----------|-----------|------------|-----------|
| LASSO   | 15.74 (4.68) | 3 (0.00)  | 3 (0.92)  | 14 (0.08)  | 7 (2.89)  |
| A-LASSO | 10.05 (3.33) | 3 (0.00)  | 2 (1.09)  | 14 (0.49)  | 4 (2.45)  |
| SCAD    | 10.84 (4.10) | 3 (0.00)  | 2 (1.24)  | 14 (0.66)  | 3 (2.94)  |
| MCP     | 10.80 (3.84) | 3 (0.00)  | 1 (1.19)  | 13 (0.95)  | 2 (2.05)  |
| HP      | 10.02 (3.82) | 3 (0.00)  | 2 (1.00)  | 14 (0.06)  | 10 (3.84) |
| G-SCAD  | 9.73 (4.00)  | 3 (0.00)  | 0 (0.67)  | 14 (0.00)  | 6 (3.39)  |
| G-MCP   | 9.55 (4.19)  | 3 (0.06)  | 0 (0.36)  | 14 (0.06)  | 6 (1.70)  |
| AHP     | 8.55 (3.27)  | 3 (0.00)  | 0 (0.64)  | 14 (0.28)  | 2 (1.60)  |
| Oracle  | 8.14 (3.79)  | 3 (0.00)  | NA        | 14 (0.00)  | NA        |

next three perform group variable selection, and AHP performs adaptive bi-level group selection. From Table 1 we see that the group variable selection methods perform significantly better than individual variable selection methods with lower $L_2$-prediction error and chose more important and less unimportant variables. However, the hierarchical penalty is not performing satisfactorily, it is selecting more groups and more unimportant variables although it has the second lowest $L_2$-prediction error. This performance has been significantly improved in the adaptive version of the penalty, resulting in lowest $L_2$-prediction error, also, the group and individual variable selection performance is very comparable with the other group selection penalties, G-SCAD and G-MCP. Nonetheless, the superiority of the adaptive hierarchical method stood out with a complex grouping structure among the covariates as shown in Table 2. Here, this penalty not only has the smallest $L_2$-prediction error but also selects significantly lower number of unimportant variables than any other group selection penalties. Hence, if there is known grouping structure available among the covariates, group selection methods are preferable over individual variable selection methods, furthermore, adaptive bi-level group selection should be considered over non-adaptive group selection method especially

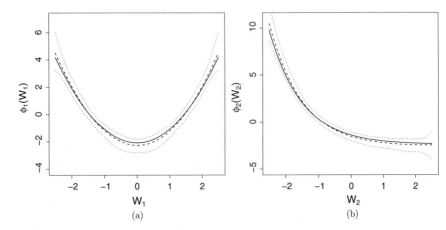

(a)                                          (b)

**Fig. 1** Estimation of $\phi(\cdot)$'s in Example 1: 95% point-wise confidence bands for $\phi(\cdot)$'s based on 500 replicates. The solid lines stand for the true curves. The dashed lines are the average estimated curves. The dot-dashed lines represent the 95% point-wise confidence bands based on 500 estimated values. (**a**) $\phi_1(\cdot)$. (**b**) $\phi_2(\cdot)$

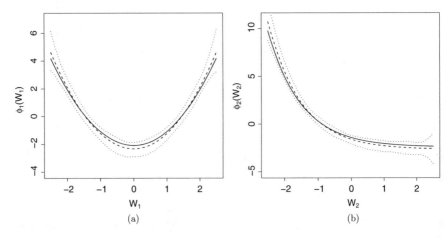

(a)                                          (b)

**Fig. 2** Estimation of $\phi(\cdot)$'s in Example 2: 95% point-wise confidence bands for $\phi(\cdot)$'s based on 500 replicates. The solid lines stand for the true curves. The dashed lines are the average estimated curves. The dot-dashed lines represent the 95% point-wise confidence bands based on 500 estimated values. (**a**) $\phi_1(\cdot)$. (**b**) $\phi_2(\cdot)$

with a complex grouping structure. The fitted curves and 95% point-wise confidence bands for $\phi_1(\cdot)$ and $\phi_2(\cdot)$ are shown in Figs. 1 and 2 for Examples 1 and 2, respectively. It is evident that the average estimated curves capture the true curves very well and that the true curves lie in the 95% point-wise confidence bands which are quite narrower.

## 4.2   Application to a Real Data Set

In this section, we illustrate application of our proposed method with a real data example. The Mayo Clinic trial in primary biliary cirrhosis (PBC) of the liver, a fatal chronic liver disease, was conducted between 1974 and 1984. The data is available in **R** package 'survival'. A total of 424 PBC patients who met eligibility criteria for the randomized placebo controlled trial of the drug D-penicillamine were referred to Mayo Clinic during that 10-year interval. At the end, a total of 312 PBC patients participated in the randomized trial of whom 158 were assigned to the drug D-penicillamine while the rest were assigned to a control group with placebo drug. During the follow-up 125 patients died due to PBC disease. The primary interest of the study was to investigate the effectiveness of D-penicillamine in curing PBC disease. Several other covariates such as age, gender, albumin etc. were recorded as baseline covariates at the beginning of the study. Detailed account of the PBC data can be found in [10].

The PBC data has been analyzed by Huang et al. [22] for group selection in PHM. We analyze this data using our proposed adaptive hierarchical penalty (AHP) to identify a smaller set of significant covariates that contribute to the hazards of dying from PBC under a PL-PHM. Our interest is on the main effects of the observed 17 risk factors using 276 complete cases in the full model. Huang et al. [22] described that these risk factors are clustered into nine categories with 10 continuous and 7 categorical variables (Table 3). We observe that age $(Z_1)$ and platelet $(Z_{17})$ are the only covariates in groups with a single continuous variable, we model their effects with nonparametric functions and perform bi-level selection in the rest of the covariates by treating them as linear covariates. We compute the maximum likelihood estimate (MLE), LASSO, A-LASSO, G-SCAD, G-MCP, HP and AHP estimates. The results are summarized in Table 4. All of the methods suggest that gender and treatment should be excluded from the final model which implies treatment (D-penicillamine) has no effect on curing PBC disease. The performance of group SCAD and group MCP is very similar. The HP selects more variables than AHP. AHP suggests deleting Groups 5 and 8 in addition to gender (Group 2) and treatment (Group 7).

The two estimated curves for $\phi_1$ (Age), $\phi_2$ (Platelet) are shown in Fig. 3, indicating nonlinear effects of age and platelet count on the hazards rate. The age effect $\hat{\phi}_1$(Age) shows that the hazards of death from PBC increases steadily up to about 66 years, and then drops sharply. PBC is a disease of middle aged people, mostly women, with a median age of disease onset is 50 years [41], which explains the increase in risk with aging. The drop in the risk for older population might be due to the fact that as the patients get older, they are more probable of dying from other causes before the incidence of liver failure [27]. On the other hand, PBC is associated with low platelet counts [1]. Since all of our participants are PBC patients, it is expected that the hazard of death will decrease as the platelet count increases, as shown in the estimated curve $\hat{\phi}_1$(Platelet). However, normal platelet count ranges from 150 to 450 (per cubic microliter/1000) (https://www.

**Table 3** PBC data analysis

| Group | Variable | Type | Definition |
|---|---|---|---|
| $G1$: Age | $Z_1$ | C | Age (years) |
| $G2$: Gender | $Z_2$ | D | Female gender (0 male and 1 female) |
| $G3$: Phenotype | $Z_3$ | D | Ascites (0 absence and 1 presence) |
| | $Z_4$ | D | Hepatomegaly (0 absence and 1 presence) |
| | $Z_5$ | D | Spiders (0 absence and 1 presence) |
| | $Z_6$ | D | Edema (0 no edema, 0.5 untreated or successfully treated and 1 edema despite diuretic therapy) |
| $G4$: Liver function damage | $Z_7$ | C | Alkaline phosphatase (units/litre) |
| | $Z_8$ | C | Sgot (liver enzyme in units/ml) |
| $G5$: Excretory function of the liver | $Z_9$ | C | Serum bilirubin (mg/dl) |
| | $Z_{10}$ | C | Serum cholesterol (mg/dl) |
| | $Z_{11}$ | C | Triglycerides (mg/dl) |
| $G6$: Liver reserve function | $Z_{12}$ | C | Albumin (g/dl) |
| | $Z_{13}$ | C | Prothrombin time (seconds) |
| $G7$: Treatment | $Z_{14}$ | D | D-Penicillamine vs. placebo (1 treatment and 2 control) |
| $G8$: Reflection | $Z_{15}$ | D | Stage (histological stage of disease, graded 1,2,3 or 4) |
| | $Z_{16}$ | C | Urine copper ($\mu$g/day) |
| $G9$: Haematology | $Z_{17}$ | C | Platelets (per cubic ml/1000) |

Dictionary of covariates

*Type* type of variable, *C* continuous, *D* discrete

hopkinsmedicine.org) and one of the reason of higher hazard beyond the normal limits is inflammatory diseases like liver cirrhosis; which explains the two tails of the curve where the hazard increases with abnormally lower or higher platelet count. Therefore, our analysis provides more detailed nonlinear profiles regarding the effects of age and platelet counts, both of which are of clinical importance.

# 5 Concluding Remarks

In this paper, we proposed a hierarchically penalized method for variable selection in the PL-PHM with diverging number of parameters. Our model allows high dimensional linear covariates and fixed low dimensional nonlinear covariates to be included in the same model to predict the hazard of failure time, which is more appealing and useful than models with only a linear term or with a large number of nonlinear functions of covariates. We modelled the nonparametric functions using B-splines and performed adaptive bi-level variable selection in the

**Table 4** Estimation results of PBC data

| Group | Covariates | MLE | LASSO | A-LASSO | G-SCAD | G-MCP | HP | AHP |
|---|---|---|---|---|---|---|---|---|
| $G_2$ | gender | −0.4458 | 0 | 0 | 0 | 0 | 0 | 0 |
| $G_3$ | asc | 0.6470 | 0.3665 | 0 | 0 | 0 | 0.4093 | 1.1869 |
| | hep | 0.0935 | 0 | 0 | 0 | 0 | 0.0208 | 0 |
| | spid | 0.2690 | 0 | 0 | 0 | 0 | 0.0973 | 0.5382 |
| | oed | 0.2482 | 0.1931 | 0.1175 | 0 | 0 | 0.2423 | 0.4513 |
| $G_4$ | alk | −0.000002 | 0 | 0 | 0 | 0 | 0 | 0 |
| | sgot | 0.0038 | 0 | 0.0015 | 0 | 0 | 0 | 0 |
| $G_5$ | bill | 0.0963 | 0.0904 | 0.1025 | 0.1289 | 0.1149 | 0.0969 | 0 |
| | chol | 0.0004 | 0 | 0 | 0.0006 | 0.0005 | 0.0006 | 0 |
| | trig | −0.0021 | 0 | 0 | −0.0011 | −0.0012 | −0.0008 | 0 |
| $G_6$ | alb | −0.7478 | −0.4189 | −0.8033 | −0.1227 | −0.9658 | −0.6672 | −0.7547 |
| | prot | 0.1784 | 0 | 0.1004 | 0.0247 | 0.2104 | 0.1126 | 0 |
| $G_7$ | trt | −0.1476 | 0 | 0 | 0 | 0 | 0 | 0 |
| $G_8$ | stage | 0.3517 | 0.1235 | 0.3232 | 0.5835 | 0.4222 | 0.3158 | 0 |
| | cop | 0.0039 | 0.0033 | 0.0038 | 0.0052 | 0.0052 | 0.0046 | 0 |

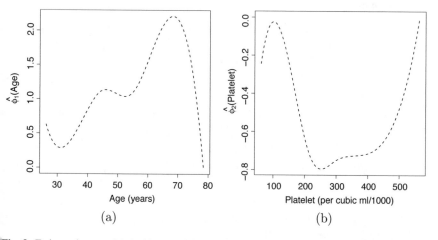

(a)          (b)

**Fig. 3** Estimated curves (**a**) $\phi_1$ ($Age$) and (**b**) $\phi_2$ ($Platelet$) in the analysis of PBC data

linear covariates. Our proposed method can effectively select important groups and important variables within a group in the linear part, and estimate both parametric and nonparametric components simultaneously. We used the theory of counting processes and martingales to establish rate of convergence, selection consistency and asymptotic normality of the proposed estimators. We developed computational algorithm for our proposed estimators and presented simulation studies along with an example of real data analyses. Numerical studies indicate that the adaptive hierarchically penalized method performs better than existing individual variable selection methods (LASSO, Adaptive LASSO, SCAD, MCP) as well as non-adaptive group variable selection methods (group SCAD, group MCP and HP), especially in the cases with a complex grouping structure among the covariates. Although our method can handle a diverging number of parameters, but it is restricted to an order of $o(n)$, i.e., $p_n = O(n^\zeta)$, for some $0 < \zeta < 1$. It would be interesting to explore the same problems in our future research when $p_n = \exp(O(n))$, which represents ultra-high dimensional data.

**Acknowledgements** The authors acknowledge with gratitude the support for this research by the Discovery Grants from Natural Sciences and Engineering Research Council (NSERC) of Canada. The authors also would like to thank the editor and the anonymous referee for their insightful and constructive comments that have helped us substantially improve the manuscript.

## Appendix

In this Appendix, we provide proofs of the lemmas, theorems, and corollaries that are presented in the paper. First, the proofs of Lemmas 1 and 2 follow those of Wang et al. [44] closely.

*Proof of Lemma 1* Let $Q^*(\lambda_\gamma, \lambda_\theta, \alpha, \gamma, \theta)$ denote the criterion that we would like to maximize in Eq. (7), let $Q^\dagger(\lambda, \alpha, \gamma, \theta)$ denote the corresponding criterion in Eq. (8), and let $(\hat{\alpha}^*, \hat{\gamma}^*, \hat{\theta}^*)$ denote a local maximizer of $Q^*(\lambda_\gamma, \lambda_\theta, \alpha, \gamma, \theta)$. We will prove that $(\hat{\alpha}^\dagger = \hat{\alpha}^*, \hat{\gamma}_g^\dagger = \lambda_\gamma \hat{\gamma}_g^*, \hat{\theta}_{(g)}^\dagger = \hat{\theta}_{(g)}^*/\lambda_\gamma)$ is a local maximizer of $Q^\dagger(\lambda, \alpha, \gamma, \theta)$.

Replacing $\gamma^* = \gamma^\dagger/\lambda_\gamma$ and $\theta^* = \theta^\dagger \lambda_\gamma$ in (7), we immediately have $Q^*(\lambda_\gamma, \lambda_\theta, \alpha, \gamma, \theta) = Q^\dagger(\lambda, \alpha, \lambda_\gamma \gamma, \theta/\lambda_\gamma)$. Since $(\hat{\alpha}^*, \hat{\gamma}^*, \hat{\theta}^*)$ is a local maximizer of $Q^*(\lambda_\gamma, \lambda_\theta, \alpha, \gamma, \theta)$, therefore, by the definition of local maximizer there exists $\delta > 0$ such that if $(\alpha', \gamma', \theta')$ satisfies $|\alpha' - \hat{\alpha}^*| + |\gamma' - \hat{\gamma}^*| + |\theta' - \hat{\theta}^*| < \delta$, then $Q^*(\lambda_\gamma, \lambda_\theta, \alpha', \gamma', \theta') \leq Q^*(\lambda_\gamma, \lambda_\theta, \hat{\alpha}^*, \hat{\gamma}^*, \hat{\theta}^*)$. We choose $\delta'$ such that $\delta'/\min(\lambda_\gamma, 1/\lambda_\gamma) \leq \delta/2$. Then, $\min(\lambda_\gamma, 1/\lambda_\gamma) \leq 1$ and $\delta' \leq \min(\lambda_\gamma, 1/\lambda_\gamma)\delta/2 \leq \delta/2$. Thus, for any $(\alpha'', \gamma'', \theta'')$ satisfying $|\alpha'' - \hat{\alpha}^\dagger| + |\gamma'' - \hat{\gamma}^\dagger| + |\theta'' - \hat{\theta}^\dagger| < \delta' \leq \delta/2$, we have, $|\alpha'' - \hat{\alpha}^\dagger| = |\alpha'' - \hat{\alpha}^*| \leq \delta/2$. Also,

$$
\left|\frac{\gamma''}{\lambda_\gamma} - \hat{\gamma}^*\right| + \left|\lambda_\gamma \theta'' - \hat{\theta}^*\right| \leq \frac{\lambda_\gamma \left|\frac{\gamma''}{\lambda_\gamma} - \hat{\gamma}^*\right| + \frac{1}{\lambda_\gamma}\left|\lambda_\gamma \theta'' - \hat{\theta}^*\right|}{\min(\lambda_\gamma, \frac{1}{\lambda_\gamma})}
$$

$$
= \frac{\left|\gamma'' - \lambda_\gamma \hat{\gamma}^*\right| + \left|\theta'' - \frac{\hat{\theta}^*}{\lambda_\gamma}\right|}{\min(\lambda_\gamma, \frac{1}{\lambda_\gamma})}
$$

$$
= \frac{|\gamma'' - \hat{\gamma}^\dagger| + |\theta'' - \hat{\theta}^\dagger|}{\min(\lambda_\gamma, \frac{1}{\lambda_\gamma})} < \frac{\delta'}{\min(\lambda_\gamma, \frac{1}{\lambda_\gamma})} \leq \frac{\delta}{2}.
$$

Therefore, $\left| \alpha'' - \hat{\alpha}^* \right| + \left| \gamma''/\lambda_\gamma - \hat{\gamma}^* \right| + \left| \lambda_\gamma \theta'' - \hat{\theta}^* \right| < \delta/2 + \delta/2 = \delta$. Hence,

$$Q^*(\lambda_\gamma, \lambda_\theta, \hat{\alpha}'', \hat{\gamma}''/\lambda_\gamma, \lambda_\gamma \hat{\theta}'') \le Q^*(\lambda_\gamma, \lambda_\theta, \hat{\alpha}^*, \hat{\gamma}^*, \hat{\theta}^*),$$

which gives us

$$Q^\dagger(\lambda, \hat{\alpha}'', \hat{\gamma}'', \hat{\theta}'') \le Q^\dagger(\lambda, \hat{\alpha}^\dagger, \hat{\gamma}^\dagger, \hat{\theta}^\dagger).$$

So, $(\hat{\alpha}^\dagger = \hat{\alpha}^*, \hat{\gamma}^\dagger = \lambda_\gamma \hat{\gamma}^*, \hat{\theta}^\dagger = \hat{\theta}^*/\lambda_\gamma)$ is a local maximizer of $Q^\dagger(\lambda, \alpha, \gamma, \theta)$.

Similarly, we can prove that for any local maximizer $(\hat{\alpha}^\dagger, \hat{\gamma}^\dagger, \hat{\theta}^\dagger)$ of $Q^\dagger(\lambda, \alpha, \gamma, \theta)$, there is a corresponding local maximizer $(\hat{\alpha}^*, \hat{\gamma}^*, \hat{\theta}^*)$ of $Q^*(\lambda_\gamma, \lambda_\theta, \alpha, \gamma, \theta)$ such that $\hat{\alpha}^* = \hat{\alpha}^\dagger$ and $\hat{\gamma}_g^* \hat{\theta}_{gj}^* = \hat{\gamma}_g^\dagger \hat{\theta}_{gj}^\dagger$. □

**Proof of Lemma 2** Suppose $(\hat{\alpha}, \hat{\gamma}, \hat{\theta})$ is a local maximizer of (8). Let $\hat{\beta}$ satisfy $\hat{\beta}_{gj} = \hat{\gamma}_g \hat{\theta}_{gj}$. It is trivial that $\hat{\gamma}_g = 0$ if and only if $\hat{\theta}_{(g)} = 0$. Hence, if $\hat{\gamma}_g \ne 0$, then $|\hat{\beta}_{(g)}| \ne 0$.

Let $(\alpha, \beta)$ be fixed at $(\hat{\alpha}, \hat{\beta})$. Then maximizing $Q^\dagger(\lambda, \alpha, \gamma, \theta)$ in (8) only depends on the penalty. For some $g$ with $|\hat{\beta}_{(g)}| \ne 0$, the corresponding penalty term is $-\gamma_g - \lambda \sum_{j=1}^{P_g} |\hat{\beta}_{gj}|/\gamma_g$, which is maximized at $\hat{\gamma}_g = (\lambda|\hat{\beta}_{(g)}|)^{1/2}$, and $\hat{\theta}_{(g)} = \hat{\beta}_{(g)}/\hat{\gamma}_g$.

Let $Q(\lambda, \alpha, \beta)$ be the corresponding criterion to be maximized in Eq. (9). By Lemma 1, the local maximizer $\hat{\alpha}$ of $\alpha$ in (7) and (8) are the same, so we only need to consider other parameters, e.g., $\beta$, and fix $\alpha$ at $\hat{\alpha}$ in both (7) and (8). We first show that $(\hat{\alpha}, \hat{\beta})$ is a local maximizer of $Q(\lambda, \alpha, \beta)$, i.e., there exists a $\delta' > 0$ such that if $|\Delta\alpha| + |\Delta\beta| < \delta'$, then $Q(\lambda, \hat{\alpha} + \Delta\alpha, \hat{\beta} + \Delta\beta) \le Q(\lambda, \hat{\alpha}, \hat{\beta})$. Particularly, taking $\Delta\alpha = 0$, it becomes $|\Delta\beta| < \delta'$, then $Q(\lambda, \hat{\alpha}, \hat{\beta} + \Delta\beta) \le Q(\lambda, \hat{\alpha}, \hat{\beta})$. Denote $\Delta\beta = \Delta\beta^{(1)} + \Delta\beta^{(2)}$, where $\Delta\beta_{(g)}^{(1)} = 0$ if $|\hat{\beta}_{(g)}| = 0$ and $\Delta\beta_{(g)}^{(2)} = 0$ if $|\hat{\beta}_{(g)}| \ne 0$. We thus have, $|\Delta\beta| = |\Delta\beta^{(1)} + \Delta\beta^{(2)}| = |\Delta\beta^{(1)}| + |\Delta\beta^{(2)}|$.

We first show $Q(\lambda, \hat{\alpha}, \hat{\beta} + \Delta\beta^{(1)}) \le Q(\lambda, \hat{\alpha}, \hat{\beta})$ for some $\delta'$. We already have $\hat{\gamma}_g = (\lambda|\hat{\beta}_{(g)}|)^{1/2}$ and $\hat{\theta}_{(g)} = \hat{\beta}_{(g)}/\hat{\gamma}_g$ if $|\hat{\gamma}_g| \ne 0$, and $\hat{\theta}_{(g)} = 0$ if $|\hat{\gamma}_g| = 0$. Let $\hat{\gamma}_g' = (\lambda|\hat{\beta}_{(g)} + \Delta\beta_{(g)}^{(1)}|)^{1/2}$ and $\hat{\theta}_{(g)}' = (\hat{\beta}_{(g)} + \Delta\beta_{(g)}^{(1)})/\hat{\gamma}_g'$ if $|\hat{\gamma}_g'| \ne 0$, and let $\hat{\gamma}_g' = 0$ and $\hat{\theta}_{(g)}' = 0$ if $|\hat{\gamma}_g| = 0$. Then we have $Q^\dagger(\lambda, \hat{\alpha}, \hat{\gamma}', \hat{\theta}') = Q(\lambda, \hat{\alpha}, \hat{\beta} + \Delta\beta^{(1)})$ and $Q^\dagger(\lambda, \hat{\alpha}, \hat{\gamma}, \hat{\theta}) = Q(\lambda, \hat{\alpha}, \hat{\beta})$. Hence, we only need to show $Q^\dagger(\lambda, \hat{\alpha}, \hat{\gamma}', \hat{\theta}') \le Q^\dagger(\lambda, \hat{\alpha}, \hat{\gamma}, \hat{\theta})$. As $(\hat{\alpha}, \hat{\gamma}, \hat{\theta})$ is a local maximizer of $Q^\dagger(\lambda, \alpha, \gamma, \theta)$, for fixed $\hat{\alpha}$, there exists a $\delta$ such that for any $(\gamma', \theta')$ satisfying $|\gamma' - \hat{\gamma}| + |\theta' - \hat{\theta}| < \delta$, we have $Q^\dagger(\lambda, \hat{\alpha}, \gamma', \theta') \le Q^\dagger(\lambda, \hat{\alpha}, \hat{\gamma}, \hat{\theta})$. Let $a = \min\left\{|\hat{\beta}_{(g)}| : |\beta_{(g)}| \ne 0, g = 1, \ldots, G\right\}, b = \max\left\{|\hat{\beta}_{(g)}| : |\beta_{(g)}| \ne 0, g = 1, \ldots, G\right\}$ and $\delta' < a/2$. It is seen that,

$$\left| |\hat{\beta}_{(g)} + \Delta\beta_{(g)}^{(1)}| - |\hat{\beta}_{(g)}| \right| \le \left| \Delta\beta_{(g)}^{(1)} \right|,$$

$$\left|(|\hat{\beta}_{(g)} + \Delta\beta_{(g)}^{(1)}|^{1/2})^2 - (|\hat{\beta}_{(g)}|^{1/2})^2\right| \leq \left|\Delta\beta_{(g)}^{(1)}\right|,$$

$$\left|(|\hat{\beta}_{(g)} + \Delta\beta_{(g)}^{(1)}|^{1/2} - |\hat{\beta}_{(g)}|^{1/2})(|\hat{\beta}_{(g)} + \Delta\beta_{(g)}^{(1)}|^{1/2} + |\hat{\beta}_{(g)}|^{1/2})\right| \leq \left|\Delta\beta_{(g)}^{(1)}\right|,$$

$$\left||\hat{\beta}_{(g)} + \Delta\beta_{(g)}^{(1)}|^{1/2} - |\hat{\beta}_{(g)}|^{1/2}\right| \leq \frac{\left|\Delta\beta_{(g)}^{(1)}\right|}{|\hat{\beta}_{(g)} + \Delta\beta_{(g)}^{(1)}|^{1/2} + |\hat{\beta}_{(g)}|^{1/2}}.$$

Since when $\min_{g}\left\{|\hat{\beta}_{(g)}|\right\} = a \neq 0$, and when $|\Delta\beta_{(g)}^{(1)}| < \delta' < a/2$, we have

$$|\hat{\beta}_{(g)} + \Delta\beta_{(g)}^{(1)}| \geq |\hat{\beta}_{(g)}| - |\Delta\beta_{(g)}^{(1)}| \geq a - \frac{a}{2} = \frac{a}{2} > 0,$$

and

$$|\hat{\beta}_{(g)} + \Delta\beta_{(g)}^{(1)}|^{1/2} + |\hat{\beta}_{(g)}|^{1/2} \geq \left(\frac{a}{2}\right)^{1/2} + a^{1/2} = (2^{-1/2} + 1)a^{1/2} \geq 2^{1/2}a^{1/2} = (2a)^{1/2}$$

Therefore,

$$\left||\hat{\beta}_{(g)} + \Delta\beta_{(g)}^{(1)}|^{1/2} - |\hat{\beta}_{(g)}|^{1/2}\right| \leq \frac{|\Delta\beta_{(g)}^{(1)}|}{(2a)^{1/2}}.$$

Hence,

$$|\hat{\gamma}_g' - \hat{\gamma}_g| = \left|(\lambda|\hat{\beta}_{(g)} + \Delta\beta_{(g)}^{(1)}|)^{1/2} - (\lambda|\hat{\beta}_{(g)}|)^{1/2}\right| \leq \frac{\lambda|\Delta\beta_{(g)}^{(1)}|}{(2\lambda a)^{1/2}}.$$

Next, if $|\hat{\gamma}_g| = 0$, then $\hat{\theta}_{(g)}' = \hat{\theta}_{(g)} = 0$, and $|\hat{\theta}_{(g)}' - \hat{\theta}_{(g)}| = 0$. If $|\hat{\gamma}_g| \neq 0$, then

$$\begin{aligned}\hat{\theta}_{(g)}' - \hat{\theta}_{(g)} &= \frac{(\hat{\beta}_{(g)} + \Delta\beta_{(g)}^{(1)})}{\hat{\gamma}_g'} - \frac{\hat{\beta}_{(g)}}{\hat{\gamma}_g}\\[2mm]&= \frac{\hat{\beta}_{(g)}\hat{\gamma}_g + \Delta\beta_{(g)}^{(1)}\hat{\gamma}_g - \hat{\beta}_{(g)}\hat{\gamma}_g'}{\hat{\gamma}_g'\hat{\gamma}_g}\\[2mm]&= \frac{\hat{\beta}_{(g)}[\hat{\gamma}_g - \hat{\gamma}_g'] + \Delta\beta_{(g)}^{(1)}\hat{\gamma}_g}{\hat{\gamma}_g'\hat{\gamma}_g}.\end{aligned} \qquad (14)$$

We already have $|\hat{\beta}_{(g)}| \leq b$ and $|\hat{\gamma}_g' - \hat{\gamma}_g| \leq \lambda|\Delta\beta_{(g)}^{(1)}|/(2\lambda a)^{1/2}$. Consider

$$\hat{\gamma}_g'\hat{\gamma}_g = (\lambda|\hat{\beta}_{(g)} + \Delta\beta_{(g)}^{(1)}|)^{1/2}(\lambda|\hat{\beta}_{(g)}|)^{1/2}.$$

Since $|\hat{\gamma}_g| = (\lambda|\hat{\beta}_{(g)}|)^{1/2} \geq \lambda^{1/2}a^{1/2}$, when $|\Delta\beta_{(g)}^{(1)}| < \delta'$ and $\delta' < a/2$, if $\hat{\gamma}_g \neq 0$, then $|\hat{\beta}_{(g)}| \neq 0$, $\Delta\beta_{(g)}^{(2)} = 0$, it implies, $|\Delta\beta_{(g)}^{(1)}| \leq |\Delta\beta^{(1)}| < \delta \Rightarrow |\Delta\beta_{(g)}^{(1)}| < \delta' < a/2$ and $|\hat{\beta}_{(g)} + \Delta\beta_{(g)}^{(1)}| \geq |\hat{\beta}_{(g)}| - |\Delta\beta_{(g)}^{(1)}| \geq a - a/2 = a/2 > 0$. Therefore, $|\hat{\gamma}_g'| = (\lambda|\hat{\beta}_{(g)} + \Delta\beta_{(g)}^{(1)}|)^{1/2} \geq \lambda^{1/2}(a/2)^{1/2}$ and $|\hat{\gamma}_g'\hat{\gamma}_g| \geq \lambda^{1/2}a^{1/2}\lambda^{1/2}(a/2)^{1/2} = \lambda a 2^{-1/2}$. From (14) we have,

$$
\begin{aligned}
|\hat{\theta}_{(g)}' - \hat{\theta}_{(g)}| &\leq \frac{|\hat{\beta}_{(g)}|}{|\hat{\gamma}_g'\hat{\gamma}_g|}|\hat{\gamma}_g' - \hat{\gamma}_g| + |\Delta\beta_{(g)}^{(1)}|\frac{|\hat{\gamma}_g|}{|\hat{\gamma}_g||\hat{\gamma}_g'|} \\
&\leq \frac{b\lambda|\Delta\beta_{(g)}^{(1)}|}{(2\lambda a)^{1/2}(\lambda a 2^{-1/2})} + |\Delta\beta_{(g)}^{(1)}|\frac{1}{\lambda^{1/2}(a/2)^{1/2}} \\
&\leq \left[\frac{b\lambda}{(2\lambda a)^{1/2}(\lambda a)2^{-1/2}} + \frac{1}{(\lambda a/2)^{1/2}}\right]|\Delta\beta_{(g)}^{(1)}| \\
&= |\Delta\beta_{(g)}^{(1)}|\left[\frac{1}{(\lambda a/2)^{1/2}} + \frac{b}{a(\lambda a)^{1/2}}\right].
\end{aligned}
$$

Therefore, we are able to choose a $\delta' > 0$ satisfying $\delta' < a/2$ such that $|\hat{\gamma}_g' - \hat{\gamma}_g| + |\hat{\theta}_g' - \hat{\theta}_g| < \delta$ when $|\Delta\beta_{(g)}^{(1)}| < \delta'$. Hence we have $Q^\dagger(\lambda, \hat{\alpha}, \hat{\gamma}', \hat{\theta}') \leq Q^\dagger(\lambda, \hat{\alpha}, \hat{\gamma}, \hat{\theta})$ due to the local maximality, that is, $Q(\lambda, \hat{\alpha}, \hat{\beta} + \Delta\beta^{(1)}) \leq Q(\lambda, \hat{\alpha}, \hat{\beta})$.

Next we show $Q(\lambda, \hat{\alpha}, \hat{\beta} + \Delta\beta^{(1)} + \Delta\beta^{(2)}) \leq Q(\lambda, \hat{\alpha}, \hat{\beta} + \Delta\beta^{(1)})$. This is trivial when $\Delta\beta^{(2)} = 0$. If $\Delta\beta^{(2)} \neq 0$, then $\Delta\beta^{(1)} = 0$ and we have

$$
\begin{aligned}
Q(\lambda, \hat{\alpha}, \hat{\beta} + \Delta\beta^{(1)} + \Delta\beta^{(2)}) - Q(\lambda, \hat{\alpha}, \hat{\beta} + \Delta\beta^{(1)}) &= (\Delta\beta^{(2)})^\top n^{-1}\frac{\partial l_n(\hat{\alpha}, \beta*)}{\partial\beta} \\
&\quad -2\sum_{g=1}^{G}(\lambda|\Delta\beta_{(g)}^{(2)}|)^{1/2},
\end{aligned}
$$

where $\beta*$ is a vector between $\hat{\beta} + \Delta\beta^{(1)} + \Delta\beta^{(2)}$ and $\hat{\beta} + \Delta\beta^{(1)}$. Since $|\Delta\beta^{(2)}| < \delta'$, for a small enough $\delta'$, the second term in the above equality dominates the first term, hence we have $Q(\lambda, \hat{\alpha}, \hat{\beta} + \Delta\beta^{(1)} + \Delta\beta^{(2)}) \leq Q(\lambda, \hat{\alpha}, \hat{\beta} + \Delta\beta^{(1)})$. Thus we have shown that there exists a $\delta' > 0$ such that if $|\Delta\beta| < \delta'$, then $Q(\lambda, \hat{\alpha}, \hat{\beta} + \Delta\beta) \leq Q(\lambda, \hat{\alpha}, \hat{\beta})$, which implies that $\hat{\beta}$ is a local maximizer of $Q(\lambda, \hat{\alpha}, \beta)$.

Similarly, we can prove that if $(\hat{\alpha}, \hat{\beta})$ is a local maximizer of $Q(\lambda, \alpha, \beta)$, then $(\hat{\alpha}, \hat{\gamma}, \hat{\theta})$ is a local maximizer of $Q^\dagger(\lambda, \alpha, \gamma, \theta)$, where $\hat{\gamma}_g = (\lambda|\hat{\beta}_{(g)}|)^{1/2}$ and $\hat{\theta}_{(g)} = \hat{\beta}_{(g)}/\hat{\gamma}_g$ if $|\hat{\beta}_{(g)}| \neq 0$, and $\hat{\gamma}_g = 0$ and $\hat{\theta}_{(g)} = 0$ if $|\hat{\beta}_{(g)}| = 0$. $\quad\square$

*Proof of Theorem 1* Let $\alpha^0 = (\alpha_1^{0\top}, \ldots, \alpha_q^{0\top})^\top$ be a $q \times K$ dimensional vector that satisfies $\left\|\phi_j^0 - \alpha_j^{0\top}B_j\right\|_\infty = O(K^{-d}), 1 \leq j \leq q$. Then, $\left\|\phi^0 - \alpha^{0\top}B\right\|_\infty = O(K^{-d})$ and $\left\|\phi^0 - \alpha^{0\top}B\right\| = O(K^{-d})$ since $q$ is fixed. Such approximation rates are possible due to our smoothness assumption (B2) and well known approximation properties of B-spline [9].

Let $\gamma_n = \sqrt{(K+p)/n} + K^{-d}$ and $u \in \mathbb{R}^{q \times K+p}$ with $\|u\| = D$, where $u = (u_1, u_2)$, $u_1$ is a $q \times K$-vector, and $u_2$ is a $p$-vector. To prove Theorem 1, we first show that $\left\| \hat{\phi} - \alpha^{0\top} B \right\| = O_p(\gamma_n)$, and $\left\| \hat{\beta} - \beta^0 \right\| = O_p(\gamma_n)$ where $\hat{\phi} = \hat{\alpha}^{0\top} B$. Then it is sufficient to show that for any $\epsilon > 0$, there exists a constant $D$ such that

$$P \left\{ \sup_{\|u\|=D} Q_n((\alpha^0, \beta^0) + \gamma_n u) < Q_n(\alpha^0, \beta^0) \right\} \geq 1 - \epsilon, \tag{15}$$

when $n$ is big enough. This implies that with probability of at least $1 - \epsilon$, there exists a local maximum in the ball $\{(\alpha^0, \beta^0) + \gamma_n u : \|u\| \leq D\}$. Hence, there exists a local maximizer such that $\left\| \hat{\phi} - \alpha^{0\top} B \right\| + \left\| \hat{\beta} - \beta^0 \right\| = O_p(\gamma_n)$.

Since $p_{\lambda_n}$ satisfies conditions (11) and (12), we have,

$$
\begin{aligned}
&Q_n((\alpha^0, \beta^0) + \gamma_n u) - Q_n(\alpha^0, \beta^0) \\
&= n^{-1} \left\{ l_n((\alpha^0, \beta^0) + \gamma_n u) - l_n(\alpha^0, \beta^0) \right\} \\
&\quad - \sum_{g=1}^{s} \left\{ p_{\lambda_n}^{(g)}(\left|\beta_{g1}^0 + \gamma_n u_{2,g1}\right|, \ldots, \left|\beta_{gs_g}^0 + \gamma_n u_{2,gs_g}\right|, \left|\beta_{g(s_g+1)}^0 + \gamma_n u_{2,g(s_g+1)}\right|, \ldots, \right. \\
&\qquad \left. \left|\beta_{gp_g}^0 + \gamma_n u_{2,gp_g}\right|) - p_{\lambda_n}^{(g)}\left(\left|\beta_{g1}^0\right|, \ldots, \left|\beta_{gs_g}^0\right|, \left|\beta_{g(s_g+1)}^0\right|, \ldots, \left|\beta_{gp_g}^0\right|\right) \right\} \\
&\quad - \sum_{g=s+1}^{G} \left\{ p_{\lambda_n}^{(g)}\left(\left|\beta_{g1}^0 + \gamma_n u_{2,g1}\right|, \ldots, \left|\beta_{gp_g}^0 + \gamma_n u_{2,gp_g}\right|\right) - p_{\lambda_n}^{(g)}\left(\left|\beta_{g1}^0\right|, \ldots, \left|\beta_{gp_g}^0\right|\right) \right\} \\
&\leq n^{-1} \left\{ l_n((\alpha^0, \beta^0) + \gamma_n u) - l_n(\alpha^0, \beta^0) \right\} \\
&\quad - \sum_{g=1}^{s} \left\{ p_{\lambda_n}^{(g)}\left(\left|\beta_{g1}^0 + \gamma_n u_{2,g1}\right|, \ldots, \left|\beta_{gs_g}^0 + \gamma_n u_{2,gs_g}\right|, \left|\beta_{g(s_g+1)}^0 + \gamma_n u_{2,g(s_g+1)}\right|, \ldots, \left|\beta_{gp_g}^0 + \gamma_n u_{2,gp_g}\right|\right) \right. \\
&\qquad \left. - p_{\lambda_n}^{(g)}\left(\left|\beta_{g1}^0\right|, \ldots, \left|\beta_{gs_g}^0\right|, \left|\beta_{g(s_g+1)}^0\right|, \ldots, \left|\beta_{gp_g}^0\right|\right) \right\} \\
&\leq n^{-1} \left\{ l_n((\alpha^0, \beta^0) + \gamma_n u) - l_n(\alpha^0, \beta^0) \right\} \\
&\quad - \sum_{g=1}^{s} \left\{ p_{\lambda_n}^{(g)}\left(\left|\beta_{g1}^0 + \gamma_n u_{2,g1}\right|, \ldots, \left|\beta_{gs_g}^0 + \gamma_n u_{2,gs_g}\right|, 0\right) - p_{\lambda_n}^{(g)}\left(\left|\beta_{g1}^0\right|, \ldots, \left|\beta_{gs_g}^0\right|, 0\right) \right\} \\
&= A - B.
\end{aligned}
$$

For $A$, denote $\omega^0 = (\alpha^0, \beta^0)$. By Taylor expansion at $\gamma_n = 0$, we have

$$n^{-1} l_n(\omega^0 + \gamma_n u) = n^{-1} l_n(\omega^0) + n^{-1} \gamma_n U(\omega^0)^\top u + (2n)^{-1} \gamma_n^2 u^\top \frac{\partial U(\omega^0)}{\partial \omega^0} u + A_n$$

$$
\begin{aligned}
A &= n^{-1} \left\{ l(\omega^0 + \gamma_n u) - l_n(\omega^0) \right\} \\
&= n^{-1} \gamma_n U(\omega^0)^\top u + (2n)^{-1} \gamma_n^2 u^\top \frac{\partial U(\omega^0)}{\partial \omega^0} u + A_n \\
&\triangleq A_1 + A_2 + A_n, \tag{16}
\end{aligned}
$$

where $A_n = (6n)^{-1} \sum_{j,k,l} (\omega_j - \omega_j^0)(\omega_k - \omega_k^0)(\omega_l - \omega_l^0)(\partial^2 U_l(\tilde{\omega})/\partial\omega_j\partial\omega_k)$, $U_l$ is the $l$-th component of $U$, and $\tilde{\omega}$ is a value between $\omega^0$ and $\omega = \omega^0 + \gamma_n u$. We first consider

$$U(\omega^0) = \sum_i \int_0^\tau \left\{ L_i - \frac{S_n^{(1)}(m_n^0, t)[L]}{S_n^{(0)}(m_n^0, t)} \right\} dN_i(t), \quad \text{where } m_n^0(R) = \alpha^{0\top} Z + \beta^{0\top} X.$$

Observe,

$$\sum_i \left\{ L_i - \frac{S_n^{(1)}(m_n^0, t)[L]}{S_n^{(0)}(m_n^0, t)} \right\} Y_i(t) \exp\left\{ \omega^\top L_i \right\} h_0(t)$$

$$= \sum_i \left\{ L_i - \frac{\sum_i L_i Y_i(t) \exp\left\{ \omega^\top L_i \right\}}{\sum_i Y_i(t) \exp\left\{ \omega^\top L_i \right\}} \right\} Y_i(t) \exp\left\{ \omega^\top L_i \right\} h_0(t)$$

$$= 0.$$

Since

$$M_i(t) = N_i(t) - \int_0^\tau Y_i(t) \exp\left\{ \omega^\top L_i \right\} h_0(t) dt,$$

this implies that,

$$U(\omega^0) = \sum_i \int_0^\tau \left\{ L_i - \frac{S_n^{(1)}(m_n^0, t)[L]}{S_n^{(0)}(m_n^0, t)} \right\} dM_i(t). \tag{17}$$

Similar to Lemma 5.3 of Huang [20], we have

$$P_{\Delta n} \left[ \frac{S_n^{(1)}(m_n^0, t)[L]}{S_n^{(0)}(m_n^0, t)} - \frac{S_n^{(1)}(m^0, t)[L]}{S_n^{(0)}(m^0, t)} \right] = P_\Delta \left[ \frac{s^{(1)}(m_n^0, t)[L]}{s^{(0)}(m_n^0, t)} - \frac{s^{(1)}(m^0, t)[L]}{s^{(0)}(m^0, t)} \right]$$

$$+ o_p(n^{-1/2}), \tag{18}$$

where $m^0(R) = \phi^0(W) + \beta^{0\top} X$. Let $s(m_n^0, t) = s^{(1)}(m_n^0, t)[L]/s^{(0)}(m_n^0, t)$ and $s(m^0, t) = s^{(1)}(m^0, t)[L]/s^{(0)}(m^0, t)$.

By Taylor series expansion, for some $\xi$ between $m^0$ and $m_n^0$ we have

$$s(m_n^0, t) - s(m^0, t) = \frac{\partial s(m^0, t)}{\partial m^0}(m_n^0 - m^0) + \frac{1}{2}\frac{\partial^2 s(\xi, t)}{\partial \xi^2}(m_n^0 - m^0)^2,$$

$$\left| s(m_n^0, t) - s(m^0, t) \right| \leq \left| \frac{\partial s(m^0, t)}{\partial m^0} d_0 \right| + \left| \frac{1}{2}\frac{\partial^2 s(\xi, t)}{\partial \xi^2} d_0^2 \right|,$$

where $d_0 = m_n^0 - m_0$. Let $W(t) = Y(t) \exp\left(m^0, t\right) / s^{(0)}(m^0, t)$. Then, by Lemma A.4 of Huang [20], we have

$$
\left| \frac{\partial s(m^0, t)}{\partial m^0} \, d_0 \right|^2 \leq |E\{W(t)h(R)d_0(R)\} - E\{W(t)h(R)\} \, E\{W(t)d_0(R)\}|^2
$$

$$
= |E[W(t)\{h(R) - E(W(t)h(R))\}\{d_0(R) - E(W(t)d_0(R))\}]|^2
$$

$$
= [E\{K_1 d_0(R) - K_1 E(K_2 d_0(R))\}]^2
$$

$$
\leq 2E\{K_1 d_0(R)\}^2 + 2E\{K_1 E(K_2 d_0(R))\}^2
$$

$$
\leq 2E\left\{K_1^2\right\} E\left\{d_0^2(R)\right\} + 2E\left\{K_3^2\right\} E\left\{d_0^2(R)\right\}
$$

$$
= K_4 E\left\{d_0^2(R)\right\}
$$

$$
= K_4 \|d_0\|^2
$$

$$
= K_4 \left\| m_n^0 - m_0 \right\|^2
$$

$$
= O_p\left(\left\| m_n^0 - m_0 \right\|^2\right).
$$

Therefore, from the approximation rate given in the beginning of the proof of Theorem 1, we have,

$$
\left| \frac{\partial s(m^0, t)}{\partial m^0} \, d_0 \right| \leq O_p\left(\left\| m_n^0 - m_0 \right\|\right) = O_p(K^{-d}).
$$

Similarly, using Lemma A.4 of Huang [20] gives us

$$
\left| \frac{1}{2} \frac{\partial^2 s(\xi, t)}{\partial \xi^2} \, d_0^2 \right| = O_p(K^{-2d}).
$$

Therefore, from (18) we have,

$$
P_{\Delta n}\left[ \frac{S_n^{(1)}(m_n^0, t)[L]}{S_n^{(0)}(m_n^0, t)} - \frac{S_n^{(1)}(m^0, t)[L]}{S_n^{(0)}(m^0, t)} \right] = O(K^{-d}) + o_p(n^{-1/2}) = O_p(K^{-d}).
$$

Consequent, from (17), we obtain

$$
U(\omega^0) = \sum_i \int_0^\tau \left\{ L_i - \frac{S_n^{(1)}(m^0, t)[L]}{S_n^{(0)}(m^0, t)} \right\} dM_i(t) + O_p\left(nK^{-d}\right)
$$

$$= \sum_i \int_0^\tau \left\{ L_i - G_n(m^0, t)[L] \right\} dM_i(t) + O_p\left(nK^{-d}\right)$$

$$= \xi_n + O_p(nK^{-d}),$$

where $\xi_n = \sum_i \int_0^\tau \left\{ L_i - G_n(m^0, t)[L] \right\} dM_i(t)$. Direct algebraic calculations show that, $E\left\{ \|\xi_n\|^2 \right\} = E\left\{ tr\left(\xi_n^\top \xi_n\right) \right\} = tr\left\{ E\left(\xi_n^\top \xi_n\right) \right\} = tr\left\{ E\left(\|\xi_n\|^2\right) \right\}$. Let

$$\xi_n = \sum_i \int_0^\tau \left\{ L_i - G_n(m^0, t)[L] \right\} dM_i(t) = \sum_i \int_0^\tau H_i(t) dM_i(t),$$

where $H_i(t) = \left\{ L_i - G_n(m^0, t)[L] \right\}$. Since $\xi_n$ is a martingale integral, we have $E(\xi_n|\mathcal{F}_t^-) = 0$, where $\mathcal{F}_t^-$ denotes the past up to the beginning of the small time interval $[t, t + dt)$, and

$$V(\xi_n|\mathcal{F}_t^-) = E(\xi_n^{\otimes 2}|\mathcal{F}_t^-)$$

$$= E(\xi_n \xi_n^\top|\mathcal{F}_t^-)$$

$$= E \sum_i \int_0^\tau \text{Var}\left\{ H_i(t) dM_i(t)|\mathcal{F}_t^- \right\}$$

$$= E \sum_i \int_0^\tau H_i(t)^{\otimes 2} d\langle M\rangle(t)$$

$$= E \int_0^\tau \sum_i \left\{ L_i - G_n(m^0, t)[L] \right\}^{\otimes 2} \Lambda_i(t) dt,$$

where $\Lambda_i(t) = h_0(t) Y_i(t) \exp\left\{ \phi^0(W) + X^\top \beta^0 \right\}$. We can show that

$$\sum_i \left\{ L_i - G_n(m^0, t)[L] \right\}^{\otimes 2} Y_i(t) \exp\left\{ m^0(R_i) \right\}$$

$$= \sum_i L_i^{\otimes 2} Y_i(t) \exp\left\{ m^0(R_i) \right\} - \sum_i G_n(m^0, t)[L]^{\otimes 2} Y_i(t) \exp\left\{ m^0(R_i) \right\}$$

$$\leq \sum_i L_i^{\otimes 2} Y_i(t) \exp\left\{ m^0(R_i) \right\}.$$

Then, $V(\xi_n|\mathcal{F}_t^-) \leq E \int_0^\tau \sum_i L_i^{\otimes 2} \Lambda_i(t) dt$. Assume $\sup_{t,W,X} |h_0(t) \exp\left\{ \phi^0(W) + \beta^{0\top} X \right\}| \leq \tilde{M}$. Therefore,

$$E\left\{\|\xi_n\|^2\right\} = \operatorname{tr}\left[E\left\{\int_0^\tau \sum_i \left(L_i - G_n(m^0, t)[L]\right)^{\otimes 2} \Lambda_i(t)dt\right\}\right]$$

$$\leq \tilde{M}\left[E\left\{\int_0^\tau \sum_i \left(L_i - G_n(m^0, t)[L]\right)^{\otimes 2} Y_i(t)dt\right\}\right]$$

$$\leq nE\left\{\operatorname{tr}L_i^{\otimes 2}Y_i(t)\right\}.$$

By condition (B4), we have,

$$\|\xi_n\| = O_p(\sqrt{n(K + p)}),$$

and

$$\left\|U(\omega^0)\right\| = O_p(\sqrt{n(K + p)} + nK^{-d}). \tag{19}$$

Consequently, from (16),

$$A_1 = \gamma_n O_p(\gamma_n) \|u\| = O_p(\gamma_n^2) \|u\|.$$

Next, for $A_2$, we already have,

$$U(\omega^0) = \sum_i \int_0^\tau \left\{L_i - \frac{S_n^{(1)}(m^0, t)[L]}{S_n^{(0)}(m^0, t)}\right\} dN_i(t)$$

$$+ O_p(nK^{-d}),$$

$$\frac{\partial U(\omega^0)}{\partial \omega^0} = -\sum_i \int_0^\tau \left[\frac{S_n^{(0)}(m^0, t)S_n^{(2)}(m^0, t)[L] - \left\{S_n^{(1)}(m^0, t)[L]\right\}^{\otimes 2}}{\left\{S_n^{(0)}(m^0, t)\right\}^2}\right] dN_i(t)$$

$$+ O_p(nK^{-d})$$

$$= -\sum_i \int_0^\tau V(m^0, t)[L] \{dM_i(t) + \lambda(t|L)dt\} + O_p(nK^{-d})$$

$$= -\left\{\sum_i \int_0^\tau V_n(m^0, t)[L]dM_i(t) + \sum_i \int_0^\tau V_n(m^0, t)[L]S_n^{(0)}(m^0, t)\lambda_0(t)dt\right\}$$

$$+ O_p(nK^{-d})$$

$$= -n\left(\vartheta_{\omega^0} + \Sigma_n\right) + O_p(nK^{-d}),$$

where $\vartheta_{\omega^0} = n^{-1}\sum_i \int_0^\tau V_n(m^0, t)[L]dM_i(t)$ and $\Sigma_n = n^{-1}\sum_i \int_0^\tau V_n(m^0, t)$ $[L]S^{(0)}(m^0, t)\lambda_0(t)dt$. Thus,

$$A_2 = -(1/2)\gamma_n^2 \left\{ u^\top \left( n^{-1} \frac{\partial U(\omega^0)}{\partial \omega^0} \right) u \right\}$$

$$= -(1/2)\gamma_n^2 \left[ u^\top \Sigma u + u^\top \left\{ (\Sigma_n - \Sigma) + \vartheta_{\omega^0} \right\} u + u^\top O(K^{-d}) u \right].$$

By Lemmas 2.3 and 4.1 of Bradic et al. [2],

$$\left\| (\Sigma_n - \Sigma) + \vartheta_{\omega^0} \right\| \le \| \Sigma_n - \Sigma \| + \left\| \vartheta_{\omega^0} \right\| = o_p(1).$$

Since $\Sigma$ is positive definite and its eigenvalues are bounded below by $O(1/K)$, we have,

$$A_2 = -(1/2)\gamma_n^2 (1/K + o_p(1) + O(K^{-d})) \|u\|^2.$$

Finally, since $\|\omega - \omega^0\|_2 \le \gamma_n$ and the average of i.i.d. terms, $n^{-1} \frac{\partial^2 U_l(\tilde{\omega})}{\partial \omega_j \partial \omega_k}$, is of order $O_p(1)$, by the Cauchy-Schwarz inequality and condition $\gamma_n (K+p)^{3/2} = O(1)$ from Theorem 1, we have $A_n = (K+p)^{3/2} O_p(\gamma_n^3) = O_p(\gamma_n^2)$.

For the penalty part, by Taylor expansion of the penalty function we have,

$$B = \sum_{g=1}^{s} \left\{ p_{\lambda_n}^{(g)} \left( |\beta_{g1}^0 + \gamma_n u_{2,g1}|, \ldots, |\beta_{gp_g}^0 + \gamma_n u_{2,gs_g}|, 0| \right) \right.$$

$$\left. - p_{\lambda_n}^{(g)} \left( |\beta_{g1}^0|, \ldots, |\beta_{gp_g}^0|, 0| \right) \right\}$$

$$= \sum_{g=1}^{s} \left\{ \sum_{j=1}^{s_g} \frac{\partial p_{\lambda_n}^{(g)} \left( |\beta_{g1}^0|, \ldots, |\beta_{gp_g}^0| \right)}{\partial |\beta_{gj}|} \mathrm{sgn}(\beta_{gj}^0) \gamma_n u_{2,gj} \right.$$

$$\left. + \frac{1}{2} \sum_{i=1}^{s_g} \sum_{j=1}^{s_g} \frac{\partial^2 p_{\lambda_n}^{(g)} \left( |\beta_{g1}^0|, \ldots, |\beta_{gPk}^0| \right)}{\partial |\beta_{gi}| \partial |\beta_{gj}|} \gamma_n^2 u_{2,gi} u_{2,gj} \right\}$$

$$+ o_p \left\{ \gamma_n^2 (u_{2,g1}^2 + \cdots + u_{2,gs_g}^2) \right\}$$

$$\le q_1^{1/2} a_n \gamma_n \|u_2\| + \frac{1}{2} \gamma_n^2 b_n \|u_2\|^2 + o_p(\gamma_n^2 \|u_2\|^2)$$

$$= q_1^{1/2} O_p(\gamma_n) \gamma_n \|u_2\| + o_p(\gamma_n^2 \|u_2\|^2) \quad \text{as} \quad b_n \to 0$$

$$= q_1^{1/2} O_p(\gamma_n^2) \|u_2\| + o_p(\gamma_n^2 \|u_2\|^2)$$

$$\triangleq B_1 + B_2,$$

where $q_1 = \sum_{g=1}^{s} s_g$.

We see that for fixed K, by choosing a sufficiently large $D$, $A_2$ dominates $A_1$, $A_n$, $B_1$, $B_2$ uniformly in $\|u\| = D$. Thus, we have shown that $\|\hat{\alpha} - \alpha^0\| + \|\hat{\beta} - \beta^0\| = O_p(\gamma_n)$. Then, $\|\hat{\phi} - \alpha^{0\top} B\| = O_p(\gamma_n)$ and $\|\hat{\beta} - \beta^0\| = O_p(\gamma_n)$. By $\|\phi^0 - \alpha^{0\top} B\|_\infty = O(K^{-d})$ and the triangle inequality, we have

$$\left\|\hat{\phi} - \phi^0\right\| \leq \left\|\hat{\phi} - \alpha^{0\top} B\right\| + \left\|\alpha^{0\top} B - \phi^0\right\|$$

$$= O_p(\gamma_n) + O(K^{-d})$$

$$= O_p(\gamma_n).$$

Hence, $\left\|\hat{\phi} - \phi^0\right\| + \left\|\hat{\beta} - \beta^0\right\| = O_p(\gamma_n)$.                                    □

*Proof of Theorem 2* Here we will prove the sparsity: $\Pr(\hat{\beta}_{\mathcal{D}} = 0) \to 1$ as $n \to \infty$. By Taylor expansion, we have

$$\frac{\partial Q_n(\hat{\alpha}, \hat{\beta})}{\partial \beta_{gj}} = n^{-1} \frac{\partial l_n(\hat{\alpha}, \beta^0)}{\partial \beta_{gj}} + \sum_{g', j'} n^{-1} \frac{\partial^2 l_n(\alpha^0, \beta^*)}{\partial \beta_{g'j'} \partial \beta_{gj}} (\hat{\beta}_{g'j'} - \beta^0_{g'j'})$$

$$- \frac{\partial p_{\lambda_n}^{(g)} \left( |\hat{\beta}_{g1}|, \ldots, |\hat{\beta}_{gp_g}| \right)}{\partial |\beta_{gj}|} \operatorname{sgn}(\hat{\beta}_{gj})$$

$$= C_1 + C_2 + C_3, \tag{20}$$

where $\beta^*$ lies between $\hat{\beta}$ and $\beta^0$. Using the result from (19), we have $|C_1| = O_p(\gamma_n)$. By the convergence rate in Theorem 1 and $n^{-1} \sum_{g', j'} \partial^2 l_n(\hat{\alpha}, \beta^*)/\partial \beta_{g'j'} \partial \beta_{gj} = O_p(1)$, we have $|\hat{\beta}_{g'j'} - \beta^0_{g'j'}| = O_p(\gamma_n)$. Thus, $|C_2| = O_p(\gamma_n)$. It follows from the definition of $\hat{\beta}_{gj}$ that, if $\hat{\beta}_{gj} \neq 0$,

$$\frac{\partial Q_n(\hat{\alpha}, \hat{\beta})}{\partial \beta_{gj}} = O_p(\gamma_n) + O_p(\gamma_n) - \frac{\partial p_{\lambda_n}^{(g)} \left( |\hat{\beta}_{g1}|, \ldots, |\hat{\beta}_{gp_g}| \right)}{\partial |\beta_{gj}|} \operatorname{sgn}(\hat{\beta}_{gj})$$

$$= \gamma_n \left\{ O_p(1) - \gamma_n^{-1} \frac{\partial p_{\lambda_n}^{(g)} \left( |\hat{\beta}_{g1}|, \ldots, |\hat{\beta}_{gp_g}| \right)}{\partial |\beta_{gj}|} \operatorname{sgn}(\hat{\beta}_{gj}) \right\}. \tag{21}$$

Next, we show that there is a contradiction in (21) if $\Pr\left\{ \beta^0_{\mathcal{D}} = 0 \right\}$ does not tend to 1 when $n \to \infty$, then there exist $(g, j) \in \mathcal{D}$, such that $\hat{\beta}_{gj} \neq 0$. By the condition given in Theorem 2, that is, $\gamma_n^{-1} \partial p_{\lambda_n}^{(g)} \left( |\hat{\beta}_{g1}|, \ldots, |\hat{\beta}_{gp_g}| \right) /\partial |\beta_{gj}| \to \infty$ with probability tending to 1 as $n \to \infty$, for an arbitrary $\epsilon > 0$, when $n$ is large we have

$$\frac{\partial Q_n(\hat{\alpha}, \hat{\beta})}{\partial \beta_{gj}} < 0, \ 0 < \hat{\beta}_{gj} < \epsilon, \quad \frac{\partial Q_n(\hat{\alpha}, \hat{\beta})}{\partial \beta_{gj}} > 0, \ -\epsilon < \hat{\beta}_{gj} < 0.$$

This is in conflict with $\partial Q_n(\hat{\alpha}, \hat{\beta})/\partial \beta_{gj} = 0$ and results in a contradiction when $\hat{\beta}_{gj} \neq 0$. Therefore, $\Pr(\hat{\beta}_{gj} = 0) \to 1$ as $n \to \infty$. $\qquad\square$

*Proof of Corollary 1* We only need to check that the conditions in Theorem 1 hold for the penalty function $p_{\lambda_n}^{(g)}(|\beta_{(g)}|) = \lambda_n(|\beta_{g1}| + \cdots + |\beta_{gp_g}|)^{1/2}$, $g = 1, \ldots, G$. For $\beta_{gj} \in \mathcal{A}$, i.e., $\beta_{gj}^0 \neq 0$, we have,

$$
\begin{aligned}
a_n &= \max_{(g,j)\in\mathcal{A}} \frac{\delta p_{\lambda_n}(|\beta_{g1}^0|, \ldots, |\beta_{gp_g}^0|)}{\delta|\beta_{gj}|} \\
&= \max_{(g,j)\in\mathcal{A}} \frac{\delta \lambda_n(|\beta_{g1}^0| + \cdots + |\beta_{gp_g}^0|)^{1/2}}{\delta|\beta_{gj}|} \\
&= \max_{(g,j)\in\mathcal{A}} \frac{1}{2}\lambda_n(|\beta_{g1}^0| + \cdots + |\beta_{gp_g}^0|)^{-1/2} \\
&\leq \frac{1}{2}\lambda_n M^{-1/2} = O_p(\gamma_n),
\end{aligned}
$$

and

$$
\begin{aligned}
b_n &= \max_{(g,j)\in\mathcal{A}} \left| \frac{\delta^2 p_{\lambda_n}(|\beta_{g1}^0|, \ldots, |\beta_{gp_g}^0|)}{\delta|\beta_{gj}|^2} \right| \\
&= \max_{(g,j)\in\mathcal{A}} \left| \frac{\delta^2 \lambda_n(|\beta_{g1}^0| + \cdots + |\beta_{gp_g}^0|)^{1/2}}{\delta|\beta_{gj}|^2} \right| \\
&= \max_{(g,j)\in\mathcal{A}} \frac{1}{4}\lambda_n(|\beta_{g1}^0| + \cdots + |\beta_{gp_g}^0|)^{-3/2} \\
&\leq \frac{1}{4}\lambda_n M^{-3/2} \to 0,
\end{aligned}
$$

where $M = \min_g(|\beta_{g1}^0| + \cdots + |\beta_{gp_g}^0|)$. Therefore, the rate of convergence follows from Theorem 1.

For sparsity, suppose there exists $(g, j) \in \mathcal{C}$ for which $\hat{\beta}_{gj} \neq 0$. Since for all $(g, j) \in \mathcal{C}$, $\beta_{gj}^0 = 0$; $j = 1, \ldots, p_g$, we have

$$\gamma_n^{-1}\frac{\partial p_{\lambda_n}\left(|\hat{\beta}_{g1}|, \ldots, |\hat{\beta}_{gp_g}|\right)}{\partial|\beta_{gj}|} = \gamma_n^{-1}\frac{\delta\lambda_n(|\hat{\beta}_{g1}| + \cdots + |\hat{\beta}_{gp_g}|)^{1/2}}{\delta|\beta_{gj}|}$$

$$= \frac{\gamma_n^{-1}\lambda_n}{2(|\hat{\beta}_{g1}| + \cdots + |\hat{\beta}_{gp_g}|)^{1/2}}.$$

According to the first conclusion of Corollary 1, there exists a $\gamma_n^{-1}$ consistent local maximizer $\hat{\beta} = (\hat{\beta}_{\mathcal{A}}^\top, \hat{\beta}_{\mathcal{B}}^\top, \hat{\beta}_{\mathcal{C}}^\top)^\top$ for the non-adaptive hierarchically penalized likelihood (9), which implies $\left\|\hat{\beta}_{\mathcal{C}} - \beta_{\mathcal{C}}^0\right\| \le M^*\gamma_n$ or for $\hat{\beta}_{gj} \ne 0$, we have $|\hat{\beta}_{gj} - \beta_{gj}^0| = |\hat{\beta}_{gj}| \le M^*\gamma_n$ for some constant $M^*$. Thus,

$$\frac{\gamma_n^{-1}\lambda_n}{2(|\hat{\beta}_{g1}| + \cdots + |\hat{\beta}_{gp_g}|)^{1/2}} \ge \frac{\gamma_n^{-1}\lambda_n}{2(M^*\gamma_n + \cdots + M^*\gamma_n)^{1/2}}$$

$$= \frac{1}{2M^{*1/2}} \times \frac{\gamma_n^{-1}\lambda_n\gamma_n^{-1/2}}{p_g^{1/2}}$$

$$\ge \frac{\gamma_n^{-3/2}\lambda_n p^{-1/2}}{2M^{*1/2}} \quad \text{(since } p \ge p_g\text{)}.$$

Therefore, for $\gamma_n^{-3/2}\lambda_n p^{-1/2} \to \infty$ when $n \to \infty$, we have, $\gamma_n^{-1}\delta\lambda_n(|\hat{\beta}_{g1}| + \cdots + |\hat{\beta}_{gp_g}|)^{1/2}/\delta|\beta_{gj}| \to \infty$, which results in a contradiction when $\hat{\beta}_{gj} \ne 0$. So, for all $(g, j) \in \mathcal{C}$, $\hat{\beta}_{gj} = 0$. □

*Proof of Theorem 3* We only need to check that the conditions in Theorem 1 hold for the penalty function $p_{\lambda_n}^{(g)}(|\beta_{(g)}|) = \lambda_n(w_{n,g1}|\beta_{g1}| + \cdots + w_{n,gp_g}|\beta_{gp_g}|)^{1/2}$.

For $\beta_{gj} \in \mathcal{A}$, i.e., $\beta_{gj}^0 \ne 0$, we have,

$$a_n = \max_{(g,j)\in\mathcal{A}} \frac{\delta p_{\lambda_n}(|\beta_{g1}^0|, \ldots, |\beta_{gp_g}^0|)}{\delta|\beta_{gj}|}$$

$$= \max_{(g,j)\in\mathcal{A}} \frac{\delta\lambda_n(w_{n,g1}|\beta_{g1}^0| + \cdots + w_{n,gp_g}|\beta_{gp_g}^0|)^{1/2}}{\delta|\beta_{gj}|}$$

$$= \max_{(g,j)\in\mathcal{A}} \frac{1}{2}\lambda_n w_{n,gj}(w_{n,g1}|\beta_{g1}^0| + \cdots + w_{n,gp_g}|\beta_{gp_g}^0|)^{-1/2}$$

$$\le \frac{1}{2}\lambda_n w_{n,\max}^{\mathcal{A}}\left(w_{n,\min}^{\mathcal{A}}\right)^{-1/2} M^{-1/2} = O_p(\gamma_n),$$

and

$$b_n = \max_{(g,j)\in\mathcal{A}} \left|\frac{\delta^2 p_{\lambda_n}(|\beta_{g1}^0|, \ldots, |\beta_{gp_g}^0|)}{\delta|\beta_{gj}|^2}\right|$$

$$
= \max_{(g,j)\in\mathcal{A}} \left| \frac{\delta^2 \lambda_n (w_{n,g1}|\beta_{g1}^0| + \cdots + w_{n,gp_g}|\beta_{gp_g}^0|)^{1/2}}{\delta|\beta_{gj}|^2} \right|
$$

$$
= \max_{(g,j)\in\mathcal{A}} \frac{1}{4}\lambda_n (w_{n,gj})^2 (w_{n,g1}|\beta_{g1}^0| + \cdots + w_{n,gp_g}|\beta_{gp_g}^0|)^{-3/2}
$$

$$
\leq \frac{1}{4}\lambda_n \left(w_{n,\max}^{\mathcal{A}}\right)^2 \left(w_{n,\min}^{\mathcal{A}}\right)^{-3/2} M^{-3/2} \to 0,
$$

where $M = \min_g(|\beta_{g1}^0| + \cdots + |\beta_{gp_g}^0|)$. Thus, the consistency follows from Theorem 1.

Next, we prove the sparsity. Assume $\hat{\beta}_{gj}$ is a local maximizer of $Q_n^w(\alpha, \beta)$ in (13) with $\left\| \hat{\beta}_{gj} - \beta_{gj}^0 \right\| = O_p(\gamma_n)$. We can find a constant $M^*$, such that $|\hat{\beta}_{gj}| \leq M^*$ for all $(g, j)$ with probability tending to 1. Then for $(g, j) \in \mathcal{D}$, i.e., $\beta_{gj}^0 = 0$, we have

$$
\gamma_n^{-1} \frac{\partial p_{\lambda_n}\left(|\hat{\beta}_{g1}|, \ldots, |\hat{\beta}_{gp_g}|\right)}{\partial|\beta_{gj}|} = \frac{\delta\lambda_n(w_{n,g1}|\hat{\beta}_{g1}| + \cdots + w_{n,gp_g}|\hat{\beta}_{gp_g}|)^{1/2}}{\delta|\beta_{gj}|}
$$

$$
= \frac{\gamma_n^{-1}\lambda_n w_{n,gj}}{2(w_{n,g1}|\hat{\beta}_{g1}| + \cdots + w_{n,gp_g}|\hat{\beta}_{gp_g}|)^{1/2}}
$$

$$
\geq \frac{\gamma_n^{-1}\lambda_n w_{n,\min}^{\mathcal{D}}}{2M^{*1/2}(w_{n,\max}^{\mathcal{A}} + w_{n,\max}^{\mathcal{D}})^{1/2}}.
$$

Therefore, when $\gamma_n^{-1}\lambda_n w_{n,\min}^{\mathcal{D}}/(w_{n,\max}^{\mathcal{A}} + w_{n,\max}^{\mathcal{D}})^{1/2} \to \infty$ as $n \to \infty$, then $\hat{\beta}_{gj} = 0$ with probability approaching to 1, and by Theorem 2, we have $\Pr(\hat{\beta}_{\mathcal{D}} = 0) \to 1$. $\square$

*Proof of Corollary 2* We only need to verify that $w_{n,gj} = |\tilde{\beta}_{n,gj}|^{-r}$ satisfy the conditions in Theorem 3. Let $A = \max_{g,j}\left\{\beta_{gj}^0\right\}$ and $B = \min_{g,j}\left\{\beta_{gj}^0 : \beta_{gj}^0 \neq 0\right\}$. Then by the consistency of $\tilde{\beta}_n$, $w_{n,\max}^{\mathcal{A}} \to B^{-r}$ and $w_{n,\min}^{\mathcal{A}} \to A^{-r}$. Thus, if $\lambda_n = \gamma_n/\log(n)$, we have $\gamma_n^{-1}\lambda_n w_{n,\max}^{\mathcal{A}}\left(w_{n,\min}^{\mathcal{A}}\right)^{-1/2} \to 0$ and $\lambda_n\left(w_{n,\max}^{\mathcal{A}}\right)^2\left(w_{n,\min}^{\mathcal{A}}\right)^{-3/2} \to 0$, as $n \to \infty$.

For each $(g, j)$ with $\beta_{n,gj}^0 = 0$, we have $\tilde{\beta}_{gj} = O_p(\gamma_n)$. Therefore, $w_{n,\min}^{\mathcal{D}}/(w_{n,\max}^{\mathcal{A}} + w_{n,\max}^{\mathcal{D}})^{1/2} = O_p(\gamma_n^{-1/2})$. Thus, for $\lambda_n = \gamma_n/\log(n)$, we have $\gamma_n^{-1}\lambda_n w_{n,\min}^{\mathcal{D}}/(w_{n,\max}^{\mathcal{A}} + w_{n,\max}^{\mathcal{D}})^{1/2} \to \infty$. $\square$

*Proof of Theorem 4* Given that $\hat{\beta}_{\mathcal{C}} = 0$ with probability tending to 1, the proof of asymptotic normality of $\hat{\beta}_{\mathcal{A}}$ is similar to that of Theorem 2 in [19], we omit the details. $\square$

# References

1. Bassendine, M., Collins, J., Stephenson, J., Saunders, P., & James, O. (1985). Platelet associated immunoglobulins in primary biliary cirrhosis: A cause of thrombocytopenia? *Gut, 26*(10),1074–1079.
2. Bradic, J., Fan, J., & Jiang, J. (2011). Regularization for Cox's proportional hazards model with NP-dimensionality. *The Annals of Statistics, 39*(6), 3092–3120.
3. Breheny, P. (2015). The group exponential lasso for bi-level variable selection. *Biometrics, 71*(3), 731–740.
4. Breheny, P., & Huang, J. (2009). Penalized methods for bi-level variable selection. *Statistics and Its Interface, 2*(3), 369–380.
5. Breiman, L. (1995). Better subset regression using the nonnegative garrote. *Technometrics, 37*(4), 373–384.
6. Cheng, G., & Wang, X. (2011). Semiparametric additive transformation model under current status data. *Electronic Journal of Statistics, 5*, 1735–1764.
7. Cox, D. R. (1972). Regression models and life-tables. *Journal of the Royal Statistical Society. Series B (Methodological), 34*(2), 187–220.
8. Cui, X., Peng, H., Wen, S., & Zhu, L. (2013). Component selection in the additive regression model. *Scandinavian Journal of Statistics, 40*(3), 491–510.
9. De Boor, C. (1978). *A practical guide to splines* (Vol. 27). New York: Springer.
10. Dickson, E. R., Grambsch, P. M., Fleming, T. R., Fisher, L. D., & Langworthy, A. (1989). Prognosis in primary biliary cirrhosis: Model for decision making. *Hepatology, 10*(1), 1–7.
11. Du, P., Ma, S., & Liang, H. (2010). Penalized variable selection procedure for Cox models with semiparametric relative risk. *The Annals of Statistics, 38*(4), 2092–2117.
12. Fan, J., Gijbels, I., & King, M. (1997). Local likelihood and local partial likelihood in hazard regression. *The Annals of Statistics, 25*(4), 1661–1690.
13. Fan, J., & Li, R. (2001). Variable selection via nonconcave penalized likelihood and its oracle properties. *Journal of the American Statistical Association, 96*(456), 1348–1360.
14. Fan, J., & Li, R. (2002). Variable selection for Cox's proportional hazards model and frailty model. *The Annals of Statistics, 30*(1), 74–99.
15. Fang, K., Wang, X., Zhang, S., Zhu, J., & Ma, S. (2015). Bi-level variable selection via adaptive sparse group lasso. *Journal of Statistical Computation and Simulation, 85*(13), 2750–2760.
16. Frank, L. E., & Friedman, J. H. (1993). A statistical view of some chemometrics regression tools. *Technometrics, 35*(2), 109–135.
17. Gray, R. J. (1992). Flexible methods for analyzing survival data using splines, with applications to breast cancer prognosis. *Journal of the American Statistical Association, 87*(420), 942–951.
18. Gui, J., & Li, H. (2005). Penalized Cox regression analysis in the high-dimensional and low-sample size settings, with applications to microarray gene expression data. *Bioinformatics, 21*(13), 3001–3008.
19. Hu, Y., & Lian, H. (2013). Variable selection in a partially linear proportional hazards model with a diverging dimensionality. *Statistics & Probability Letters, 83*(1), 61–69.
20. Huang, J. (1999). Efficient estimation of the partly linear additive Cox model. *The Annals of Statistics, 27*(5), 1536–1563.
21. Huang, J., Horowitz, J. L., & Wei, F. (2010). Variable selection in nonparametric additive models. *The Annals of Statistics, 38*(4), 2282–2313.
22. Huang, J., Liu, L., Liu, Y., & Zhao, X. (2014). Group selection in the Cox model with a diverging number of covariates. *Statistica Sinica, 24*(4), 1787–1810.
23. Huang, J., Ma, S., Xie, H., & Zhang, C.-H. (2009). A group bridge approach for variable selection. *Biometrika, 96*(2), 339–355.
24. Kai, B., Li, R., & Zou, H. (2011). New efficient estimation and variable selection methods for semiparametric varying-coefficient partially linear models. *The Annals of Statistics, 39*(1), 305–332.

25. Kanehisa, M., & Goto, S. (2000). Kegg: Kyoto encyclopedia of genes and genomes. *Nucleic Acids Research, 28*(1), 27–30.
26. Kim, J., Sohn, I., Jung, S.-H., Kim, S., & Park, C. (2012). Analysis of survival data with group lasso. *Communications in Statistics-Simulation and Computation, 41*(9), 1593–1605.
27. Kubota, J., Ikeda, F., Terada, R., Kobashi, H., Fujioka, S.-i., Okamoto, R., et al. (2009). Mortality rate of patients with asymptomatic primary biliary cirrhosis diagnosed at age 55 years or older is similar to that of the general population. *Journal of Gastroenterology, 44*(9), 1000–1006.
28. Lian, H., Li, J., & Tang, X. (2014). Scad-penalized regression in additive partially linear proportional hazards models with an ultra-high-dimensional linear part. *Journal of Multivariate Analysis, 125,* 50–64.
29. Liang, H., & Li, R. (2009). Variable selection for partially linear models with measurement errors. *Journal of the American Statistical Association, 104*(485), 234–248.
30. Liu, J., Zhang, R., & Zhao, W. (2014). Hierarchically penalized additive hazards model with diverging number of parameters. *Science China Mathematics, 57*(4), 873–886.
31. Lv, J., Yang, H., & Guo, C. (2016). Variable selection in partially linear additive models for modal regression. http://dx.doi.org/10.1080/03610918.2016.1171346
32. Ma, S., & Du, P. (2012). Variable selection in partly linear regression model with diverging dimensions for right censored data. *Statistica Sinica, 22*(3), 1003–1020.
33. Ma, S., & Huang, J. (2007). Combining clinical and genomic covariates via Cov-TGDR. *Cancer Informatics, 3,* 371–378.
34. Ma, S., Song, X., & Huang, J. (2007). Supervised group lasso with applications to microarray data analysis. *BMC Bioinformatics, 8*(60), 1–17.
35. Ni, X., Zhang, H. H., & Zhang, D. (2009). Automatic model selection for partially linear models. *Journal of Multivariate Analysis, 100*(9), 2100–2111.
36. O'Sullivan, F. (1993). Nonparametric estimation in the Cox model. *The Annals of Statistics, 21*(1), 124–145.
37. Park, M. Y., & Hastie, T. (2007). L1-regularization path algorithm for generalized linear models. *Journal of the Royal Statistical Society: Series B (Statistical Methodology), 69*(4), 659–677.
38. Shen, X., & Ye, J. (2002). Adaptive model selection. *Journal of the American Statistical Association, 97*(457), 210–221.
39. Simon, N., Friedman, J., Hastie, T., & Tibshirani, R. (2011). Regularization paths for Cox's proportional hazards model via coordinate descent. *Journal of Statistical Software, 39*(5), 1–13.
40. Simon, N., Friedman, J., Hastie, T., & Tibshirani, R. (2013). A sparse-group lasso. *Journal of Computational and Graphical Statistics, 22*(2), 231–245.
41. Talwalkar, J. A., & Lindor, K. D. (2003). Primary biliary cirrhosis. *The Lancet, 362*(9377), 53–61.
42. Tibshirani, R. (1997). The lasso method for variable selection in the Cox model. *Statistics in Medicine, 16*(4), 385–395.
43. Wang, L., Liu, X., Liang, H., & Carroll, R. J. (2011). Estimation and variable selection for generalized additive partial linear models. *The Annals of Statistics, 39*(4), 1827–1851.
44. Wang, S., Nan, B., Zhu, N., & Zhu, J. (2009). Hierarchically penalized Cox regression with grouped variables. *Biometrika, 96*(2), 307–322.
45. Xia, X., & Yang, H. (2016). Variable selection for partially time-varying coefficient error-in-variables models. *Statistics, 50*(2), 278–297.
46. Xie, H., & Huang, J. (2009). Scad-penalized regression in high-dimensional partially linear models. *The Annals of Statistics, 37*(2), 673–696.
47. Yang, J., Lu, F., & Yang, H. (2017). Quantile regression for robust estimation and variable selection in partially linear varying-coefficient models. http://dx.doi.org/10.1080/02331888.2017.1314482

48. Yuan, M., & Lin, Y. (2006). Model selection and estimation in regression with grouped variables. *Journal of the Royal Statistical Society: Series B (Statistical Methodology), 68*(1), 49–67.
49. Yuan, M., & Lin, Y. (2007). On the non-negative garrotte estimator. *Journal of the Royal Statistical Society: Series B (Statistical Methodology), 69*(2), 143–161.
50. Zhang, H. H., & Lu, W. (2007). Adaptive lasso for Cox's proportional hazards model. *Biometrika, 94*(3), 691–703.
51. Zhao, P., & Xue, L. (2010). Variable selection for semiparametric varying coefficient partially linear errors-in-variables models. *Journal of Multivariate Analysis, 101*(8), 1872–1883.
52. Zhao, P., & Yu, B. (2006). On model selection consistency of lasso. *Journal of Machine Learning Research, 7*, 2541–2563.
53. Zhou, N., & Zhu, J. (2010). Group variable selection via a hierarchical lasso and its oracle property. *Statistics and Its Interface, 3*(4), 557–574.
54. Zou, H. (2006). The adaptive lasso and its oracle properties. *Journal of the American Statistical Association, 101*(476), 1418–1429.
55. Zou, H. (2008). A note on path-based variable selection in the penalized proportional hazards model. *Biometrika, 95*(1), 241–247.

# Inference of Transition Probabilities in Multi-State Models Using Adaptive Inverse Probability Censoring Weighting Technique

Ying Zhang and Mei-Jie Zhang

**Abstract** Inverse probability censoring weighting (IPCW) technique is often used to adjust for right censoring or recover information for censored individuals in survival analysis and in multi-state modeling. A simple IPCW (SIPCW) technique which does not consider the intermediate states, has been proposed for analyzing multi-state data. However, our simulation studies show that the SIPCW technique may lead to biased estimates when being applied in complex multi-state models. We thereby propose a model-specific, state-dependent adaptive IPCW (AIPCW) technique for estimating transition probabilities in multi-state models. Intensive simulation results verified that the proposed AIPCW technique improves the accuracy of transition probability estimates compared to the SIPCW technique and leads to asymptotic unbiased estimates. We applied the proposed technique to a real-world hematopoietic stem cell transplant (HSCT) data to assess the acute and chronic graft-versus-host disease (GVHD) effects on disease relapse rates and mortality rates.

**Keywords** Inverse probability censoring weighting · IPCW · Probability · Stem cells · Stem cell transplant · Graft-versus-host disease · AIPCW

## 1 Introduction

Multi-state models are often used to analyze complicated event history data, where the health history for the $i$th individual are represented by $\{\Gamma_i(t), t \geq 0\}$ which gives the state for the $i$th individual at time $t$, and the final states are represented by $\delta_i =$

Y. Zhang (✉)
Merck & Co., Kenilworth, NJ, USA
e-mail: ying.zhang25@merck.com

M.-J. Zhang
Medical College of Wisconsin, Milwaukee, WI, USA
e-mail: meijie@mcw.edu

© Springer Nature Switzerland AG 2020
Y. Zhao, D.-G. (Din) Chen (eds.), *Statistical Modeling in Biomedical Research*, Emerging Topics in Statistics and Biostatistics,
https://doi.org/10.1007/978-3-030-33416-1_19

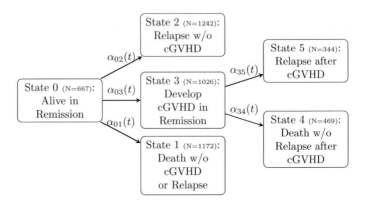

**Fig. 1** Events after HSCT in a three-level six-state model

$\Gamma_i(\infty)$. The transition intensities $\alpha_{hj}(t)$ represent the instantaneous risk of moving from state $h$ to state $j$ at time $t$, and the transition probabilities are $P_{hj}(s, t) = P\{\Gamma(t) = j | \Gamma(s) = h\}$, for $s \leq t$. States can be either transient or absorbing, if no transitions can emerge from the state (for example, death). Our motivation for this study is to gain insights into the effect of GVHD on clinical outcomes after HSCT for leukemia patients. Although HSCT is a life-saving procedure for many cancer patients, GVHD after HSCT is one of the major causes of treatment-related mortality. On the other hand, GVHD may have beneficial graft-verse-leukemia (GVL) effect which helps to reduce the cancer relapse rate. Clinically, it is critical to estimate and summarize the clinical outcomes with and without GVHD. The clinical outcomes after HSCT can be described with multi-state models. For example, the data from an allogeneic HSCT study [11] can be represented by a three-level six-state model (see Fig. 1): Patients who undergo transplantation for hematological malignancies may experience death (State 1) or relapse (State 2) before developing chronic GVHD (cGVHD) (State 3), or experience death (State 4) or relapse (State 5) after the occurrence of cGVHD. Moreover, investigators can always construct the model as needed depending on their research interests. For instance, researchers may be interested in investigating the effects of both acute GVHD (aGVHD) and cGVHD on treatment-related mortality and relapse rate. In such a case, a four-level twelve-state model can be employed to model aGVHD and cGVHD effects separately (see Fig. 2).

The non-cyclical and non-reversible multi-state models are considered in this study. The standard approach to estimating transition probabilities is the product-integral method which estimates all transition intensities based on Nelson-Aalen estimates [1, 12, 13] and then combines them into transition probabilities by product integration of the transition intensities [2]. Recently, Datta and Satten [6, 7] showed that the Aalen and Johansen [2] product limit estimator of transition probabilities is valid for non-Markov models as well as under state-dependent censoring. Andersen et al. [3] provided the estimates for the variance and covariances of

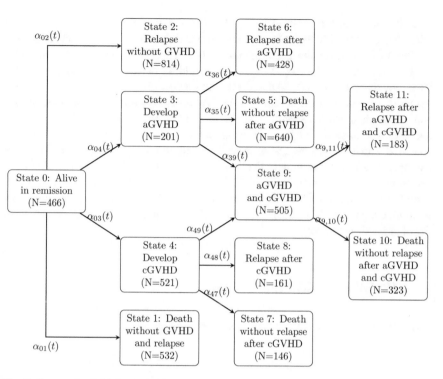

**Fig. 2** Events after HSCT in a four-level twelve-state model

transition probabilities. The variance estimates are relatively complicated, especially when being used to estimate the variances of composite endpoints [10].

Recently, Scheike and Zhang [15] and Scheike et al. [16] considered an alternative approach for estimating and modelling all the transition probabilities based on binomial outcomes using IPCW technique. The key with their approach is to adjust the binomial responses by the corresponding censoring distributions which are estimated by the Kaplan-Meier estimators assuming they are independent of covariates. To estimate the censoring distributions used in the weighting process, Scheike and Zhang [15] considered individuals in all transient states at the end of study as censored individuals. We refer their approach as simple IPCW (SIPCW) technique. However, they pointed out the estimated transition probabilities are not identical to the standard product-integral estimates, and the estimated transition probabilities do not add up to 1. Our simulation studies also showed that the transition probabilities estimates based on the SIPCW technique can be severely biased. Scheike and Zhang [15] suggested to consider state-dependent censoring weighting approaches, but without a detailed study of the potential bias introduced by the SIPCW technique.

In this work, we adopted their idea of state-dependent censoring and proposed using an adaptive IPCW (AIPCW) technique to estimate the transition probabilities directly for non-Markov models which takes the model structures into account when being applied to estimate the censoring distributions. We conduct simulation studies to investigate the performance of our proposed method. The simulation studies indicate that the SIPCW estimates could be biased for complicated multi-state models, and the AIPCW-based estimates are virtually unbiased. In Sect. 2, we demonstrate how to construct such an AIPCW for estimating transition probabilities and derive their variance estimators. Since the construction of AIPCW is model-specific, we chose to illustrate the construction procedure in two models that we specified above (Fig. 1 as an example for a three-level model and Fig. 2 as an example for a four-level model). Section 3 includes summaries of simulation studies for comparing the performance of AIPCW with SIPCW, and for evaluating the overall performance of the AIPCW technique. In Sect. 4, we apply the proposed method to the real HSCT data [11]. Finally, Sect. 5 concludes this work and presents the planned future works.

## 2 AIPCW in Multi-State Models

The SIPCW technique estimates the transition probability to absorbing state $k$ by

$$\widehat{P}_{0k}(0, t) = \widehat{F}_k^{\text{SIPCW}}(t) = \frac{1}{n} \sum_{i=1}^{n} \frac{I(T_i \leq t, \Gamma_i(t) = k)}{\widehat{G}_C(T_i)},$$

where $T_i$ is the observed time and $1/\{n\widehat{G}_C(T_i)\}$ is the weight carried by individual $i$ at time $t$. The SIPCW technique combines all transient states and calculates the censoring survival distributions $G_C(t)$ by Kaplan-Meier estimators where individuals in all transient states by the end of study are treated as censored (see Fig. 3). Although the calculation is simple, the SIPCW approach fails to consider

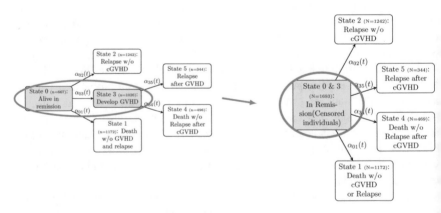

**Fig. 3** Illustrate simple IPCW technique for estimating censoring distributions

the complex transition paths and will lead to biased estimates: Since the HSCT model is not reversible, the transition probability of $P_{03}(t)$ can be considered as a competing event when we estimate $P_{01}(t)$ and $P_{02}(t)$, thus individuals who have already entered state 3 are no longer in the 'risk set' in estimating the censoring weight and should not be considered as censored.

Thus, we propose the AIPCW technique where the censoring distributions are model- and state-dependent, to potentially reduce the bias introduced by the SIPCW technique. The states of multi-state models can be categorized into distinct levels according to their transition paths and the number of states traveled. For instance, the six-state multi-state model can be dissected into three levels: level I is 'being alive' at state 0, level II is staying in state 1, 2, or 3, and level III is entered states 4 and 5. The key with the AIPCW approach is to estimate the censoring distributions distinctively for individuals at different levels of states, since their risk sets are different.

The AIPCW weights are derived based on the following conditional probabilities, which is essential to achieve asymptotic unbiased estimators: $E\{R_{i,k}(t)/W_{i,k}(t)\} = P_{0k}(t)$, where $R_{i,k}(t)$ is the indicator of individual $i$ being in state $k$ at time $t$, and $W_{i,k}(t)$ is the state- and time-dependent weight function corresponding to individual $i$. When the weight function $W_{i,k}(t)$ is known, the transition probability $P_{0k}(t)$ can be estimated by $\sum_i R_{i,k}(t)/n W_{i,k}(t)$. Thus individual $i$ carries a weight of $1/\{n W_{i,k}(t)\}$ at time $t$ if $R_{i,k}(t) = 1$.

Since the AIPCW weights depend on the model and the states of interests, there is no general formula for estimating the weights. Therefore, we focused on illustrating the construction of the AIPCW technique in a three-level model (see Fig. 1) using the six-state HSCT model as an example, and briefly extended the AIPCW technique to a four-level model (see Fig. 2), and similar weighting technique can be extended to a more complicated higher level multi-state model.

## 2.1   Estimate Transition Probabilities For a Three-Level Model

Let $C_i$ denote the censoring time, $T_{i,k}^*$ denote the transition time to state $k$ and assume $C_i$ to be independent of $\Gamma_i(t)$. Let $T_{i,123}^* = (T_{i,1}^* \wedge T_{i,2}^* \wedge T_{i,3}^*)$ for $\delta_i \geq 1$. For $\delta_i = 0$, set $T_{i,123}^* = C_i$ , which is the end of follow-up time. The transition probability $P_{0k}(0, t)$ can be estimated by

$$\widehat{P}_{0k}^{\text{AIPCW}}(0, t) = \frac{1}{n} \sum_{i=1}^{n} \frac{R_{i,k}(t)}{\widehat{G}_{C_{00}}(T_{i,123}^*)}, \tag{1}$$

where $R_{i,0}(t) = I(\Gamma_i(t) = 0)I(C_i > t)$, $R_{i,k}(t) = I(T_{i,k}^* \leq t, \Gamma_i(T_{i,k}^*) = k)I(C_i > T_{i,k}^*)$ for $k = 1, 2$, and the censoring survival distribution $G_{C_{00}}$ is estimated by a Kaplan-Meier estimator using observations $I\{(C_i \wedge T_{i,123}^*), \Delta_{C_{00},i} = I(C_i \leq T_{i,123}^*), i = 1, \ldots, n\}$. Zhang et al. [17] showed that $\widehat{P}_{0k}^{\text{AIPCW}}(0, t)$ is identical to the corresponding Kaplan-Meier estimator for $k = 0$ and is identical to the Aalen-Johansen estimator for $k = 1, 2$.

For $k = 3$, $P_{03}(0, t)$ is the probability of being in state 3 at time $t$. Let $T^*_{i,45} = (T^*_{i,4} \wedge T^*_{i,5})$ for $\delta_i \geq 4$ and $T^*_{i,45} = C_i$ for $\delta_i = 3$. Individuals in state 3 are censored if $\{\delta_i \geq 3, T^*_{i,3} \leq C_i < T^*_{i,45}\}$. The indicator of being in state 3 at time $t$ is

$$R_{i,3}(t) = I(\Gamma_i(t) \in \{3\})I(C_i > t) = I(T^*_{i,3} \leq t < T^*_{i,45}, \delta_i \geq 3)I(C_i > t)$$

$$= I(T^*_{i,3} \leq t < T^*_{i,45}, \delta_i \geq 3)I(T^*_{i,3} \leq t < C_i, \delta_i \geq 3).$$

Since $E\{I(T^*_{i,3} \leq t < T^*_{i,45}, \delta_i \geq 3)\} = P_{03}(0, t)$ and

$$E\{I(T^*_{i,3} \leq t < C_i, \delta_i \geq 3)\} = E[E\{I(T^*_{i,3} \leq t < C_i, \delta_i \geq 3)|T^*_{i,3} \leq t, \delta_i \geq 3\}]$$

$$= E[(C_i > T^*_{i,3}, \delta_i \geq 3)E\{I(C_i > t)|T^*_{i,3} \leq t, \delta_i \geq 3\}]$$

$$= G_{C_{00}}(T^*_{i,3})G_{C_{33}}(t),$$

where $T^*_{i,3}$ is observed only when $\delta_i \geq 3$. We can estimate $P_{03}(0, t)$ by:

$$\widehat{P}^{\text{AIPCW}}_{03}(0, t) = \frac{1}{n}\sum_{i=1}^{n}\frac{R_{i,3}(t)}{\widehat{G}_{C_{00}}(T^*_{i,3})\widehat{G}_{C_{33}}(t)}. \tag{2}$$

We can understand this estimator from a redistribution-to-the-right (RTR) perspective where individuals in state 3 at time $t$ carry a weight of $1/\{nG_{C_{00}}(T^*_{i,3}) G_{C_{33}}(t)\}$. Individuals with $I(T^*_{i,3} \leq t, \delta_i \geq 3)$ carry initial weights of $w^3_i = 1/\{n\widehat{G}_{C_{00}}(T^*_{i,3})\}$ when they enter state 3 at time $T^*_{i,3}$ and the subsequent conditional censoring probability $G_{C_{33}}(t) = P(C_i > t|T^*_{i,3} \leq t, \delta_i \geq 3)$ can be estimated by

$$\widehat{G}_{C_{33}}(t) = \prod_{v \leq t}\left\{1 - \frac{dN^{C_{33}}_{\bullet}(v)}{Y^{C_{33}}_{\bullet}(v)}\right\},$$

where

$$N^{C_{33}}_{\bullet}(v) = \sum_{i=1}^{n}N^{C_{33}}_i(v) = \sum_{i=1}^{n}I(T^*_{i,45} \leq v, \delta_i = 3)w^3_i$$

$$Y^{C_{33}}_{\bullet}(v) = \sum_{i=1}^{n}Y^{C_{33}}_i(v) = \sum_{i=1}^{n}I(T^*_{i,3} \leq v \leq T^*_{i,45}, \delta_i \geq 3)w^3_i.$$

Similarly, the indicators of being in state 4 or 5 at time $t$ are

$$R_{i,k}(t) = I(T^*_{i,45} \leq t, \delta_i = k)I(C_i > T^*_{i,45}) = I(T^*_{i,45} \leq t, \delta_i = k)I(T^*_{i,3} \leq t, C_i >$$

$$T^*_{i,45}, \delta_i \geq 3)$$

$$E\{I(T^*_{i,3} \leq t, C_i > T^*_{i,45}, \delta_i \geq 3)\} = G_{C_{00}}(T^*_{i,3})G_{C_{33}}(T^*_{i,45})$$

The weights carried by those individuals when they enter state 4 or 5 at time $T^*_{i,45}$ are $1/\{nG_{C_{00}}(T^*_{i,3})G_{C_{33}}(T^*_{i,45})\}$. Thus we estimate of $P_{0k}(0, t)$ by:

$$\widehat{P}^{AIPCW}_{0k}(0, t) = \frac{1}{n}\sum_{i=1}^{n} \frac{R_{i,k}(t)}{\widehat{G}_{C_{00}}(T^*_{i,3})\widehat{G}_{C_{33}}(T^*_{i,45})}, \quad \text{for } k = 4, 5. \tag{3}$$

Under regularity conditions [8, 9, 15], it can be shown that

$$\sqrt{n}\left\{\widehat{P}^{AIPCW}_{0k}(0, t) - P_{0k}(0, t)\right\} = n^{-1/2}\sum_{i} W_{i,0k}(t) + o_P(1),$$

which converges in distribution to a mean zero Gaussian process with asymptotic variance that can be estimated by

$$\widehat{\Sigma}_{0k}(t) = n^{-1}\sum_{i}\left\{\widehat{W}_{i,0k}(t)\right\}^2,$$

where explicit expressions for $W_{i,0k}(t)$ and $\widehat{W}_{i,0k}(t)$ can be found in the Appendix. The variance estimators contain two parts: the first part is from the transition probability estimator itself as if the censoring distributions are known; the second part is from the uncertainty of the estimated censoring distributions. In most of our simulation settings, the second part is negligible.

## 2.2   Estimate Transition Probabilities For a Four-Level Model

If we are interested in estimating $P_{0,10}(0, t)$ or $P_{0,11}(0, t)$, and if we are interested in estimating all transition probabilities simultaneously, we need to derive the AIPCW technique for a four-level model (Fig. 2). In this section, we only illustrate the AIPCW estimators for the fourth-level transition probabilities $P_{0k}(0, t), k = 9, 10, 11$, because other transition probabilities can be estimated analogous to a three-level model.

Let $T^*_{i,L_4} = (T^*_{i,10} \wedge T^*_{i,11})$ for $\delta_i \geq 10$ and $T_{i,L_4} = C_i$ for $\delta_i = 9$. Let $\eta_{i,3}$ and $\eta_{i,4}$ be the indicators of transiting from state 3 and 4 respectively. For $k = 9$, the binary outcomes of subject $i$ entered and remaining in state 9 at time $t$ are

$$R_{i,9}(t) = I\{\Gamma_i(t) \in 9\}I\{C_i > t\} = I\{T^*_{i,9} \leq t < T^*_{i,L_4}, \delta_i \geq 9\}I\{C_i > t\}$$

$$= I\{T^*_{i,9} \leq t < (T^*_{i,L_4} \wedge C_i), \delta_i \geq 9\}$$

$$= R_{i,39}(t) + R_{i,49}(t),$$

where $R_{i,s9}(t) = I\{\Gamma_i(t) \in 9, \eta_{i,s} = 1\}I\{C_i > t\}$ for $s = 3, 4$.

Individuals entered in state 9 carry initial weights of $w_{i;9,3} = 1/\{n\widehat{G}_{C_{00}}(T^*_{i,3})$ $\widehat{G}_{C_{33}}(T^*_{i,9})\}$ if they enter from 3, and $w_{i;9,4} = 1/\{n\widehat{G}_{C_{00}}(T^*_{i,4})\widehat{G}_{C_{44}}(T^*_{i,9})\}$ if they enter from 4. Let $G_{C_{99,s}}(t)$ for $s = 3, 4$ be the conditional censoring process in state 9, so $G_{C_{99,s}}(t) = P\{C_i > t | (T^*_{i,9} \leq t, \delta_i \geq 9, \eta_{i,s} = 1)\}$ and the Kaplan-Meier estimate for $G_{C_{99,s}}(t)$ can be written as

$$\widehat{G}_{C_{99,s}}(t) = \prod_{v \leq t} \left\{ 1 - \frac{dN_\bullet^{C_{99,s}}(v)}{Y_\bullet^{C_{99,s}}(v)} \right\}$$

where

$$N_\bullet^{C_{99,s}}(v) = \sum_{i=1}^n N_i^{C_{99,s}}(v) = \sum_{i=1}^n I(T^*_{i,L_4} \leq v, \delta_i = 9, \eta_{i,s} = 1)w_{i;9,s}$$

$$Y_\bullet^{C_{99,s}}(v) = \sum_{i=1}^n Y_i^{C_{99,s}}(v) = \sum_{i=1}^n I(T^*_{i,9} \leq v \leq T^*_{i,L_4}, \delta_i \geq 9, \eta_{i,s} = 1)w_{i;9,s}$$

The censoring distributions are $\{G_{C_{00}}(T^*_{i,3})G_{C_{33}}(T^*_{i,9})G_{C_{99,3}}(t)\}$ for individuals who enter in state 9 from state 3, and $\{G_{C_{00}}(T^*_{i,4})G_{C_{44}}(T^*_{i,9})G_{C_{99,4}}(t)\}$ for individuals who enter state 9 from state 4. The transition probabilities to state 9 can be estimated by

$$\widehat{P}^{\text{AIPCW}}_{09}(0, t) = \frac{1}{n} \sum_{i=1}^n \left\{ \frac{R_{i,39}(t)}{\widehat{G}_{C_{00}}(T^*_{i,3})\widehat{G}_{C_{33}}(T^*_{i,9})\widehat{G}_{C_{99,3}}(t)} \right.$$
$$\left. + \frac{R_{i,49}(t)}{\widehat{G}_{C_{00}}(T^*_{i,4})\widehat{G}_{C_{44}}(T^*_{i,9})\widehat{G}_{C_{99,4}}(t)} \right\}$$

For $k = 10, 11, s = 3, 4$, the binary outcomes are also specified according to their transition paths:

$$R_{i,sk}(t) = I\{T^*_{i,L_4} \leq t, \eta_{i,s} = 1, \delta_i = k\}I\{C_i > T^*_{i,L_4}\} = I\{T^*_{i,L_4} \leq t, \eta_{i,s} = 1, \delta_i = k\}.$$

The transition probabilities $P_{0k}(0, t), k = 10, 11$ can be estimated by

$$\widehat{P}^{\text{AIPCW}}_{0k}(0, t) = \frac{1}{n} \sum_{i=1}^n \left\{ \frac{R_{i,3k}(t)}{\widehat{G}_{C_{00}}(T^*_{i,3})\widehat{G}_{C_{33}}(T^*_{i,9})\widehat{G}_{C_{99,3}}(T^*_{i,L_4})} \right.$$
$$\left. + \frac{R_{i,4k}(t)}{\widehat{G}_{C_{00}}(T^*_{i,4})\widehat{G}_{C_{44}}(T^*_{i,9})\widehat{G}_{C_{99,4}}(T^*_{i,L_4})} \right\}.$$

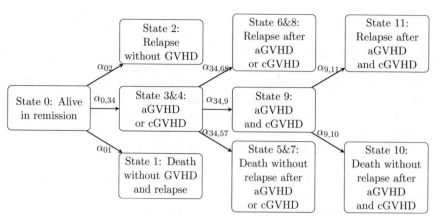

**Fig. 4** Reconfigure the twelve-state model

Depend on the state of interest, one may reconstruct the model to simplify the estimates. For instance, a simpler way to estimate $P_{0k}(0, t), k = 9, 10, 11$, is to reconfigure the data and combine state 3 and 4 as a single transient state (see Fig. 4) before applying the AIPCW technique.

Under regularity conditions [8, 9, 15], the variance of $\sqrt{n} \{ \widehat{P}_{0k}^{\text{AIPCW}}(0, t) - P_{0k}(0, t) \}$, for $k = 9, 10, 11$, can be estimated by

$$\widehat{\Sigma}_{0k}(t) = n^{-1} \sum_i \{ \widehat{W}_{i,0k}(t) \}^2 ,$$

where explicit expressions for $\widehat{W}_{i,0k}(t)$ can be found in the Appendix.

# 3 Simulation Studies and Results

## 3.1 Compare SIPCW and AIPCW

In this section, two scenarios are considered to compare the transition probability estimates and their variances obtained using the SIPCW and AIPCW techniques. The data were generated in a setting of the six-state HSCT model. The event and censoring times were assumed to follow independent exponential distributions with constant transition intensities $\alpha_{hk}(t)$. Due to the similarities of state 1 and 2, 4 and 5, we only present the simulation results for state $\{0, 1, 3, 4\}$. The simulation results are based on 1000 samples each with sample size $N = 300$.

We created scenarios A and B with the same transition intensities but different censoring rates. The pre-specified transition intensities are (0.08, 0.03, 0.15, 0.08, 0.03) respectively for states 1–5. In scenario A, the two-piece constant censoring rates are set to be 0.01 at state 0, and 0.10 at state 3, so that the overall censoring percentage is 30%. In scenario B, the censoring rates are set to be 0.05 and 0.20, so that the overall censoring percentage reaches 50%. The average number of patients in state 0–5 by the end of study are {11, 90, 33, 80, 63, 24} and {48, 78, 29, 93, 38, 14} for scenario A and B, respectively. The average of estimated transition probabilities, their standard deviations (SD), average of estimated standard errors (SE), bias, and 95% coverage probabilities at four different time points $t = (5, 7, 10, 16)$ are shown in Table 1. In Table 1, $T$ denotes the time points, $P_{hj}(t)$ denotes the true transition probabilities, $K$ is the estimable number among 1000 samples. $S$ and $A$ indicate that the results are based on the SIPCW and AIPCW estimators, respectively. The coverage probabilities are based on 95% confidence intervals with respect to the log transformation of transition probabilities [4, 5].

Table 1 shows that the estimates obtained using the SIPCW technique overall have larger bias compared to those obtained using the AIPCW technique in both scenarios with 30% and 50% censoring. Due to similarity, simulation results for $P_{02}(t)$ and $P_{05}(t)$ are not showing here. In the meantime, the SIPCW technique turns out to overestimate $P_{00}(t)$, $P_{01}(t)$ and their variances, while underestimating $P_{03}(t)$, $P_{04}(t)$ and their variances. This result is not surprising, because the SIPCW technique underestimates the censoring probabilities that are being used to estimate $P_{00}(t)$, $P_{01}(t)$ and vice versa. We also observed that the 95% coverage probabilities of SIPCW estimates are not close to 0.95 in most cases, especially for $P_{01}(t)$ and $P_{03}(t)$.

On the other hand, the bias is much smaller when the AIPCW technique was applied, the estimated SEs are close to the SDs, and the coverage probabilities are reasonably around 0.95. In conclusion, the AIPCW technique reduces bias and improves the accuracy of variance estimates compare to the SIPCW technique. Although the bias is larger when the censoring proportion gets higher, the scale of the bias is small and reasonable when using the AIPCW technique.

## 3.2   Evaluate the Performance of AIPCW

We further conduct intensive simulation studies with various sample size (100, 500, 1200, 1500) and different censoring proportions (30% vs. 50%) to evaluate the performance of the AIPCW technique in estimating the transition probabilities and their variances. Only the results for state {0, 1, 3, 4} are presented. The pre-specified transition intensities are set to be (0.05, 0.02, 0.15, 0.02, 0.02) respectively for states 1–5. The two-piece constant censoring rates are set to be 0.01 at state 0, 0.03 at state 3 to achieve 30% overall censoring, and 0.04 at state 0, 0.06 at state 3 to reach 50% overall censoring.

Table 2 shows the simulation results with sample size 100 and 500. Table 3 shows the simulation results with sample size 1200 and 1500. The simulation results in Tables 2 and 3 show that the bias of AIPCW estimates are small in all scenarios regardless of the sample size and censoring proportion.

**Table 1** SIPCE vs. AIPCW for estimating transition probabilities with 30% and 50% censoring

| $(h, j)$ | $T$ | $P_{hj}$ | $K$ | $\widehat{P}^S_{hj}(SD)$ | Bias$^S$ | SE | Cov.p$^S$ | $K$ | $\widehat{P}^A_{hj}(SD)$ | Bias$^A$ | SE | Cov.p$^A$ |
|---|---|---|---|---|---|---|---|---|---|---|---|---|
| *30% censoring and sample size = 300* | | | | | | | | | | | | |
| (0, 0) | 5 | 0.273 | 1000 | 0.307 (0.029) | 0.034 | 0.035 | 0.868 | 1000 | 0.272 (0.026) | −0.001 | 0.026 | 0.943 |
| (0, 0) | 7 | 0.162 | 1000 | 0.199 (0.026) | 0.037 | 0.035 | 0.844 | 1000 | 0.161 (0.022) | −0.001 | 0.022 | 0.950 |
| (0, 0) | 10 | 0.074 | 1000 | 0.108 (0.023) | 0.034 | 0.035 | 0.868 | 1000 | 0.074 (0.016) | −0.001 | 0.016 | 0.945 |
| (0, 0) | 16 | 0.016 | 1000 | 0.034 (0.016) | 0.018 | 0.034 | 0.946 | 1000 | 0.015 (0.007) | 0.000 | 0.007 | 0.981 |
| (0, 1) | 5 | 0.224 | 1000 | 0.233 (0.025) | 0.009 | 0.025 | 0.932 | 1000 | 0.225 (0.025) | 0.002 | 0.024 | 0.945 |
| (0, 1) | 7 | 0.258 | 1000 | 0.273 (0.027) | 0.015 | 0.027 | 0.924 | 1000 | 0.260 (0.026) | 0.002 | 0.026 | 0.942 |
| (0, 1) | 10 | 0.285 | 1000 | 0.309 (0.029) | 0.024 | 0.029 | 0.881 | 1000 | 0.287 (0.026) | 0.002 | 0.026 | 0.942 |
| (0, 1) | 16 | 0.303 | 1000 | 0.340 (0.030) | 0.037 | 0.031 | 0.777 | 1000 | 0.305 (0.027) | 0.002 | 0.027 | 0.945 |
| (0, 3) | 5 | 0.304 | 1000 | 0.270 (0.027) | −0.035 | 0.015 | 0.425 | 1000 | 0.308 (0.028) | 0.004 | 0.031 | 0.966 |
| (0, 3) | 7 | 0.301 | 1000 | 0.263 (0.029) | −0.038 | 0.016 | 0.425 | 1000 | 0.308 (0.029) | 0.007 | 0.034 | 0.972 |
| (0, 3) | 10 | 0.259 | 1000 | 0.224 (0.030) | −0.035 | 0.017 | 0.483 | 1000 | 0.270 (0.031) | 0.011 | 0.034 | 0.957 |
| (0, 3) | 16 | 0.156 | 1000 | 0.138 (0.028) | −0.019 | 0.019 | 0.725 | 1000 | 0.171 (0.030) | 0.014 | 0.033 | 0.946 |
| (0, 4) | 5 | 0.084 | 1000 | 0.077 (0.017) | −0.007 | 0.016 | 0.929 | 1000 | 0.081 (0.018) | −0.003 | 0.017 | 0.938 |
| (0, 4) | 7 | 0.133 | 1000 | 0.119 (0.020) | −0.014 | 0.020 | 0.892 | 1000 | 0.127 (0.022) | −0.005 | 0.021 | 0.937 |
| (0, 4) | 10 | 0.200 | 1000 | 0.178 (0.024) | −0.023 | 0.025 | 0.862 | 1000 | 0.192 (0.026) | −0.008 | 0.027 | 0.934 |
| (0, 4) | 16 | 0.299 | 1000 | 0.264 (0.030) | −0.035 | 0.031 | 0.797 | 1000 | 0.288 (0.033) | −0.011 | 0.034 | 0.942 |

(continued)

**Table 1** (continued)

| $(h, j)$ | $T$ | $P_{hj}$ | $K$ | $\widehat{P}_{hj}^{S}(SD)$ | Bias$^S$ | SE | Cov.p$^S$ | $K$ | $\widehat{P}_{hj}^{A}(SD)$ | Bias$^A$ | SE | Cov.p$^A$ |
|---|---|---|---|---|---|---|---|---|---|---|---|---|
| 50% censoring and sample size = 300 | | | | | | | | | | | | |
| (0, 0) | 5 | 0.273 | 1000 | 0.329 (0.033) | 0.056 | 0.038 | 0.706 | 1000 | 0.272 (0.028) | −0.001 | 0.028 | 0.953 |
| (0, 0) | 7 | 0.162 | 1000 | 0.225 (0.033) | 0.063 | 0.041 | 0.634 | 1000 | 0.162 (0.024) | −0.001 | 0.024 | 0.949 |
| (0, 0) | 10 | 0.074 | 1000 | 0.134 (0.033) | 0.059 | 0.045 | 0.683 | 1000 | 0.074 (0.018) | 0.000 | 0.018 | 0.957 |
| (0, 0) | 16 | 0.016 | 997 | 0.050 (0.034) | 0.034 | 0.055 | 0.785 | 997 | 0.016 (0.010) | 0.000 | 0.009 | 0.949 |
| (0, 1) | 5 | 0.224 | 1000 | 0.237 (0.028) | 0.013 | 0.027 | 0.910 | 1000 | 0.225 (0.026) | 0.001 | 0.025 | 0.936 |
| (0, 1) | 7 | 0.258 | 1000 | 0.281 (0.030) | 0.023 | 0.030 | 0.884 | 1000 | 0.259 (0.027) | 0.001 | 0.027 | 0.949 |
| (0, 1) | 10 | 0.285 | 1000 | 0.322 (0.033) | 0.037 | 0.033 | 0.805 | 1000 | 0.286 (0.029) | 0.001 | 0.028 | 0.948 |
| (0, 1) | 16 | 0.303 | 997 | 0.362 (0.040) | 0.060 | 0.038 | 0.670 | 997 | 0.304 (0.030) | 0.001 | 0.029 | 0.945 |
| (0, 3) | 5 | 0.304 | 1000 | 0.247 (0.030) | −0.058 | 0.017 | 0.231 | 1000 | 0.311 (0.029) | 0.006 | 0.040 | 0.990 |
| (0, 3) | 7 | 0.301 | 1000 | 0.236 (0.034) | −0.065 | 0.020 | 0.268 | 1000 | 0.314 (0.034) | 0.013 | 0.046 | 0.988 |
| (0, 3) | 10 | 0.259 | 1000 | 0.198 (0.037) | −0.060 | 0.024 | 0.389 | 1000 | 0.280 (0.038) | 0.021 | 0.053 | 0.983 |
| (0, 3) | 16 | 0.156 | 997 | 0.122 (0.045) | −0.035 | 0.032 | 0.702 | 997 | 0.189 (0.052) | 0.032 | 0.067 | 0.934 |
| (0, 4) | 5 | 0.084 | 1000 | 0.073 (0.016) | −0.011 | 0.017 | 0.928 | 1000 | 0.080 (0.018) | −0.004 | 0.019 | 0.965 |
| (0, 4) | 7 | 0.133 | 1000 | 0.112 (0.021) | −0.021 | 0.022 | 0.851 | 1000 | 0.123 (0.024) | −0.009 | 0.025 | 0.941 |
| (0, 4) | 10 | 0.200 | 1000 | 0.165 (0.028) | −0.036 | 0.028 | 0.756 | 1000 | 0.185 (0.031) | −0.015 | 0.033 | 0.926 |
| (0, 4) | 16 | 0.299 | 997 | 0.242 (0.040) | −0.057 | 0.040 | 0.693 | 997 | 0.278 (0.049) | −0.022 | 0.050 | 0.908 |

Note: $^S$: SIPCW; $^A$: AIPCW; $K$: number of estimable samples; Cov.p: 95% coverage probability

**Table 2** Results from scenarios in the six-state model

| $(h, j)$ | $T$ | $P_{hj}$ | $K$ | $\hat{P}_{hj}(SD)$ | Bias | $\bar{\sigma}$ | $\bar{\sigma}^M$ | Cov.p | Cov.p$^M$ | $K$ | $\hat{P}_{hj}(SD)$ | Bias | $\bar{\sigma}$ | $\bar{\sigma}^M$ | Cov.p | Cov.p$^M$ |
|---|---|---|---|---|---|---|---|---|---|---|---|---|---|---|---|---|
| | | | *30% censoring and sample size = 100* | | | | | | | *30% censoring and sample size = 500* | | | | | | |
| (0, 0) | 5 | 0.333 | 1000 | 0.333 (0.045) | 0.000 | 0.048 | 0.049 | 0.961 | 0.963 | 1000 | 0.332 (0.021) | 0.000 | 0.021 | 0.022 | 0.954 | 0.958 |
| (0, 0) | 7 | 0.214 | 1000 | 0.216 (0.040) | 0.001 | 0.042 | 0.043 | 0.959 | 0.967 | 1000 | 0.214 (0.018) | 0.000 | 0.019 | 0.019 | 0.958 | 0.963 |
| (0, 0) | 10 | 0.111 | 998 | 0.110 (0.033) | −0.001 | 0.032 | 0.033 | 0.944 | 0.948 | 1000 | 0.111 (0.014) | 0.000 | 0.014 | 0.015 | 0.963 | 0.967 |
| (0, 0) | 16 | 0.030 | 994 | 0.029 (0.018) | −0.001 | 0.016 | 0.017 | 0.904 | 0.904 | 1000 | 0.030 (0.008) | 0.000 | 0.008 | 0.008 | 0.957 | 0.964 |
| (0, 1) | 5 | 0.152 | 1000 | 0.154 (0.036) | 0.003 | 0.036 | 0.036 | 0.951 | 0.951 | 1000 | 0.152 (0.016) | 0.001 | 0.016 | 0.016 | 0.950 | 0.950 |
| (0, 1) | 7 | 0.179 | 1000 | 0.182 (0.040) | 0.003 | 0.039 | 0.039 | 0.942 | 0.943 | 1000 | 0.179 (0.017) | 0.001 | 0.017 | 0.017 | 0.954 | 0.954 |
| (0, 1) | 10 | 0.202 | 998 | 0.207 (0.042) | 0.005 | 0.041 | 0.041 | 0.940 | 0.940 | 1000 | 0.203 (0.018) | 0.001 | 0.018 | 0.018 | 0.946 | 0.946 |
| (0, 1) | 16 | 0.221 | 994 | 0.225 (0.044) | 0.004 | 0.042 | 0.043 | 0.935 | 0.935 | 1000 | 0.221 (0.020) | 0.001 | 0.019 | 0.019 | 0.936 | 0.937 |
| (0, 3) | 5 | 0.405 | 1000 | 0.404 (0.048) | −0.001 | 0.052 | 0.053 | 0.963 | 0.966 | 1000 | 0.406 (0.022) | 0.001 | 0.023 | 0.024 | 0.965 | 0.968 |
| (0, 3) | 7 | 0.451 | 1000 | 0.450 (0.052) | −0.001 | 0.054 | 0.057 | 0.953 | 0.962 | 1000 | 0.452 (0.023) | 0.001 | 0.024 | 0.025 | 0.955 | 0.969 |
| (0, 3) | 10 | 0.466 | 998 | 0.466 (0.052) | 0.000 | 0.056 | 0.061 | 0.967 | 0.983 | 1000 | 0.469 (0.023) | 0.003 | 0.025 | 0.027 | 0.961 | 0.973 |
| (0, 3) | 16 | 0.415 | 994 | 0.417 (0.054) | 0.002 | 0.058 | 0.067 | 0.963 | 0.986 | 1000 | 0.420 (0.024) | 0.005 | 0.026 | 0.030 | 0.962 | 0.990 |
| (0, 4) | 5 | 0.025 | 1000 | 0.024 (0.016) | −0.001 | 0.014 | 0.014 | 0.864 | 0.864 | 1000 | 0.025 (0.008) | 0.000 | 0.007 | 0.007 | 0.943 | 0.943 |
| (0, 4) | 7 | 0.042 | 1000 | 0.042 (0.021) | 0.000 | 0.020 | 0.020 | 0.960 | 0.960 | 1000 | 0.042 (0.010) | 0.000 | 0.009 | 0.009 | 0.945 | 0.946 |
| (0, 4) | 10 | 0.070 | 998 | 0.069 (0.026) | −0.001 | 0.026 | 0.026 | 0.949 | 0.950 | 1000 | 0.068 (0.012) | −0.002 | 0.012 | 0.012 | 0.941 | 0.942 |
| (0, 4) | 16 | 0.123 | 994 | 0.122 (0.035) | −0.002 | 0.036 | 0.036 | 0.956 | 0.957 | 1000 | 0.120 (0.016) | −0.003 | 0.016 | 0.016 | 0.942 | 0.945 |

(continued)

**Table 2** (continued)

| $(h, j)$ | T | $P_{hj}$ | K | $\hat{P}_{hj}(SD)$ | Bias | $\hat{\sigma}$ | $\bar{\hat{\sigma}}^M$ | Cov.p | Cov.p$^M$ | K | $\hat{P}_{hj}(SD)$ | Bias | $\hat{\sigma}$ | $\bar{\hat{\sigma}}^M$ | Cov.p | Cov.p$^M$ |
|---|---|---|---|---|---|---|---|---|---|---|---|---|---|---|---|---|
| | | | | *50% censoring and Sample size = 100* | | | | | | | *50% censoring and sample size = 500* | | | | | |
| (0, 0) | 5 | 0.333 | 1000 | 0.333 (0.050) | 0.000 | 0.050 | 0.054 | 0.949 | 0.958 | 1000 | 0.333 (0.023) | 0.000 | 0.022 | 0.024 | 0.951 | 0.966 |
| (0, 0) | 7 | 0.214 | 999 | 0.213 (0.045) | −0.002 | 0.044 | 0.048 | 0.950 | 0.965 | 1000 | 0.214 (0.021) | 0.000 | 0.020 | 0.022 | 0.944 | 0.965 |
| (0, 0) | 10 | 0.111 | 997 | 0.110 (0.036) | −0.001 | 0.035 | 0.039 | 0.953 | 0.973 | 1000 | 0.111 (0.017) | 0.000 | 0.016 | 0.017 | 0.938 | 0.959 |
| (0, 0) | 16 | 0.030 | 986 | 0.029 (0.022) | 0.000 | 0.019 | 0.021 | 0.786 | 0.793 | 1000 | 0.030 (0.010) | 0.000 | 0.010 | 0.011 | 0.965 | 0.973 |
| (0, 1) | 5 | 0.152 | 1000 | 0.153 (0.037) | 0.002 | 0.037 | 0.037 | 0.957 | 0.957 | 1000 | 0.152 (0.016) | 0.000 | 0.017 | 0.017 | 0.953 | 0.955 |
| (0, 1) | 7 | 0.179 | 999 | 0.182 (0.041) | 0.003 | 0.040 | 0.041 | 0.958 | 0.959 | 1000 | 0.179 (0.017) | 0.001 | 0.018 | 0.018 | 0.958 | 0.959 |
| (0, 1) | 10 | 0.202 | 997 | 0.206 (0.044) | 0.004 | 0.043 | 0.044 | 0.956 | 0.959 | 1000 | 0.203 (0.019) | 0.000 | 0.019 | 0.020 | 0.953 | 0.959 |
| (0, 1) | 16 | 0.221 | 986 | 0.223 (0.046) | 0.003 | 0.045 | 0.046 | 0.952 | 0.957 | 1000 | 0.221 (0.020) | 0.000 | 0.020 | 0.021 | 0.958 | 0.960 |
| (0, 3) | 5 | 0.405 | 1000 | 0.405 (0.052) | 0.001 | 0.057 | 0.060 | 0.977 | 0.985 | 1000 | 0.406 (0.023) | 0.002 | 0.026 | 0.027 | 0.969 | 0.976 |
| (0, 3) | 7 | 0.451 | 999 | 0.451 (0.056) | 0.000 | 0.060 | 0.067 | 0.964 | 0.984 | 1000 | 0.453 (0.025) | 0.002 | 0.027 | 0.030 | 0.965 | 0.981 |
| (0, 3) | 10 | 0.466 | 997 | 0.469 (0.056) | 0.002 | 0.064 | 0.077 | 0.974 | 0.993 | 1000 | 0.471 (0.027) | 0.005 | 0.030 | 0.034 | 0.978 | 0.992 |
| (0, 3) | 16 | 0.415 | 986 | 0.419 (0.061) | 0.004 | 0.068 | 0.095 | 0.970 | 0.998 | 1000 | 0.423 (0.028) | 0.008 | 0.032 | 0.042 | 0.962 | 0.998 |
| (0, 4) | 5 | 0.025 | 1000 | 0.025 (0.017) | 0.000 | 0.015 | 0.015 | 0.861 | 0.861 | 1000 | 0.025 (0.008) | 0.000 | 0.007 | 0.007 | 0.944 | 0.944 |
| (0, 4) | 7 | 0.042 | 999 | 0.043 (0.022) | 0.000 | 0.021 | 0.021 | 0.950 | 0.950 | 1000 | 0.042 (0.010) | −0.001 | 0.010 | 0.010 | 0.950 | 0.951 |
| (0, 4) | 10 | 0.070 | 997 | 0.068 (0.028) | −0.002 | 0.028 | 0.029 | 0.958 | 0.960 | 1000 | 0.068 (0.013) | −0.002 | 0.013 | 0.013 | 0.959 | 0.960 |
| (0, 4) | 16 | 0.123 | 986 | 0.119 (0.042) | −0.004 | 0.041 | 0.042 | 0.930 | 0.937 | 1000 | 0.120 (0.018) | −0.004 | 0.019 | 0.019 | 0.945 | 0.951 |

Note: Sample size for each scenario is 1000; $K$: estimable number of simulations; Cov.p: 95% coverage probabilities; $M$: estimates are based on the main-part estimators

**Table 3** Results from scenarios with sample size $N = 1200$ vs. $N = 1500$

| $(h, j)$ | T | $P_{hj}$ | Sample size = 1200 | | | | | Sample size = 1500 | | | | |
|---|---|---|---|---|---|---|---|---|---|---|---|---|
| | | | K | $\widehat{P}_{hj}(SD)$ | Bias | $\widehat{\overline{\sigma}}^M$ | Cov.p$^M$ | K | $\widehat{P}_{hj}(SD)$ | Bias | $\widehat{\overline{\sigma}}^M$ | Cov.p$^M$ |
| *30% censoring* | | | | | | | | | | | | |
| (0, 0) | 5 | 0.333 | 1000 | 0.333 (0.014) | 0.000 | 0.014 | 0.958 | 1000 | 0.333 (0.013) | 0.000 | 0.013 | 0.951 |
| (0, 0) | 7 | 0.214 | 1000 | 0.214 (0.012) | 0.000 | 0.012 | 0.958 | 1000 | 0.215 (0.011) | 0.000 | 0.011 | 0.957 |
| (0, 0) | 10 | 0.111 | 1000 | 0.111 (0.009) | 0.000 | 0.010 | 0.957 | 1000 | 0.111 (0.008) | 0.000 | 0.009 | 0.953 |
| (0, 0) | 16 | 0.030 | 1000 | 0.030 (0.005) | 0.000 | 0.005 | 0.960 | 1000 | 0.030 (0.004) | 0.000 | 0.005 | 0.968 |
| (0, 1) | 5 | 0.152 | 1000 | 0.152 (0.010) | 0.001 | 0.010 | 0.953 | 1000 | 0.152 (0.009) | 0.000 | 0.009 | 0.958 |
| (0, 1) | 7 | 0.179 | 1000 | 0.179 (0.011) | 0.001 | 0.011 | 0.950 | 1000 | 0.179 (0.010) | 0.000 | 0.010 | 0.959 |
| (0, 1) | 10 | 0.202 | 1000 | 0.203 (0.012) | 0.001 | 0.012 | 0.954 | 1000 | 0.202 (0.010) | 0.000 | 0.011 | 0.949 |
| (0, 1) | 16 | 0.221 | 1000 | 0.221 (0.012) | 0.001 | 0.012 | 0.953 | 1000 | 0.221 (0.011) | 0.000 | 0.011 | 0.945 |
| (0, 3) | 5 | 0.405 | 1000 | 0.405 (0.014) | 0.000 | 0.015 | 0.959 | 1000 | 0.405 (0.013) | 0.000 | 0.014 | 0.967 |
| (0, 3) | 7 | 0.451 | 1000 | 0.452 (0.015) | 0.000 | 0.016 | 0.962 | 1000 | 0.452 (0.013) | 0.001 | 0.015 | 0.970 |
| (0, 3) | 10 | 0.466 | 1000 | 0.468 (0.015) | 0.002 | 0.018 | 0.979 | 1000 | 0.468 (0.013) | 0.002 | 0.016 | 0.976 |
| (0, 3) | 16 | 0.415 | 1000 | 0.418 (0.016) | 0.003 | 0.019 | 0.982 | 1000 | 0.418 (0.014) | 0.004 | 0.017 | 0.989 |
| (0, 4) | 5 | 0.025 | 1000 | 0.025 (0.005) | 0.000 | 0.005 | 0.948 | 1000 | 0.025 (0.004) | 0.000 | 0.004 | 0.945 |
| (0, 4) | 7 | 0.042 | 1000 | 0.042 (0.006) | 0.000 | 0.006 | 0.951 | 1000 | 0.042 (0.005) | 0.000 | 0.005 | 0.952 |
| (0, 4) | 10 | 0.070 | 1000 | 0.069 (0.008) | −0.001 | 0.008 | 0.954 | 1000 | 0.069 (0.007) | −0.001 | 0.007 | 0.947 |
| (0, 4) | 16 | 0.123 | 1000 | 0.121 (0.011) | −0.002 | 0.011 | 0.932 | 1000 | 0.121 (0.009) | −0.002 | 0.009 | 0.934 |

(continued)

**Table 3** (continued)

| | | | Sample size = 1200 | | | | | Sample size = 1500 | | | | |
|---|---|---|---|---|---|---|---|---|---|---|---|---|
| $(h, j)$ | T | $P_{hj}$ | $K$ | $\widehat{P}_{hj}(SD)$ | Bias | $\bar{\widehat{\sigma}}^M$ | Cov.p$^M$ | $K$ | $\widehat{P}_{hj}(SD)$ | Bias | $\bar{\widehat{\sigma}}^M$ | Cov.p$^M$ |
| *50% censoring* | | | | | | | | | | | | |
| (0, 0) | 5 | 0.333 | 1000 | 0.333 (0.015) | 0.000 | 0.016 | 0.964 | 1000 | 0.333 (0.013) | 0.000 | 0.014 | 0.974 |
| (0, 0) | 7 | 0.214 | 1000 | 0.215 (0.013) | 0.000 | 0.014 | 0.965 | 1000 | 0.215 (0.011) | 0.000 | 0.013 | 0.975 |
| (0, 0) | 10 | 0.111 | 1000 | 0.111 (0.011) | 0.000 | 0.011 | 0.964 | 1000 | 0.111 (0.009) | 0.000 | 0.010 | 0.965 |
| (0, 0) | 16 | 0.030 | 1000 | 0.030 (0.006) | 0.000 | 0.007 | 0.965 | 1000 | 0.030 (0.006) | 0.000 | 0.006 | 0.964 |
| (0, 1) | 5 | 0.152 | 1000 | 0.152 (0.010) | 0.000 | 0.011 | 0.961 | 1000 | 0.151 (0.009) | 0.000 | 0.010 | 0.966 |
| (0, 1) | 7 | 0.179 | 1000 | 0.179 (0.011) | 0.000 | 0.012 | 0.955 | 1000 | 0.179 (0.010) | 0.000 | 0.011 | 0.961 |
| (0, 1) | 10 | 0.202 | 1000 | 0.202 (0.012) | 0.000 | 0.013 | 0.956 | 1000 | 0.202 (0.011) | 0.000 | 0.011 | 0.950 |
| (0, 1) | 16 | 0.221 | 1000 | 0.221 (0.013) | 0.000 | 0.013 | 0.954 | 1000 | 0.221 (0.011) | 0.000 | 0.012 | 0.946 |
| (0, 3) | 5 | 0.405 | 1000 | 0.406 (0.015) | 0.001 | 0.017 | 0.977 | 1000 | 0.406 (0.014) | 0.001 | 0.016 | 0.982 |
| (0, 3) | 7 | 0.451 | 1000 | 0.453 (0.016) | 0.002 | 0.019 | 0.988 | 1000 | 0.453 (0.014) | 0.002 | 0.017 | 0.988 |
| (0, 3) | 10 | 0.466 | 1000 | 0.470 (0.017) | 0.004 | 0.022 | 0.991 | 1000 | 0.470 (0.016) | 0.004 | 0.020 | 0.988 |
| (0, 3) | 16 | 0.415 | 1000 | 0.422 (0.018) | 0.007 | 0.027 | 0.995 | 1000 | 0.422 (0.016) | 0.007 | 0.024 | 0.996 |
| (0, 4) | 5 | 0.025 | 1000 | 0.025 (0.005) | 0.000 | 0.005 | 0.957 | 1000 | 0.025 (0.004) | 0.000 | 0.004 | 0.948 |
| (0, 4) | 7 | 0.042 | 1000 | 0.042 (0.006) | −0.001 | 0.006 | 0.948 | 1000 | 0.042 (0.006) | −0.001 | 0.006 | 0.947 |
| (0, 4) | 10 | 0.070 | 1000 | 0.068 (0.008) | −0.002 | 0.009 | 0.960 | 1000 | 0.068 (0.008) | −0.002 | 0.008 | 0.949 |
| (0, 4) | 16 | 0.123 | 1000 | 0.120 (0.012) | −0.004 | 0.012 | 0.944 | 1000 | 0.120 (0.011) | −0.003 | 0.011 | 0.944 |

Note: Sample size for each scenario is 1000; $K$: estimable number of simulations; Cov.p: 95% coverage probabilities; $M$: estimates are based on the main-part estimators

In Table 2, we present two types of variance estimates for each transition probability: $\bar{\bar{\sigma}}$ is the full standard error estimate, while $\bar{\bar{\sigma}}^M$ is the main-part standard error estimate which assumes the censoring distributions are known. According to the simulation results, the main-part variance $\bar{\bar{\sigma}}^M$ are slightly conservative compare to $\bar{\bar{\sigma}}$, and the 95% coverage probabilities based on $\bar{\bar{\sigma}}^M$ are bigger than its 95% nominal range [0.9365, 0.9635] in transient states 3.

In Table 3, only the simulation results based on $\bar{\bar{\sigma}}^M$ are presented for larger sample size 1200 and 1500. The coverage probabilities based on $\bar{\bar{\sigma}}^M$ are still slightly larger for the transient state. The reasons are possibly the higher flowability in the transient states and the bias of K-M estimators of censoring distributions. Further studies are desirable to determine the actual reasons for this observed phenomenon. Despite that $\bar{\bar{\sigma}}^M$ are larger in transient states, the difference between $\bar{\bar{\sigma}}$ and $\bar{\bar{\sigma}}^M$ are generally negligible for large sample size and small censoring proportion, moreover, the computation time can be significantly reduced by using the main-part variance when sample size is large.

We notice that several coverage probabilities are much smaller than 0.95 when sample size is small, such as $P_{00}(t = 16)$, and $P_{04}(t = 5)$ when sample size is 100. The reason is that the corresponding true probabilities are very small ($P_{00}(t = 16) = 0.03$, $P_{04}(t = 5) = 0.025$), it is difficult to obtain accurate tail estimates because of the lack of enough events and 'at risk' subjects to make inferences.

By comparing the coverage probabilities from scenarios with different censoring proportions, we observed that the coverage probabilities are closer to 0.95 in scenarios with less censoring. This observation is rational because we do expect more accurate estimates with more information. Moreover, when the sample size gets larger, those coverage probabilities also get closer to 0.95. Based on these results, we argue that a sample size less than 500 is maybe too small to provide accurate estimates for the transition probabilities in this specified six-state model when the censoring proportion is relatively high.

## 3.3 Evaluate the Performance of AIPCW in a Four-Level Twelve-State Model

We conduct simulation studies to evaluate the performance of the proposed AIPCW technique in the specified four-level twelve-state model. We create simulation scenarios with different sample sizes (300, 500, 1000, 1500) and 30% censoring. The transition intensities $\alpha_{01} - \alpha_{08}$, $\alpha_{39}$, $\alpha_{49}$, $\alpha_{9,10}$, $\alpha_{9,11}$ are set to be (0.02, 0.03, 0.10, 0.15, 0.03, 0.04, 0.02, 0.03, 0.10, 0.05, 0.03, 0.05), and the censoring intensities for transient states 0, 3, 4, 9 are set to be (0.02, 0.03, 0.03, 0.03) respectively to meet the desired percentage of censoring. The average number of patients in state 0–11 by the end of study are {19, 19, 28, 14, 33, 14, 19, 21, 33, 27, 27, 46}, {31, 32, 47, 23, 54, 24, 31, 36, 54, 46, 46, 76}, {63, 63, 94, 47, 108, 46, 62, 72, 108,

92, 92, 153}, and {94, 94, 141, 71, 161, 70, 94, 108, 162, 138, 138, 229}, for N = 300, 500, 1000 and 1500, respectively. We only report results for transition probabilities $P_{09}(0, t)$, $P_{0,10}(0, t)$, $P_{0,11}(0, t)$. Only the main-part variances and the corresponding coverage probabilities are considered for large simple size of 1000 and 1500 to reduce the computation time.

Table 4 summarizes the simulation results. Overall, the estimated biases are relatively small, the variance estimates are consistent, and the estimated standard errors are close to the standard deviations. The coverage probabilities fall into the nominal range [0.9365, 0.9635] for almost all the cases. Specifically, the biases of estimated transition probabilities of $P_{09}(0, t)$ are slightly larger than bias of estimating $P_{0,10}(0, t)$ and $P_{0,11}(0, t)$, however, the biases get reduced when the sample size gets larger. In summary, the AIPCW technique performs well in estimating transition probabilities in complex multi-state models.

# 4 Real Data Example: The HSCT Data

In this section, we study the cumulative incidences of relapse and death with or without development of chronic GVHD (cGVHD) by analyzing the real data from the HSCT study [11]. The data were initially collected to compare the survival outcomes of patients with high-risk acute myeloid leukemia or myelodysplasia when they were treated with myeloablative (MA) procedures versus reduced-intensity conditioning or nonmyeloablative (RIC/NMA) conditioning regimens. Primary endpoints were hematopoietic recovery, GVHD, treatment related mortality (TRM), clinical disease relapse (hematological or extramedullary), overall survival and disease-free survival (DFS). TRM was defined as death during continuous complete remission without relapse after transplant. Relapse was defined as clinical or hemotological recurrence. For the purposes of the analysis, the date of the transplant was the starting time point, and surviving patients were censored at the date of last contact. The data contain a total of 5179 patients who received an HLA-identical sibling or an unrelated HCT transplant (3731 MA and 1448 RIC/NMA) procedures performed at 217 centers between 1997 and 2004. For illustrative purposes, we consider a cohort of 4920 patients with complete information.

## 4.1 Quantify Transition Probabilities

In a multi-state framework, the data from [11] can be configured into a six-state model (see Fig. 1). In the following contents, we estimate the transition probabilities and explore the cGVHD effect within this model applying the proposed AIPCW technique. The transition probabilities at every 12 months are summarized in Table 5. From the analysis output, we learn that the 1-year cGVHD and relapse-free survival (cGRFS) is $P_{00}(12) = 0.180$, the DFS is $P_{00}(12) + P_{03}(12) = 0.449$,

**Table 4** Results from scenarios with 30% censoring in the twelve-state model

| $(h, j)$ | T | $P_{hj}$ | Sample size = 300 | | | | | | Sample size = 500 | | | | | |
|---|---|---|---|---|---|---|---|---|---|---|---|---|---|---|
| | | | $\hat{P}_{hj}(SD)$ | Bias | $\bar{\hat{\sigma}}$ | $\bar{\hat{\sigma}}^M$ | Cov.p | Cov.p$^M$ | $\hat{P}_{hj}(SD)$ | Bias | $\bar{\hat{\sigma}}$ | $\bar{\hat{\sigma}}^M$ | Cov.p | Cov.p$^M$ |
| (0, 9) | 5 | 0.095 | 0.094 (0.017) | 0.000 | 0.020 | 0.018 | 0.968 | 0.958 | 0.094 (0.013) | 0.000 | 0.016 | 0.014 | 0.965 | 0.960 |
| (0, 9) | 10 | 0.173 | 0.175 (0.025) | 0.002 | 0.030 | 0.026 | 0.978 | 0.962 | 0.175 (0.019) | 0.002 | 0.025 | 0.020 | 0.976 | 0.963 |
| (0, 9) | 15 | 0.186 | 0.193 (0.026) | 0.007 | 0.036 | 0.030 | 0.982 | 0.974 | 0.193 (0.020) | 0.007 | 0.029 | 0.023 | 0.988 | 0.973 |
| (0, 9) | 20 | 0.165 | 0.176 (0.028) | 0.011 | 0.039 | 0.032 | 0.970 | 0.963 | 0.176 (0.022) | 0.011 | 0.032 | 0.025 | 0.978 | 0.963 |
| (0, 10) | 5 | 0.006 | 0.006 (0.005) | 0.000 | 0.005 | 0.005 | 0.960 | 0.957 | 0.006 (0.004) | 0.000 | 0.004 | 0.004 | 0.980 | 0.980 |
| (0, 10) | 10 | 0.027 | 0.026 (0.010) | −0.001 | 0.010 | 0.010 | 0.958 | 0.956 | 0.026 (0.008) | −0.001 | 0.008 | 0.008 | 0.955 | 0.953 |
| (0, 10) | 15 | 0.054 | 0.053 (0.015) | −0.001 | 0.015 | 0.015 | 0.952 | 0.953 | 0.053 (0.011) | −0.002 | 0.012 | 0.011 | 0.956 | 0.955 |
| (0, 10) | 20 | 0.081 | 0.079 (0.019) | −0.002 | 0.019 | 0.019 | 0.947 | 0.941 | 0.079 (0.014) | −0.002 | 0.015 | 0.015 | 0.957 | 0.951 |
| (0, 11) | 5 | 0.010 | 0.010 (0.006) | 0.000 | 0.006 | 0.006 | 0.979 | 0.977 | 0.009 (0.005) | 0.000 | 0.004 | 0.004 | 0.980 | 0.980 |
| (0, 11) | 10 | 0.045 | 0.043 (0.013) | −0.002 | 0.013 | 0.013 | 0.947 | 0.947 | 0.043 (0.010) | −0.002 | 0.010 | 0.010 | 0.957 | 0.954 |
| (0, 11) | 15 | 0.091 | 0.088 (0.020) | −0.003 | 0.019 | 0.019 | 0.941 | 0.938 | 0.089 (0.015) | −0.002 | 0.015 | 0.015 | 0.949 | 0.951 |
| (0, 11) | 20 | 0.135 | 0.133 (0.024) | −0.002 | 0.025 | 0.024 | 0.950 | 0.952 | 0.133 (0.018) | −0.002 | 0.019 | 0.019 | 0.959 | 0.958 |

(continued)

**Table 4** (continued)

| $(h, j)$ | T | $P_{hj}$ | $\hat{P}_{hj}(SD)$ | Bias | $\bar{\hat{\sigma}}$ | $\bar{\hat{\sigma}}^M$ | Cov.p | Cov.p$^M$ | $\hat{P}_{hj}(SD)$ | Bias | $\bar{\hat{\sigma}}$ | $\bar{\hat{\sigma}}^M$ | Cov.p | Cov.p$^M$ |
|---|---|---|---|---|---|---|---|---|---|---|---|---|---|---|
| | | | Sample size = 1000 | | | | | | Sample size = 1500 | | | | | |
| (0, 9) | 5 | 0.095 | 0.094 (0.010) | 0.000 | | 0.010 | | 0.956 | 0.094 (0.008) | −0.001 | | 0.008 | | 0.959 |
| (0, 9) | 10 | 0.173 | 0.174 (0.014) | 0.001 | | 0.014 | | 0.952 | 0.174 (0.011) | 0.001 | | 0.012 | | 0.966 |
| (0, 9) | 15 | 0.186 | 0.192 (0.014) | 0.006 | | 0.016 | | 0.963 | 0.192 (0.012) | 0.005 | | 0.013 | | 0.957 |
| (0, 9) | 20 | 0.165 | 0.176 (0.016) | 0.011 | | 0.018 | | 0.936 | 0.175 (0.012) | 0.010 | | 0.014 | | 0.925 |
| (0, 10) | 5 | 0.006 | 0.006 (0.002) | 0.000 | | 0.002 | | 0.972 | 0.006 (0.002) | 0.000 | | 0.002 | | 0.951 |
| (0, 10) | 10 | 0.027 | 0.026 (0.006) | −0.001 | | 0.005 | | 0.939 | 0.026 (0.005) | −0.001 | | 0.004 | | 0.937 |
| (0, 10) | 15 | 0.054 | 0.053 (0.008) | −0.002 | | 0.008 | | 0.950 | 0.053 (0.007) | −0.002 | | 0.007 | | 0.937 |
| (0, 10) | 20 | 0.081 | 0.079 (0.010) | −0.002 | | 0.010 | | 0.962 | 0.079 (0.008) | −0.002 | | 0.008 | | 0.943 |
| (0, 11) | 5 | 0.010 | 0.010 (0.003) | 0.000 | | 0.003 | | 0.951 | 0.010 (0.003) | 0.000 | | 0.003 | | 0.950 |
| (0, 11) | 10 | 0.045 | 0.043 (0.007) | −0.001 | | 0.007 | | 0.944 | 0.044 (0.006) | −0.001 | | 0.006 | | 0.935 |
| (0, 11) | 15 | 0.091 | 0.088 (0.010) | −0.002 | | 0.010 | | 0.946 | 0.088 (0.008) | −0.002 | | 0.008 | | 0.955 |
| (0, 11) | 20 | 0.135 | 0.133 (0.013) | −0.002 | | 0.013 | | 0.943 | 0.132 (0.010) | −0.003 | | 0.011 | | 0.959 |

Note: The estimable number $K = 1000$ at all the time points for both scenarios

$M$ indicates that the variance estimates and the coverage probabilities are estimated by the main-part only

Cov.p: 95% coverage probabilities

**Table 5** Estimated transition probabilities at every 12 months

| Month | $\widehat{P}_{jk}(t)(se)$ | | | | | |
|---|---|---|---|---|---|---|
| | $\widehat{P}_{00}(t)$ | $\widehat{P}_{03}(t)$ | $\widehat{P}_{01}(t)$ | $\widehat{P}_{04}(t)$ | $\widehat{P}_{02}(t)$ | $\widehat{P}_{05}(t)$ |
| 12 | 0.180 (0.075) | 0.269 (0.081) | 0.229 (0.078) | 0.052 (0.057) | 0.235 (0.078) | 0.036 (0.052) |
| 24 | 0.134 (0.072) | 0.246 (0.082) | 0.236 (0.078) | 0.075 (0.062) | 0.250 (0.079) | 0.059 (0.059) |
| 36 | 0.120 (0.074) | 0.229 (0.085) | 0.240 (0.078) | 0.089 (0.065) | 0.254 (0.079) | 0.068 (0.061) |
| 48 | 0.111 (0.078) | 0.211 (0.091) | 0.242 (0.079) | 0.103 (0.068) | 0.258 (0.080) | 0.074 (0.063) |

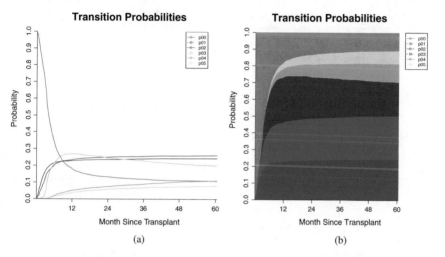

(a)  (b)

**Fig. 5** Estimated transition probabilities. (**a**) Transition probability curves. (**b**) Proportions of transition probabilities

and the incidence of cGVHD at 1-year is $P_{03}(12) + P_{04}(12) + P_{05}(12) = 0.357$. The estimated transition probabilities are also plotted in Fig. 5a, b. Figure 5b illustrates the proportion of each transition probability at all time points. We observe that most of the TRM and relapse happen at the early stage after transplant without developing cGVHD, this is partially because cGVHD typically occurs after 100 days from transplant.

The transition probabilities of relapse and TRM are plotted and compared in Fig. 6. The upper plots show the cumulative incidence functions of disease relapse with and without cGVHD ($P_{02}(t)$ vs. $P_{05}(t)$), and the lower plots show the cumulative incidence functions of TRM with and without cGVHD ($P_{01}(t)$ vs. $P_{04}(t)$). These plots provide direct perceptions of TRM and relapse incidences from both transition paths. At 48-month after transplant, the proportion of disease relapse after cGVHD is 22.3% ($0.074/(0.074 + 0.258)$) of the total relapse, and the proportion of treatment-related mortality after cGVHD is 29.9% ($0.103/(0.103 + 0.242)$) of the total treatment-related mortality.

In addition, the transition probabilities of adverse events with and without cGVHD are plotted and compared in Fig. 7. The upper plots show the cumulative

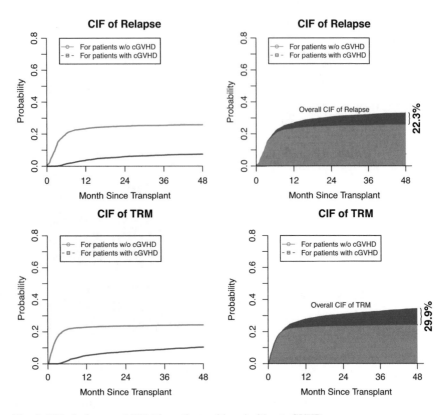

**Fig. 6** CIF of relapse and TRM for patients with and without cGVHD

incidence functions of TRM and Relapse ($P_{01}(t)$ vs. $P_{02}(t)$) among patients without cGVHD, and the lower plots show TRM and Relapse ($P_{04}(t)$ vs. $P_{05}(t)$) among patients with cGVHD. These plots provide direct perceptions of proportions of adverse events with and without cGVHD. The results show that, at 48-month after transplant, relapse counts for 51.6% ($0.258/(0.258 + 0.242)$) of total observed adverse events among patients without cGVHD, while this percentage is only 41.8% ($0.074/(0.074 + 0.103)$) among patients with cGVHD. These results indicate that cGVHD has graft-verse-leukemia (GVL) effect to reduce the cancer recurrence rate. Also, these results are useful for disease prognostic. Given whether a patient has developed cGVHD or not at a certain time after transplantation, we can predict the mortality or relapse rate.

Moreover, we have discussed earlier that the same dataset can be represented by different multi-state models depending on the research interests. If both aGVHD and cGVHD are considered, the data from [11] can be re-configured into a four-level of a twelve-state model (see Fig. 2). We want to investigate the TRM and relapse probabilities under different health conditions after transplant, thereby we estimated and presented the TRM probabilities to state 1 (without GVHD), state 5

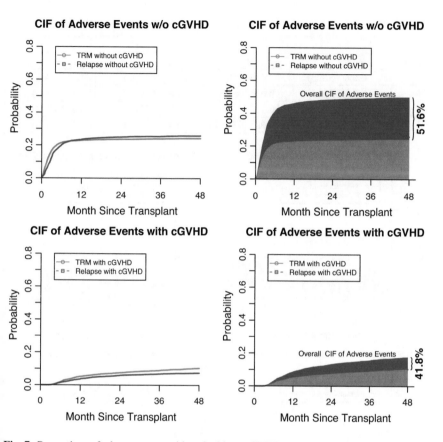

**Fig. 7** Proportions of adverse events with and without cGVHD

**Table 6** Estimated TRM probability from different transition paths at every 12 months

| Month | $\widehat{P}_{jk}(t)(se)$ | | | |
|---|---|---|---|---|
| | $\widehat{P}_{01}(t)$ | $\widehat{P}_{05}(t)$ | $\widehat{P}_{07}(t)$ | $\widehat{P}_{0,10}(t)$ |
| 12 | 0.100 (0.066) | 0.129 (0.069) | 0.013 (0.041) | 0.038 (0.003) |
| 24 | 0.106 (0.066) | 0.131 (0.070) | 0.023 (0.047) | 0.051 (0.003) |
| 36 | 0.108 (0.067) | 0.132 (0.070) | 0.027 (0.049) | 0.062 (0.004) |
| 48 | 0.110 (0.067) | 0.132 (0.070) | 0.033 (0.053) | 0.070 (0.004) |

(with the only aGVHD), state 7 (with only cGVHD), and state 10 (with both types of GVHD) at every 12 months in Table 6, and the relapse probabilities to state 2 (without GVHD), state 6 (with the only aGVHD), state 8 (with the only cGVHD), and state 11 (with both types of GVHD) at every 12 months in Table 7.

The analysis results show that at 48-month after transplant, the total relapse probability is 33.2% (0.169 + 0.089 + 0.035 + 0.039). The proportion of relapse among patients with the only aGVHD is 26.8% (0.089/0.332) of the total relapse;

**Table 7** Estimated relapse probability from different transition paths at every 12 months

| Month | $\widehat{P}_{jk}(t)(se)$ | | | |
|---|---|---|---|---|
| | $\widehat{P}_{02}(t)$ | $\widehat{P}_{06}(t)$ | $\widehat{P}_{08}(t)$ | $\widehat{P}_{0,11}(t)$ |
| 12 | 0.152 (0.005) | 0.083 (0.004) | 0.014 (0.002) | 0.021 (0.002) |
| 24 | 0.163 (0.005) | 0.086 (0.004) | 0.025 (0.002) | 0.034 (0.003) |
| 36 | 0.167 (0.005) | 0.088 (0.004) | 0.031 (0.002) | 0.037 (0.003) |
| 48 | 0.169 (0.005) | 0.089 (0.004) | 0.035 (0.003) | 0.039 (0.003) |

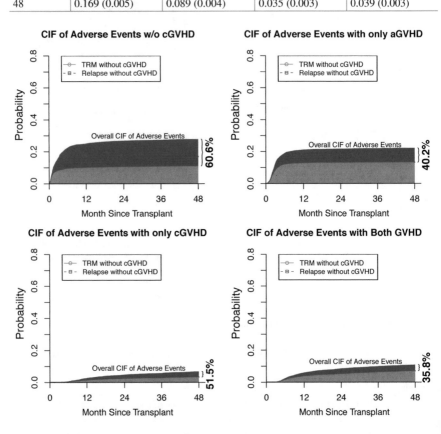

**Fig. 8** Proportion of adverse events under different disease conditions

this proportion among patients with the only cGVHD is 10.5% (0.035/0.332), and among patients with both types of GVHD is 11.7% (0.039/0.332).

On the other hand, relapse counts for 60.6% (0.169/(0.169 + 0.110)) of all adverse events among patients without any type of GVHD; this proportion is 40.2% (0.089/(0.089+0.132)) among patients with only aGVHD, 51.5% (0.035/(0.035+ 0.033)) among patients with only cGVHD, and 35.8% (0.039/(0.039 + 0.070)) among patients with both types of GVHD (also see Fig. 8). Simultaneously, relapse counts for 41.0% (0.163/0.398) among patients with any type of GVHD. These results may show that both aGVHD and cGVHD have GVL effect and patients experienced both type of GVHD has strongest GVL effect.

# 5 Discussion

This work has been committed to investigate the estimation of the transition probabilities in multi-state models using the proposed AIPCW. Simulation studies show that the proposed AIPCW technique provides more accurate estimates for the censoring distributions which lead to asymptotic unbiased estimates of the transition probabilities. The proposed AIPCW technique can be extended to more complicated multi-level models, and it can be applied to directly model the transition probabilities. More detailed study will be needed to study the performance of estimates for the regression parameters using the AIPCW technique in direct binomial modeling.

The drawback of any inverse probability censoring weighting approach is that one needs to estimate the censoring distribution for each individual. Beside, one additional disadvantage of our proposed AIPCW method is the lack of universal formulas for constructing the censoring distributions, because they are model- and state-specific. We did not explore the scenarios with covariate-dependent censoring in this work, but previous studies have indicated that regression modeling of the censoring distributions may further improve the efficiency of the AIPCW estimating procedures [9, 14, 16], even when the censoring is independent of covariates. Proper regression adjustments for the censoring distributions may be worth pursuing in future work.

In addition, we only studied using AIPCW method for analyzing right censored multi-state model data. Application of AIPCW method in left-truncated and right censored multi-state model data, and in data with other types of censoring, like interval censoring and current status, may be worth pursuing in future works.

# Appendix 1

Large sample property of IPCW-based estimator has been studied extensively [8, 9, 16]. We present a brief derivation for the variance estimations. Let $T_{i,123} = (T_{i,123}^* \wedge C_i)$, $N_i^{C_{00}}(t) = I(T_{i,123} \leq t, \Delta_{C_{00},i} = 1)$, $Y_i^{C_{00}}(t) = I(T_{i,123} \geq t)$, and $Y_{\bullet}^{C_{00}}(t) = \sum_i Y_i^{C_{00}}(t)$. Under regularity condition [9], we have that

$$\widehat{G}_{C_{00}}(T_{i,k}^* \wedge t) - G_{C_{00}}(T_{i,k}^* \wedge t) \approx_p -\widehat{G}_{C_{00}}(T_{i,k}^* \wedge t) \sum_{j=1}^{n} \int_0^{T_{i,k}^* \wedge t} \frac{d\widehat{M}_j^{C_{00}}(u)}{Y_{\bullet}^{C_{00}}(u)}$$

$$d\widehat{M}_j^{C_{00}}(t) = dN_j^{C_{00}}(t) - Y_j^{C_{00}}(t)d\widehat{\Lambda}_{C_{00}}(t)$$

$$d\widehat{\Lambda}_{C_{00}}(t) = \sum_j \frac{dN_j^{C_{00}}(t)}{Y_{\bullet}^{C_{00}}(t)}$$

Thus, variance of $\left\{ \widehat{P}_{0k}^{\text{AIPCW}}(0, t) - P_{0k}(0, t) \right\}$, for $k = 0, 1, 2$, can be estimated by

$$\widehat{\Sigma}_{P_{0k}}(t) = \frac{1}{n^2} \sum_{i=1}^{n} \left\{ \widehat{W}_{i,0k}(t) \right\}^2, \tag{4}$$

where

$$\widehat{W}_{i,00}(t) = \left\{ \frac{R_{i,0}(t)}{\widehat{G}_{C_{00}}(t)} - \widehat{P}_{00}^{\text{AIPCW}}(0, t) \right\} + \left\{ \sum_{j=1}^{n} \frac{R_{j,0}(t)}{\widehat{G}_{C_{00}}(t)} \right\} \int_0^t \frac{d\widehat{M}_i^{C_{00}}(u)}{Y_{\bullet}^{C_{00}}(u)}$$

$$\widehat{W}_{i,0k}(t) = \left\{ \frac{R_{i,k}(t)}{\widehat{G}_{C_{00}}(T_{i,k}^*)} - \widehat{P}_{0k}^{\text{AIPCW}}(0, t) \right\}$$

$$+ \int_0^t \left\{ \sum_{j=1}^{n} \frac{R_{j,k}(t)}{\widehat{G}_{C_{00}}(T_{j,k}^*)} I\{u \leq T_{j,k}^* \leq t\} \right\} \frac{d\widehat{M}_i^{C_{00}}(u)}{Y_{\bullet}^{C_{00}}(u)}, \text{ for } k = 1, 2.$$

For the variance of $P_{03}^{\text{AIPCW}}(0, t)$, since

$$\sqrt{n} \left\{ \widehat{P}_{03}^{\text{AIPCW}}(0, t) - P_{03}(0, t) \right\}$$

$$= \frac{1}{\sqrt{n}} \sum_{i=1}^{n} \left\{ \frac{R_{i,3}(t)}{G_{C_{00}}(T_{i,3}^*) G_{C_{33}}(t)} - P_{03}(0, t) \right\}$$

$$+ \frac{1}{\sqrt{n}} \sum_{i=1}^{n} \frac{R_{i,3}(t)}{\widehat{G}_{C_{33}}(t)} \left\{ \frac{1}{\widehat{G}_{C_{00}}(T_{i,3}^*)} - \frac{1}{G_{C_{00}}(T_{i,3}^*)} \right\}$$

$$+ \frac{1}{\sqrt{n}} \sum_{i=1}^{n} \frac{R_{i,3}(t)}{G_{C_{00}}(T_{i,3}^*)} \left\{ \frac{1}{\widehat{G}_{C_{33}}(t)} - \frac{1}{G_{C_{33}}(t)} \right\}$$

$$\approx_p \frac{1}{\sqrt{n}} \sum_{i=1}^{n} \left\{ \frac{R_{i,3}(t)}{G_{C_{00}}(T_{i,3}^*) G_{C_{33}}(t)} - P_{03}(0, t) \right\}$$

$$+ \frac{1}{\sqrt{n}} \sum_{i=1}^{n} \int_0^t \left\{ \sum_{j=1}^{n} \frac{R_{j,3}(t)}{G_{C_{00}}(T_{j,3}^*) G_{C_{33}}(t)} I\{u \leq T_{j,3}^* \leq t\} \right\} \frac{dM_i^{C_{00}}(u)}{Y_{\bullet}^{C_{00}}(u)}$$

$$+ \frac{1}{\sqrt{n}} \sum_{i=1}^{n} \left\{ \sum_{j=1}^{n} \frac{R_{j,3}(t)}{G_{C_{00}}(T_{j,3}^*) G_{C_{33}}(t)} \right\} \int_0^t \frac{dM_i^{C_{33}}(u)}{Y_{\bullet}^{C_{33}}(u)},$$

where $M_i^{C_{33}}(u)$ can be estimated by

$$d\widehat{M}_i^{C_{33}}(u) = dN_i^{C_{33}}(u) - Y_i^{C_{33}}(u)d\widehat{\Lambda}^{C_{33}}(u)$$

$$d\widehat{\Lambda}^{C_{33}}(u) = \sum_j \frac{dN_j^{C_{33}}(u)}{Y_\bullet^{C_{33}}(u)}.$$

Then, variance of $\left\{\widehat{P}_{03}^{\text{AIPCW}}(0, t) - P_{03}(0, t)\right\}$ can be estimated by

$$\widehat{\Sigma}_{P_{03}}(t) = \frac{1}{n^2} \sum_{i=1}^n \left\{\widehat{W}_{i,03}(t)\right\}^2, \tag{5}$$

where

$$\widehat{W}_{i,03}(t) = \left\{\frac{R_{i,3}(t)}{\widehat{G}_{C_{00}}(T_{i,3}^*)\widehat{G}_{C_{33}}(t)} - \widehat{P}_{03}^{\text{AIPCW}}(0, t)\right\}$$

$$+ \int_0^t \left\{\sum_{j=1}^n \frac{R_{j,3}(t)}{\widehat{G}_{C_{00}}(T_{j,3}^*)\widehat{G}_{C_{33}}(t)} I\{u \le T_{j,3}^* \le t\}\right\} \frac{d\widehat{M}_i^{C_{00}}(u)}{Y_\bullet^{C_{00}}(u)}$$

$$+ \left\{\sum_{j=1}^n \frac{R_{j,3}(t)}{\widehat{G}_{C_{00}}(T_{j,3}^*)\widehat{G}_{C_{33}}(t)}\right\} \int_0^t \frac{d\widehat{M}_i^{C_{33}}(u)}{Y_\bullet^{C_{33}}(u)}.$$

Similarly for $k = 4, 5$, variance of $\left\{\widehat{P}_{0k}^{\text{AIPCW}}(0, t) - P_{0k}(0, t)\right\}$ can be estimated by

$$\widehat{\Sigma}_{P_{0k}}(t) = \frac{1}{n^2} \sum_{i=1}^n \left\{\widehat{W}_{i,0k}(t)\right\}^2, \tag{6}$$

where

$$\widehat{W}_{i,0k}(t) = \left\{\frac{R_{i,k}(t)}{\widehat{G}_{C_{00}}(T_{i,3}^*)\widehat{G}_{C_{33}}(T_{i,45}^*)} - \widehat{P}_{0k}^{\text{AIPCW}}(0, t)\right\}$$

$$+ \int_0^t \left\{\sum_{j=1}^n \frac{R_{j,k}(t)}{\widehat{G}_{C_{00}}(T_{j,3}^*)\widehat{G}_{C_{33}}(T_{j,45}^*)} I\{u \le T_{j,3}^* \le t\}\right\} \frac{d\widehat{M}_i^{C_{00}}(u)}{Y_\bullet^{C_{00}}(u)}$$

$$+ \int_0^t \left\{\sum_{j=1}^n \frac{R_{j,k}(t)}{\widehat{G}_{C_{00}}(T_{j,3}^*)\widehat{G}_{C_{33}}(T_{j,45}^*)} I\{u \le T_{j,45}^* \le t\}\right\} \frac{d\widehat{M}_i^{C_{33}}(u)}{Y_\bullet^{C_{33}}(u)}.$$

The derived moment-type variance estimates have two parts. For example, there are two parts in $\widehat{W}_{i,00}(t) = \widehat{W}_{i1,00}(t) + \widehat{W}_{i2,00}(t)$ for estimating variance of $P_{00}^{\text{AIPCW}}(0, t)$. The second part

$$\widehat{W}_{i2,00}(t) = \left\{ \sum_{j=1}^{n} \frac{R_{j,0}(t)}{\widehat{G}_{C00}(t)} \right\} \int_0^t \frac{d\widehat{M}_i^{C00}(u)}{Y_\bullet^{C00}(u)} \tag{7}$$

is needed due to the estimation of the censoring distributions. In other words, when the censoring distributions are known, $\widehat{W}_{i2,00}(t)$ becomes zero, and $\widehat{W}_{i,00}(t)$ reduces to

$$\widehat{W}_{i1,00}(t) = \left\{ \frac{R_{i,0}(t)}{\widehat{G}_{C00}(t)} - \widehat{P}_{00}^{\text{AIPCW}}(0, t) \right\}. \tag{8}$$

In most situations, $\widehat{W}_{i2,00}(t)$ is negligible. The variance estimates estimated from $\widehat{W}_{i,00}(t)$ are close to that estimated from $\widehat{W}_{i1,00}(t)$ alone, but not necessarily larger, because the covariance of $W_{i1,00}(t)$ and $W_{i2,00}(t)$ are not necessarily positive. Similar arguments are true for the variances of transition probabilities to other states. We presented both variance estimates in the simulation studies.

## Appendix 2

For a four-level twelve-state model, we here only present the variance estimates of $P_{09}(t)$, $P_{0,10}(t)$, $P_{0,11}(t)$, one can refer to Appendix 1 for the variance of other transition probabilities. We have

$$\sqrt{n} \left\{ \widehat{P}_{09}^{\text{AIPCW}}(0, t) - P_{09}(0, t) \right\}$$

$$= \frac{1}{\sqrt{n}} \sum_{i=1}^{n} \left\{ \frac{R_{i,39}(t)}{\widehat{G}_{C00}(T_{i,3}^*)\widehat{G}_{C33}(T_{i,9}^*)\widehat{G}_{C99,3}(t)} + \frac{R_{i,49}(t)}{\widehat{G}_{C00}(T_{i,4}^*)\widehat{G}_{C44}(T_{i,9}^*)\widehat{G}_{C99,4}(t)} \right.$$

$$\left. - P_{09}(0, t) \right\}$$

$$= \frac{1}{\sqrt{n}} \sum_{i=1}^{n} \left\{ \frac{R_{i,39}(t)}{G_{C00}(T_{i,3}^*)G_{C33}(T_{i,9}^*)G_{C99,3}(t)} + \frac{R_{i,49}(t)}{G_{C00}(T_{i,4}^*)G_{C44}(T_{i,9}^*)G_{C99,4}(t)} \right.$$

$$\left. - P_{09}(0, t) \right\}$$

$$+ \frac{1}{\sqrt{n}} \sum_{i=1}^{n} \left\{ \frac{R_{i,39}(t)}{\widehat{G}_{C00}(T_{i,3}^*)\widehat{G}_{C33}(T_{i,9}^*)\widehat{G}_{C99,3}(t)} - \frac{R_{i,39}(t)}{G_{C00}(T_{i,3}^*)G_{C33}(T_{i,9}^*)G_{C99,3}(t)} \right\}$$

$$+ \frac{1}{\sqrt{n}} \sum_{i=1}^{n} \left\{ \frac{R_{i,49}(t)}{\widehat{G}_{C00}(T_{i,4}^*)\widehat{G}_{C44}(T_{i,9}^*)\widehat{G}_{C99,4}(t)} - \frac{R_{i,49}(t)}{G_{C00}(T_{i,4}^*)G_{C44}(T_{i,9}^*)G_{C99,4}(t)} \right\}$$

$$\approx_p \frac{1}{\sqrt{n}} \sum_{i=1}^{n} \left\{ \frac{R_{i,39}(t)}{G_{C00}(T_{i,3}^*)G_{C33}(T_{i,9}^*)G_{C99,3}(t)} + \frac{R_{i,49}(t)}{G_{C00}(T_{i,4}^*)G_{C44}(T_{i,9}^*)G_{C99,4}(t)} \right.$$

$$\left. - P_{09}(0,t) \right\}$$

$$+ \frac{1}{\sqrt{n}} \sum_{i=1}^{n} \int_0^t \left\{ \sum_{j=1}^{n} \frac{R_{j,39}(t)}{G_{C00}(T_{j,3}^*)G_{C33}(T_{j,9}^*)G_{C99,3}(t)} I\{u \le T_{j,3}^* \le t\} \right\} \frac{dM_i^{C00}(u)}{Y_{\bullet}^{C00}(u)}$$

$$+ \frac{1}{\sqrt{n}} \sum_{i=1}^{n} \int_0^t \left\{ \sum_{j=1}^{n} \frac{R_{j,39}(t)}{G_{C00}(T_{j,3}^*)G_{C33}(T_{j,9}^*)G_{C99,3}(t)} I\{u \le T_{j,9}^* \le t, \eta_{j,3} = 1\} \right\}$$

$$\frac{dM_i^{C33}(u)}{Y_{\bullet}^{C33}(u)}$$

$$+ \frac{1}{\sqrt{n}} \sum_{i=1}^{n} \left\{ \sum_{j=1}^{n} \frac{R_{j,39}(t)}{G_{C00}(T_{j,3}^*)G_{C33}(T_{j,9}^*)G_{C99,3}(t)} I\{u \le T_{j,9}^* \le t, \eta_{j,3} = 1\} \right\}$$

$$\int_0^t \frac{dM_i^{C99,3}(u)}{Y_{\bullet}^{C99,3}(u)}$$

$$+ \frac{1}{\sqrt{n}} \sum_{i=1}^{n} \int_0^t \left\{ \sum_{j=1}^{n} \frac{R_{j,49}(t)}{G_{C00}(T_{j,4}^*)G_{C44}(T_{j,9}^*)G_{C99,4}(t)} I\{u \le T_{j,4}^* \le t\} \right\}$$

$$\frac{dM_i^{C00}(u)}{Y_{\bullet}^{C00}(u)}$$

$$+ \frac{1}{\sqrt{n}} \sum_{i=1}^{n} \int_0^t \left\{ \sum_{j=1}^{n} \frac{R_{j,49}(t)}{G_{C00}(T_{j,4}^*)G_{C44}(T_{j,9}^*)G_{C99,4}(t)} I\{u \le T_{j,9}^* \le t, \eta_{j,4} = 1\} \right\}$$

$$\frac{dM_i^{C44}(u)}{Y_{\bullet}^{C44}(u)}$$

$$+ \frac{1}{\sqrt{n}} \sum_{i=1}^{n} \left\{ \sum_{j=1}^{n} \frac{R_{j,49}(t)}{G_{C00}(T_{j,4}^*)G_{C44}(T_{j,9}^*)G_{C99,4}(t)} I\{u \le T_{j,9}^* \le t, \eta_{j,4} = 1\} \right\}$$

$$\int_0^t \frac{dM_i^{C99,4}(u)}{Y_{\bullet}^{C99,4}(u)},$$

where $M_i^{C_{99,s}}(u)$, for $s = 3, 4$ can be estimated by

$$d\widehat{M}_i^{C_{99,s}}(u) = dN_i^{C_{99,s}}(u) - Y_i^{C_{99,s}}(u)d\widehat{\Lambda}^{C_{99,s}}(u)$$

$$d\widehat{\Lambda}^{C_{99,s}}(u) = \frac{dN_\bullet^{C_{99,s}}(u)}{Y_\bullet^{C_{99,s}}(u)}.$$

Thus, the variance of $\sqrt{n}\left\{\widehat{P}_{09}^{\mathrm{AIPCW}}(0,t) - P_{09}(0,t)\right\}$ can be estimated by

$$\widehat{\Sigma}_{P_{09}}(t) = \frac{1}{n}\sum_{i=1}^{n}\left\{\widehat{W}_{i,09}(t)\right\}^2, \tag{9}$$

where

$$\widehat{W}_{i,09}(t) = \left\{\frac{R_{i,39}(t)}{\widehat{G}_{C_{00}}(T_{i,3}^*)\widehat{G}_{C_{33}}(T_{i,9}^*)\widehat{G}_{C_{99,3}}(t)} + \frac{R_{i,49}(t)}{\widehat{G}_{C_{00}}(T_{i,4}^*)\widehat{G}_{C_{44}}(T_{i,9}^*)\widehat{G}_{C_{99,4}}(t)}\right.$$

$$\left. - \widehat{P}_{09}^{\mathrm{AIPCW}}(0,t)\right\}$$

$$+ \int_0^t\left\{\sum_{j=1}^{n}\frac{R_{j,39}(t)}{\widehat{G}_{C_{00}}(T_{j,3}^*)\widehat{G}_{C_{33}}(T_{j,9}^*)\widehat{G}_{C_{99,3}}(t)}I\{u \le T_{j,3}^* \le t\}\right\}\frac{d\widehat{M}_i^{C_{00}}(u)}{Y_\bullet^{C_{00}}(u)}$$

$$+ \int_0^t\left\{\sum_{j=1}^{n}\frac{R_{j,39}(t)}{\widehat{G}_{C_{00}}(T_{j,3}^*)\widehat{G}_{C_{33}}(T_{j,9}^*)\widehat{G}_{C_{99,3}}(t)}I\{u \le T_{j,9}^* \le t, \eta_{j,3} = 1\}\right\}$$

$$\frac{d\widehat{M}_i^{C_{33}}(u)}{Y_\bullet^{C_{33}}(u)}$$

$$+ \left\{\sum_{j=1}^{n}\frac{R_{j,39}(t)}{\widehat{G}_{C_{00}}(T_{j,3}^*)\widehat{G}_{C_{33}}(T_{j,9}^*)\widehat{G}_{C_{99,3}}(t)}I\{u \le T_{j,9}^* \le t, \eta_{j,3} = 1\}\right\}$$

$$\int_0^t\frac{d\widehat{M}_i^{C_{99,3}}(u)}{Y_\bullet^{C_{99,3}}(u)}$$

$$+ \int_0^t\left\{\sum_{j=1}^{n}\frac{R_{j,49}(t)}{\widehat{G}_{C_{00}}(T_{j,4}^*)\widehat{G}_{C_{44}}(T_{j,9}^*)\widehat{G}_{C_{99,4}}(t)}I\{u \le T_{j,4}^* \le t\}\right\}$$

$$\frac{d\widehat{M}_i^{C_{00}}(u)}{Y_\bullet^{C_{00}}(u)}$$

$$+ \int_0^t \left\{ \sum_{j=1}^n \frac{R_{j,49}(t)}{\widehat{G}_{C_{00}}(T_{j,4}^*)\widehat{G}_{C_{44}}(T_{j,9}^*)\widehat{G}_{C_{99,4}}(t)} I\{u \le T_{j,9}^* \le t, \eta_{j,4} = 1\} \right\}$$

$$\frac{d\widehat{M}_i^{C_{44}}(u)}{Y_\bullet^{C_{44}}(u)}$$

$$+ \left\{ \sum_{j=1}^n \frac{R_{j,49}(t)}{\widehat{G}_{C_{00}}(T_{j,4}^*)\widehat{G}_{C_{44}}(T_{j,9}^*)\widehat{G}_{C_{99,4}}(t)} I\{u \le T_{j,9}^* \le t, \eta_{j,4} = 1\} \right\}$$

$$\int_0^t \frac{d\widehat{M}_i^{C_{99,4}}(u)}{Y_\bullet^{C_{99,4}}(u)}$$

Similarly, for $k = 10, 11$, the variance of $\sqrt{n}\left\{\widehat{P}_{0k}^{\text{AIPCW}}(0, t) - P_{0k}(0, t)\right\}$ can be estimated by:

$$\widehat{\Sigma}_{P_{0k}}(t) = \frac{1}{n} \sum_{i=1}^n \left\{\widehat{W}_{i,0k}(t)\right\}^2.$$

where

$$\widehat{W}_{i,0k}(t) = \left\{ \frac{R_{i,3k}(t)}{\widehat{G}_{C_{00}}(T_{i,3}^*)\widehat{G}_{C_{33}}(T_{i,9}^*)\widehat{G}_{C_{99,3}}(T_{i,L_4}^*)} \right.$$

$$\left. + \frac{R_{i,4k}(t)}{\widehat{G}_{C_{00}}(T_{i,4}^*)\widehat{G}_{C_{44}}(T_{i,9}^*)\widehat{G}_{C_{99,4}}(T_{i,L_4}^*)} - \widehat{P}_{0k}^{\text{AIPCW}}(0, t) \right\}$$

$$+ \int_0^t \left\{ \sum_{j=1}^n \frac{R_{j,3k}(t)}{\widehat{G}_{C_{00}}(T_{j,3}^*)\widehat{G}_{C_{33}}(T_{j,9}^*)\widehat{G}_{C_{99,3}}(T_{j,L_4}^*)} I\{u \le T_{j,3}^* \le t\} \right\}$$

$$\frac{d\widehat{M}_i^{C_{00}}(u)}{Y_\bullet^{C_{00}}(u)}$$

$$+ \int_0^t \left\{ \sum_{j=1}^n \frac{R_{j,3k}(t)}{\widehat{G}_{C_{00}}(T_{j,3}^*)\widehat{G}_{C_{33}}(T_{j,9}^*)\widehat{G}_{C_{99,4}}(T_{j,L_4}^*)} I\{u \le T_{j,9}^* \le t, \eta_{j,3} = 1\} \right\}$$

$$\frac{d\widehat{M}_i^{C_{33}}(u)}{Y_\bullet^{C_{33}}(u)}$$

$$+ \int_0^t \left\{ \sum_{j=1}^n \frac{R_{j,3k}(t)}{\widehat{G}_{C_{00}}(T_{j,3}^*)\widehat{G}_{C_{33}}(T_{j,9}^*)\widehat{G}_{C_{99,3}}(T_{j,L_4}^*)} I\{u \le T_{j,L_4}^* \le t, \eta_{j,3} = 1\} \right\}$$

$$\frac{d\widehat{M}_i^{C_{99,3}}(u)}{Y_\bullet^{C_{99,3}}(u)}$$

$$+ \int_0^t \left\{ \sum_{j=1}^n \frac{R_{j,4k}(t)}{\widehat{G}_{C_{00}}(T_{j,4}^*)\widehat{G}_{C_{44}}(T_{j,9}^*)\widehat{G}_{C_{99,4}}(T_{j,L_4}^*)} I\{u \le T_{j,4}^* \le t\} \right\}$$

$$\frac{d\widehat{M}_i^{C_{00}}(u)}{Y_\bullet^{C_{00}}(u)}$$

$$+ \int_0^t \left\{ \sum_{j=1}^n \frac{R_{j,4k}(t)}{\widehat{G}_{C_{00}}(T_{j,4}^*)\widehat{G}_{C_{44}}(T_{ij,9}^*)\widehat{G}_{C_{99,4}}(T_{j,L_4}^*)} I\{u \le T_{j,9}^* \le t, \eta_{j,4} = 1\} \right\}$$

$$\frac{d\widehat{M}_i^{C_{44}}(u)}{Y_\bullet^{C_{44}}(u)}$$

$$+ \int_0^t \left\{ \sum_{j=1}^n \frac{R_{j,4k}(t)}{\widehat{G}_{C_{00}}(T_{j,4}^*)\widehat{G}_{C_{44}}(T_{j,9}^*)\widehat{G}_{C_{99,4}}(T_{j,L_4}^*)} I\{u \le T_{j,L_4}^* \le t, \eta_{j,4} = 1\} \right\}$$

$$\frac{d\widehat{M}_i^{C_{99,4}}(u)}{Y_\bullet^{C_{99,4}}(u)}.$$

# References

1. Aalen, O. (1978). Nonparametric inference for a family of counting processes. *The Annals of Statistics, 6*, 701–726.
2. Aalen, O., & Johansen, S. (1978). An empirical transition matrix for non-homogeneous Markov chains based on censored observations. *Scandinavian Journal of Statistics, 5*, 141–150.
3. Andersen, P. K., Borgan, O., Gill, R. D., & Keiding, N. (1993). *Statistical models based on counting processes*. New York: NY Springer.
4. Bie, O., Borgan, Ø., & Liestøl, K. (1987). Confidence intervals and confidence bands for the cumulative hazard rate function and their small sample properties. *Scandinavian Journal of Statistics, 14*, 221–233.
5. Borgan, Ø., & Liestøl, K. (1990). A note on confidence intervals and bands for the survival function based on transformations. *Scandinavian Journal of Statistics, 17*, 35–41.
6. Datta, S., & Satten, G. A. (2001). Validity of the Aalen–Johansen estimators of stage occupation probabilities and Nelson–Aalen estimators of integrated transition hazards for non-Markov models. *Statistics & Probability Letters, 55*(4), 403–411.
7. Datta, S., & Satten, G. A. (2002). Estimation of integrated transition hazards and stage occupation probabilities for non-Markov system under stage dependent censoring. *Biometrics, 58*, 792–802.
8. Fine, J. P., & Gray, R. J. (1999). A proportional hazards model for the subdistribution of a competing risk. *Journal of the American Statistical Association, 94*(446), 496–509.

9. He, P., Eriksson, F., Scheike, T. H., & Zhang, M.-J. (2015). A proportional hazards regression model for the subdistribution with covariates-adjusted censoring weight for competing risks data. *Scandinavian Journal of Statistics, 43*, 103–122.

10. Klein, J. P., Szydlo, R. M., Craddock, C., & Goldman, J. M. (2000). Estimation of current leukaemia-free survival following donor lymphocyte infusion therapy for patients with leukaemia who relapse after allografting: Application of a multistate model. *Statistics in Medicine, 19*(21), 3005–3016.

11. Luger, S. M., Ringdén, O., Zhang, M.-J., Pérez, W. S., Bishop, M. R., Bornhauser, M., et al. (2012). Similar outcomes using myeloablative vs reduced-intensity allogeneic transplant preparative regimens for AML or MDS. *Bone Marrow Transplantation, 47*(2), 203–211.

12. Nelson, W. (1969). Hazard plotting for incomplete failure data. *Journal of Quality Technology, 1*(1), 27–52.

13. Nelson, W. (1972). Theory and applications of hazard plotting for censored failure data. *Technometrics, 14*(4), 945–966.

14. Robins, J. M., & Rotnitzky, A. (1992). Recovery of information and adjustment for dependent censoring using surrogate markers. In *AIDS epidemiology* (pp. 297–331). Boston: Birkhäuser.

15. Scheike, T., & Zhang, M. J. (2007). Direct modelling of regression effects for transition probabilities in multistate models. *Scandinavian Journal of Statistics, 34*(1), 17–32.

16. Scheike, T. H., Zhang, M. J., & Gerds, T. A. (2008). Predicting cumulative incidence probability by direct binomial regression. *Biometrika, 95*(1), 205–220.

17. Zhang, X., Zhang, M. J., & Fine, J. P. (2009). A mass redistribution algorithm for right-censored and left-truncated time to event data. *Journal of Statistical Planning and Inference, 139*(9), 3329–3339.

# Index

Printed in the United States
by Baker & Taylor Publisher Services